The Physiology of Health and Illness

with related anatomy

Judy Hubbard
School of Health and Policy Studies
University of Central England
Birmingham, UK

and

Derek Mechan
Department of Biology
Brentwood School
formerly of the
Institute of Medical and Health Care
Hong Kong Polytechnic

Illustrated by Derek Mechan

Stanley Thornes (Publishers) Ltd

First published in 1997 by:
Stanley Thornes (Publishers) Ltd
Ellenborough House
Wellington Street
CHELTENHAM
GL50 1YW
United Kingdom

97 98 99 00 01 / 10 9 8 7 6 5 4 3 2 1

A catalogue record for this book is available from the British Library

ISBN 0-7487-3173-3

Designed and formatted by Geoffrey Wadsley and Marion H Wadsley
Printed and bound in Spain by Mateu Cromo

Contents

Preface

This book has been written for students either already working in, or preparing for work in, a variety of health care fields such as nursing, occupational therapy, physiotherapy, podiatry, radiography and speech therapy. It is suitable for both diploma and degree level health courses.

Although readers are likely to have studied some science before, for some it may have been some time ago. The first chapter, therefore, provides a synopsis of biological molecules, chemical reactions and units of measurement used in the rest of the book and referred to by margin boxes.

We have entitled the book *Physiology of Health and Illness* to emphasize that the content applies across the range of states of health that students encounter in their studies and health-care practice. We have, however, not used the terms 'normal' and 'abnormal physiology' because they imply that *different* physiological mechanisms operate in health from those in illness. We present examples which demonstrate that the same cause-and-effect mechanisms are operating, within the framework of homoeostasis, across the range of states of health.

While the emphasis of the book is clearly on physiological mechanisms, the anatomical frameworks in which the physiological mechanisms operate are also covered.

As far as possible, colour has been used consistently in the illustrations so that particular organs, tissues, organelles and ions are generally the same colours. For example, the liver is brown, connective tissue is green, mitochondria are brown and Na^+ ions are purple.

Judy Hubbard and Derek Mechan

Acknowledgements

Students, especially those working in the health-care fields, have undoubtedly been the greatest stimulus for writing this book. Their readiness to ask questions and discuss their practice in class has shaped both the teaching curriculum and the contents of this book.

We should like to thank our colleagues Stuart Brand, Roy Smith and Marion Thompson at UCE and Mike Chambers at Brentwood School for their encouragement and forbearance, especially during the final stages of preparation of this book, when it took up a large part of our time. We thank Carol Reeves and Pauline Wilkins at Brentwood School for their practical help and Mike Filby, Head of the School of Health and Policy Studies at UCE, for his support. Annis and Jonathan Mechan contributed some interesting suggestions, which we have incorporated into the text.

The development of teaching applied physiology has been a major interest at UCE and colleagues from other disciplines have also stimulated and influenced our thinking, particularly Linda Jones, currently at the Department of Health and Social Welfare at the Open University, and Madeline Stafford in the School of Nursing and Community Health at UCE.

Our thanks are also due to David Quincey at Bournemouth University and David Smith, formerly at UCE, who took photographs of tissues for us. Andrew Payne at Queen Margaret College, Edinburgh gave us detailed comments and constructive advice on each chapter.

We should like to thank the publishing team, especially our editor Rosemary Morris, whose enthusiasm has sustained us throughout, and Dominic Ricaldin for writing the Lecturer's Resource Pack for the book.

Most of all, we owe an enormous debt of gratitude to our partners John and Ruth for their love and support.

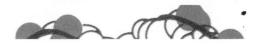
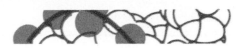
Molecules, ions and units

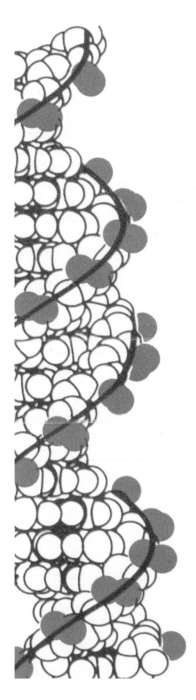

Atoms, molecules and elements

A **molecule** is a collection of elements, present in fixed proportions, which are joined together by chemical 'bonds'. Sodium chloride (common salt) is a molecule that consists of only two elements, sodium and chloride, which are present in equal proportions. Glucose contains three elements: carbon, hydrogen and oxygen, in the proportions 6:12:6.

An **element** is a 'pure' chemical substance, in the sense that it is made up of a number of identical units. These units are called atoms.

An **atom** is the smallest part of an element that still retains all of the physical and chemical properties of the element.

Chemical symbols

Elements and molecules are generally identified by the use of abbreviations or chemical symbols. These abbreviations are usually the first one or two letters of the word so that, for example, the symbol for hydrogen is H, for oxygen O and for carbon, C. In some cases, the letters of the equivalent Latin term are used, rather than the English. Thus the symbol for sodium is Na (from *natrium*) and that for potassium is K (*kalium*). This avoids any confusion between atoms which begin with the same letter: S is the symbol for sulphur and P for phosphorus (Table 1.1).

Table 1.1 Chemical symbols, atomic numbers and masses of the major elements found in the body

Element	Number	Mass	Symbol
Hydrogen	1	1	H
Helium	2	4	He
Lithium	3	7	Li
Carbon	6	12	C
Nitrogen	7	14	N
Oxygen	8	16	O
Sodium	11	23	Na (Latin, *natrium*)
Magnesium	12	24	Mg
Phosphorus	15	31	P
Sulphur	16	32	S
Chlorine	17	35.5	Cl
Potassium	19	39	K (Latin, *kalium*)
Calcium	20	40	Ca
Iron	26	56	Fe (Latin, *ferrum*)
Copper	29	63	Cu (Latin, *cuprum*)
Iodine	53	127	I

A molecule of a substance contains a number of atoms of different elements. These atoms are always present in particular proportions, which are indicated by a subscript, so that glucose (each molecule of which contains six carbon atoms, 12 hydrogen atoms and six oxygen atoms) is represented by the formula $C_6H_{12}O_6$. Sodium chloride (one atom of sodium and one of chlorine) is represented as NaCl.

Atomic structure

Atoms consist of three fundamental particles: **protons, neutrons** and **electrons**. Protons and neutrons have the same mass (for convenience taken to be 1), while the electron is much smaller, with a mass about one-2000th of that of a proton/neutron. Protons and electrons carry equal but opposite electrical charges; that of the proton is positive, while the electron carries a negative charge. Neutrons, as the name implies, do not carry any charge at all.

An atom has equal numbers of protons and electrons and is therefore electrically neutral.

Within any atom, the subatomic particles are always arranged in the same way (Figure 1.1).

Protons and neutrons are located within a central **nucleus** while the electrons orbit at fixed distances from the nucleus (rather in the same way as the planets orbit around the Sun in the Solar System). Each electron orbit, or shell, is able to contain a maximum number of particles. The innermost shell is able to accept only two electrons and when it is 'full' (in the element helium) a third electron is placed in a new shell (in the element lithium). The second shell can take eight electrons, so that in an atom of neon there are 10 electrons arranged 2:8. The third shell is also filled by eight electrons, so that the 19 electrons of the next element (potassium) are arranged 2:8:8:1. In larger atoms there are additional shells.

Atomic number

Since the atoms of different elements possess different numbers of

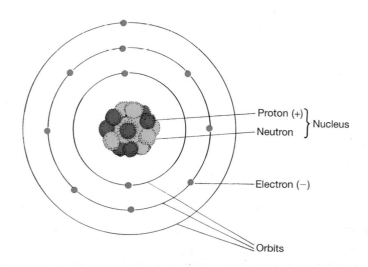

Proton (+) ⎫
            ⎬ Nucleus
Neutron ⎭

Electron (−)

Orbits

Figure 1.1 Diagrammatic representation of a sodium atom showing a central nucleus containing protons (positive charge) and neutrons (neutral) surrounded by three concentric orbits containing electrons (negative charge).

protons, neutrons and electrons, they are allotted numbers to assist in their identification. The atomic number of an element is determined by the number of its protons (and hence electrons). Thus hydrogen, with a single proton, has the atomic number 1; helium has the number 2 and so on (Table 1.1).

Atomic mass

The masses of individual atoms are almost infinitesimally small and so cannot be measured in kilograms or grams. Instead, a relative scale is used, so that the lightest atom, hydrogen, has an atomic mass of 1, carbon has a mass of 12 and so on. Atomic mass is determined by adding the number of protons to the number of neutrons present. Atomic mass is, therefore, a comparative rather than an absolute measure.

Isotopes

Although a particular element has a specific atomic number, all of its

Figure 1.2 The two isotopes of chlorine: chlorine-35 (^{35}Cl) and chlorine-37 (^{37}Cl). Both isotopes have 17 protons and 17 electrons but differ in their number of neutrons.

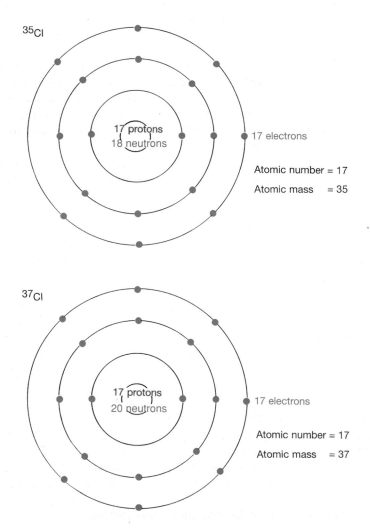

^{35}Cl

17 protons
18 neutrons

17 electrons

Atomic number = 17
Atomic mass   = 35

^{37}Cl

17 protons
20 neutrons

17 electrons

Atomic number = 17
Atomic mass   = 37

atoms do not necessarily have the same atomic mass. This is because, although the number of protons and the number of electrons are always fixed, the number of neutrons in the nucleus may vary (Figure 1.2).

Chlorine has the atomic number 17 and its atomic mass is 35.5. Each atom of chlorine has 17 protons and 17 electrons and, it would appear, 18.5 neutrons. Since an atom cannot contain fractions of neutrons, there must be an alternative explanation.

In fact, two types of chlorine atoms are found. 75% of chlorine atoms contain 17 protons and 18 neutrons (atomic mass 35) and 25% contain 17 protons and 20 neutrons (atomic mass 37).

$$\text{Thus } 3 \times 35 = 105$$
$$1 \times 37 = 37$$
$$\text{Total} = 142$$
$$\text{Mean value} = 142/4 = 35.5.$$

Atoms of the same element that contain different numbers of neutrons are called isotopes. Chlorine therefore has two isotopes, chlorine-35 (^{35}Cl) and chlorine-37 (^{37}Cl). The masses of individual elements recorded in tables are the relative mean isotopic masses.

RADIOISOTOPES

Radioisotopes are unstable and break down, giving off a number of particles including alpha-particles (α-particles), beta-particles (β-particles), gamma-rays (γ-rays) and neutrinos. Alpha-particles are actually helium nuclei, with two protons and two neutrons, whereas beta-particles are either negatively charged 'negatrons' or positively charged 'positrons'; each has the same mass as an electron. Gamma-rays are a type of electromagnetic radiation like light or X-rays (see *Electromagnetic radiation*, below). Neutrinos are particles without a charge and with no measurable mass.

Clinical applications of radioisotopes

Some of the particles given off by radioactive substances are destructive to tissues and can therefore be used as radiotherapeutic agents in the treatment of cancer, in which there is uncontrolled tissue growth.

Cobalt-60 is used as a source of gamma-rays, which are employed in the treatment of cancer, and also as an immunosuppressant following organ transplantation. In addition, radioisotopes can be used as tracers which accumulate in particular tissues or organs and provide valuable information about the target site. Iodine-131, for example, is used to study the thyroid gland, as well as treat hyperthyroidism and thyroid cancer.

Combination of atoms to form molecules

In forming compounds atoms join together by rearranging their electrons. In doing so one atom donates or shares one or more of its electrons and fills the outer shell(s) of the atom(s) to which it is bonding. The atom(s) donating or sharing electrons also achieves a 'filled' outer shell(s).

Two types of bond can be formed, ionic and covalent.

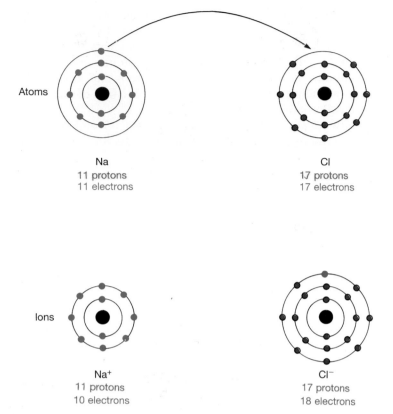

Atoms

Na
11 protons
11 electrons

Cl
17 protons
17 electrons

Ions

Na⁺
11 protons
10 electrons

Cl⁻
17 protons
18 electrons

Figure 1.3 Ionic bonding. The sodium atom donates the electron (negative) from its outer shell to the chlorine atom, giving rise to sodium (Na⁺) and chloride (Cl⁻) ions.

IONIC BONDS

When sodium chloride forms, a sodium atom (which has the electron shell pattern 2:8:1) transfers its outer electron to chlorine (2:8:7) (Figure 1.3).

Thus sodium now has 10 electrons in a pattern 2:8 and has a new outer shell, which is filled. The chlorine atom now has 18 electrons in a pattern 2:8:8 and it too has a filled outer shell. However, sodium still has 11 positively-charged protons, while chlorine has 17. Sodium therefore has an excess of one positive charge and chlorine has one extra negative charge. The two atoms are held together by an electrostatic or ionic bond. Clearly the NaCl molecule will be electrically neutral.

COVALENT BONDS

Some elements form compounds by sharing, rather than donating or receiving electrons. Carbon has four electrons in its outer shell and in order to fill the shell it must obtain four more electrons. It could, for example, link with four hydrogen atoms, in which case it would 'borrow' one electron from each atom while 'lending' each hydrogen atom one of its own electrons. Thus the carbon would have an outer shell with eight electrons and each hydrogen atom would have two electrons. The resulting molecule is methane (CH_4) (Figure 1.4).

Alternatively the carbon atom could combine with oxygen. An oxygen atom has six electrons in its outer shell, so each one requires two

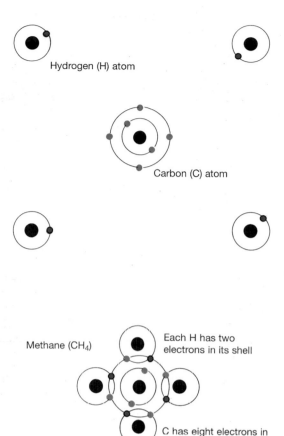

Hydrogen (H) atom

Carbon (C) atom

Methane (CH₄)

Each H has two electrons in its shell

C has eight electrons in its outer shell

Figure 1.4 Covalent bonding. Four hydrogen atoms combine with a single carbon atom. The single electron of each hydrogen is shared with the carbon so that the carbon atom has eight shared electrons in its outer shell; each hydrogen borrows an electron from the carbon so that it has two electrons in its outer shell.

electrons from the carbon. The carbon requires four extra electrons to fill its outer shell. This can be achieved by combining two oxygen atoms with one carbon atom to form the compound carbon dioxide (CO_2) (Figure 1.5).

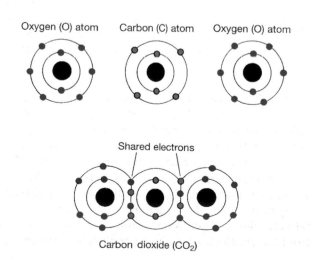

Oxygen (O) atom   Carbon (C) atom   Oxygen (O) atom

Shared electrons

Carbon dioxide (CO_2)

Figure 1.5 Covalent bonding. Two oxygen atoms combine with a single carbon atom. Each oxygen atom shares two of its electrons with the carbon atom, so that the carbon atom has eight electrons in its outer shell; each oxygen borrows two electrons from the carbon so that both also have eight electrons in their outer shells.

Carbonic acid, which has the formula H_2CO_3 and which breaks down (dissociates) into H^+ and HCO_3^- includes both covalent and ionic bonds.

VALENCY

The number of electrons in the outermost shell of an atom determines its chemical combining power. When atoms combine to form molecules they do so in a way that fills (or empties) their outer electron shells. Thus carbon, which has four outer electrons, can combine with four hydrogen atoms, each of which has one electron in its outer shell. The combining 'power' of an atom is known as its valency. Carbon has a valency of 4, hydrogen has a valency of 1. Oxygen, which has six outer electrons, has a valency of 2 and can combine with two hydrogen atoms, forming H_2O (water).

Ions

When molecules containing ionic bonds dissolve in water they dissociate into their constituent ions so that, for example, NaCl dissociates into Na^+ (a sodium atom with an excess of one proton) and Cl^- (a chlorine atom

Table 1.2 Chemical symbols and valencies of the major ions (electrolytes) in body fluids

Name	Chemical symbol	Valency
Cations		
Hydrogen	H^+	1
Sodium	Na^+	1
Potassium	K^+	1
Ammonium	NH_4^+	1
Calcium	Ca^{2+}	2
Magnesium	Mg^{2+}	2
Iron (ferrous)	Fe^{2+}	2
Iron (ferric)	Fe^{3+}	3
Anions		
Chloride	Cl^-	1
Bicarbonate (hydrogen carbonate)	HCO_3^-	1
Nitrate	NO_3^-	1
Dihydrogen phosphate	$H_2PO_4^-$	1
Sulphate	SO_4^{2-}	2
Hydrogen phosphate	HPO_4^{2-}	2
Phosphate	PO_4^{3-}	3

with an excess of one electron). Thus solutions of ionic substances contain ions or electrolytes rather than molecules. Such electrolytes are major constituents of body fluids. Positively charged ions are known as **cations**, whereas negatively charged ions are called **anions**.

Some ions contain more than one atom (**polyatomic ions** or **radicals**). Thus nitric acid (HNO_3) consists of a hydrogen ion (H^+) and a nitrate ion (NO_3^-). The latter includes one atom of nitrogen and three of oxygen. Table 1.2 lists the chemical symbols of the major ions found in body fluids.

The valency of an ion is indicated by the number of positive or negative charges, which is dependent upon the number of electrons lost or gained. Thus Na^+ has a valency of 1 (monovalent), SO_4^{2-} has a valency of 2 (divalent) (Table 1.2).

Ions are described as **polar** as they always carry a charge, and **hydrophilic** as they dissolve in water. Substances dissolved in water are known as **solutes**.

Units

SI units

In 1960, the 11th General Conference on Weights and Measures formulated a new international system of units. Since the conference was held in France, the system is known as the Système Internationale d'Unités (SI units).

Six base units were defined:

- **Length:** metre (m)
- **Mass:** kilogram (kg)
- **Time:** second (s)
- **Electric current:** ampere (A)
- **Temperature:** kelvin (K)
- **Light intensity:** candela (cd)

A number of units are derived from those listed above. Table 1.3 gives those commonly used in physiology.

Multiples and submultiples of the base units are frequently used when referring to very large or small measures. Thus one-100th (10^{-2}) of a metre is known as a centimetre, whereas 1000 (10^3) metres is known as a kilometre. Table 1.4 lists the prefixes and accompanying symbols used in the SI system.

Concentration

Concentration is a measure of the density of particles (solutes) in solution, expressed as mass per unit volume, e.g. kg/m^3, g/L or mg/100 mL. By international convention, concentration is expressed as moles/litre (mol/L). (The litre (L), though in common use, is not an SI unit. It is equivalent to $1000\,cm^3$.)

One **mole** is equal to the relative molecular mass (molecular weight) of a compound expressed in grams. To determine relative molecular

Table 1.3 SI-derived units used in this book

Quantity	Unit	Symbol
Area	square metre	m^2
Volume	cubic metre or litre	m^3 or L
Velocity	metre/second	m/s
Acceleration	metre/second/second	m/s^2
Force	newton (kilogram/metre/second/second)	N
Pressure	pascal (newton/square metre)	Pa
Energy	joule (newton metre)	J
Frequency	hertz (per second)	Hz
Electrical voltage	volt	V
Loudness	decibel	dB
Concentration	mole	mol

Table 1.4 Prefixes and their symbols in the SI system

Prefix	Symbol	Multiplier	
tera	T	10^{12}	1 000 000 000 000
giga	G	10^9	1 000 000 000
mega	M	10^6	1 000 000
kilo	k	10^3	1 000
hecto	h	10^2	100
deca	da	10^1	10
deci	d	10^{-1}	$\dfrac{1}{10}$
centi	c	10^{-2}	$\dfrac{1}{100}$
milli	m	10^{-3}	$\dfrac{1}{1\,000}$
micro	μ	10^{-6}	$\dfrac{1}{1\,000\,000}$
nano	n	10^{-9}	$\dfrac{1}{1\,000\,000\,000}$
pico	p	10^{-12}	$\dfrac{1}{1\,000\,000\,000\,000}$

mass, the chemical formula and the atomic weights (relative molecular masses) of the constituent elements of the compound are needed.

For common salt, sodium chloride, the chemical formula is NaCl. Using Table 1.1, the relative atomic mass of Na is 23 and the relative atomic mass of Cl is 35.5. Adding these two together gives the relative molecular mass of NaCl as $23 + 35.5 = 58.5$. One mole of NaCl would therefore be 58.5 g.

One mol/L of NaCl would be made by weighing out 58.5 g of salt and dissolving it in water (the solvent) to make up a final volume of one litre.

To calculate the relative molecular mass of glucose ($C_6H_{12}O_6$):

relative atomic mass of C = 12
relative atomic mass of H = 1
relative atomic mass of O = 16

therefore the relative atomic mass of $C_6H_{12}O_6$

$$= (12 \times 6) + (1 \times 12) + (16 \times 6) = 180.$$

One mole of glucose would therefore be 180 g.

As the relative atomic mass scale takes into account the differing atomic masses of the elements, then it follows that relative molecular masses reflect the differing masses of molecules. One mole of a substance contains the same number of molecules as one mole of any other substance. One mole actually contains 6.0222×10^{23} molecules (Avogadro's constant).

Expressing concentration in mol/L, therefore, is a reflection of the number of molecules present in solution.

The concentration of ions can be expressed in terms of **equivalents** per litre, rather than moles per litre. In this case, the chemical combining powers of ions in solution can be compared. The equivalent weight of a substance is equal to its relative molecular mass divided by its valency. The equivalent weight of Ca^{2+}, for example, is 40/2 or 20 g, whereas that of Na^+, which has a valency of 1, is the same as its atomic weight, 23 g. In body fluids the concentrations of ions are very low, so that it is usual to measure them in milliequivalents/litre (meq/L).

To convert concentration in mmol/L to meq/L, multiply by the valency of the ion.

Example:

Ion	Concentration in mmol/L	Concentration in meq/L
Na^+	10	$10 \times 1 = 10$
Ca^{2+}	5	$5 \times 2 = 10.$

In the example given there are twice as many Na^+ as Ca^{2+} in the same volume of solution. Each Ca^{2+} is twice as potent chemically as Na^+, however, because it has a valency of 2, so that, for example, one Ca^{2+} can combine with two Cl^-, whereas one Na^+ can combine with only one Cl^-. If the valency of the two ions is taken into account, then the concentration in meq/L becomes the same, because it takes half as many Ca^{2+} as Na^+ to combine with the same number of Cl^-.

Pressure

Pressure is defined as force per unit area and is measured in pascals (Pa), after the 17th-century French philosopher Blaise Pascal. One **pascal** is equal to a force of one newton (after Sir Isaac Newton) exerted over an area of one square metre (N/m^2). Since the newton is a very small quantity the kilopascal, or kPa (defined as $1000\,N$, or one kilonewton per square metre, $1\,kN/m^2$), is a much more useful unit.

When considering pressure, both force and area must be taken into account. Thus, wooden floors are unlikely to be damaged by the heels of flat shoes, whereas high-heeled shoes may leave marks. Clearly a person's weight does not alter when changing shoes and neither does the overall force exerted on the floor. The pressure on the floor exerted by the heels changes, however, because the area of the heel in contact with the floor is much smaller than that of a flat shoe.

The atmosphere itself exerts a pressure due to the molecules of gas moving randomly and colliding with each other. 'Standard' **atmospheric pressure** at sea level, at 25°C, is defined as exactly 101.321 kPa. At the top of a mountain, because the weight of the atmosphere is much less than it is at sea level, the pressure is lower, while at the bottom of a mine it is higher. When blood and other pressures are measured, the values obtained are always additional to atmospheric pressure and are known as 'gauge' pressures, rather than 'absolute' pressures.

For most purposes, the kilopascal is the unit used to measure pressure; it is used in respiratory physiology, for example. However, when discussing blood pressure, millimetres of mercury (mmHg) are used instead. This is mainly because existing devices for blood pressure measurement are calibrated in mmHg.

Temperature

Temperature is the measure of 'hotness' and 'coldness'. The SI unit of measurement is the **kelvin** (**K**). The scale has its zero point at absolute zero, where all atomic motion ceases, and is therefore not very useful when studying body temperature. Temperature is usually measured instead using a thermometer calibrated in degrees **Celsius** (also called **Centigrade °C**), rather than K. By definition, the temperature of pure melting ice is identified as 0°C (273.15 K), and pure boiling water has a temperature of 100°C (373.15 K).

As temperature rises atoms and molecules move about more quickly. As a result of this, chemical reactions proceed more rapidly at higher temperatures. This is the case for reactions that take place both inside and outside the body. However such reactions are usually catalysed (speeded up) by enzymes (proteins), which are easily destroyed at high temperatures. As a result, the reactions which take place within living cells only increase their rate up to a temperature of about 40°C. Body temperature is maintained at around 37°C.

Diffusion

Diffusion is the net movement of molecules from a region where their density is higher to a region where it is lower, i.e. from a region of higher concentration to a region of lower concentration. The process thereby results in a more even distribution of molecules. It results from the thermal energy (kinetic energy) of the molecules themselves, which causes them to move randomly, collide with each other and change direction. Where molecules are densely packed such collisions occur more often and cause them to move away from the higher concentration towards a region of lower concentration. Diffusion occurs over short distances, relatively quickly in gases, in which molecules are able to move quite freely, less quickly in liquids and hardly at all in solids.

In the body, cell membranes separate solutions of different concentrations. Figure 1.6 illustrates the diffusion of non-electrolytes across cell membranes.

Figure 1.6(a) shows two solutions separated by a membrane that is permeable to both solute and water. In compartment 1 there is a strong solution (i.e. one which contains a high concentration of solute), and in compartment 2 a weak one. Molecules of solute, moving randomly due to their own kinetic energy, pass from 1 to 2 as well as from 2 to 1. However, since there are more molecules of solute in 1 there is a much greater chance that solutes will travel from 1 to 2 than from 2 to 1. Over a period of time there will be net movement of solutes (diffusion) across the membrane from 1 to 2. Eventually an equilibrium is established when equal numbers of molecules pass between the two sides.

When there are more solute molecules on one side of the membrane than on the other a **concentration gradient** exists, which promotes diffusion from high to low concentration (down the concentration gradient).

The diffusion of electrolytes (ions) is governed not only by the concentration gradient, but also by electrical forces operating across the cell membrane. Ions diffuse down an electrochemical gradient. This is explained in relation to Na^+ and K^+ in *The resting potential*, in Chapter 4. Molecules of gas also move within the body by diffusion – between the lungs and the blood, and between the blood and the tissues. The concentration of gases is expressed as partial pressures. Gases, therefore, diffuse down a partial pressure gradient.

Osmosis

In Figure 1.6(b), if the membrane separating 1 and 2 is selectively permeable, so that solute molecules are not able to penetrate but water molecules can, then a different result is produced. In this case, side 1 contains more solute molecules than side 2, but side 2 contains more water molecules than side 1. Since only water molecules can pass through the membrane then they diffuse down their gradient into 1,

Figure 1.6 **(a)** Diffusion. Solute molecules (●) move randomly in both directions between compartments. As there are more solutes in compartment 1 than in compartment 2, more solutes diffuse from compartment 1 to compartment 2. **(b)** Osmosis. Water molecules (▲) move randomly in both directions between compartments, separated by a membrane permeable only to water. As there are more water molecules in compartment 2 than in compartment 1, the net effect is the movement of water (osmosis) from compartment 2 into compartment 1.

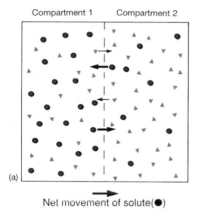

(a)

Net movement of solute(●)

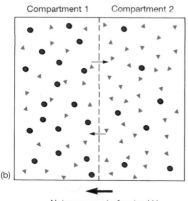

(b)

Net movement of water (▲)

diluting it and increasing its volume. This specialized form of water diffusion is known as **osmosis.**

Cell membranes are permeable both to water and solutes (as in Figure 1.6(a)); as a result, osmosis and diffusion usually occur at the same time.

Osmotic pressure

A solution with a higher concentration of solute is said to have a higher osmotic pressure than the weaker one. This is actually the pressure that must be applied to the membrane to stop osmosis from occurring, and depends upon the number of osmotically active molecules in the solution. The size of the solute molecules is irrelevant, so that one albumin molecule (molecular weight 70 000) has the same osmotic effect as one of glucose (molecular weight 180). Further, a molecule that dissociates into two ions, e.g. NaCl into Na^+ and Cl^-, exerts twice as much osmotic influence as one that does not.

Osmotic pressure is measured in **osmoles** (osmol), one osmole being defined as one gram molecule of a non-ionizable substance. A substance which ionizes gives rise to more particles in solution than one which does not and therefore exerts a greater osmotic effect. Thus 180 g of glucose (which does not ionize) dissolved in water to make one litre of solution exerts an osmotic pressure of 1.0 osmol/L, while 58.5 g of sodium chloride (each molecule of which dissociates into Na^+ and Cl^-) in the same volume of solution exerts a pressure of 2.0 osmol/L. The two solutions have an **osmolarity** of 1 and 2 osmol/L, respectively. If the solutions were made up by dissolving the compounds in 1 kg of water, rather than making the final volume up to 1 L, they would have an **osmolality** of 1 and 2 osmol/kg H_2O.

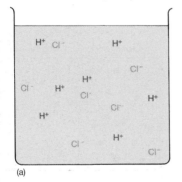

(a)

Acids and bases

Acids are substances that yield hydrogen ions (H^+) in solution. Their strength depends upon the quantity of H^+ liberated so that a solution of a strong acid contains a great deal of free ion, while that of a weak acid contains very little (Figure 1.7).

This is because a strong acid dissociates to a much greater extent than a weak one. Thus, for example, hydrochloric acid (HCl) dissociates almost completely so that in solution there would be large quantities of H^+ and Cl^- and almost no HCl molecules. In a solution of a weak acid such as carbonic acid (H_2CO_3) there would be large numbers of acid molecules but relatively few H^+ and HCO_3^- ions. The strength of an acid is measured in SI units as the concentration of H^+ expressed as millimoles per litre (mmol/L) of solution.

Bases are substances that accept H^+. Thus ammonia (NH_3) is a base because it takes up H^+ to become the ammonium ion (NH_4^+). Many bases produce hydroxyl (OH^-) ions in solution. Again the strength of a base is determined by the extent to which it dissociates (Figure 1.8). Sodium hydroxide (NaOH) is a strong base and ammonium hydroxide (NH_4OH) is a weak one.

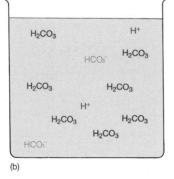

(b)

Figure 1.7 **(a)** A solution of the strong acid, hydrochloric acid, consists of dissociated H^+ and Cl^- ions. **(b)** A solution of the weak acid carbonic acid contains large numbers of H_2CO_3 molecules and a small number of H^+ and HCO_3^- ions.

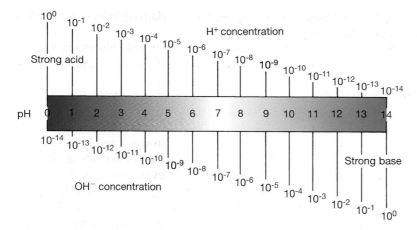

Figure 1.9 The relationship between the concentrations of H⁺ and OH⁻ (mol/L) and the pH scale. For each concentration of H⁺, the pH value is the negative logarithm to the base 10 of that concentration ($-\log_{10}[\text{H}^+]$). A neutral solution that has equal concentrations of H⁺ and OH⁻ (10^{-7} mol/L) has a pH of 7. The total concentration of H⁺ and OH⁻ always equals 10^{-14} mol/L, so that as the concentration of one increases that of the other decreases. Increasing the concentration of OH⁻ makes the solution basic (alkaline) (pH > 7) whereas increasing the concentration of H⁺ makes the solution acid (pH < 7).

The pH scale

Although acidity (and basicity) is now expressed as mol/L in SI units, a more traditional measure, which is still in common usage, is the 14-point pH scale (Figure 1.9).

The strength of an acid or a base is defined as its pH ('power of Hydrogen'). The pH scale is based upon the formula

$$pH = -\log_{10}[\text{H}^+]$$

where [H⁺] is the hydrogen ion concentration in mol/L.

Expressing the concentration in this way gives rise to whole numbers, so that the $-\log_{10}$ of a solution containing 10^{-5} mol/L of H⁺ is 5, one with 10^{-9} is 9, and so on. A litre of water contains 10^{-7} moles of H⁺ and 10^{-7} moles of OH⁻; the pH of water is thus $-\log_{10}[10^{-7}] = 7$. Since the product of the concentrations of H⁺ and OH⁻ in any aqueous solution is always 10^{-14} (i.e. [H⁺] x [OH⁻]) then an increase in H⁺ means a decrease in OH⁻ and vice versa. A substance with a larger amount of H⁺ than water will have more than 10^{-7} moles of H⁺ and thus a lower pH. Thus, for example, 10^{-4} represents more H⁺ than is found in water and the pH will be 4; in this solution there would be 10^{-10} moles of OH⁻ ions. A substance which gives rise to less H⁺ (and therefore more OH⁻) than water will have a higher pH (e.g. 10^{-9} represents less H⁺ than is found in water and the pH will be 9). Such a solution would be alkaline.

Buffers

There are molecules in the body fluids and inside cells which are able to take up H⁺ or OH⁻ ions, thereby effectively removing them from solution and maintaining a constant pH (Figure 1.10).

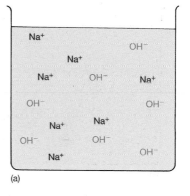

(a)

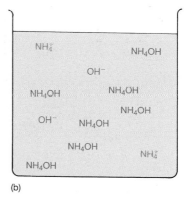

(b)

Figure 1.8 **(a)** A solution of the strong base, sodium hydroxide, consists of dissociated Na⁺ and OH⁻ ions. **(b)** A solution of the weak base ammonium hydroxide contains large numbers of NH₄OH molecules and a small number of NH₄⁺ and OH⁻ ions.

Figure 1.10 Buffer action. As hydrochloric acid is added to a solution of sodium bicarbonate (sodium hydrogen carbonate), free H^+ ions are taken up by the HCO_3^- forming the weak carbonic acid. H^+ is thus effectively removed from the solution.

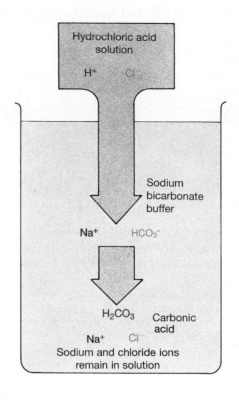

Table 1.5 Major buffers in the blood	
Buffer (H⁺) accepter	*Weak acid*
HCO_3^-	H_2CO_3
HPO_4^{2-}	$H_2PO_4^-$
Hb^-	HHb
Protein⁻	HProtein

The constant pH of the blood at 7.4 is largely dependent, in the first instance, upon the presence of chemicals that 'buffer' acids and alkalis. Major blood buffers are hydrogen carbonate (bicarbonate) ion (HCO_3^-), hydrogen phosphate ion (HPO_4^{2-}), plasma proteins and haemoglobin.

A buffer combines with H^+ (or OH^-), and converts it into a weak acid (or base) (Table 1.5).

HCl, for example, dissociates almost completely into H^+ and Cl^- and is therefore very acid. If HCl is added to a solution of NaHCO₃, H^+ combines with HCO_3^- and forms H_2CO_3, which hardly dissociates at all. The strong acid is therefore converted to a weak acid and H^+ is effectively removed from solution.

$$H^+ \quad Cl^- \quad + \quad HCO_3^- \longrightarrow H_2CO_3$$
$$\text{Strong acid} \qquad \text{Buffer} \qquad \text{Weak acid}$$

Biological molecules

Living cells contain a relatively small number of different elements with carbon, hydrogen, oxygen and nitrogen making up about 99% of the cell mass. The chemicals that make up living matter all include carbon atoms and are termed 'organic' compounds. The carbon atom has four electrons in its outer shell and is able to form strong covalent bonds with up to four other atoms. Carbon is therefore able to form chains and rings with other carbon atoms and still have the capacity to join with other elements. As a result carbon compounds may be extremely large and complex and are able to carry out a variety of biological functions.

A few chemical groups form part of many biological compounds. These include methyl (–CH₃), **hydroxyl** (–OH), **carboxyl** (–COOH) and **amino** (–NH₂).

There are four principal classes of organic compounds found in living material: carbohydrates, lipids, proteins and nucleotides.

Carbohydrates

Carbohydrates are used as sources of energy (1 gram liberates 17.22 kJ of energy), are found as constituents of nucleic acids and cell membranes and are constituents of plant cell walls. They are composed of one or more units called monosaccharides, each of which contains between three and six carbon atoms.

MONOSACCHARIDES

All monosaccharides contain the atoms carbon, hydrogen and oxygen in the proportion $C_nH_{2n}O_n$.

The most common monosaccharides in the diet are the **hexoses**, which contain six carbon atoms, giving a general formula of $C_6H_{12}O_6$. The commonest hexoses are **glucose**, **fructose** and **galactose**.

In Figure 1.11, it can be seen that four or five of the carbon atoms form a ring with one of the oxygen atoms, and the remaining atoms form side groups, projecting upwards or downwards from the ring. Glucose and galactose differ only in the orientation of the hydrogen (H) and hydroxyl (OH) groups on carbon 4 (C4).

The atoms that constitute monosaccharides are arranged in a number of different configurations (isomers). Monosaccharides are denoted

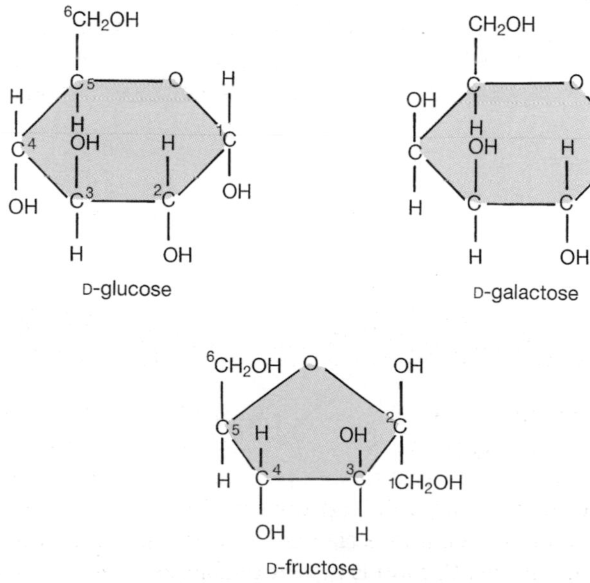

Figure 1.11 Structures of monosaccharide hexoses: glucose, galactose and fructose.

D-glucose

D-galactose

D-fructose

dextro- (D) or laevo- (L) forms according to the orientation of the H and CH$_2$OH groups on C5. Alpha and beta forms are determined by the orientation of H and OH on C1.

Pentoses have five carbon atoms per molecule. Two such molecules, ribose and deoxyribose, are found as constituents of nucleic acids (Figure 1.12).

The diet contains relatively few free monosaccharides; most of them are incorporated into larger molecules.

Figure 1.12 Structures of monosaccharide pentoses: ribose and deoxyribose.

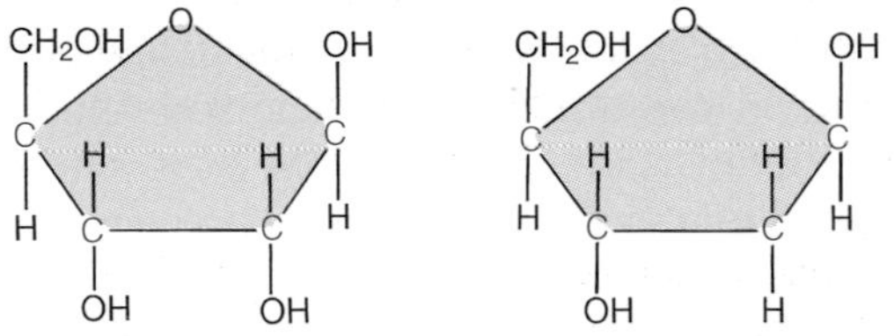

Ribose

Deoxyribose

Figure 1.13 Structures of disaccharides: sucrose, maltose and lactose.

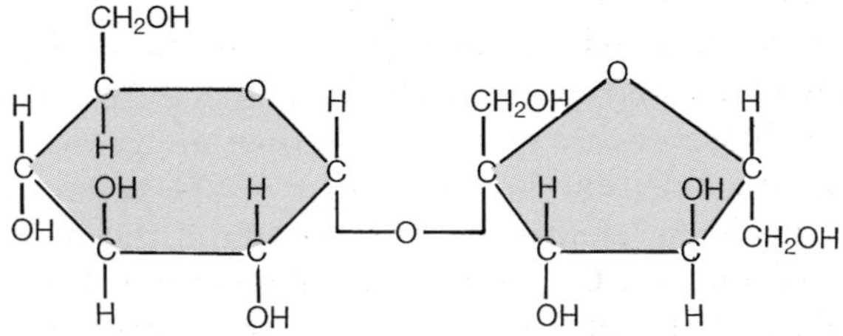

Sucrose
(α-D-glucosyl-β-D-fructoside)

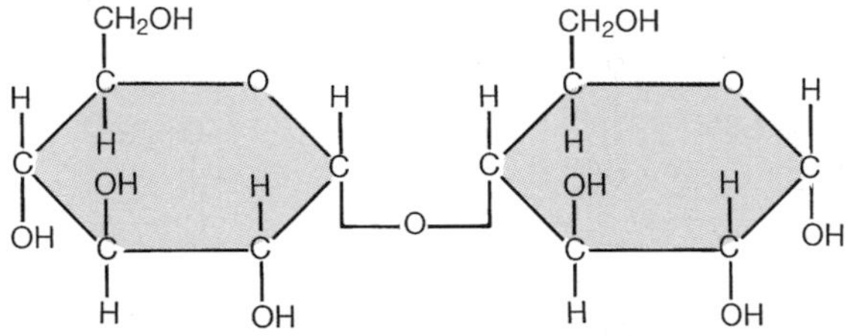

Maltose
(α-D-glucosyl-1, 4 D-glucose)

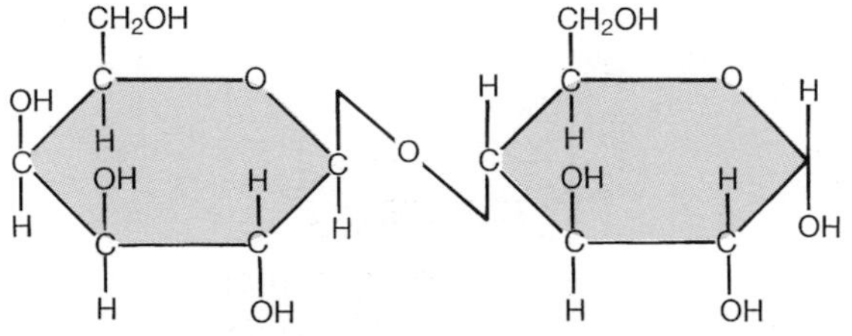

Lactose
(β-D-galactosyl-1, 4 D-glucose)

DISACCHARIDES

Disaccharides are formed from two monosaccharide subunits (called 'residues' since they are not complete molecules). Dietary disaccharides include sucrose (the principal one), **lactose** and **maltose**. Their structures are shown in Figure 1.13.

Polysaccharides

Polysaccharides are the largest carbohydrates and can contain many thousands of monosaccharide residues. They include **starch**, **glycogen** and **cellulose**. All of these molecules are polymers of glucose. Monosaccharides are joined together by removing H and OH from two adjacent molecules to make water (a condensation reaction). Figure 1.14 shows how this results in three different types of link found in starch, cellulose and glycogen.

Starch is the main dietary source of carbohydrate and is stored by plants in granules. These are insoluble in water, unless they are cooked. Starch is composed of glucose chains formed by two different linkages. The α-1,4 links form straight chains of 25–2000 glucose residues, called **amylose**, and this makes up about 20% of the starch molecule. The remaining 80% of starch is made up of **amylopectin**, which is a branched chain: 25–30 glucose molecules are joined by α-1,4 links and then an α-1,6 link occurs, which gives a branch point.

Glycogen resembles amylopectin, but the branch points occur more frequently. This is the storage form of carbohydrate found in the liver and muscles of animals. **Cellulose**, a component of plant cell walls, is a straight chain polymer of some 3000 glucose residues joined by α-1,4 links.

Figure 1.14 Types of linkages formed in disaccharides and polysaccharides: **(a)** α-1,4 link, as in maltose, amylose in starch; **(b)** β-1,4 link, as in cellulose; **(c)** α-1,6 link as in amylopectin in starch, glycogen.

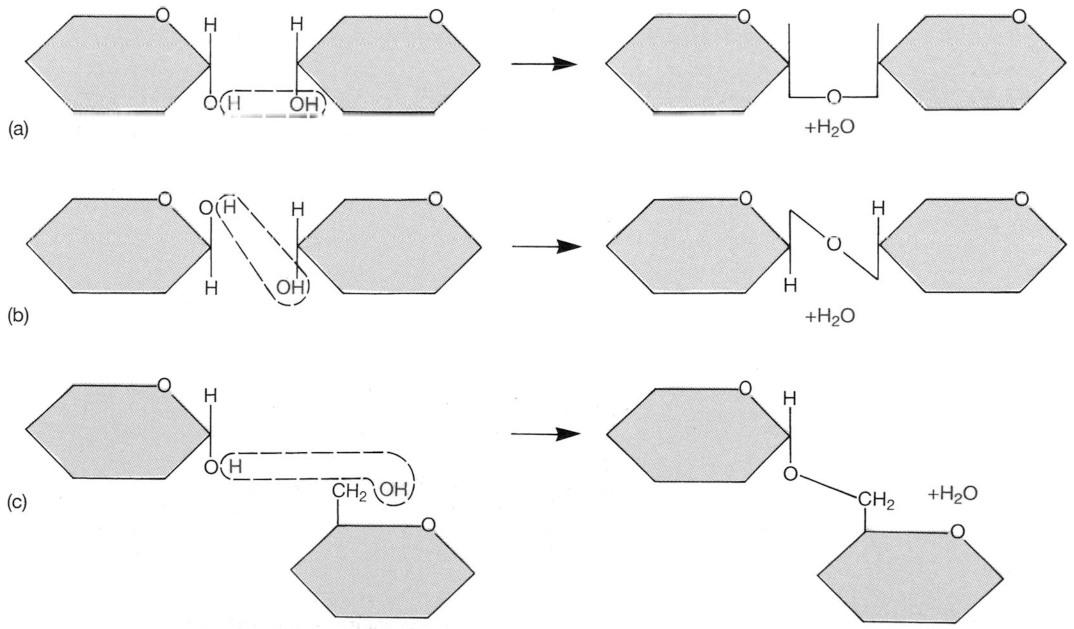

GLYCOPROTEINS AND GLYCOLIPIDS

Carbohydrates also combine with proteins, forming glycoproteins, and lipids, forming glycolipids, both of which are found in cell membranes.

Lipids

Lipids are major constituents of cell membranes and some hormones. They are stored in adipose tissues and oxidized in the tissues, which liberates more than twice as much energy (39.06 kJ/g) as the equivalent amount of glucose. In addition to its role as a stored form of energy, adipose tissue forms an insulating layer beneath the skin and also provides physical protection to some organs, such as the kidneys and eyes.

TRIGLYCERIDES

The majority of dietary fat, as well as the fat stored in subcutaneous adipose tissue, is in the form of **triglycerides** (triacylglycerols). A triglyceride consists of an alcohol, glycerol, linked to three (usually different) fatty acid residues (Figure 1.15). Butter, for example, contains butyric acid, oleic acid and stearic acid linked to glycerol.

Fatty acids comprise a hydrocarbon chain and an acidic carboxyl group (−COOH). There are over 40 different fatty acids, although only three, stearic, oleic and palmitic acids, are common. Altogether, 16 different fatty acids are incorporated into triglycerides in adipose tissue, with oleic acid, palmitic acid and linoleic acid constituting some 80% of the total.

Fatty acids can be subdivided into **saturated** or **unsaturated** types. The former, present in animal fats, are molecules within which all the available sites on the hydrocarbon chain are occupied by hydrogen atoms (Figure 1.16). Unsaturated fatty acids, which are the type found in plants and fish (and present in other animals too, as well as the saturated fats), have one or more double bonds present in the hydrocarbon chain and therefore contain less hydrogen.

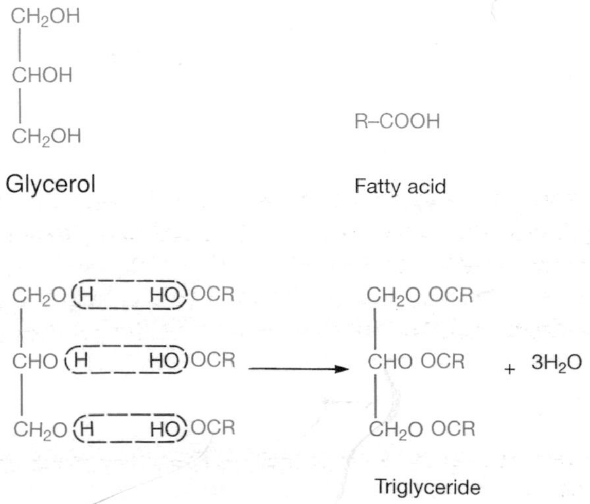

Figure 1.15 Structure of a triglyceride molecule formed from glycerol and three fatty acids with the exclusion of water.

CH_2OH
|
$CHOH$
|
CH_2OH

Glycerol

R–COOH

Fatty acid

CH_2O (H —— HO) OCR CH_2O OCR
| |
CHO (H —— HO) OCR ⟶ CHO OCR + $3H_2O$
| |
CH_2O (H —— HO) OCR CH_2O OCR

Triglyceride

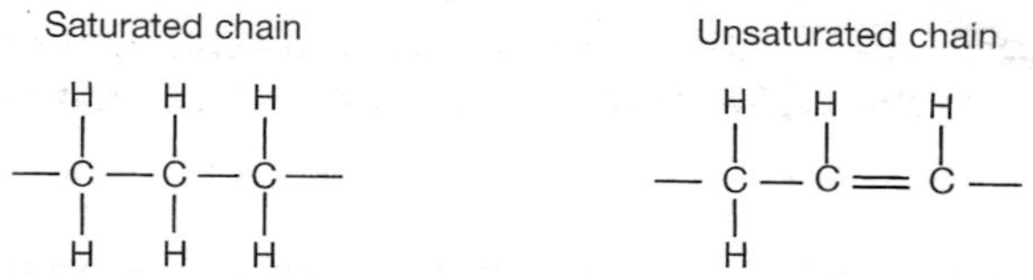

Saturated chain

Unsaturated chain

Saturated fatty acids $C_nH_{2n+1}COOH$

    butyric, C_3H_7COOH
    stearic, $C_{17}H_{35}COOH$
    palmitic, $C_{15}H_{31}COOH$

Unsaturated fatty acids

One double bond, C_nH_{2n-1}
e.g. oliec acid, $C_{17}H_{33}COOH$

Two double bonds, C_nH_{2n-3}
e.g. linoleic acid, $C_{17}H_{31}COOH$

Three double bonds, C_nH_{2n-5}
e.g. linolenic acid, $C_{17}H_{29}COOH$

Four double bonds, C_nH_{2n-7}
e.g. arachidonic acid, $C_{19}H_{31}COOH$

Figure 1.16 Classes of fatty acid molecules.

Lipids containing a high proportion of unsaturated fatty acids are liquid at room temperature (**oils**); those with a high proportion of saturated fatty acids are solid at room temperature (**fats**).

PHOSPHOLIPIDS

Phospholipid molecules are composed of glycerol, two fatty acid residues and a phosphate group which is attached to a nitrogenous group such as choline, serine or ethanolamine (Figure 1.17).

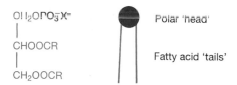

$CH_2OPO_3^-X^-$

$CHOOCR$

CH_2OOCR

Polar 'head'

Fatty acid 'tails'

Figure 1.17 General structure of a phospholipid molecule, consisting of glycerol [green] joined to two fatty acid residues [blue], phosphate (negative charge) and a nitrogenous group X (positive charge). R = hydrocarbon chain. The nitrogenous group may be choline (in lecithins), serine or ethanolamine. The fatty acid residues form a hydrophobic two-pronged 'tail', while the charged groups form a polar 'head'.

The fatty acid chains are **hydrophobic** (repel water) while the 'head' region is **hydrophilic** (attracts water). The head of a phospholipid molecule is polar and usually carries both positive and negative charges; as a result it may be electrically neutral. Phospholipid molecules can combine to form flat sheets and two such sheets are major constituents of cell membranes.

STEROIDS

Steroids are complex lipids, with a hydrocarbon ring structure as shown in Figure 1.18.

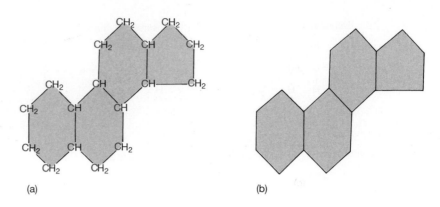

(a)

(b)

(c)

Figure 1.18 Steroid nucleus **(a)**, its abbreviated form **(b)** and the structure of cholesterol **(c)**.

They are found in cell membranes and also form some hormones; the adrenal cortical and sex hormones. **Cholesterol** is a steroid that is found in foods derived from animals, particularly eggs and prawns. Bile salts are derived from cholesterol.

Proteins

Proteins are major constituents of cytoplasm and of cell membranes. Enzymes, which catalyse all the biochemical reactions that take place within living organisms, are also proteins. Although they are used less than carbohydrates or fats, they may also be broken down to liberate energy; one gram of protein releases 22.68 kJ of energy.

Like polysaccharides, proteins are polymers, but in this case the repeating units are **amino acids**. These are named because of the presence of an amino group (–NH_2) and an acid carboxyl group (–COOH) in the molecules (Figure 1.19).

Amino acids are classified as 1) acidic, if there are two carboxyl groups; 2) basic, if there are two basic groups; or 3) neutral, if there is one carboxyl and one amino group. Approximately 20 different amino acids are found in the diet.

Peptide chains are built up of amino acid residues linked by peptide bonds (Figure 1.19) and the final proteins may consist of only one polypeptide chain or as many as four of them, linked together at various

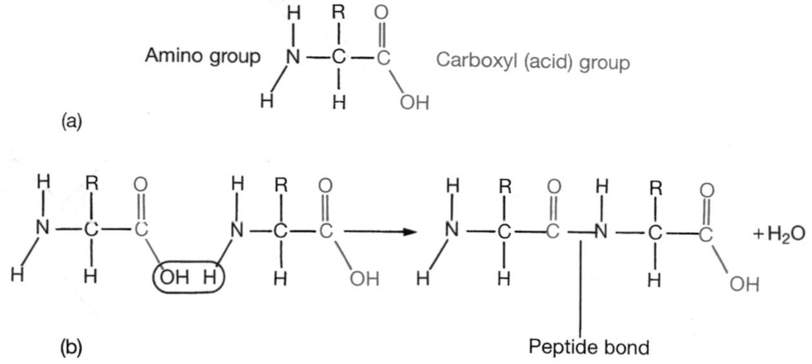

(a)

(b)

Figure 1.19 General structure of (a) an amino acid and (b) the formation of a peptide bond (–CO–NH–) between the carboxyl group of one amino acid and the amino group of a second amino acid, with the formation of water.

points. The chains may be folded in a complex three-dimensional arrangement, the shape of which is important for the function of the particular protein. **Globular proteins** are so-named because the peptide chains are coiled and folded into a globular shape. These proteins are water-soluble and include albumin, globulins, haemoglobin and most cellular enzymes.

Other proteins are classified as **fibrous**, because their polypeptide chains are elongated and the separate chains are linked together to form bundles. Such proteins include collagen and elastin in connective tissue, actin and myosin in muscle and keratins in skin, nails and hair.

Conjugated proteins are those which are combined with non-protein substances e.g. nucleoproteins (nucleic acid and protein), proteo-glycans or mucoproteins (protein and polysaccharide), lipoproteins (lipid and protein) and phosphoproteins (phosphorus and protein).

A linear chain of 30 amino acids or less is generally classified as a peptide. Single linear chains of more than 30 but less than 1000 amino acids are called **polypeptides**, whereas molecules that are folded into tertiary structures and/or consist of two polypeptide chains or more are described as **proteins**, no matter what their size. Thus, the hormone insulin, which contains 51 amino acids, is usually classified as a protein because it has two chains, whereas growth hormone, with 191 amino acids arranged in a single chain is called a polypeptide.

ENZYMES

The chemical reactions that take place in the cells are all driven by enzymes. Enzymes are biological catalysts, that is they speed up chemical reactions without themselves being altered. An enzyme-catalysed reaction may be 10 million times faster than the equivalent non-catalysed reaction.

Enzymes are large globular protein molecules which are often anchored to particular structures within the cell. In most cases there is a series of enzymes that bring about a series of chemical reactions; a single cell may contain up to 4000 different enzymes. In addition to these intracellular enzymes, others are extracellular, being secreted by cells into the surrounding environment: e.g. the cells of the pancreas secrete several digestive enzymes into the duodenum.

Enzymes are used in the synthesis and the breakdown of substances (substrates) within the cell and the same enzyme may catalyse a reaction in either direction. In both cases the enzyme combines with the substrate(s) to form a complex. The unstable complex then rearranges to give rise to an unaltered enzyme molecule and the reaction product(s) (Figure 1.20). In a synthetic reaction the enzyme speeds up the reaction by combining with the reactants so that they are brought together.

Figure 1.20 Enzyme function. **1**. Breakdown reaction. The substrate (carbonic acid) combines with the enzyme molecule to form a complex. The complex then rearranges and gives rise to the reaction products (water and carbon dioxide). **2**. Synthetic reaction. The reverse of the breakdown reaction.

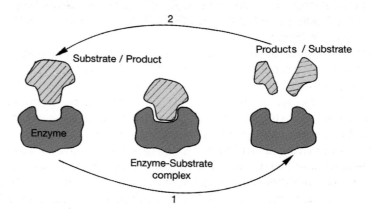

Enzymes are usually named according to their substrate, the suffix '-ase' indicating their enzymatic nature. Thus ATPase catalyses the breakdown of ATP to ADP while sucrase breaks down sucrose to glucose and fructose.

The reaction between water and carbon dioxide is accelerated by the enzyme **carbonic anhydrase**, which is present inside erythrocytes and gastric and renal tubular cells. The product is carbonic acid, a weak acid and therefore only a small proportion of the acid dissociates into hydrogen and bicarbonate ions.

$$\text{carbonic anhydrase}$$
$$H_2O + CO_2 \;\rightleftharpoons\; H_2CO_3 \;\rightleftharpoons\; H^+ + HCO_3^-$$

Many enzymes require additional, non-protein, substances in order to function effectively. These are called **cofactors** and are of two types: 1) ions, such as Fe^{2+}, Ca^{2+} or Mg^{2+}; or 2) **coenzymes**, derived from vitamins, which transfer molecular fragments from one substrate to another. Nicotinamide adenine dinucleotide (NAD^+), derived from niacin (a B vitamin) and flavin adenine dinucleotide (FAD), derived from riboflavin (vitamin B_2) transfer electrons from one substrate to another in oxidative phosphorylation. Coenzyme A (CoA) transfers the 2-C acetyl molecule in the citric acid cycle.

Each enzyme molecule can be re-used many times and a single molecule may catalyse up to 10 000 reactions per second. They vary in the specificity that they exhibit so that some enzymes will only react with one molecule while others react with a whole range of similar molecules. Enzyme reactions are temperature-dependent, the rate doubling for every 10°C rise. Enzyme molecules are easily destroyed by temperatures above 40°C, however, and they usually only function within a narrow pH range.

Enzyme inhibition

Enzymes can be inhibited in two principal ways: competitively and non-competitively.

Competitive inhibition. Molecules which are similar in structure to the usual substrate may combine with the enzyme's active site and prevent the binding of the substrate. This is called competitive inhibition and is reversible (Figure 1.21).

Sometimes the products of a series of enzyme reactions inactivate the first enzyme in the sequence and prevent the build up of product. This is an example of negative feedback. Some poisons act as enzyme inhibitors. Cyanide, for example, inhibits oxidative phosphorylation by inhibiting cytochrome oxidase (the last enzyme of the electron transport chain). As a result ATP synthesis ceases and the affected cells die.

Non-competitive inhibition. Heavy metal ions such as those of lead, mercury and arsenic all combine with secondary sites on enzyme molecules, causing distortion of the active site and inactivation (Figure 1.21). In this case, since the inhibitor is combining with an alternative site, inhibition is non-competitive and irreversible.

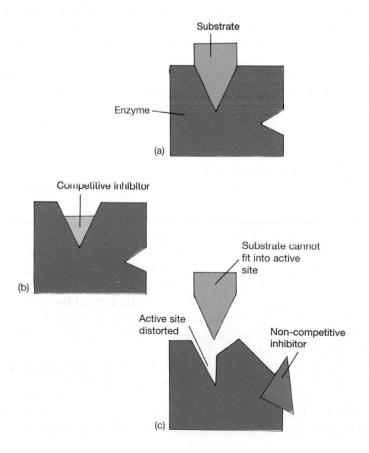

Figure 1.21 **(a)** The usual relationship between an enzyme and its substrate: the substrate combines with the active site on the enzyme. **(b)** Competitive inhibition: an inhibitor with a similar shape to the substrate combines with the active site and temporarily blocks it. **(c)** Non-competitive inhibition: an inhibitor combines with a different site on the enzyme, causing it to change its shape permanently so that it will no longer accept the substrate.

Nucleotides

Nucleotides are the structural components of deoxyribonucleic and ribonucleic acids (DNA and RNA). The nucleotide phosphate adenosine triphosphate (ATP) acts as an energy carrier within cells while cyclicadenosine monophosphate (-cAMP) is an intracellular messenger. Some nucleotides combine with other chemical groups to form coenzymes such as coenzyme A, nicotinamide adenine dinucleotide (NAD^+) and flavin adenine dinucleotide (FAD).

There are five different nucleotides, each of which is composed of a nitrogenous base linked to a sugar (either **ribose** or **deoxyribose**) and a phosphate group (Figure 1.22). The five bases are adenine, guanine (both purines), **cytosine**, **thymine** and **uracil** (pyrimidines) (Figure 1.23).

Each base links with a sugar to give rise to a **nucleoside** – adenosine, guanosine, cytidine, uridine and thymidine – and then with a phosphate group to create a nucleotide. Adenosine, guanosine, cytidine and thymidine are all constituents of the DNA molecule, while in RNA thymidine is replaced by uridine.

Figure 1.22 Structure of a nucleotide. P = phosphate; Sugar = ribose or deoxyribose; Base = adenine, cytosine, guanine, thymine or uracil.

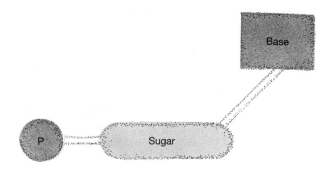

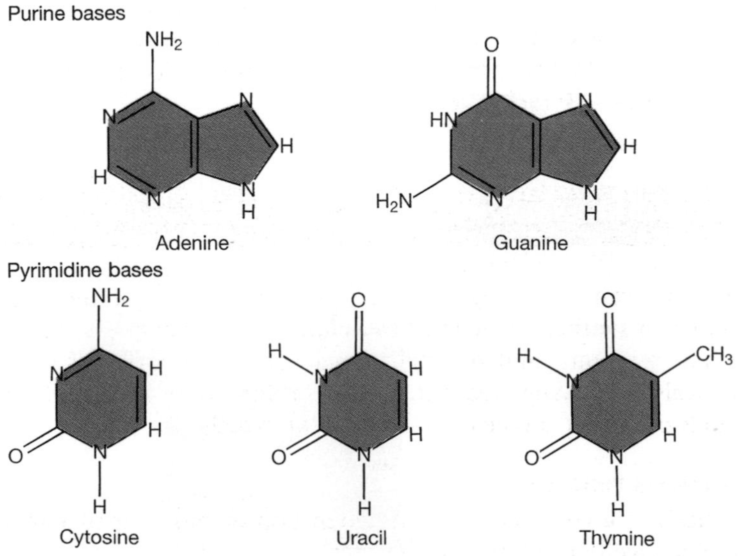

Figure 1.23 Structures of the five bases found in nucleotides.

Purine bases

Adenine

Guanine

Pyrimidine bases

Cytosine

Uracil

Thymine

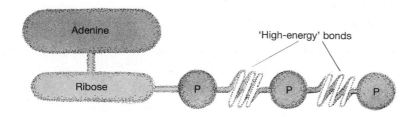

Figure 1.24 Diagrammatic representation of ATP structure. When a phosphate group is split off from the molecule, energy is released as if it were stored in the 'high-energy' bond.

The combination of adenine and ribose (adenosine) with one or more phosphate groups gives rise to a group of compounds that are concerned with energy storage and transfer. ATP stores energy (Figure 1.24); this energy is released when it is broken down to adenosine diphosphate (ADP) and phosphate (P).

The conversion of ATP to ADP liberates 30.6 kJ of energy per mole of ATP. cAMP is an important signalling compound within cells and is used as a 'second messenger' (i.e. it transfers the hormone's 'message' from the cell's surface into the cytoplasm) by many hormones.

$$ATP \xrightarrow{\text{ATPase}} ADP + P + ENERGY$$

$$ATP \xrightarrow{\text{Adenylate cyclase}} cAMP + P + P + ENERGY$$

ATP is formed when glucose molecules are broken down during cellular respiration. Glucose is oxidized (see Oxidation below), giving rise to water and carbon dioxide molecules and releasing energy which is stored as ATP.

$$C_6H_{12}O_6 + 6O_2 \longrightarrow 6CO_2 + H_2O + ATP$$

This equation is a summary of a complex series of enzyme-driven processes constituting cellular respiration (oxidation). The energy released from the breakdown of a single glucose molecule can be used to synthesize 38 ATP molecules.

Chemical reactions

Chemicals can react together in a number of ways: by combining together in synthesis reactions; by splitting into smaller parts in decomposition reactions; and by exchanging parts of themselves with other chemicals in exchange reactions. Of major importance in cellular metabolism is oxidation, a type of decomposition reaction.

Synthesis reactions

Synthesis of a compound occurs when two or more smaller molecules combine together to form a larger one.

$$A + B \longrightarrow AB$$

Such reactions occur in the body when, for example, amino acids join together to form proteins, or when glucose molecules link up to form glycogen. These reactions occur when food is stored in the liver and in fatty tissues and when the body is growing.

Within cells, the synthesis of larger compounds by the joining together of smaller ones is known as **anabolism**. These reactions require energy from the breakdown of ATP and are catalysed by enzymes.

Decomposition reactions

When a large molecule breaks down to form smaller units, decomposition is said to have taken place. Thus, when glycogen is broken down in the liver to release glucose into the blood, a decomposition reaction has taken place. This is also known as **catabolism**. The molecules that constitute food are catabolized by digestive enzymes. Catabolism also occurs in cellular oxidation when food molecules are broken down.

$$AB \longrightarrow A + B$$

OXIDATION/REDUCTION REACTIONS

Oxidation of a molecule occurs when it either gains oxygen (rare in biological systems) or loses hydrogen; conversely a molecule is reduced by the loss of oxygen (again rare) or the gain of hydrogen. When glucose is broken down within cells it can be said to be oxidized, since it loses hydrogen atoms; oxygen is, on the other hand, reduced since it gains hydrogen and forms water.

Oxidation by the removal of H is the commonest means of oxidation in cells; it is called **dehydrogenation**. The process usually involves coenzymes, which accept the H atoms and themselves become reduced. An example of this involves the coenzyme flavin adenine dinucleotide (FAD):

$$\underset{\text{coenzyme}}{FAD} + \underset{\text{hydrogen atoms}}{2H} \longrightarrow \underset{\text{reduced coenzyme}}{FADH_2}$$

Reduction is the reverse of this reaction, since reduced coenzyme supplies hydrogen atoms to the molecule (the substrate) which is itself being reduced. As a consequence the coenzyme is oxidized.

$$\underset{\substack{\text{reduced} \\ \text{coenzyme}}}{FADH_2} + \underset{\text{substrate}}{X} \longrightarrow \underset{\substack{\text{reduced} \\ \text{substrate}}}{XH_2} + \underset{\substack{\text{oxidized} \\ \text{coenzyme}}}{FAD}$$

Oxygen gain/hydrogen loss are not the only ways that molecules can be oxidized. It can also happen through the transfer of electrons from one molecule or atom to another. In this case the one that loses electrons (electron donor) is said to be oxidized, while the one which receives them (electron acceptor) is reduced. It is clear from this that such reactions occur when ionic compounds are formed. A simple example of reduction occurs in the stomach when ferric iron (Fe^{3+}) gains an electron to form ferrous iron (Fe^{2+}) which is more easily absorbed through the wall of the small intestine. Ferrous iron could be oxidized again by giving up its electron.

Exchange reactions

In this case part of one molecule is exchanged with, or is displaced by, a part of another molecule.

$$AB + CD \longrightarrow AD + BC$$

When glucose reacts with ATP, the latter loses its terminal phosphate group and transfers it to the glucose:

$$Glucose + ATP \longrightarrow Glucose\ phosphate + ADP.$$

Energy

Energy is defined as the ability to do work. It has two principal forms: kinetic and potential. **Kinetic energy** is the energy of movement, e.g. the movement of molecules in a gas or a liquid or the movement of muscles. **Potential energy** is, on the other hand, stored energy; a glucose molecule is high in potential energy because only when it breaks down will it release kinetic energy that drives cellular processes.

The concentration and electrical gradients across cell membranes provide examples of potential energy, because the presence of large numbers of molecules or ions on one side of a membrane create a driving force that will enable them to pass to the other side. Such gradients are themselves dependent upon active transport mechanisms, which use chemical energy. Thus, kinetic energy is employed to create a potential energy gradient.

All metabolic activities either use or liberate energy. Warm-blooded animals generate large quantities of heat, which is ultimately dispersed by radiation or conduction from the body's surface.

Energy is expressed as **joules** (J) or kilojoules (kJ). One joule is the quantity of potential energy released when a force of one Newton moves through a distance of one metre. 4.2 J of energy is the amount required to raise the temperature of 1 g of water by 1°C (4.2 kJ raises the temperature of 1 kg of water by the same amount). The amount of energy in food can be determined by burning it completely and using the heat to raise the temperature of a known volume of water. Knowledge of the energy content of the diet then enables estimates of energy requirements to be made; an active man may require approximately 14 000 kJ of energy per day.

Energy can neither be created nor destroyed, only converted from one form to another. In muscles and nerves, for example, chemical (potential) energy is converted into electrical and mechanical (kinetic) energy so that a nerve impulse is transmitted or a muscle shortens.

Ultimately all of the energy in all living organisms derives from the light emitted by the Sun. Green plants use the energy of sunlight to make sugars, thereby storing it as chemical energy. The plants are consumed by herbivorous animals, which are then eaten by carnivores. Some of the chemical energy is used for cellular activities and some is converted into chemical, mechanical or thermal energy. When organisms die their bodies are decomposed by organisms such as bacteria and fungi and so some of the energy is passed on.

Electromagnetic radiation

If electrons gain energy, they jump to a higher orbit within the atom. When they return to their original orbit, they emit energy as waves of electromagnetic radiation. In such waves, the electromagnetic disturbance is at right angles to the direction of motion of the wave (Figure 1.25).

The distance between equivalent points on two adjacent waves is known as the **wavelength** (measured in metres) and is equal to one complete cycle (Figure 1.26).

The **amplitude** of the wave is its 'height', while the **frequency** (measured in Hertz, Hz) is the number of waves generated by the source every second. Radiation with a short wavelength therefore has a higher frequency.

Figure 1.25 Electromagnetic waves.

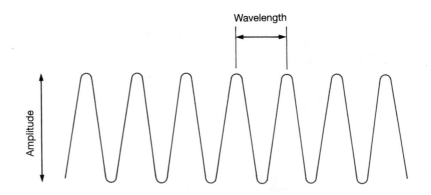

All electromagnetic waves travel at the same velocity (3×10^8 m/s) but there is a wide range of wavelengths from $< 10^{-10}$ m to $> 10^{-4}$ m, giving rise to an electromagnetic spectrum which covers a range from **gamma-rays, X-rays, visible light rays** and **infra-red waves** to **radio waves** (Figure 1.26).

Figure 1.26 The electromagnetic spectrum (not to scale).

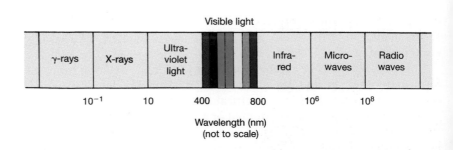

2

Cells and the internal environment

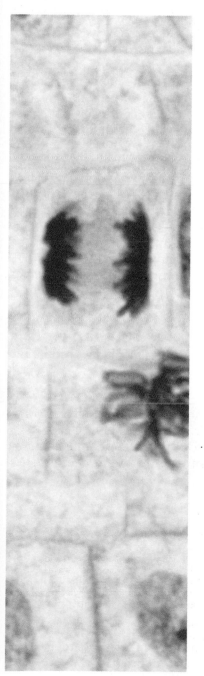

Body fluids

Water constitutes about 60% of the body mass of adult men of average weight. This is a composite figure, since different tissues vary in the amount of water they contain; thus fat-free tissue contains about 72 mL/100 g of water, whereas fatty (adipose) tissue contains practically none. It therefore follows that the greater the proportion of fat in the body, the lower will be the percentage composition of water. Women generally have a higher percentage of adipose tissue than men and thus a lower overall water content, about 50%. There is, however, a tremendous variation in the amount of adipose tissue present in both sexes. It is the convention therefore, rather than refer to water content as a percentage of whole body weight, to refer to the amount in fat-free tissue (72 mL/100 g) or as a percentage of lean body mass (72%).

During development from babyhood to adulthood there is a progressive reduction in the amount of extracellular fluid in the tissues. In the newborn baby fat-free tissue contains about 82 mL/100 g. A newborn baby has about 16% adipose tissue, which is approximately the same proportion as is found in an adult male. However, since the baby's tissues contain more water, the overall content is about 69% of total body mass. The water content of the lean body mass of a new-born baby falls from about 82% to about 72% in the adult.

In a 70 kg adult male the amount of fat-free tissue present is of the order of 58 kg. Since this 58 kg includes approximately 72% water (i.e. 60% of total body mass) then 42 L of body fluids is present. This is distributed between intracellular and extracellular 'compartments', roughly in the proportion 2:1, so that 28 L is found inside the cells and 14 L outside (Figure 2.1). Extracellular fluid is further subdivided into the fluid which surrounds and bathes the cells, interstitial fluid, which together with lymph constitutes some 11 L; and plasma within the cardiovascular system makes up the remaining 3 L.

Figure 2.1 The distribution of body fluids between intracellular, interstitial and plasma compartments. Values assume a gross body weight of 70 kg.

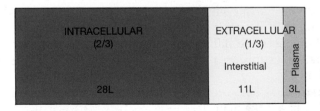

Composition and exchange of constituents between compartments

The composition of intracellular fluid varies in different cells, but there are consistent qualitative differences between it and extracellular fluid (Table 2.1).

Intracellular fluid contains a high proportion of soluble proteins, consisting mostly of enzymes. Although they are relatively mobile, the large size of proteins effectively traps them within the cell. Since these

Units of concentration are explained in **Concentration** (page 9), in Ch. 1, Molecules, Ions and Units.

Table 2.1 Electrolyte composition of body fluids (meq/L)

Substance	Intracellular	Interstitial	Serum
Cations			
Na$^+$	10	140	142
K$^+$	150	4	4
Ca^{2+}	2	5	5
Mg^{2+}	30	2	2
Anions			
Cl$^-$	10	110	100
HCO$_3^-$	10	28	27
HPO$_4^{2-}$/H$_2$PO$_4^-$	100	2	2
SO$_4^{2-}$	20	1	1
Protein	60	1	16

molecules carry negative charges, they make a major contribution to the total amount of intracellular anion and contribute to the uneven distribution of ions between the inside and outside of cells. Cl$^-$ and HCO$_3^-$ are present in small quantities compared with extracellular fluid, but the amount of PO$_4^{3-}$ is relatively high. K$^+$ is the most abundant cation in intracellular fluid, followed by Mg^{2+}, whereas Na$^+$ predominates in extracellular fluid. Differences in composition between intracellular and interstitial fluids are maintained by active transport systems operating across the cell membrane (see *Movement of substances across the cell membrane*, below).

Overall there are slightly more anions inside the cell than outside. This produces a small difference in charge between the inside and the outside of cells which is known as the **membrane potential**. This charge influences the diffusion of ions across cell membranes. Further consideration of this, in relation to Na$^+$ and K$^+$, is given in *The resting potential*, in Chapter 4.

Interstitial fluid is the largest component of extracellular fluid, i.e. about 11 L in a 70 kg man. This fluid lies between cells, usually held in a gel of polymerized hyaluronic acid. Dissolved materials pass between the cells and through the gel by diffusion.

Plasma volume averages about 3 L (with about 2 L of cells, total blood volume is around 5 L).

Plasma and interstitial fluid have a similar composition (Table 2.1) but plasma has a much higher protein content. Serum is the fluid which exudes from a clot. Its composition is the same as plasma, except that it lacks the protein fibrinogen (which forms the clot). As the movement of constituents between plasma and interstitial fluid is by diffusion across the capillary walls, it is understandable that the composition of the two

Plasma (page 325), in Ch. 11, Blood, Lymphoid Tissue and Immunity.

See **Formation and reabsorption of interstitial fluid** (page 409), in Ch. 12, Circulation of Blood and Lymph.

fluids is similar. Protein is retained largely within the blood vessels because of its large molecular size.

Every day, 20 or more litres of fluid filters out from the blood capillaries into the tissue spaces as interstitial fluid and, while about 90% of this fluid is normally reabsorbed, some drains away through the lymphatic system. Lymph is therefore derived from blood and is also ultimately returned to it.

Homoeostasis

The mineral and organic compositions of the plasma and interstitial fluid are maintained within very narrow limits by a variety of physiological mechanisms. This 'constant internal environment' is a necessary condition of life, an observation made by **Claude Bernard** in 1857. 'It is the constancy of the internal environment which is the condition of free and independent life. All vital mechanisms, however varied they may be, have only one object, that of preserving constant the conditions of life in the internal environment.' Later, in 1929, **Walter Cannon** coined the

Table 2.2   Contribution to homoeostasis made by the major body systems

System	Major activities	Effects on blood/interstitial fluid composition
Cardiovascular	Regulation of blood pressure	Maintenance of plasma composition and flow to the tissues
Digestive	Uptake of nutrients, water and ions; elimination of wastes	Maintenance of nutrient, water and ion concentrations; metabolite levels
Endocrine	Water and ion retention/elimination; control of plasma nutrient concentrations; sex drive	Maintenance of fluid volume; ion and nutrient concentrations
Locomotor	Release/addition of Ca^{2+} and PO_4^{3-} from/to bone; blood cell production; support/protection of internal organs; reflex and voluntary movement	Maintenance of Ca^{2+} and PO_4^{3-} concentrations; blood cell count; reflex and voluntary withdrawal from sources of damage/danger
Nervous	Regulation of cardiovascular, digestive, respiratory, locomotor systems and some endocrine organs; sensory processes; consciousness; mental processes; hunger and thirst	See other systems
Renal	Retention/elimination of water and solutes	Maintenance of fluid volume and composition
Respiratory	Intake of oxygen and elimination carbon dioxide	Maintenance of O_2, CO_2, H^+ concentrations

term homoeostasis to denote the constant and optimal internal environment (of interstitial fluid) resulting from the many varied regulatory mechanisms involved. Physiology is largely concerned with how these mechanisms operate within the body.

The term 'system' has been used traditionally to describe the group of organs that are associated with a particular physiological function, e.g. the nervous system, the digestive system. Table 2.2 provides an indication of the contribution to the maintenance of homoeostasis made by the systems of the body.

Cells

The observation that all living organisms are made of cells was first made by Robert Hooke in 1665. In 1839 the two German scientists Matthias Schleiden and Theodor Schwann postulated that the cell was the fundamental unit of which all living things are made. A little later, in 1858, Rudolph Virchow put forward the hypothesis that all cells arise from other pre-existing cells.

An understanding of cell structure and function is of fundamental importance in the analysis of body functions. The biochemical reactions that take place within cells determine their activities, and such reactions are under the control of the genetic material housed within the cell's nucleus. Cellular activity in turn affects the composition of the internal environment and therefore the health of the individual. An altered state of health, whether it is in the direction of illness or fitness, usually involves a change in the internal environment and therefore has a cellular basis. Drugs used in the treatment of illness act at the cellular level.

The smallest free-living single-celled organisms are the mycoplasmas, which are about 100 nm in diameter. The smallest bacteria are about 500 nm in diameter, while the majority of plant and animal cells vary between about 20 and 30 µm or 20 000–30 000 nm in diameter.

In the human body the majority of cells are grouped together with cells of similar types to form tissues.

Tissues are then grouped to form organs, the functional units of the body.

Before discussing cell and tissue structure and function, it is useful to consider some of the methods used to visualize them. Since cells are so small a magnifying system must be used in order to see them. While the light microscope allows cells and tissues to be observed at relatively low magnification (less than ×2000), it does not generally permit an examination of the internal structures of cells. This is because the resolution (the smallest distance between two points that can be differentiated) of the optical microscope is proportional to the wavelength of light used. Since the electron microscope employs a beam of electrons instead of light and such a beam has a very short wavelength, then the resolution of the electron microscope is correspondingly greater and allows much greater magnification (potentially up to ×several million).

> An account of the different types of tissue found in the body is given in Ch. 3, Tissues.

Optical microscopy

The basic components of the optical or light microscope are a light source, and objective and eyepiece lenses. Light passes through the specimen and is collected and focussed by the objective lens to create a real image. The latter is then viewed by the eyepiece lens, which produces an enlarged virtual image that is projected on to the retina of the eye (Figure 2.2).

The modern light microscope normally has, in addition to the above, a built-in light source, condenser lenses, which focus light on to the specimen, and compound objective and eyepiece lenses, which eliminate the chromatic and spherical aberrations produced by single lenses.

It is evident that, if light is to pass through the specimen, then the specimen must be transparent or at least translucent. For this reason only thin sections of tissues and organs and in some cases smears or squashes, can be studied. In addition, since most tissues, in section, are not only transparent but also colourless, they must be stained in order to be seen at all.

A wide variety of techniques exists for the **preparation of materials for optical microscopy** and tissues may be examined fresh, frozen or fixed. The most common technique requires the preparation of thin sections of fixed (preserved) material and it is this which is described here.

It is important, if an accurate picture of tissue structure is to be achieved, that tissue is removed from the body, either living, as in a biopsy, or as soon as possible after death. A small piece of tissue is taken and placed in a fixative solution (e.g. one that includes formaldehyde). This not only kills the tissue, but also preserves it. After several hours, or in some cases days, the fixative is washed away and the tissue is dehydrated by replacing the water held within its structure by an organic agent (e.g. alcohol). The tissue is then impregnated with a substance which can be made to set hard. Molten paraffin wax may be used for this, but since it is not miscible with alcohol some intermediate or 'clearing' agent must be employed prior to wax impregnation.

Once the tissue is fully impregnated with wax, it is allowed to cool and harden. The tissue is now fully embedded within a wax block and is hard enough that thin sections (usually less than $60\,\mu m$) can be cut with a microtome.

The tissue sections are floated out on to the surface of a warm water bath from which they are collected on to glass slides. After drying, the wax is removed with an organic solvent and the section is hydrated again, by reversing the dehydration procedure. This is followed by a staining procedure, which may be simple, involving one stain only, or complex, involving several different stains. A vast range of chemical dyes is available for this purpose and they may be used in combination to differentiate the components of cells and tissues. One of the simplest combinations uses haematoxylin (an acid blue dye) and eosin (a basic pink dye) to differentiate purple nuclei from pink cytoplasm.

Once again the tissue is dehydrated and then cleared by treating it with a solvent which is miscible with the medium used to mount the final product.

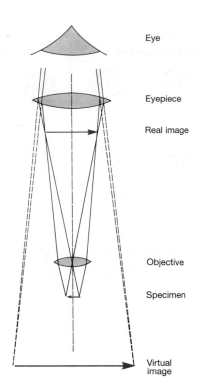

Eye

Eyepiece

Real image

Objective

Specimen

Virtual image

Figure 2.2 Principle of the optical microscope.

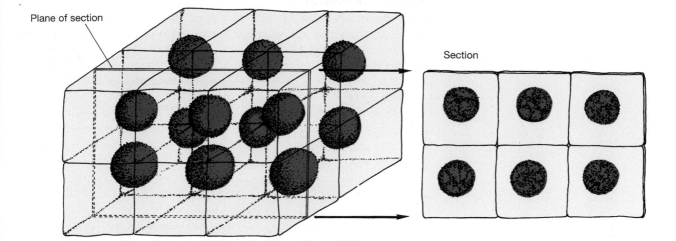

Section

The prepared section is now ready to be viewed through the microscope. Clearly, what is being observed is quite different from the original specimen. The tissue is no longer alive, it has been thoroughly soaked in a series of organic solvents and its structure is incomplete, since the section only represents a thin slice of the original (Figure 2.3). Nevertheless it is possible, by cutting many such sections, to create a three-dimensional picture of the tissue's original structure; this is called micro-reconstruction.

Newer methods use hard-setting plastics and resins rather than paraffin wax and are capable of generating images with finer detail.

Frozen sections are prepared when speed is important but quality less so. They are used, for example, during surgery for the identification of cancerous cells.

Figure 2.3 Removal of a thin section from a block of tissue.

Electron microscopy

Most intracellular structures are too small to be visualized with the long wavelengths employed by the optical microscope. For this reason the transmission electron microscope is used, since it uses a beam of electrons of very short wavelength. This beam is fired down a column and transmitted through a thin section of tissue before striking a fluorescent plate upon which an image is produced. The electron beam is focussed by a series of magnets which are analogous to the glass lenses in the optical microscope (Figure 2.4).

The **preparative techniques** are also similar to those employed by light microscopists. Fresh tissue is taken and fixed, then embedded, sectioned and stained. In this case very small pieces are taken to facilitate the rapid penetration of fixative.

After fixation the tissue is dehydrated and then mounted in a plastic or resin (not wax), which is hardened by the addition of chemical hardeners and the application of heat. The block, which is much harder than the wax blocks employed by optical microscopists, is sectioned on an ultramicrotome, which includes an extremely sharp glass or diamond knife. Sections of less than 150 nm thick are normally cut.

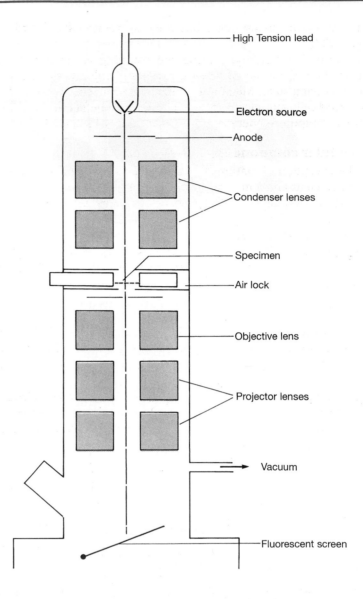

Figure 2.4 Structure of the transmission electron microscope.

The sections are stained by the addition of heavy metal ions, which show up in the electron beam. The stained sections, each of which is probably less than 1 mm square, are introduced into the electron beam. The latter passes down to the specimen, which freely transmits the electrons through unstained areas while heavy metal ions that have been deposited in the section absorb electrons, the amount of absorption being proportional to the amount of stain. At the bottom of the column is a fluorescent screen, which is excited by the transmitted electrons such that a 'shadow picture' is produced. Thus, the images produced by the electron microscope are black and white and have very high magnification and a much higher definition than those obtained by optical microscopy (see Figures 8.4, 14.9).

If pressed, electron microscopists might admit that the internal structure of the cell does not have the appearance of an electron micrograph when it is in the living state, but they conventionally describe it as though it did!

An alternative technique, using the scanning electron microscope, produces three-dimensional images, perhaps giving a better representation of the living state. Metal ions are deposited on the surfaces of intact or fractured cells and electrons are reflected off the surface and used to produce a computer-generated image (see Figures 14.7, 8.24).

Intracellular components

With the exception of mature red blood cells, all human cells contain at least one nucleus and a mass of surrounding **cytoplasm** (Figure 2.5).

The latter is made up of the **cytosol**, a watery gelatinous mass that constitutes about half the bulk of most cells, and a variety of small components or **organelles**. In addition, the cell may also contain temporary structures, or inclusions, such as excretory vesicles or glycogen deposits. No cell contains every type of cytoplasmic organelle or inclusion and some cells contain very few of them.

NUCLEUS

Not only is the nucleus normally the most evident organelle within a cell, it is also of great importance because it regulates all the functions of the cell by controlling enzyme synthesis. It also plays a central role in cell division.

The contents of the nucleus are separated from the cytoplasm by a double nuclear membrane. The two layers are fused at some points, giving rise to nuclear pores, which are thought to allow molecules to pass between nucleus and cytoplasm (Figures 2.5, 2.6).

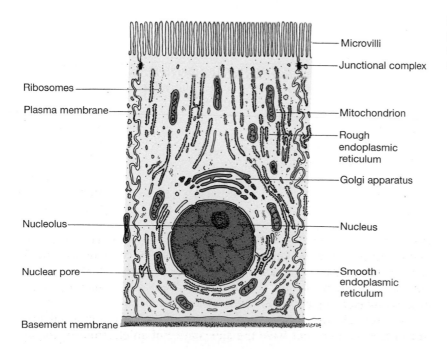

Ribosomes

Plasma membrane

Microvilli

Junctional complex

Mitochondrion

Rough endoplasmic reticulum

Golgi apparatus

Nucleolus

Nucleus

Nuclear pore

Smooth endoplasmic reticulum

Basement membrane

Figure 2.5 Section through a cell of striated epithelium to show some of the common intracellular organelles.

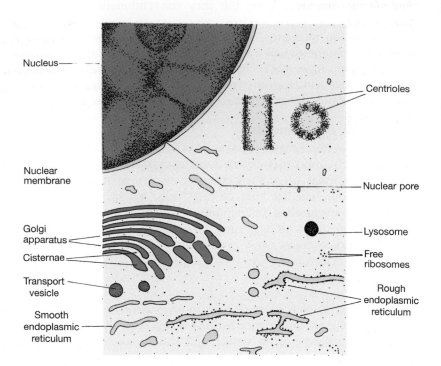

Figure 2.6 Section through the cytoplasm close to the nucleus to show the centrioles and Golgi apparatus.

Electron micrographs reveal irregular masses of a heavily stained material in the nucleus. This is called **chromatin** and is a mixture of protein, **deoxyribonucleic acid (DNA)** and some **ribonucleic acid (RNA)**. When the cell reproduces itself the chromatin condenses to form 46 small threads, the **chromosomes**.

Normally one or two areas appear to be especially condensed: these are the **nucleoli**, which are rich in RNA. The nucleoli disappear during cell replication and then reappear in the daughter cells.

The nucleus is the repository of genetic information for the whole body. However, while each cell contains identical genetic information, in any one cell most of it will not be functional, i.e. it will be 'switched off'. In cells of the same type, the same part of the message will be 'switched on' but in different types of cells, different parts will be 'switched on'. The nature of this genetic information and the way in which it functions is described in the sections on *Chromosomes* and *Protein synthesis,* below.

CYTOPLASM

Cytosol

The cytosol represents approximately 50% of the cell's volume. It is a watery, gelatinous substance containing about 20% protein, much of which is arranged in strands or fibrils. There are also thousands of enzyme molecules present so that the cytosol is metabolically very active.

Endoplasmic reticulum

The endoplasmic reticulum is usually one of the more obvious cytoplasmic organelles. It is composed of a series of interconnecting membrane-bound tubules or channels and is found in the cytoplasm of all nucleated cells (Figures 2.5, 2.6). Very small amounts of endoplasmic reticulum may be present, or the cytoplasm may be almost completely filled as, for example, in pancreatic cells. Endoplasmic reticulum is always being destroyed and reformed and the amount is not constant in any one particular cell.

The membranes of the endoplasmic reticulum may have a smooth or granular appearance (**smooth endoplasmic reticulum** or **rough endoplasmic reticulum**). The latter is due to the presence of minute RNA-rich particles called **ribosomes**, which are attached to the membrane surface.

Smooth endoplasmic reticulum is involved in the synthesis of lipids, including those required for the synthesis of membrane. In liver cells it contains the enzymes that catalyse glycogen breakdown. It may also be associated with the detoxification of drugs.

Rough endoplasmic reticulum synthesizes protein molecules, most of which are to be secreted by the cell. For example, the cells of the pancreas synthesize digestive enzymes. Molecules pass into the cavities of the endoplasmic reticulum and are transported towards the Golgi apparatus. **Transport vesicles** containing the protein are pinched off from the endoplasmic reticulum and then travel to and fuse with the Golgi apparatus. Most protein for intracellular use is assembled on the free ribosomes in the cytosol. Free ribosomes become attached to the endoplasmic reticulum and thus become part of the rough endoplasmic reticulum only when they are synthesizing secretory proteins.

Golgi apparatus

The Golgi apparatus (Golgi body or complex) is similar in appearance to smooth endoplasmic reticulum. It consists of several flattened sacs or cisternae, which are usually arranged in a cup-like configuration. The 'cup' may face towards the nucleus, but more often it faces away.

The Golgi apparatus receives membrane-bound protein, in the form of transport vesicles from the rough endoplasmic reticulum, on its convex surface (Figure 2.6). Vesicles then pass from cisterna to cisterna within the Golgi apparatus, undergoing biochemical changes. Finally they are pinched off from the concave surface and pass into the cytoplasm. These vesicles may be of the secretory type, in which case they will pass to the edge of the cell and the contents will be discharged, or they may form lysosomes.

Carbohydrates may be added to the protein within the Golgi apparatus to form glycoproteins, and mucus is also formed in this area.

Lysosomes

Lysosomes are small, membrane-bound bodies about 0.5 μm in diameter that are formed from vesicles separated off from the Golgi apparatus. Typically they appear darkly stained in electron micrographs and they are present in varying numbers in all of the nucleated cells of the human body.

Lysosomes contain about 40 different enzymes, including **hydrolases**, which can break down all types of macromolecules, and **lysozyme**, which digests the cell walls of bacteria.

Their function is thus primarily digestive. In damaged tissues they break open and cause the digestion of adjacent cells; at other times they may simply cause the breakdown of individual organelles. In this case the organelle becomes surrounded by a membrane, forming an isolation body. The lysosome then combines with this body and the contents are broken down (see Figure 2.14).

In phagocytic cells, which ingest foreign or waste material, the lysosome combines with the phagocytic vesicle and the digestion products are absorbed into the cytoplasm, leaving the undigested residue behind. Pinocytic vesicles are also digested by lysosomes (see also *Endocytosis and exocytosis*, below).

Peroxisomes

Peroxisomes are small, membrane-bound bodies similar in appearance to lysosomes. They are different in function, however, in that they contain **catalase**, which causes the breakdown of **hydrogen peroxide**. The latter is formed by some of the metabolic reactions of the cell and is extremely toxic. The peroxisomes remove the molecules as they are formed and thus prevent damage to the cell.

Mitochondria

Mitochondria are found in varying numbers in all nucleated cells. They may be distributed evenly throughout the cytoplasm or concentrated in areas of high energy requirement; for example they lie between the fibrils of muscle fibres, where they produce energy for contraction.

Mitochondria are small bodies, which may be round or filamentous and may be less than 1 µm wide and up to 9 µm long; they are sometimes found to be branched. Mitochondrial form is not necessarily fixed and may change, depending upon external factors acting upon the cell. Each mitochondrion is bounded by a smooth outer membrane, which is separated by a small space of between 10 and 20 nm from a folded inner membrane. These folds are called **cristae** (Figure 2.7) and are studded with minute mushroom-like particles.

Figure 2.7 Structure of a typical mitochondrion.

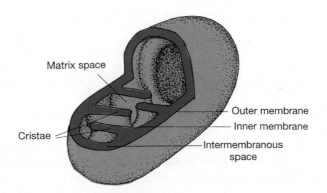

Both inner and outer membranes, the space between them, the membrane-bound particles and the inner matrix all contain enzymes.

Some enzymes oxidize (break down) nutrients into carbon dioxide and water, with the release of energy. Other enzymes enable part of this energy to be 'trapped' within **adenosine triphosphate** (ATP) molecules.

The remaining energy released during oxidation is lost as heat.

ATP is used as a source of energy in cells for activities such as active transport, muscle contraction and synthesis of molecules. The energy stored within the ATP molecule is released when it loses one phosphate group and becomes adenosine diphosphate (ADP). This reaction is catalysed by the enzyme ATPase, which is found at many sites within cells.

Mitochondria contain their own DNA, which directs the synthesis of mitochondrial protein. In addition, mitochondria are able to replicate themselves. When cells divide, the original number of mitochondria are distributed between the two daughter cells. These mitochondria later replicate themselves so that each daughter cell has roughly the same number as the parent. It has been suggested that mitochondria are actually bacteria that have become incorporated into the cells of animals and plants. This supposition is supported by the fact that mitochondrial DNA is circular and closely resembles that found in bacteria.

Actin filaments, microtubules and intermediate filaments

Within the cytoplasm of the cell there are a number of filaments and tubules which give rise to a supporting network, the **cytoskeleton**.

Actin filaments are about 7 nm in diameter and are linked by cross-bridges to form three-dimensional networks. An especially dense network beneath the cell membrane provides mechanical strength to the cell surface. Filaments extend up into and provide mechanical strength for the microvilli that project from the surface of cells that, for example, line the gut.

Actin is capable, in association with myosin, of causing cellular movement and shape changes.

Like microfilaments, **microtubules** contribute to the maintenance of cell shape and are found, for example, as neurofibrils in the axons of nerve fibres. They provide a framework for the attachment of cytoplasmic organelles and pathways for the movement of some of them. In addition, they also constitute the motile structures of cilia and flagellae and form the spindle of dividing cells.

In the majority of cells microtubules develop from the centrosome (Figure 2.8).

Microtubules are larger than actin filaments, having a diameter of about 25 nm, and are more highly organized, being composed of 13 **protofilaments** arranged so as to form a hollow cylinder. The protofilaments are themselves composed of assemblies of the globular protein **tubulin**. They grow out by the addition of tubulin subunits until they reach a cytoplasmic structure, to which they become attached. Microtubules which are not 'capped' in this way continually break down and re-form so that there is a constant turnover of microtubules and tubulin within the cell.

The structure of ATP is described in **Nucleotides** (page 26) in Ch. 1, Molecules, Ions and Units.

The processes by which ATP is synthesized are described in **Metabolic fate of absorbed food** (page 594), in Ch. 15, Digestion and Absorption of Food.

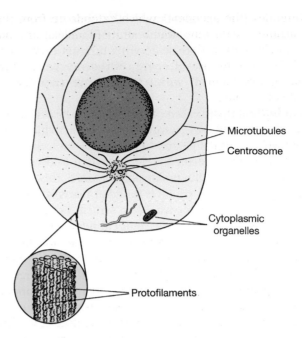

Figure 2.8 Microtubules develop from the centrosome and become attached to cytoplasmic organelles (**Inset** – short section of a microtubule comprising 13 protofilaments of the protein tubulin).

The molecular components of **intermediate filaments** are fibrous in nature. The filaments formed from these subunits are thicker than actin filaments (about 10 nm in diameter) and provide mechanical support to the plasma and nuclear membranes. There are at least four different types of intermediate filament, which are specific to particular tissues, e.g. desmin is found only in muscle cells.

Centrioles

Two short cylindrical bodies, the centrioles (approximately 0.7 μm long and 0.2 μm in diameter), lie close to the nucleus, usually at right angles to one another. They lie at the centre of a small volume of cytoplasm which is identified as the **centrosome**, the cell 'centre'. Each centriole contains nine sets of triple microtubules (Figure 2.6).

The centrioles assist in cell division, since they give rise to the spindle fibres (which are, in fact, microtubules) that pull the daughter chromatids apart.

Centrioles are self-replicating and in the early stages of cell division they separate slightly and reproduce themselves. Thus, for a while, the dividing cell has two sets of centrioles.

Cilia and flagella

Both cilia and flagella are thread-like processes, 0.2 μm in diameter, which protrude from the apical surfaces of some cells. Flagella are normally quite long, up to 200 μm, while cilia are much shorter, being less than 10 μm in length. Flagella are normally present in small numbers; for example, the male human spermatozoon has only one. Cilia, on the other hand, are more numerous and the free surfaces of the epithelial cells that line the upper respiratory tract are covered by them.

Both types of thread have the same internal structure, having a core of microtubules (the axoneme) which extends up from the basal body and are arranged with nine double units (doublets) around the outside and two single ones in the centre. This 'nine plus two' organization is slightly different from the 'nine plus zero' structure of centrioles (Figure 2.9). During development the doublets arise from only two of the tubules of each triplet.

A **basal body** lies at the base of each cilium, having a 'nine plus zero' structure like that of centrioles. Some basal bodies are attached to rootlets which anchor the cilia in the cytoplasm.

Both types of organelle are able to move due to the sliding of adjacent doublets against one another. The doublets are linked by large protein complexes (**dynein**), which project from the microtubules and have ATPase activity. The dynein heads enable the doublets to interact in much the same way as actin and myosin in muscle contraction.

Flagella move the cell to which they are attached through the surrounding liquid medium. Cilia, on the other hand, tend to move the medium over the cell surface.

Cilia have a stiff, rapid effective stroke and a slower, flexible recovery stroke. All the cilia at a given site beat in the same direction, and commonly in epithelial tissues the beat is metachronal. This means that all the cilia in each successive row start their cycle slightly later than those in the one before, so that a wave sweeps over the surface. The effect of this activity in the respiratory tract, for example, is that a sheet of mucus is propelled towards the pharynx. Such cilia are strictly called

See **Ciliated cells** (page 75), in Ch. 3, Tissues.

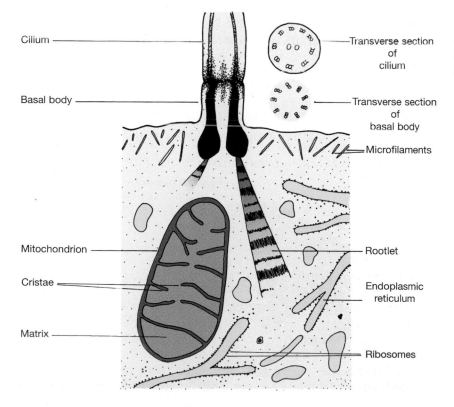

Cilium

Basal body

Transverse section of cilium

Transverse section of basal body

Microfilaments

Mitochondrion

Cristae

Matrix

Rootlet

Endoplasmic reticulum

Ribosomes

Figure 2.9 Section through the cytoplasm near the surface of the cell to show the base of a cilium and a mitochondrion.

kinocilia to distinguish them from stereocilia, which are nonmobile and resemble long microvilli.

Membranes

STRUCTURE

In an electron micrograph of an animal cell, darkly-stained membrane structures usually form the most obvious features. The cell is bounded by a membrane, variously called the cell membrane, plasma membrane or plasmalemma. The nucleus is bounded by the nuclear membrane and the cytoplasmic organelles e.g. endoplasmic reticulum, Golgi apparatus and mitochondria are all membrane-bound structures. Membranes regulate the entry and exit of molecules between the cytoplasm and the surrounding medium and perform vital functions within the cell.

Lipid constitutes approximately 50% of the mass of the plasma membrane; the remainder is protein, with a relatively small amount of carbohydrate. There is, however, considerable variation in the relative proportions of lipid and protein at different sites and the inner membranes of mitochondria, for example, are about 80% protein and 20% lipid. A study of the penetration of various substances into cells indicates that the lipid extends over all, or almost all, of the cell surface. Much of the lipid is in the form of **phospholipid** molecules, which have a charged 'head' region and a pair of hydrocarbon 'tails'. One end of the molecule, the 'head', is **hydrophilic** (has an affinity for water) and the other end is **hydrophobic** (does not mix with water) (see Figure 1.17). Although there may be approximately equal masses of protein and lipid, because of the small size of the phospholipid molecules there are about 50 phospholipid molecules for each one protein molecule.

Singer and Nicolson, in 1972, put forward the '**fluid-mosaic**' model of the cell membrane in which the protein molecules 'float' in a two-layered 'sea' of phospholipid (Figure 2.10).

The double layer of phospholipid molecules has the hydrophilic 'heads' next to the water and the hydrophobic 'tails' sandwiched in the middle. The 'fluid-mosaic' model is asymmetrical so that the phospholipid molecules in one layer may differ from those in the other and

Figure 2.10 The fluid-mosaic model of the cell membrane.

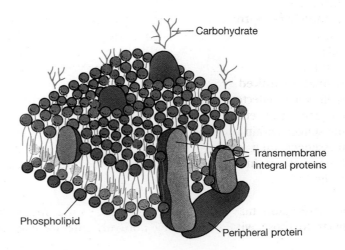

molecules do not readily exchange between the two layers. In addition, some proteins lie in one lipid layer, some in the other, while **trans-membrane (integral) proteins** extend right through the membrane. Some of these proteins are known as permeases and are thought to act as channels or 'pores' for the passage of water and small solutes. According to this model, proteins can move about within the lipid layer, although it is suggested that cholesterol (which is also part of the membrane) is able to restrict this movement. Furthermore, some proteins are anchored to underlying microtubules and/or filaments, which restricts their movement. Other proteins (**peripheral proteins**) are found only on the inner surface of the cell membrane, while carbo-hydrate molecules are attached to proteins and lipids only on the outer surface. This sparse carbohydrate layer on the outer surface of the cell membrane is called the **glycocalyx**.

MEMBRANE RECEPTORS

One of the activities of the cell membrane is that it receives information from other cells. Communication between cells takes the form of chem-ical messages and there are receptors on the cell surface that are able to detect these messages. There are specific proteins incorporated into the plasma membrane which are able to 'recognize' water-soluble substances, such as protein hormones and neurotransmitters and also some lipids.

Receptor proteins may be scattered over the surface of a cell or they may be confined to small areas; there may be between 500 and 100 000 on any one cell.

There are three types of receptor found: 1) channel-linked, 2) catalytic and 3) G protein-linked receptors.

1. **Channel-linked receptors** are found on the surfaces of nerve cell bodies and dendrites (in synapses) and effectors such as muscles, glands and the heart. They combine with ('recognize') neurotransmitter substances such as acetylcholine and noradrena-line and the combination opens channels that enable ions to pass into or out of the target cell. This then initiates, or in some cases prevents, the generation of an action potential in the effector cell membrane.

2. **Catalytic receptors**, such as tyrosine-specific protein kinases, are transmembrane proteins that are activated by the signalling mole-cule and then catalyse a reaction within the cytoplasm. The hormone insulin is a signalling molecule for this type of receptor.

3. **G protein-linked receptors** take up the signalling molecule and then, via an effector protein, influence either an ion channel or an enzyme. The enzyme catalyses the production of a second messenger within the cytoplasm (cyclic AMP or Ca^{2+}). The second messenger then catalyses specific intracellular reactions. Many hormones act in this way, causing an increase in intracellular cyclic AMP.

Second messengers are discussed in **Cellular mechanisms of hormone action** (page 612), in Ch. 16, Endocrine Physiology.

Membrane receptors may not be totally specific, so that molecules that are similar to those with which they normally interact may become

See **The thyroid gland** (page 623), in Ch. 16, Endocrine Physiology.

The principles of diffusion are described in **Diffusion** (page 13), in Ch. 1, Molecules, Ions and Units.

bound to them. In hyperthyroidism, for example, an antibody (LATS – long acting thyroid stimulator) binds to the TSH (thyroid stimulating hormone) sites on the cells of the thyroid gland. The latter then react as though they had been stimulated by TSH and produce large quantities of thyroxine.

MOVEMENT OF SUBSTANCES ACROSS THE CELL MEMBRANE

The cell membrane separates the intracellular and interstitial compartments. There is continual movement of water and solutes between the two compartments brought about by a variety of mechanisms. Substances may pass down a concentration gradient (i.e. from a region of high concentration to a region of low concentration) using their own inherent kinetic energy. This process is known as simple diffusion and is generally employed by small ions or molecules and lipids.

Large solutes generally cross the membrane attached to a carrier molecule (a protein in the membrane). When such transport is from a high to a low concentration it is known as **facilitated diffusion**.

A different transport mechanism employs energy derived from the breakdown of ATP so that molecules can be taken against the concentration gradient. This is **carrier-mediated active transport**.

Molecules may also enter or leave the cell by a mechanism which involves a physical change in the structure of the membrane. **Phagocytosis** or **pinocytosis** literally means 'cell eating' or 'cell drinking' and involves the uptake of relatively large amounts of particulate matter or fluid. **Exocytosis** is the reverse of this and involves the elimination of material from the cell.

Simple diffusion

Intracellular and interstitial fluid compartments are separated by a cell membrane, which is permeable, to a variable extent (selectively), to most solutes. The unequal distribution of each solute between compartments gives rise to a concentration gradient which promotes the diffusion of solute towards the lower concentration.

The selective nature of membrane permeability affects the ease with which particular solutes diffuse across the cell membrane. Lipid solubility, particle size and ionic charge are the major **factors affecting diffusion**. (Figure 2.11).

Molecules of high lipid solubility pass through the membrane more easily than those with low lipid solubility. When lipid solubilities are identical small molecules pass more easily than large ones. Lipids and lipid soluble substances diffuse through the phospholipid bilayer.

Electrolytes, which are water-soluble, pass through less easily than non-electrolytes. The greater the charge the more difficult it becomes for molecules to pass; thus Ca^{2+} will enter a cell less easily than Na^+. Ionic size is a further regulating factor in that small ions will pass more easily than large ions of the same charge. Size in this case, however, does not necessarily just mean ionic size, for ions tend to collect water molecules, which travel with them. Na^+ is a smaller ion than K^+, but Na^+ gathers more water molecules around itself than does K^+. Therefore the 'hydrated radius' of Na^+ is larger and it passes less easily than K^+. Water-

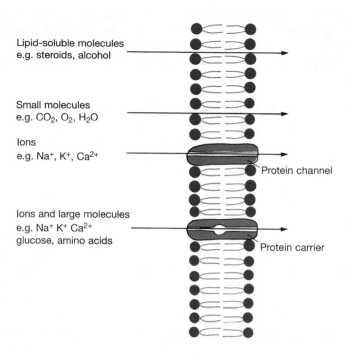

Lipid-soluble molecules
e.g. steroids, alcohol

Small molecules
e.g. CO_2, O_2, H_2O

Ions
e.g. Na^+, K^+, Ca^{2+}

Protein channel

Ions and large molecules
e.g. Na^+ K^+ Ca^{2+}
glucose, amino acids

Protein carrier

Figure 2.11 Factors affecting membrane transport.

soluble substances such as ions pass through protein channels in the membrane; such channels are generally specific to particular ions.

Although the concentration gradient is the principal driving force for the diffusion of ions, the presence of a potential difference (electrical gradient) across the surface membrane of all cells also affects their movement. If there is a concentration gradient promoting the diffusion of anions into the cell, for example, the negative intracellular charge acts as a force impeding their entry, so that the number diffusing into the cell is reduced. If, however, the concentration gradient for cations promotes diffusion into the cell, the electrical gradient facilitates their entry.

The combined effects of a concentration gradient and an electrical gradient (**electrochemical gradient**), therefore, control the diffusion of ions across the cell membrane.

The permeability of the membrane to various substances is not necessarily fixed and in the activated nerve axon, for example, the permeability for Na^+ is markedly raised above its resting value.

Osmosis

Water moves through the cell membrane by osmosis when there is a concentration gradient. Water diffuses from a region where there is more water to a region of less water. Since the solution with more water molecules is the one with fewer solute molecules, it is usually considered to be the 'weaker' one; osmosis can therefore also be defined as the passage of water from a 'weak' solution to a 'strong' one.

As water molecules are small and do not carry a charge, they are able to pass through the lipid layers of the membrane.

Generation of action potentials is described in **Cellular basis of the nerve impulse** (page 114), in Ch. 4, Cellular Mechanisms of Neural Control.

The principles of osmosis are described in **Osmosis** (page 13), in Ch. 1, Molecules, Ions and Units.

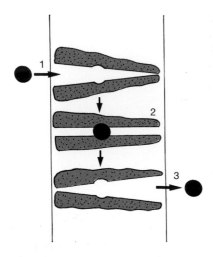

Figure 2.12 Active transport through the cell membrane. (1) A molecule passes into the space within the carrier molecule in the membrane, and (2) attaches to a binding site. (3) The carrier molecule then alters its configuration so that the binding site will release the transported molecule into the cytoplasm.

Active transport and facilitated diffusion

Most solutes are transported actively across the cell membrane, thereby maintaining the difference in composition between intracellular and extracellular fluids. Glucose enters most cells by the process of facilitated diffusion, but in some sites by secondary active transport.

Active transport and facilitated diffusion both depend upon the presence of **carrier molecules** in the membrane. Since there are a finite number of such molecules, both processes are liable to saturation, i.e. a maximum rate of transfer may be achieved.

The two processes differ in that active transport requires metabolic energy (from ATP breakdown) and moves solutes **up a concentration gradient**; facilitated diffusion is a passive process and requires only the kinetic energy of the molecules to move them **down a concentration gradient**.

In both active transport and facilitated diffusion the carrier molecules are proteins. In both cases the molecule to be transported is taken up on one side of the membrane by the carrier which then undergoes a structural (conformational) change.

In active transport the carrier is either an enzyme or a molecule that is enzyme-linked. The carrier for both Na$^+$ and K$^+$ is the enzyme **ATPase**, so that it catalyses the release of energy from ATP at the same time as it transports K$^+$ into the cell and Na$^+$ out. This process is known as the **sodium–potassium 'pump' (Na$^+$–K$^+$ pump)**.

Figure 2.12 shows a possible mechanism for the carrier-assisted transport of materials through a membrane.

More than one molecule may be transported at a time. Glucose is transported coupled with Na$^+$ in specific sites such as the epithelial lining of the small intestine and the proximal tubule of the nephron (Figure 2.13).

Figure 2.13 Secondary active transport (cotransport). Na$^+$ is actively transported out of the cell, thereby maintaining a low intracellular concentration. Na$^+$ diffuses into the cell down its concentration gradient attached to a carrier to which glucose is also bound. The uptake of glucose is therefore secondary to the active transport of Na$^+$ out of the cell.

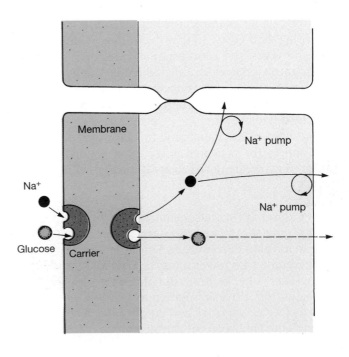

In this case glucose can be taken against a concentration gradient because it links to the same carrier as Na$^+$, which is passing down a gradient. Na$^+$ is then removed from the cell by active transport, which maintains a low level of Na$^+$ within the cell and thus preserves the gradient. The glucose transport mechanism is known as **secondary active transport** or **cotransport**. The mechanism by which Na$^+$ is extruded from the cell is called **primary active transport**.

The brain damage that follows acute oxygen deprivation may be due to the inactivation of the Na$^+$–K$^+$ pump, which leads to the accumulation of Na$^+$ inside the cells, a raised osmotic pressure and consequently cellular swelling.

Endocytosis and exocytosis

Endocytosis is cellular uptake of fluid (pinocytosis) or particles (phagocytosis) by invagination of the cell's membrane forming membrane-bound vesicles or vacuoles (Figure 2.14).

Exocytosis is the reverse of endocytosis, in which the contents of vacuoles are released from the cell and the vacuolar membrane fuses with the cell membrane. Both mechanisms require cellular energy, which is derived from ATP.

Small amounts of extracellular fluid are taken up continuously by most cells by **pinocytosis** ('cell drinking'). This process is non-selective, so that the contents of the vesicles so formed are in the same proportions as in extracellular fluid.

Receptor-mediated endocytosis, on the other hand, is a highly selective process by which specific molecules bind to the cell membrane which invaginates and takes in extracellular fluid and the bound molecules.

Figure 2.14 Endocytosis and exocytosis. **(a)** Phagocytosis: pseudopodia engulf the particle and fuse to enclose the particle in a vesicle. **(b)** The fate of particulate matter. The particle is taken into the cytoplasm (1) and is carried to a lysosome (3) with which it fuses (4). The lysosome has been formed by the Golgi apparatus (2). The particle is digested by the lysosomal enzymes and the waste material is ejected by exocytosis (5). **(c)** Pinocytosis: a small channel forms in the surface membrane (1), it deepens (2) and pinches off at the bottom to form a vesicle (3).

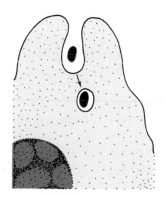

(a)

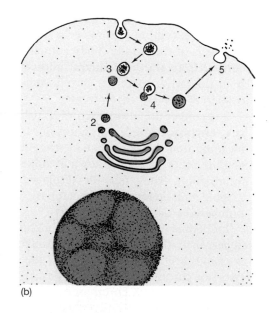

(b)

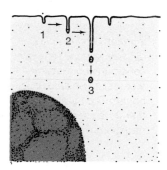

(c)

Large particles such as bacteria and cellular debris are absorbed by **phagocytosis** ('cell eating'). In this process the cell normally puts out large cytoplasmic extensions or **pseudopodia**, which surround and engulf the particle, forming a phagosome (diameter > 250 nm), which is then digested by lysosomal enzymes. The mechanism by which pseudopodia are formed is actin-dependent. Cells in which phagocytosis is a major activity are known as **phagocytes**; they include neutrophils and macrophages.

Phagocytosis only occurs in the presence of 'foreign' material. Receptors on the cell surface bind with the molecules/objects to be ingested. Thus, for example, receptors on the surface of a neutrophil recognize antibodies on the surface of a foreign cell. Receptor–antibody binding then induces phagocytosis.

Large molecules, such as proteins and those of neurotransmitters, hormones and mucus, to which the cell membrane is impermeable, are passed out of the cell by a process of **exocytosis**.

Stimulation of the cell causes a rise in intracellular Ca^{2+}, either by influx from extracellular fluid or from intracellular storage sites. This Ca^{2+} activates an intracellular protein, usually **calmodulin**, which activates or inhibits intracellular enzymes (e.g. protein kinases). This causes the movement of vesicles along microtubules to the surface membrane, with which they fuse; they then release their contents.

When phagocytosis/pinocytosis occurs plasma membrane is removed from the cell surface as part of it is used to form the membrane-bound phagosome/pinosome. In the case of exocytosis the surface membrane area increases as the membrane binding the secretory vesicle is incorporated into the cell's surface. Most cells carry out constant removal and replacement of portions of plasma membrane so that a relatively constant surface area is maintained.

Chromosomes

With the exception of some cells in the ovaries and testes, all the nucleated cells of the human body contain 46 chromosomes; 23 of these are derived from the individual's mother (maternal chromosomes) and 23 from the father (paternal chromosomes). The cells are therefore said to contain 23 pairs of chromosomes.

It is conventional to describe 22 pairs of '**autosomes**' and one pair of **sex chromosomes**. All autosomes are described as **homologous**, meaning that they are alike in size and shape, but since one is maternal and the other paternal, they may differ in the expression of their genetic information. They may be displayed in a **karyotype**, when photographic enlargements of metaphase chromosomes are arranged in a numbered sequence (Figure 2.15).

Individual chromosomes are identified according to their size and appearance; the autosomes are numbered from 1–22 and the sex chromosomes are identified as XX (in the female) or XY (in the male). The two sex chromosomes of a male are exceptional in that they are not homologous. The X chromosome is maternal in origin, while the Y chromosome derives from the father.

Chromosomes contain the information that governs all cellular activi-

See **Cells involved in innate immunity** (page 355), in Ch. 11, Blood, Lymphoid Tissue and Immunity.

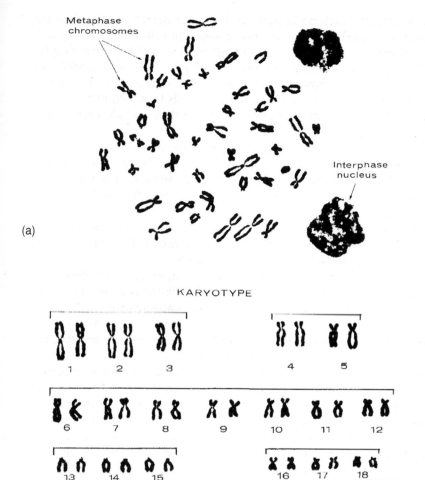

Metaphase
chromosomes

Interphase
nucleus

(a)

KARYOTYPE

6 7 8 9 10 11 12

13 14 15 16 17 18

19 20 21 22 X Y

(b)

Figure 2.15 **(a)** Photomicrograph of human metaphase chromosomes. **(b)** The human karyotype constructed by cutting out the chromosomes from such a photograph and arranging them in groups according to their size, and the location of the primary constriction. The 22 pairs of autosomes are identified by number, and the sex chromosomes by X and Y. (Reproduced with permission from Fawcett, D. W. (1993) *Bloom and Fawcett: A Textbook of Histology*, Chapman & Hall, London.)

ties. Reproductive cells contain complete blueprints, which will enable new individuals to be formed; every other cell contains the same information, but only the part required for that particular cell to function is 'switched on'. This information is encoded in DNA molecules in the form of **genes**. Each gene consists of a part of a DNA molecule that regulates a specific function within a cell; the code incorporated in a gene is a blueprint that determines the synthesis of an RNA molecule or a polypeptide (see *Protein synthesis*, below). There are about 100 000 genes on the 46 chromosomes found in the nuclei of human cells; each chromosome therefore contains a large number of genes.

Chromosomes are not visible, even with a microscope, in a nondividing ('resting') cell. Instead the nuclear material is in the form of chromatin, long, extremely fine threads of DNA and protein. At the commencement of cell division these threads condense, coiling up tightly to become visible (with appropriate stains) as chromosomes.

INHERITANCE

A great many structural, functional and behavioural characteristics are inherited by children from their parents. The expression of such an inherited characteristic is called its **phenotype**: hair colour, eye colour, height and blood group are all examples of phenotypes. The underlying genetic constitution which gives rise to a particular phenotype is called the **genotype** and is dependent upon the genes, themselves long sequences of bases on DNA molecules, which are present on the chromosomes.

Since chromosomes are paired there are at least two copies of each gene (one on each chromosome) regulating each characteristic. A gene usually exists in more than one form, each of which is called an **allele**. The two alleles which code for a particular characteristic occupy thc same position (**locus**) on each of the two chromosomes of an homologous pair. The gene that codes for the ABO blood group system, for example, has three alleles, which can be designated A, B and O. If the loci on the two chromosomes are occupied by the same alleles (e.g. A and A), then the person is said to be **homozygous**, if the two are different (e.g. A and O) then the person is **heterozygous**.

Both the A and B genes are '**dominant**' to the O gene, which is therefore said to be '**recessive**', but not to each other. This means that, for example, the possession of one A gene in combination with an O gene always produces group A, because the A gene effectively suppresses the O gene. Therefore possession of the genotypes AA and AO both give blood group A (i.e. phenotype A) and BB and BO give group B. However the genotype AB gives only blood group AB and group O only derives from the genotype OO.

During formation of spermatozoa and ova the chromosome pairs split so that each reproductive cell receives only one from each pair (see *Meiosis*, below). When fertilization occurs, the fertilized ovum, or **zygote**, again contains pairs of chromosomes, one from each parent. A father who is blood group B, but who is heterozygous (genotype BO) produces spermatozoa half of which have the B gene and half the O gene (Figure 2.16).

See **ABO blood groups** (page 338), in Ch. 11, Blood, Lymphoid Tissue and Immunity.

Figure 2.16 The inheritance of the ABO blood group. A heterozygous group B father and a heterozygous group A mother could have children with any of the four blood groups.

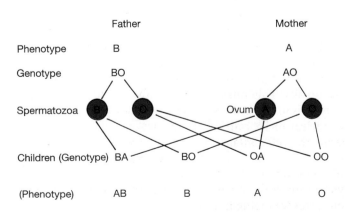

A mother who is heterozygous for group A (genotype AO) produces an ovum which has an equal chance of possessing either an A or an O gene. Fertilization is random, so there is an equal chance of either sperm type fertilizing the ovum. As a consequence there is an equal chance that a child will have any of the four blood groups.

CELL DIVISION

It is the chromosomes which play the leading part in the division (replication) of cells.

There are two mechanisms by which nucleated cells may replicate themselves. Most cells of the body replicate by **mitosis**, giving rise to two daughter cells that are identical to the parent cell and to each other. Reproductive cells undergo **meiosis**, in which four dissimilar cells are formed, each containing only half of the parental chromosome number. Cells containing 23 pairs of chromosomes are said to be **diploid** whereas cells containing half this number, i.e. 23 single chromosomes, are **haploid**.

Mitosis

Immediately before a cell undergoes mitotic division, before condensation of the DNA threads, each chromosome replicates itself. Therefore, when the chromosomes appear, each one is in the form of two **chromatids** and therefore appears X-shaped. Each chromatid, at the end of mitosis, becomes a new chromosome and is, at this time, a single thread.

For convenience mitosis may be divided into four phases even though it is a continuous process (Figure 2.17).

The initial appearance of the chromatids signals the beginning of **prophase**. The replicated chromosomes appear as fine threads which become thicker as the genetic material condenses more and more. Each pair of chromatids are attached only at one point, the **centromere**.

Outside the nuclear membrane, the centrioles replicate and begin to migrate to the opposite poles of the cell.

The end of prophase and the beginning of **metaphase** occurs when the nuclear membrane disappears. The chromosomes are cast free in the cytoplasm and migrate towards the equator of the cell. The centrioles, which have by now moved to opposite poles of the cell, give rise to a number of radiating microtubules, the other ends of which are attached to the centromeres of the chromosomes lying at the equator of the cell. These microtubules form what is known as the **spindle**.

The spindle tubules begin to contract so that the two chromatids derived from each of the original chromosomes are pulled apart as the centromere breaks. This phase, which involves the physical movement of the chromatids towards the poles of the cell, is called **anaphase**.

Finally, nuclear membranes form around the chromosomes so that for a short period the cell contains two nuclei. This is **telophase** and it ends when the new chromosomes disappear and the cytoplasm becomes pinched off to form two new cells (**cytokinesis**).

This type of division occurs when tissues grow and also when they repair themselves following injury.

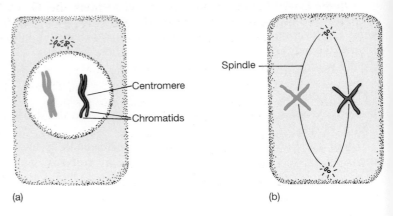

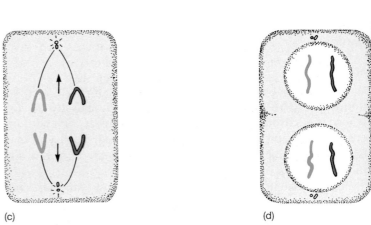

Figure 2.17 Mitosis – only two chromosomes are shown.
(a) Prophase – chromosomes, already in the form of pairs of chromatids, appear in the nucleus.
(b) Metaphase – the chromatids move to the equator of the cell.
(c) Anaphase – the spindle contracts and pulls the chromatids apart.   **(d)** Telophase – nuclear membranes reform prior to division of the cytoplasm.

Cell cycle
Mitosis usually occupies less than 10% of the life of the cell. The period of the cell's life between divisions is known as **interphase**; this can be broken down into three distinct phases (Figure 2.18).

Figure 2.18 The cell cycle.

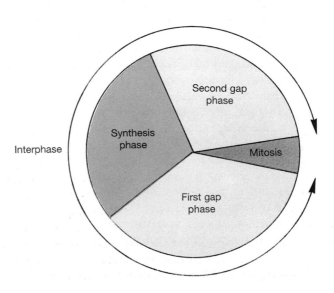

Immediately following division the cell enters the G_1 or **first gap phase** and this is then followed by the **S phase**, during which DNA is synthesized. A **second gap (G_2) phase** then precedes the next **M (mitotic) phase**.

The S and M phases are both initiated by activators within the cell and the four phases of mitosis are brought about by a cascade of reactions resulting from activation by M-phase promoting factor.

Some cells, such as those found lining the gut, divide frequently, about twice a day, while those of the liver divide only once every 1–2 years; nerve cells do not divide at all. Cells with long cycles have very long G_1 phases but, once DNA has been replicated, mitosis follows shortly after. In some cases external stimuli are required to promote mitosis, e.g. epithelial cells in the vicinity of a wound proliferate and bring about wound repair.

Meiosis

The first stage of the reproductive process involves the fertilization of a female cell (ovum) by a male cell (spermatozoon). The resulting zygote then divides and differentiates to form an embryo.

Clearly, if the cells of the embryo are to contain the diploid number of chromosomes (46) then the ovum and spermatozoon must both be haploid and contain 23 chromosomes. If this were not so there would be a doubling of the chromosome number in each generation.

Meiosis, or reduction division, avoids this eventuality, since it consists of two consecutive cell divisions but only one chromosomal replication. Thus four daughter haploid cells are formed (Figure 2.19).

Each division may be separated into the same four phases as mitosis. However, **prophase** of the first division is extended to include reassortment of genetic material between homologous chromosomes. For this reason it is conventional to recognize five subphases in the first phase of the first division.

The first of these subphases is **leptotene**, when the chromosomal threads first become visible within the nucleus. Replication has already occurred, so that each chromosome consists of two chromatids. However, these chromatids are so tightly wrapped around one another that the chromosomes have the appearance of single threads.

In the second subphase, **zygotene**, homologous chromosomes pair up and form bivalents. At this stage the nucleus contains 23 pairs of chromosomes, each pair consisting of four chromatids. The chromosomes shorten and thicken during the third subphase, **pachytene** and in the fourth, **diplotene**, they begin to pull apart from one another. At this point individual chromatids are visible, still held together at the centromere. The chromatids of homologous chromosomes are also held together at a variable number of other points or **chiasmata** (Figure 2.19). At such points chromatids may break and the broken portions may join up with breakage points on the homologous chromatids. This process is called **crossing-over** and it allows reciprocal exchange of genetic information between maternal and paternal chromosomes. Although no new genetic information appears at this time, the remixing of information from two different sources is a means of achieving genetic

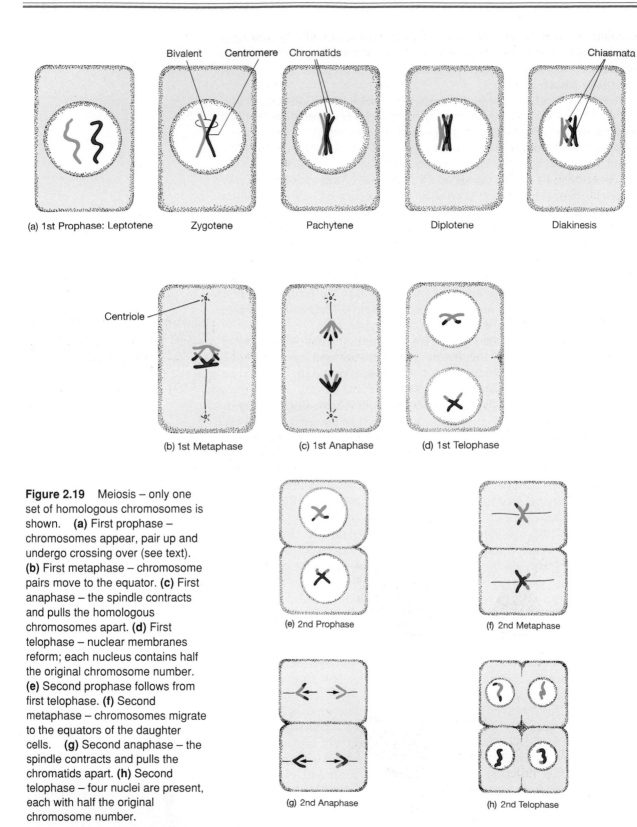

Figure 2.19 Meiosis – only one set of homologous chromosomes is shown. **(a)** First prophase – chromosomes appear, pair up and undergo crossing over (see text). **(b)** First metaphase – chromosome pairs move to the equator. **(c)** First anaphase – the spindle contracts and pulls the homologous chromosomes apart. **(d)** First telophase – nuclear membranes reform; each nucleus contains half the original chromosome number. **(e)** Second prophase follows from first telophase. **(f)** Second metaphase – chromosomes migrate to the equators of the daughter cells. **(g)** Second anaphase – the spindle contracts and pulls the chromatids apart. **(h)** Second telophase – four nuclei are present, each with half the original chromosome number.

variability at each generation and makes everyone genetically unique. Only identical twins, who both derive from a single fertilized egg, are exceptions to this rule.

The final stage, **diakinesis**, occurs when the centromeres of each pair of chromosomes start to pull apart when the spindle tubules contract.

The end of prophase and beginning of **metaphase** is marked by the disappearance of the nuclear membrane. The chromosomes then move to the centre of the cell and arrange themselves at the equator so that their centromeres lie equidistant on either side.

In **anaphase**, homologous chromosomes move apart (in contrast to mitosis, in which it is the chromatids that separate).

Telophase follows anaphase and is then followed immediately by a second prophase. Each nucleus, at this stage, contains 23 chromosomes, each one composed of two chromatids. In the second division these chromatids separate, without further replication, giving rise to four nuclei, each of which contains 23 genetically different single-threaded chromosomes.

DEOXYRIBONUCLEIC ACID (DNA)

DNA is a deceptively simple molecule consisting of four nucleotides, each of which contains a simple sugar (**deoxyribose**), a **phosphate** group and one of four different nitrogenous **bases**.

Two of these bases, **adenine** and **guanine**, are purines and have similar structures. The other two, **thymine** and **cytosine**, are pyrimidines (Figure 2.20).

Again, the two pyrimidines are very similar to each other but differ from the purines. In any DNA molecule the concentration of adenine is equal to that of thymine, while the amount of guanine present equals the amount of cytosine.

> **Nucleotides** are described on page 26, in Ch. 1, Molecules, Ions and Units.

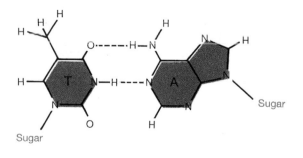

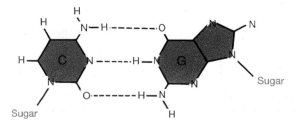

Figure 2.20 The four bases of DNA. Adenine (A) always joins to thymine (T) and cytosine (C) always joins to guanine (G).

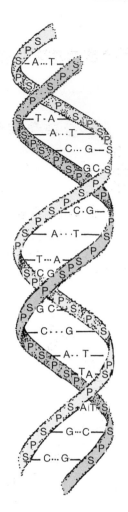

Figure 2.21 The Watson–Crick model of DNA. P = phosphate; S = sugar (deoxyribose); A = adenine; G = guanine; T = thymine; C = cytosine.

For many years scientists attempted to understand how the nucleotides could be arranged in such a way as to produce a molecule complicated enough to determine the structure of all the proteins in a cell. Furthermore, the molecule had to be capable of replicating itself so accurately that a daughter cell would be identical to its parent.

In 1953, **James Watson** and **Francis Crick** proposed a model for DNA consisting of a molecule with two backbones, each with alternating sugar and phosphate groups. Each backbone is twisted around the other to produce a **double helix** (Figure 2.21).

To each sugar is bonded a purine or a pyrimidine which projects inwards between the backbones and links to the opposite unit of the other chain, a purine always being linked with a pyrimidine. Linking is specific so that adenine is always joined to thymine and guanine to cytosine, which explains why the amount of adenine in the molecule is always equal to the amount of thymine, and guanine is always equal to cytosine. The combined diameters of adenine–thymine and cytosine–guanine are identical which explains why the two sugar–phosphate backbones are parallel to each other.

Chromosomes are made up of a mixture of proteins (histones) and nucleic acids, mostly deoxyribonucleic acid (DNA) with small amounts of ribonucleic acid (RNA). The exact arrangement of the DNA and protein components of chromosomes is not fully understood. It is suggested that the histones are grouped into a globular complex around which is wrapped a DNA double helix. These 'beads' are then linked together by a 'string' of DNA (Figure 2.22).

DNA molecules are extremely long and it has been estimated that the total length of those present in the nucleus of a human cell may be up to 1.8 m. Within the chromosomes the molecules are therefore extensively folded in a very complex manner.

The DNA is able to reproduce itself (replication) by splitting the parent molecule so that the two backbones separate. On to each backbone, nucleotides are then built up in the correct sequence, i.e. adenine links with thymine and guanine with cytosine (Figure 2.23).

Replication occurs during interphase prior to mitosis or meiosis. The daughter DNA strands correspond to the chromatids which will separate in cell division.

RIBONUCLEIC ACID (RNA)

RNA has a similar structure to a single strand of DNA: the sugar ribose replaces deoxyribose and the pyrimidine thymine is replaced by uracil. Several different forms of RNA exist within the nucleus and cytoplasm.

RNA is found within ribosomes attached to the surfaces of the rough endoplasmic reticulum, as well as free in the cytoplasm. Each ribosome is made of two subunits, the smaller one consisting of a single molecule of **ribosomal RNA** and 33 proteins. The larger unit contains three molecules of ribosomal RNA and more than 40 proteins. These RNA molecules are formed in the nucleus on a DNA template.

In addition to ribosomal RNA, two other forms are found in the cell. The original DNA message which determines the structure of a protein is transferred to a **messenger RNA (mRNA)** molecule, which then passes out into the cytoplasm where it associates with one or more ribosomes. Amino acids are transported to the mRNA on the ribosomes by another type of RNA, known as **transfer RNA** or **tRNA**. The latter are able to form bridges between the amino acids and mRNA.

tRNA is a short chain molecule of between about 75 and 90 nucleotides (Figure 2.24), synthesized in the nucleus.

The molecule is only partially coiled and some of the free nucleotides at the end are able to form attachments with amino acids. There are many more different types of tRNA than amino acids and it appears therefore that there may be several for each amino acid. A triplet of unpaired bases also exists in each tRNA which is able to 'recognize' a corresponding triplet on the mRNA. Again, there are several mRNA triplets known to code for each amino acid.

PROTEIN SYNTHESIS

Enzymes determine the size, shape and physiological functions of a cell by regulating its internal biochemical activities. Each gene, which is the functional unit of the chromosome, is responsible for the formation of a single enzyme.

Protein synthesis, a large part of which is enzyme synthesis, is carried out in the cytoplasm and, while DNA governs the process, it is not itself directly involved. The relevant section of the genetic message is copied and taken into the cytoplasm in the form of an mRNA molecule.

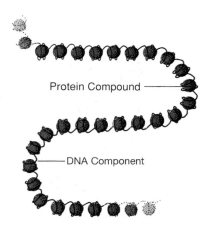

Figure 2.22 Possible arrangement of DNA and protein in chromosomes.

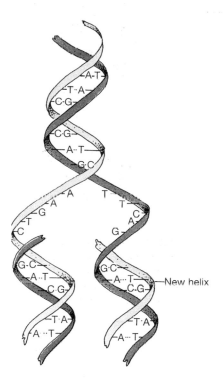

Figure 2.23 Replication of DNA The DNA splits open and new helices are built up on the original ones.

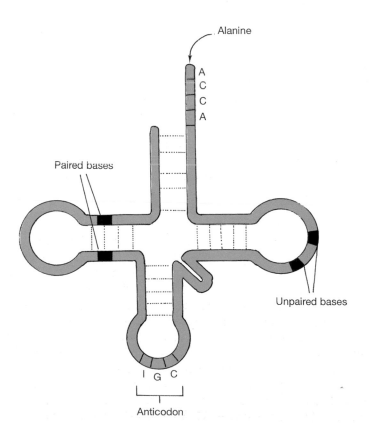

Figure 2.24 Outline structure of alanine transfer RNA Paired bases are joined by dotted lines (I = inosine, a base variant found only in transfer RNA).

It has long been established that the **genetic code** is a triplet code, i.e. each group of three nucleotides on one chain of the DNA molecule is responsible for the placement of one amino acid into a protein chain.

The process of protein synthesis begins when a portion of DNA splits open and one strand (the sense strand) acts as a template for mRNA formation. Nucleotides are then assembled on this template, with cytosine on the DNA linking with guanine on the RNA and adenine linking with uracil, and so on until a complete mirror image of the DNA base sequence is created. This process, which is regulated by enzyme action, is called **transcription**.

The mRNA then passes out into the cytoplasm, where the base sequence is translated into an amino acid sequence, with the assistance of tRNA.

DNA molecules contain sequences of triplets which do not code for specific amino acids; such sequences are called **introns**. The DNA that makes up introns is thought by some scientists to be redundant but others believe that it does have a function, and there is a growing body of experimental evidence to support this view. It may, for example, help to determine the three-dimensional arrangement of DNA within the chromosomes.

Introns may occur in the middle of the base sequences which make up genes. In this case they are edited out by enzymes during the transcription process and the sequences that code for amino acids (**exons**) are joined together. The presence of introns in a gene does not, therefore, affect the process of protein synthesis.

Each triplet of nucleotides on the mRNA that encodes a single amino acid is called a **codon** and the mirror image on the tRNA is known as an **anticodon**. The nucleotides which make up each codon (64 are known, representing all the possible combinations of the four bases) are known and appear to be universal in all living organisms (Table 2.3).

Each amino acid is able to link, with the assistance of appropriate enzymes, with one of a small group of tRNAs; each of these is then able to recognize one of a small group of mRNA codons. Thus, while the code is not strictly amino acid–codon-specific, it is specific enough to ensure that the correct amino acid is placed in the correct position within a protein molecule.

Once the mRNA is in position, threaded through a ribosome, **translation** of the genetic code can begin (Figure 2.25).

The ribosome appears to move along the mRNA, 'reading' the message as it progresses. As a particular codon passes through the ribosome, the appropriate tRNA, with an amino acid in tow, is picked up and the mRNA codon and tRNA anticodon link up. A ribosome has two positions into which tRNAs can be slotted. One of these is occupied by a newly arrived tRNA while the other contains a tRNA that anchors the growing polypeptide chain. The chain is then attached to the newly arrived amino acid and the now freed tRNA passes out of the ribosome, which moves along to occupy the next position. A new codon is now available for the next tRNA–amino acid complex to slot into.

Thus, as the ribosome moves along the length of the mRNA a polypeptide chain is formed, its structure being determined by the RNA

Table 2.3 The genetic code: sequences of three bases on mRNA which are read by the ribosome and bring about the incorporation of the corresponding amino acid into a protein molecule (TERM = terminating codons; signals the end of an amino acid sequence)

	U	C	A	G	
U	UUU UUC } Phe UUA UUG } Leu	UCU UCC UCA UCG } Ser	UAU UAC } Tyr UAA UAG } TERM	UGU UGC } Cys UGA TERM UGG Trp	U C A G
C	CUU CUC CUA CUG } Leu	CCU CCC CCA CCG } Pro	CAU CAC } His CAA CAG } Gln	CGU CGC CGA CGG } Arg	U C A G
A	AUU AUC AUA } Ile AUG Met	ACU ACC ACA ACG } Thr	AAU AAC } Asn AAA AAG } Lys	AGU AGC } Ser AGA AGG } Arg	U C A G
G	GUU GUC GUA GUG } Val	GCU GCC GCA GCG } Ala	GAU GAC } Asp GAA GAG } Glu	GGU GGC GGA GGG } Gly	U C A G

base sequence. Sometimes an mRNA may be threaded through several ribosomes and each individual ribosome will still produce a protein. In addition to this a single mRNA can be 'read' several times by a single ribosome. It is evident that a single messenger RNA molecule can be responsible for the formation of many protein molecules, although exactly how this facet of protein synthesis is governed is not fully understood.

All RNA messages commence with the sequence AUG, the code for the amino acid methionine. Thus, initially, all proteins start with methionine. In many cases, however, the amino acid is removed enzymatically before the protein molecule is folded into its final shape. There are also three codons which serve to terminate a protein: UAA, UAG and UGA.

As a protein molecule grows and detaches from the ribosome it folds to assume a secondary and then tertiary shape. This folding is determined by the amino acid sequence of the protein chain and the tertiary structure of the protein molecule plays an important part in determining its function.

Benign and malignant tumours

If cell division proceeds in a rapid and uncoordinated manner, a cell mass or tumour (**neoplasm**) results. Such a tumour may remain as a single mass within a tissue, in which case it is described as **benign**; alternatively it may invade other tissues, in which case it is **malignant**

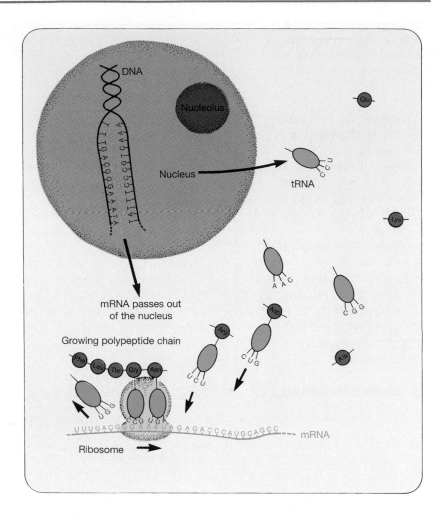

Figure 2.25   Protein synthesis. An RNA copy of the nuclear DNA message passes into the cytoplasm where it associates with a ribosome. The ribosome then moves along the mRNA, reading the message as it progresses. As a particular codon passes through the ribosome, the appropriate tRNA, with an amino acid in tow, is picked up, and the mRNA codon and tRNA anticodon link up. A ribosome has two positions into which tRNA can be slotted. One of these is occupied by a newly arrived tRNA while the other contains a tRNA that anchors the growing polypeptide chain. The chain is then attached to the newly arrived amino acid and the now freed tRNA passes out of the ribosome, which moves along to occupy the next position. As the ribosome passes along the mRNA new amino acids are continually incorporated into the growing protein molecule.

(cancer). The cells of malignant tumours often escape from the cell mass and enter the lymphatic system or blood stream, passing to other parts of the body and establishing new colonies or **metastases**.

Most tumours probably develop initially from a single primary cell whose DNA has undergone an alteration (**mutation**). This single cell may give rise to a colony of 'altered' cells. It is believed, however, that in order to develop into a tumour, the cells must undergo further alterations. This is supported by the observation that the rate of tumour formation increases with age. Clearly, the greater the period of time elapsed since an initial mutation the greater the chance that further mutations will have occurred.

There are two possible mutational routes by which tumours can arise. A single stimulatory gene (**proto-oncogene**) may mutate into a hyperactive form (**oncogene**); this gene would be dominant and therefore only one of a homologous pair would be needed. Secondly, an inhibitory gene may itself be inhibited. In this case the mutation would be recessive so that both copies of the gene would need to be altered in order to give rise to a tumour cell. Alternatively, a virus may be incorporated into the cell's DNA, thereby altering it.

Mutations may involve a relatively small change in the DNA sequence in a gene, due to an error in DNA replication prior to cell division. Alternatively, there may be a transfer of genetic material between non-homologous chromosomes (**translocation**); this will occur during cell division itself. In either case abnormal proteins will be produced by the cell.

Mutations may be caused by the exposure of cells to **carcinogens**. These may be chemicals or radiation (X-rays, UV light, etc.).

Tumours may take many years to develop following exposure to the mutagenic substance. A **tumour initiator** may bring about tissue changes, but will not itself directly promote the development of a tumour. This may only occur when a, possibly unrelated, **tumour promoter** is applied. Clearly it is very difficult to identify the precise cause of cancer.

Treatment of malignant tumours may involve surgical excision and/or treatment with drugs and/or radiation. The drugs used in chemotherapy are designed to, as far as possible, stop cell division and therefore destroy the tumour. Unfortunately, the drugs stop all division and therefore produce unpleasant side-effects such as hair loss. Radiation treatment also interferes with cell division but it is usually more specific since it can be focused upon the tumour itself, or the area from which the tumour has been removed.

ALTERATIONS IN CHROMOSOME NUMBER OR STRUCTURE

Nearly 2500 conditions that can be traced to alterations in inherited material have been described in humans. They may be due to: 1) a change in the number of chromosomes; 2) alterations in the gross structure of chromosomes; or 3) a change in the arrangement of bases in DNA. Table 2.4 lists the types of alteration and gives examples of some resultant conditions.

1. **A change in the number of chromosomes**. During the formation of the gametes, during first meiotic division, chromosomes sometimes fail to separate, so that one nucleus contains more than the expected number of chromosomes while another contains fewer. This phenomenon is known as **non-disjunction**. After fertilization, therefore, the zygote will contain more of less than the usual number of 46 chromosomes.

   Non-disjunction is very often lethal, since an individual cannot survive if large amounts of genetic information are missing from his/her cells, or if there is a great excess. Those who do survive are disabled to a greater or lesser extent. In **Klinefelter's syndrome**, for example, there is an extra sex chromosome (XXY), which produces male characteristics, infertility and usually mental retardation. In **Turner's syndrome**, on the other hand, there is a single X chromosome, which produces an infertile individual with female characteristics. An extra chromosome 21 (trisomy 21) gives rise to **Down's syndrome** or mongolism, in which there is again mental retardation, as well as a number of physical changes.

2. **Alterations in the gross structure of chromosomes**. Chromosome structure may be altered in a number of ways,

Table 2.4 Major types of chromosomal alterations and examples of their outcomes

Chromosomal alteration	Outcome
Change in the number of chromosomes	
↑Chromosome number	Down's syndrone Klinefelter's syndrome
↓Chromosome number	Turner's syndrome
Loss or relocation of part of chromosome	
Loss of part of chromosome	Cri du chat syndrome Wolf's syndrome
Translocation	Abortion
Balanced translocation	No change
Alterations in single genes	
Autosomal dominant	Achondroplasia (dwarfism) Huntington's chorea
Autosomal recessive	Cystic fibrosis Sickle cell anaemia
Sex-linked recessive	Colour blindness Haemophilia

including loss of part of a chromosome or translocation of a segment of one chromosome to another.

Loss of the short arm of chromosome 5 (Figure 2.15) results, for example, in **'cri du chat' syndrome**, which is characterized by a mewing, cat-like cry. Loss of so much genetic material leads to severe mental retardation and cardiac anomalies, which result in poor survival rates.

In translocation, if all of the relocated material is intact, the individual is phenotypically unchanged.

3. **A change in the arrangement of bases in DNA.** Alterations in single genes can occur during DNA replication: an extra nucleotide may be inserted in one of the new chains (insertion), or one may be lost (deletion); alternatively, lengths of DNA may become inverted. Such 'mutations' are likely to be fatal.

If a dominant gene gives rise to a genetic condition then it is present in both homozygous dominant and heterozygous individuals. In many instances, however, the presence of two dominant genes is incompatible with life. There are approximately 750 **autosomal dominant conditions** known, including achondroplasia (dwarfism) and Huntington's chorea.

Recessive genes only give expression in homozygous individuals; heterozygotes do not have the condition themselves but are said to be 'carriers'. Most recessive conditions are characterized by an enzyme deficiency, which leads to a biochemical disorder. Such conditions are often referred to as **inborn errors of metabolism**. Cystic fibrosis and sickle cell anaemia are examples of **autosomal recessive conditions**.

In **sickle cell anaemia**, a single base change (uracil replaces adenine) in the RNA sequence that codes for the beta-chain of haemoglobin leads to the replacement of the amino acid glutamic acid by valine. This alters the haemoglobin molecule sufficiently that it crystallizes when oxygen tension falls, and the erythrocytes deform. Possession of a single gene leads to **sickle cell trait**, in which only one gene codes for the abnormal haemoglobin S and the other for the normal haemoglobin A, and usually produces no symptoms. Possession of both genes for haemoglobin S leads to full-blown sickle cell anaemia. Although the condition is often lethal, the fact that heterozygotes survive means that it does not die out; it is present as sickle trait in about 10% of British people of Afro-Caribbean origin, while about 1 in 400 of them have sickle cell anaemia.

Alterations in single genes on the X-chromosome can also lead to a number of conditions. These are said to be 'sex-linked' and, because males only have a single X chromosome, they are much more common in males than females, because in males the recessive altered gene cannot be 'hidden' by a normal dominant gene. Haemophilia and red–green colour blindness are examples of **sex-linked genetic conditions**.

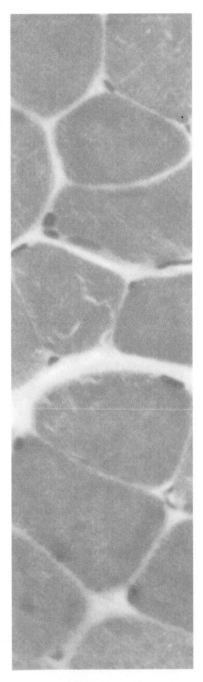

Tissues

3

Tissues, organs and body systems

A **tissue** is a collection of structurally similar cells together with an intercellular matrix or ground substance which may contain fibres. Collections of tissues form organs such as the heart, stomach and skin; these may then be linked to form anatomical **body systems**. Thus, for example, the heart and blood vessels form the cardiovascular system, while the stomach, the small and large intestines and associated glands constitute the digestive system.

It is usual to classify tissues into four primary groups:

- epithelium
- connective tissue (including blood, cartilage and bone)
- muscle tissue
- nervous tissue

Attachments between cells

There are several ways by which cells are held together on their lateral borders. Such attachments are observed in many tissues but are particularly well developed in epithelia. Some cells (such as those lining the alimentary tract) have interlocking projections forming a jigsaw-like structure. Columnar epithelial cells frequently have a collection of structures called a **junctional complex** just below their free surfaces. Some of these join the cells together while others function as communication routes. They are illustrated in Figure 3.1.

The uppermost region is called the **zonula occludens**, or tight junction; here the adjacent membranes appear to fuse in a belt which passes all round each cell. This type of junction prevents fluid from passing from the cavity above the epithelium, between the cells and into the underlying tissues.

The middle section is known as the **zonula adhaerens** (adherent junction), in which the membranes are reinforced by fine filaments. Again the structure is belt-like, but it differs from the tight junction in

Figure 3.1   A junctional complex.

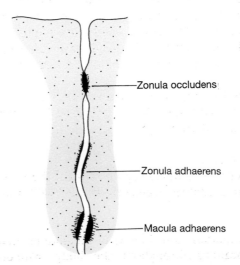

that adjacent cells do not touch. Similar, but more extensive structures, the fascia adhaerens, form the intercalated discs that are characteristic of cardiac muscle.

The lower region is known as the **macula adhaerens** or **desmosome**; the membranes are attached to a feltwork of fine filaments in a matrix, and filaments from the cytoplasm anchor to the structure. Desmosomes are button-like and also occur in other tissues, in the absence of the other types of cellular attachments. They act as a focus for cytoskeletal microfilaments.

A fourth type of structure, the **gap junction** or **nexus** is also found in some tissues. There is a narrowing of the intercellular gap, but no fusion. These appear to be sites of intercellular communication.

Epithelium

Epithelial tissues are composed of cells which are tightly packed together, forming a continuous sheet or membrane, and are found covering the outer surface of the body and lining all internal cavities and ducts. In addition, secretory epithelium is found in some glands.

All epithelial tissues are supported by a **basement membrane**, or basal lamina, consisting principally of a glycoprotein, laminin, and a network of collagen fibrils, some of which are anchored to the underlying connective tissue.

Epithelia are classified according to the number of layers of cells present, the shapes of the cells in longitudinal section (i.e. in a section cut at right angles to the basement membrane) and the presence of surface specializations. Epithelia may therefore be described as **simple** (one cell thick) or **stratified** (several cells thick), while individual cells are either **squamous** (flat), **cuboidal** or **columnar** and their surfaces may bear cilia or microvilli. Thus, for example, epithelium which forms the alveoli in the lungs is described as simple squamous epithelium and that which lines the oviducts is simple ciliated columnar epithelium.

A summary of the different types of epithelia, together with their locations, is given in Table 3.1 and photomicrographs in Figure 3.2.

Simple epithelium consists of a single layer of cells, which are variously specialized for secretion, absorption or transport of substances over their surface.

Stratified epithelium, on the other hand, is many cells thick and consequently protects underlying structures against chemical or mechanical damage or dehydration.

BLOOD SUPPLY

Epithelia do not have a blood supply as such: the cells exchange water and solutes with capillaries in adjacent tissue, by diffusion.

Membranes

Epithelia are important constituents of membranes that are found at a number of locations throughout the body. **Mucous membranes**

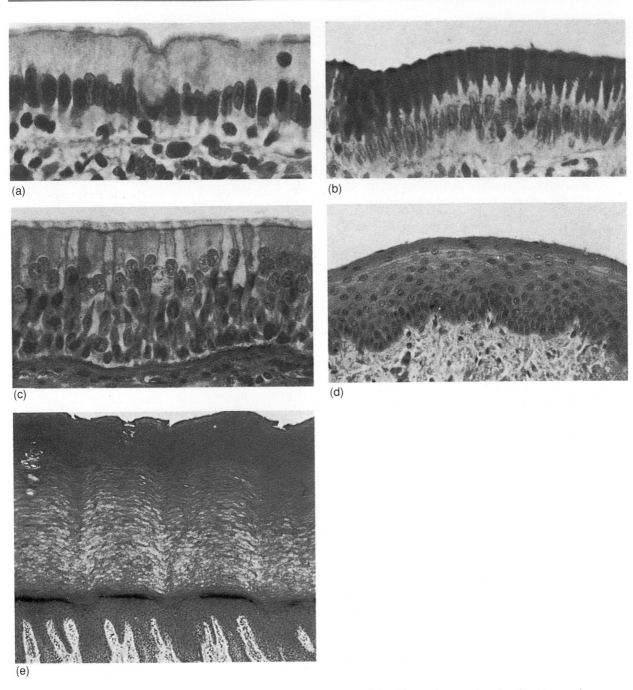

Figure 3.2 Photomicrographs of various types of epithelium. **(a)** Simple columnar epithelium: brush border and goblet cells. **(b)** Simple columnar epithelium: mucous cells. **(c)** Ciliated pseudostratified columnar epithelium. **(d)** Stratified squamous epithelium. **(e)** Keratinized stratified squamous epithelium of the epidermis. (Reproduced with permission from Fawcett, D. W. (1993) *Bloom and Fawcett: A Textbook of Histology*, Chapman & Hall, London.)

Table 3.1 Classification and distribution of epithelia

Type	Name	Distribution
Simple	Squamous	Lining all blood vessels (endothelium); nephron of kidney; ear; small ducts in glands; pleurae; peritoneum; lining cavities (mesothelium)
	Cuboidal	Covering ovaries; pigment layer of retina; secretory parts of glands
	Columnar	Brush border – lining intestine and gall bladder Ciliated – lining fallopian tubes Mucous – lining stomach, small intestine and digestive glands Pseudostratified ciliated – lining nasal cavity, trachea; auditory tube and tympanic cavity; central canal of spinal cord and ventricles of brain
Stratified	Squamous	Keratinized – skin Non-keratinized – lining of mouth, oesophagus; anal canal and vagina; covering cornea of eye
	Transitional	Lining urinary tract
	Cuboidal	Sweat glands; ovarian follicles; ducts of salivary glands and pancreas
	Columnar	Conjunctiva

(**mucosae**) are found lining the respiratory, alimentary and reproductive tracts. They comprise a layer of epithelium together with connective tissue (**lamina propria**) beneath. **Serous membranes (serosae)** are smooth and moist; they include the peritoneum, pericardium and pleurae. They consist of thin layers of connective tissue covered by simple squamous epithelium, which at these sites is known as **mesothelium**.

Simple squamous epithelium

In longitudinal section, simple squamous cells appear to be extremely thin, down to 0.1 µm thickness, except where the nucleus causes a bulge (Figure 3.3).

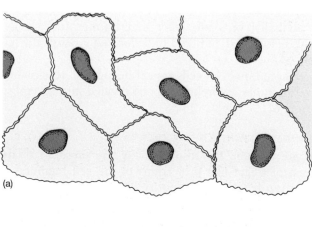

(a)

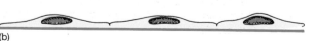

(b)

Figure 3.3 Simple squamous (pavement) epithelium **(a)** in transverse and **(b)** longitudinal section.

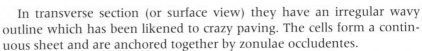

In transverse section (or surface view) they have an irregular wavy outline which has been likened to crazy paving. The cells form a continuous sheet and are anchored together by zonulae occludentes.

This extremely thin tissue is found appropriately in the alveoli of the lungs, where rapid diffusion of oxygen and carbon dioxide takes place through and between the cells. Simple squamous epithelium also lines the whole of the cardiovascular and lymphatic systems, where it is called **endothelium**. The smoothness of endothelium facilitates blood flow and reduces clotting.

Other sites where this tissue is found include: parts of the kidney nephron (the outer layer of Bowman's capsule and thin part of the loop of Henle); in the ear (covering the tympanum on the middle ear side and lining the membranous labyrinth); small ducts in glands; and lining cavities as mesothelium.

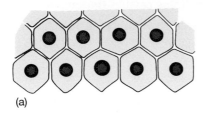

(a)

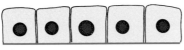

(b)

Figure 3.4 Simple cuboidal epithelium in **(a)** transverse and **(b)** longitudinal section.

Simple cuboidal epithelium

These cells appear square in longitudinal section, but in transverse section and surface view they are polygonal, usually hexagonal (Figure 3.4).

Much of the nephron of the kidney is composed of simple cuboidal epithelium. The proximal convoluted tubule is primarily engaged in reabsorption of solutes and water from the tubular lumen. The relative thinness of the tissue is appropriate for the rapid transfer of materials across it but, compared with squamous cells, there are many more mitochondria and therefore a greater capacity for active transport. The luminal surfaces of the cells project, forming **microvilli**, which increase the surface area available for absorption.

Cuboidal epithelium covers the ovaries, where it is known as germinal epithelium, and forms the pigment layer of the retina. The excretory ducts, as well as the secretory parts of many glands, are also composed of cuboidal cells.

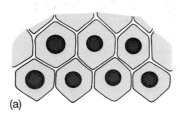

(a)

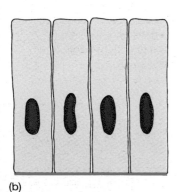

(b)

Figure 3.5 Simple columnar epithelium in **(a)** transverse and **(b)** longitudinal section.

Simple columnar epithelium

Columnar epithelial cells are taller and thinner than cuboidal cells. Nuclei are also elongated and tend to be located towards the bases of the cells (Figure 3.5).

In cross section, however, cells appear hexagonal, resembling cuboidal epithelium. Columnar epithelium can be divided into several specialized types (Figure 3.6).

STRIATED OR BRUSH BORDER CELLS

These cells are adapted for absorption by the presence of **microvilli**, which consist of finger-like projections of the cell membrane between 0.5 and 1.0 µm in length. The majority of cells comprising the epithelial covering of the intestinal villi are of this type. They are also found lining the gall bladder, in which bile is concentrated by the absorption of salts and water.

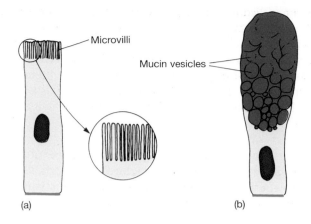

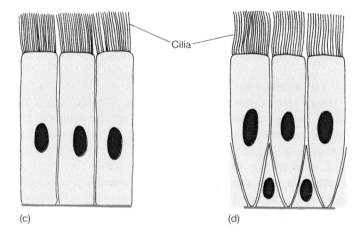

Figure 3.6 Specializations of columnar epithelium. **(a)** Brush border cell **(b)** Goblet cell. **(c)** Ciliated epithelium. **(d)** Pseudostratified epithelium.

CILIATED CELLS

The free, or luminal, surfaces of some epithelial cells are covered by **cilia**. All the cilia on an epithelial surface beat in the same direction in such a way that a wave sweeps over the surface.

In the respiratory tract, for example, this action propels a sheet of mucus towards the pharynx.

Two types of ciliated epithelium are found: **simple** and **pseudostratified**. Simple ciliated epithelium is characteristic of the female reproductive tract and is found lining part of the uterus and oviducts. Pseudostratified ciliated columnar epithelium is much more common; it lines the trachea and larger bronchi, the paranasal sinuses and lacrimal sac, the auditory tube and part of the tympanic cavity. In addition, it is found in the central canal of the spinal cord and the ventricles of the brain.

MUCOUS CELLS

The epithelial lining of the stomach is made up of mucous cells which secrete mucin into the lumen of the stomach. The chief cells of the

Cilia are described in **Cilia and flagella** (page 44), in Ch. 2, Cells and the Internal Environment.

The role of cilia in the respiratory tract is described in **The conducting airways (anatomical dead space)** (page 429), in Ch. 13, Respiration.

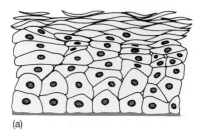

(a)

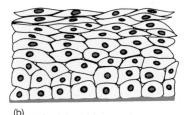

(b)

Figure 3.7 Stratified squamous epithelium. **(a)** Keratinized. **(b)** Non-keratinized.

Skin structure is described in **The skin** (page 306), in Ch. 10, The Skin and the Regulation of Body Temperature.

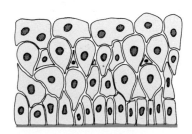

Figure 3.8 Transitional epithelium.

gastric glands are also a secretory form of columnar epithelium. In this case the secretory product is pepsinogen. The mucous cells, interspersed with the brush border cells covering the intestinal villi, have expanded apices, distended with mucin. These cells are known as **goblet** or **chalice cells** and they are also found in the mucous membrane lining the respiratory tract.

PSEUDOSTRATIFIED EPITHELIUM

In this tissue, a false impression of more than one layer of cells is given by the nuclei which lie at more than one level. Although all the bases of the cells lie on the basement membrane, their heights vary, and so do the positions of the nuclei. Such a tissue is afforded strength by the packing of the cells, and is found in the male urethra and some large excretory ducts. In the upper respiratory tract, the taller cells are ciliated and columnar (pseudostratified ciliated columnar epithelium). Some of the smaller cells divide and replenish the other cells and some grow into the taller cells.

Stratified squamous epithelium

Stratified epithelium contains several layers of cells. The superficial layers of cells are squamous in longitudinal section, whereas the basal cells are usually cuboidal. Intermediate cells show progressive flattening towards the surface (Figure 3.7).

The basal cells divide and push the cells above them towards the surface. The surface cells are continually sloughed off.

Because of its relative thickness, simple stratified epithelium has a protective role. It may be keratinized or non-keratinized. **Keratinized stratified squamous epithelium** constitutes the epidermis of the skin.

Non-keratinized stratified squamous epithelium is found on wet surfaces which are subject to a lot of wear and tear, such as the lining of the mouth, pharynx and oesophagus and the covering of the cornea.

Transitional epithelium

Transitional epithelium is so named because it was, at one time, considered to be intermediate in structure between stratified squamous and stratified columnar epithelium. It contains cells with a variety of shapes. The superficial cells are large, often binucleate and umbrella-shaped. Beneath this layer are pear-shaped cells, which have their apices pointing downwards and the rounded part fits into the concavity of the outer layer of cells. Between the tapering cells are a third type of smaller cell (Figure 3.8). A characteristic of this tissue is that it will withstand stretching, in which case the superficial cells flatten and the pear-shaped cells shorten and thicken; the integrity of the tissue is maintained.

Transitional epithelium is found lining the excretory passages of the urinary tract: the ureters, bladder and proximal urethra. At all these sites the tissues are stretched when urine is stored or passed.

Stratified cuboidal and columnar epithelium

Stratified cuboidal or columnar epithelium is found in relatively few sites. These include the larger ducts of the salivary glands and the pancreas; the ducts of sweat glands; the fornix of the conjunctiva; the cavernous urethra and ovarian follicles.

Glands

Glands of epithelial origin are usually found in connective tissue underlying the surface membrane from which they have developed. **Exocrine glands** retain their connection with the surface by means of a duct, whereas **endocrine glands** lose their connection and are therefore an island of cells from which the secretion passes into the blood, rather than into a duct.

Exocrine glands may be unicellular, such as goblet cells, or, more usually, multicellular. If the secretory part of the gland opens directly on to the surface, or indirectly via a single duct, then it is designated **simple**; whereas if the duct is branched the gland is described as **compound**.

The shape of the secretory units may be **tubular, acinar** (spherical) or **alveolar** (flask-shaped). Figure 3.9 illustrates various types of gland.

> Exocytosis is described in **Endocytosis and exocytosis** (page 51), in Ch. 2, Cells and the Internal Environment.

Figure 3.9 Diagrammatic representation of the principal types of simple and compound glands. **(a)** Simple tubular (e.g. intestinal crypt of Lieberkühn). **(b)** Simple coiled tubular (e.g. sweat gland). **(c)** Simple branched tubular (e.g. gastric gland). **(d)** Compound tubular (e.g. mucous gland in oral cavity). **(e)** Compound acinar (e.g. salivary gland).

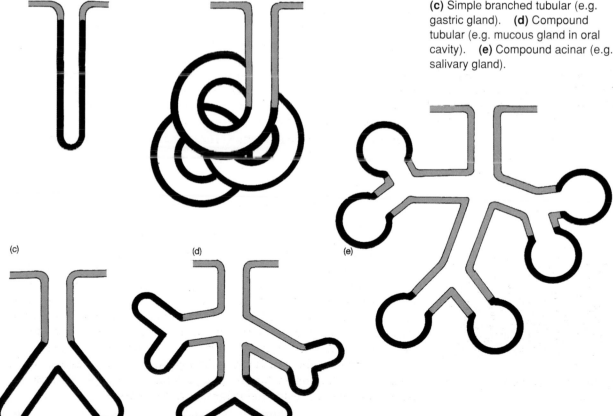

Sweat glands are described on page 313, in Ch. 10, The Skin and the Regulation of Body Temperature.

Repair of skin is described in **Regeneration and healing of skin** (page 316), in Ch. 10, The Skin and the Regulation of Body Temperature.

Villi are described on page 576, in Ch. 15, Digestion and Absorption of Food.

The functional units of the liver are described in **Structure of the liver** (page 564), in Ch. 15, Digestion and Absorption of Food.

Blood and lymph are covered in Ch.11, Blood, Lymphoid Tissue and Immunity and Ch. 12, Circulation of Blood and Lymph.

In large glands containing connective tissue and secretory cells, the former tissue (the supporting framework) is known as **stroma**, while the glandular tissue (the functional part) is called **parenchyma**.

Glands may be classified according to their mode of secretion. Most glands release their secretions by exocytosis, in which case they are classified as **merocrine glands**.

Sebaceous glands secrete their product, sebum, in a different way. The oil accumulates in the cells until they rupture. The sebum that is delivered into the sebaceous duct, therefore, consists of this oil plus debris from the ruptured cells. Sebaceous glands are the only example of **holocrine** secretion found in humans.

A third type of secretion occurs in **apocrine glands**, in which the tip of the gland is pinched off. The occurrence of this type of secretion in humans is somewhat controversial. Some histologists classify mammary glands as apocrine, others as merocrine. One group of sweat glands is described as apocrine, although their mode of secretion is now thought to be by exocytosis, which would reclassify them as merocrine.

Regeneration of epithelium

The replenishment of lost or damaged epithelial cells is a particularly strong feature of tissues in this group. The basal cells of stratified epithelium continually divide mitotically and replenish the more superficial cells.

The surface cells of villi in the small intestine are replenished by cell division in the intestinal glands (crypts of Lieberkühn).

Damage to liver cells is followed by production of replacement cells, not always, however, organized into the same functional units as before.

Connective tissue

Connective tissues provide structural support for the other tissues and organs throughout the body. They differ from other tissues in that they have a high proportion of intercellular substance so that the cells are relatively widely spaced. It is usual to subdivide the many diverse tissues included in this group into five types:

1. connective tissue proper;
2. adipose tissue;
3. cartilage;
4. bone;
5. blood and lymph.

With the exception of blood and lymph, the intercellular material consists of an amorphous **ground substance**, which contains extracellular fluid and fibres. It is this intercellular material that largely determines the characteristics of the different types of connective tissue. The ground substance of loose connective tissue, for example, is the site of

Table 3.2 Classification and distribution of connective tissue

Type	Name	Distribution
Connective tissue proper	Areolar (loose)	Supports linings of gastrointestinal, respiratory and urinary tracts; skin; eyelids; around blood vessels and nerves; interstitial packing in all tissues
	Dense regular	Tendons, ligaments, fascia; cornea
	Dense irregular	Periosteum of bone; perichondrium around cartilage; dura mater; pericardium; sclera of eye
	Elastic	Small arteries; vocal cords; ligamenta flava of vertebral column
Adipose tissue	White	Under skin; omenta; mesenteries; orbit of eye; palms of hands and soles of feet
	Brown	In newborn, reduced amounts in adults, – between shoulder blades, around kidneys, axillae, mediastinum, along thoracic aorta
Cartilage	Hyaline	Foetal skeleton; nose; larynx, trachea and bronchi; articular surfaces and epiphysial plates of bones: ventral ends of ribs
	Fibrocartilage	Intervertebral discs; pubic symphyses; attachments of tendons
	Elastic	External ear, auditory meatus and tube; epiglottis and laryngeal cartilages
Bone	Compact	Surfaces of bones
	Cancellous	Interiors of bones

various defence mechanisms involved in combating infection or tissue damage. The closely packed fibres found in the intercellular material of dense connective tissue, on the other hand, impart the property of mechanical strength. The calcified ground substance found in bone imparts rigidity and, again, mechanical strength.

The different types of connective tissue, together with their distribution, are shown in Table 3.2.

BLOOD SUPPLY

The blood supply to connective tissue itself is not extensive, though many vessels may be seen *en route* to adjacent tissues. Lymphatic vessels are, on the other hand, frequently abundant.

Connective tissue proper

Connective tissue proper contains three types of fibre called **collagen, elastin** and **reticulin**. The quantity and arrangement of these fibres gives rise to a further classification of the tissue. Thus, loose connective tissue contains loosely woven fibres whereas dense connective tissue contains large quantities of fibres, which may be arranged either regularly or irregularly.

The principal types of connective tissue proper include areolar (loose connective tissue) and two types of dense connective tissue; regular (white fibrous) and irregular. Adipose tissue and elastic tissue may also be included in this group although some classifications separate them.

Figure 3.10 Loose (areolar) connective tissue. A clear matrix contains collagen, elastic and reticular fibres and a variety of cells.

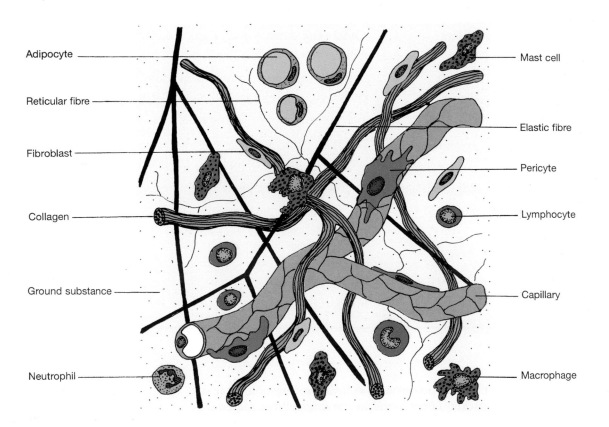

It is useful to study areolar connective tissue first because it contains all the characteristic components of connective tissue.

Areolar (loose) connective tissue

Areolar connective tissue (Figure 3.10) is soft and transparent and contains loosely arranged collagen fibres separated by relatively large open spaces filled with ground substance.

The collagen fibres are interlaced with elastin fibres, and these impart strength and elasticity, respectively, to the tissue.

The ground substance of areolar connective tissue, which appears structureless under the light microscope, contains extracellular fluid and several protein–polysaccharide complexes (**proteoglycans**). The two principal proteoglycans are chondroitin sulphate and hyaluronic acid. The presence of these substances makes the intercellular material viscous, which holds it in place; it also limits the movement of microorganisms through the tissue. Some bacteria, however, secrete the enzyme hyaluronidase, which changes the structure of hyaluronic acid and reduces the viscosity of the ground substance around it. Such bacteria are therefore able to move more easily through the tissue. The proteoglycans also have the property of binding water, which is important for the diffusion of materials between the capillaries and connective tissue cells.

The collagen or white fibres are usually found in bundles running in various directions. Each fibre is made up of individual fibrils, which show cross-striations in electron micrographs. The striations result from the way the molecules of the constituent protein tropocollagen are aligned (Figure 3.11).

Reticular fibres are finer than typical collagen fibres, and they stain black with silver salts. They are usually found arranged as a network supporting fine structures such as the basement membranes of epithelial tissues. They are now known to be composed of tropocollagen molecules and are thus more properly classified as specialized collagen fibres.

Elastic fibres are thinner than collagen fibres and are not arranged in bundles. As their name suggests, their main property is elasticity. They are composed of the protein elastin and the fibres can be stretched up to about 150% of their original length without damage. Electron micrographs show that the fibres have an amorphous core surrounded by microfibrils.

There are a variety of cells present in areolar connective tissue. Fibroblasts, which may be regarded as the cells characteristic of connective tissue, are usually the most numerous. In addition, there are also mast cells and fat cells (adipocytes) and a variable population of macrophages, lymphocytes, neutrophils, eosinophils and plasma cells

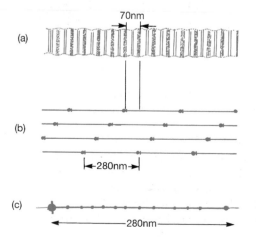

Figure 3.11 **(a)** Collagen fibre. **(b)** Collagen fibre with tropocollagen components separated to show the overlapping arrangement. **(c)** Single tropocollagen molecule.

which have migrated from the blood and whose numbers may dramatically increase in inflammation.

Fibroblasts are flattened, spindle-shaped cells which may have several processes. They are usually found in close proximity to the fibres which they synthesize (Figure 3.12).

These cells both produce and maintain the extracellular material. In the repair of wounds fibroblasts produce new connective tissue (granulation tissue and scar tissue).

The appearance of **macrophages** (histiocytes) varies according to whether they are stationary ('fixed') or mobile ('free'). When stationary, they appear irregular, whereas they adopt a rounded shape as they move through the matrix. The nucleus is indented and the cytoplasm contains granules and lysosomes. The name 'macrophage' reflects the highly developed phagocytic ability of the cells, which is used to ingest cell debris, bacteria and other foreign matter. The lysosomes then break down the ingested material. When tissue is damaged or invaded by microorganisms the 'fixed' macrophages are stimulated to move and their numbers are supplemented by monocytes leaving the blood and transforming into macrophages in the connective tissue. In some instances, where there is a large amount of material to be phagocytosed, several macrophages fuse together to form giant cells around the object. Macrophages play an important role in immune responses by activating lymphocytes.

Mast cells are ovoid, with a small, round nucleus. They contain basophilic granules containing histamine and heparin. The cells are disrupted by tissue damage or infection, releasing the active agents, thereby increasing the blood supply and facilitating the migration of white cells from the blood. Mast cells are implicated in the tissue changes occurring in allergic and hypersensitivity reactions. It is possible that heparin prevents extravascular clotting of protein which leaks out of the

Granulation and scar formation is described in **Regeneration and healing of skin** (page 316), in Ch. 10, The Skin and the Regulation of Body Temperature.

Lymphocyte activation is described in **Acquired (specific) immunity** (page 360), in Ch. 11, Blood, Lymphoid Tissue and Immunity.

Figure 3.12 Micrograph of fibroblast and collagen bundles in a developing tendon. Small groups of fibrils can be seen within narrow recesses in the cell surface (at arrows). Larger bundles are partially or completely surrounded by fibroblast processes (at asterisk). (Reproduced with permission from Fawcett, D. W. (1993) *Bloom and Fawcett: A Textbook of Histology*, Chapman & Hall, London.)

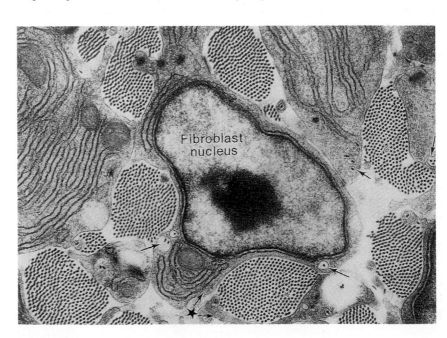

capillaries in inflammatory states. There is a great similarity between mast cells in the tissue and basophils in the blood, but it is probable that they are independent cell types.

Some cells in the connective tissue are specialized for the synthesis and storage of fats. These **adipocytes** may be present singly or in groups. Their appearance varies according to the amount of fat present. When empty, the cells resemble fibroblasts, whereas when full of fat they become spherical, with the centre filled with fat and only a thin rim of cytoplasm visible around the periphery. The nucleus is flattened and displaced.

Neutrophils, eosinophils and lymphocytes derive from the blood and are all involved in different ways in combating infection and tissue damage.

The connective tissue population of these cells increases in inflammatory states.

Neutrophils have a lobed nucleus and fine granules which take up acid and basic dyes, giving them a lilac appearance. They are quickly attracted to the site of tissue damage and are phagocytic.

Eosinophils are not very numerous in most connective tissue, but they are found particularly in the lamina propria of the small intestine, in the interstitial connective tissue of the lungs, in the omentum and in the stroma of mammary glands. The cells have a bilobed nucleus and coarse granules containing hydrolytic enzymes, which stain red with the dye eosin. Eosinophils have been shown to phagocytose antigen–antibody complexes and they have a probable role in combating parasitic infections. Their numbers are increased in some hypersensitivity states.

Lymphocytes have a large nucleus and normally appear rounded and, although they are capable of amoeboid movement, they are not phagocytic. These cells are concerned with the production of antibodies. When stimulated by specific antigens they are capable of transforming into larger cells, which divide and some of which differentiate to form plasma cells. It is the plasma cells that synthesize antibody against antigen. Plasma cells have an eccentrically placed nucleus and they are found in greater numbers underneath the epithelial membranes lining the respiratory and alimentary tracts, where microorganisms are liable to gain entry to the body.

Areolar connective tissue is extensively distributed throughout the body. It supports the epithelial linings of the gastrointestinal, respiratory and urinary tracts, is found in the deeper layers of the skin and also in areas that lack subcutaneous fat, such as the eyelids. It surrounds blood vessels and nerves and also provides loose interstitial packing in virtually all tissues and organs. The open nature of the tissue enables the various reactions that constitute inflammation to take place; areolar connective tissue is synthesized in the repair of wounds.

See also **White blood cells (leucocytes)** (page 341), in Ch. 11, Blood, Lymphoid Tissue and Immunity.

Regular dense (white fibrous) connective tissue

The name of this tissue derives from the preponderance of bundles of collagen fibres, which have fibroblasts (which produce the collagen) lying between them (Figure 3.13). This tissue has great strength and its locations reflect this function.

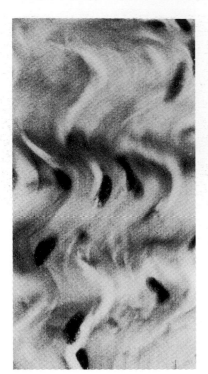

Figure 3.13 Photomicrograph of regular dense (white fibrous) connective tissue. Abundant collagen fibres are arranged in wavy bundles. (Reproduced with permission from Fawcett, D. W. (1993) *Bloom and Fawcett: A Textbook of Histology*, Chapman & Hall, London.)

The arrangement of the tendon of the superior oblique muscle of the eye is described in **Rotational movements of the eyeballs** (page 233), in Ch. 8, The Special Senses.

In the dense, regular connective tissue of tendons, the bundles of collagen run parallel. In ligaments, the arrangement is similar, but slightly less regular. Other sites where regular connective tissue is found include fasciae, tendons and aponeuroses and the cornea. In these sites the tissue is built up in sheets and in each sheet the fibres run parallel; however, the orientation of the sheets may be different.

LIGAMENTS

Ligaments are bands of regular dense connective tissue which link bones together. They reinforce joint articulations, as in the elbow and other synovial joints. They may form part of the joint capsule itself as thickened bands of tissue, or they may lie outside the capsule as extracapsular ligaments. Some ligaments, e.g. those of the knee, lie within the cavity of the joint.

TENDONS

Tendons are composed of dense regular connective tissue and are much stronger than the muscles to which they are attached. A tendon is therefore much thinner and/or flatter than its muscle and at sites where several muscles are attached to bone the overall bulk of the tendons is relatively small.

The strength and pressure-withstanding properties of tendons make them particularly valuable in situations where muscle passes over bone. They can also be used to change the direction of pull of a muscle, by passing around a hook of bone. This unusual arrangement is found in the superior oblique muscle of the eye.

Tendons may be strap-like or flattened, generally depending upon the shape of their muscle. Very flat, thin tendons are referred to as **aponeuroses** (*sing.* **aponeurosis**).

Tendons are flexible, but offer resistance to the pulling action of muscle and will recoil after being stretched. For example, the tendons of the lower limb are stretched when the ball of the foot makes contact with the ground in running; when they recoil to their original length, the energy stored within them is used to push the foot off the ground and begin the next step.

Irregular dense connective tissue

In some sites, the arrangement of collagen bundles is irregular and has more of a woven appearance (Figure 3.14). Such fibrous membranes are found surrounding some organs; as periosteum surrounding bones and perichondrium surrounding cartilage; as the dura mater, one of the meninges surrounding the central nervous system; as the fibrous pericardium surrounding the heart; and as the sclera of the eye.

Elastic tissue

Elastic tissue is a type of dense connective tissue that contains a particularly high proportion of elastic fibres (Figure 3.15), which have flattened fibroblasts between them.

The abundance of elastic fibres confers a yellow coloration. This type of tissue is not widely distributed; it is found in sites where its ability to

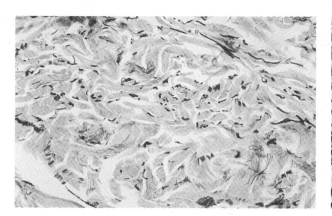

Figure 3.14 Photomicrograph of irregular dense connective tissue. Collagen fibres are arranged in irregular bundles which give a woven appearance to the tissue. (Reproduced by courtesy of D. R. Smith.)

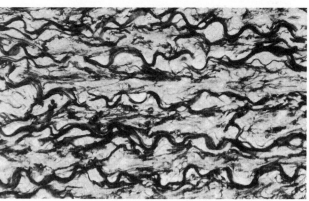

Figure 3.15 Photomicrograph of elastic tissue (carotid artery). Dark-stained elastic fibres are arranged in concentric sheets. (Reproduced by courtesy of D. R. Smith.)

be stretched and then regain its original configuration is important. In small arteries, for example, the elastic tissue forms a sheet of tissue called the internal elastic lamina. The vocal cords are composed of elastic tissue, as are the ligamenta flava of the vertebral column.

Adipose tissue

This tissue contains cells which are specialized for the synthesis, storage and release of fat, and they are under hormonal and nervous control. The most widespread type of adipose tissue is known as **white adipose tissue**.

The cells (**adipocytes**) can be very large (up to 120 µm diameter) and are basically spherical, although, in section, they may appear polyhedral because they are squashed by their neighbours (Figure 3.16).

The fat is usually stored as a single droplet, in which case the cells are described as **unilocular**. As well as being the primary cells of adipose tissue, single or small groups of adipocytes are also found in areolar connective tissue.

This type of tissue is present in the superficial fasciae under the skin. The distribution is different in the two sexes, so that in men, in whom it typically constitutes about 20% of the body weight of an adult, the main sites are overlying the cervical vertebrae and the deltoid and triceps muscles, the lumbosacral region and the buttocks. In women adipose tissue is about 25% of total body weight; it is found principally in the breasts, thighs and buttocks. Both sexes have stores of fat in the omentum and mesenteries.

The quantity of fat from all these areas will diminish with prolonged fasting, when the fat is released and used by other cells. In some sites, however, the fat has primarily a protective function and is not released

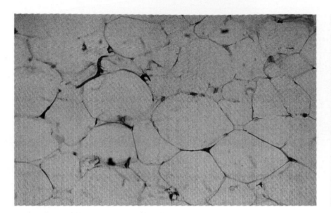

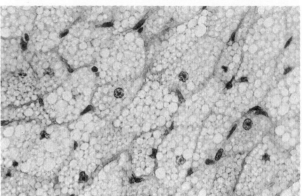

Figure 3.16 Photomicrograph of white adipose tissue. Large adipocytes, each of which consists of a single fat droplet surrounded by a narrow rim of cytoplasm, are squashed into polyhedral shapes by their neighbours. (Reproduced by courtesy of D. R. Smith.)

Figure 3.17 Photomicrograph of brown adipose tissue. Adipocytes contain numerous tiny fat droplets. (Reproduced by courtesy of D. R. Smith.)

so readily for metabolic functions. Such sites include the tissue in the orbit of the eye, in the joints and on the palms of the hands and the soles of the feet.

The cells of **brown adipose tissue** contain large numbers of mitochondria. The cells are described as **multilocular** because the fat is present as many droplets rather than one large one. The cells are smaller than those found in white fat (Figure 3.17).

Brown adipose tissue is found in new-born babies, but only in small quantities in adults. Its function appears to be primarily one of heat generation. Mitochondrial oxidation of the fat results in the energy being released as heat, rather than partly as ATP, which is the usual pattern in cells. The oxidation is stimulated by the sympathetic nervous system and the hormone noradrenaline.

Brown fat is found between the shoulder blades, around the kidneys, in the axillae, mediastinum and along the aorta in the thorax.

Cartilage

The cells of cartilage (**chondrocytes**) are present in spaces (lacunae) in the intercellular matrix (Figure 3.18).

The matrix is firm and solid and can therefore withstand pressure, tension and torsion. The type and quantity of fibres present affects the nature of the intercellular material and gives rise to three types of cartilage: hyaline (meaning 'glassy') cartilage, fibrocartilage and elastic cartilage.

The ground substance and the fibres are produced by small immature cells called **chondroblasts**. They have a round or oval nucleus and are usually flattened and irregular in shape. As the matrix is formed, the cells are separated from each other by it, although cell division often

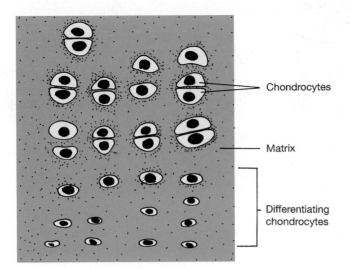

Chondrocytes

Matrix

Differentiating chondrocytes

Figure 3.18 The principal components of cartilage. Chondrocytes are observed in small cavities, or lacunae, in the clear matrix. Differentiating cells give rise to small groups of isogenous chondrocytes.

results in several isogenous cells lying together in a lacuna. The mature chondrocytes have a more rounded shape.

The matrix contains glycosaminoglycans, which are a mixture of hyaluronic acid and a number of other proteoglycans.

BLOOD SUPPLY

Nutrition of chondrocytes occurs largely, if not entirely, by diffusion of substances from blood vessels in adjacent tissue, or from synovial fluid in the case of articular cartilage. Cartilage itself does not have a blood or a lymph supply of its own, although vessels may pass through it *en route* to other tissues.

Hyaline cartilage

The matrix of hyaline cartilage appears pearly and translucent and has some flexibility. Collagen fibres are present in the form of fine, interlacing fibrils which cannot be seen with the light microscope (Figure 3.19).

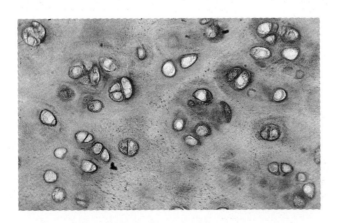

Figure 3.19 Photomicrograph of hyaline cartilage (trachea). (Reproduced by courtesy of D. R. Smith.)

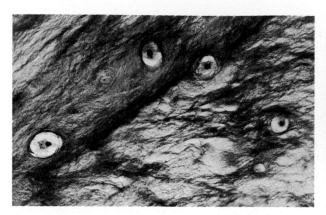

Figure 3.20 Photomicrograph of fibrocartilage (intervertebral disc). It is characterized by thick bundles of collagen fibres. (Reproduced by courtesy of D. R. Smith.)

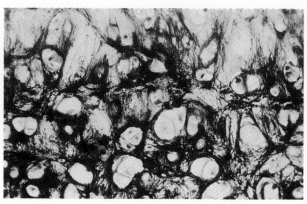

Figure 3.21 Photomicrograph of elastic cartilage (epiglottis). Chondrocytes are present either singly or in isogenous groups surrounded by dark-staining elastic fibres. (Reproduced by courtesy of D. R. Smith.)

The foetal skeleton is laid down as hyaline cartilage, most of which is subsequently replaced by bone. The cartilage persists in the costal cartilages of the ribs, in the nose, larynx, trachea and bronchi. In long bones, hyaline cartilage persists until adolescence as epiphysial cartilage plates, which, because of their capacity for interstitial growth, enable the bones to increase in length (see Figure 3.26). Hyaline cartilage is found covering articular surfaces where the smoothness of the tissue enables the bones to move easily against each other.

Fibrocartilage

The principal structural feature of fibrocartilage is thick bundles of collagen fibres running parallel with each other. The chondrocytes lie in lacunae between the fibres and there is little matrix present (Figure 3.20). This structure makes the tissue rigid and very strong, although it still has some flexibility.

The tissue is found in the intervertebral discs, the pubic symphysis, the attachments of some tendons and the linings of tendon grooves in long bones. Fibrocartilage is continuous with the dense connective tissue in joint capsules and ligaments and has no perichondrium around it.

Elastic cartilage

Elastic cartilage is yellow, opaque and, as the name indicates, elastic. It contains branching and anastomosing elastic fibres, which are continuous with those in the surrounding perichondrium. There are some fine collagen fibres present as well. The chondrocytes in lacunae are present singly or in isogenous groups of two or four cells (Figure 3.21).

Elastic cartilage will withstand deformation and return to its original shape. It is found in the external ear, external auditory meatus and auditory tube, in the epiglottis and in some laryngeal cartilages.

GROWTH AND REPAIR OF CARTILAGE

Growth of cartilage occurs in two ways, from within (**interstitial**) or by the addition of new tissue to the outer edges (**appositional**). The latter occurs when chondrocytes differentiate from connective tissue cells in the perichondrium that surrounds cartilage (except at articular surfaces).

If cartilage is damaged, repair can take place by fibroblasts in the perichondrium invading the damaged area to form granulation tissue. The fibroblasts may then transform into cartilage cells. Except in young children, however, the repair of cartilage only occurs with difficulty and is often incomplete.

Bone

Bone has the characteristic components of connective tissues, that is cells, ground substance and fibres, but its principal distinguishing feature is that the intercellular material is calcified. The tissue has, therefore, high tensile and compressive strength, coupled with some degree of flexibility. The structure of bones renders them remarkably lightweight in view of the composition of the tissue. Complete bones are composed of two types of tissue, **compact** and **cancellous bone**. The former, as its name suggests, is dense and ivory-like and forms the outer layer of bones; whereas cancellous bone has a honeycomb-like structure and is found in the middle of bones (Figure 3.22).

Long bones, such as the humerus and tibia of the limbs, have rounded ends or **epiphyses** which are composed of cancellous bone with a thin peripheral layer of compact bone (Figure 3.23).

A covering of hyaline cartilage at the articular surfaces prevents the ends of bone from rubbing together in joints. In children and young

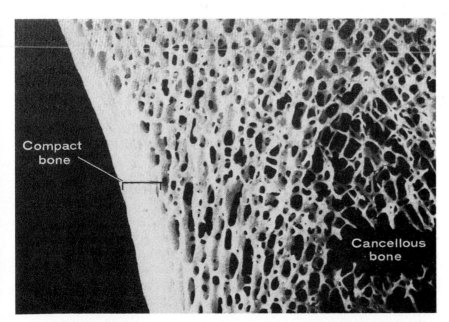

Compact
bone

Cancellous
bone

Figure 3.22 A section of the tibia, illustrating the outer layer of compact bone surrounding a lattice of trabeculae of cancellous bone. (Reproduced with permission from Fawcett, D. W. (1993) *Bloom and Fawcett: A Textbook of Histology*, Chapman & Hall, London.)

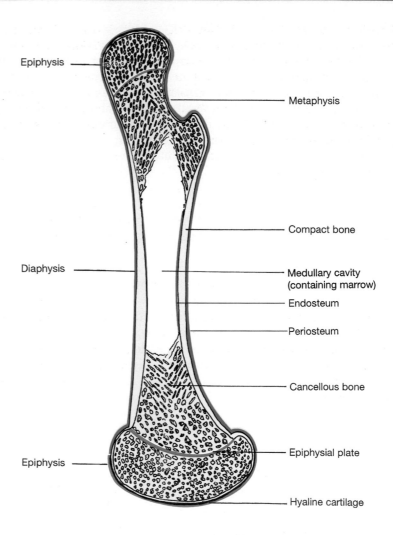

Epiphysis

Metaphysis

Compact bone

Diaphysis

Medullary cavity
(containing marrow)

Endosteum

Periosteum

Cancellous bone

Epiphysis

Epiphysial plate

Hyaline cartilage

Figure 3.23 Longitudinal section through a long bone.

adults, who are still growing, a cartilage disc called the **epiphysial plate** is present next to each epiphysis. The latter is connected to the shaft of the bone (**diaphysis**) by columns of spongy bone in a region called the **metaphysis**. The diaphysis is a thick-walled tube of compact bone with a central **medullary cavity** containing marrow.

Flat bones, such as those of the skull, are composed of a layer of cancellous bone (diploe) sandwiched between two layers of compact bone.

Bones are surrounded (except at the articular surfaces) by a layer of connective tissue called **periosteum**, which has the potential to form bone-producing cells (osteogenic potency). Cavities in bone are lined by **endosteum**, which consists of a thin layer of squamous cells, which also have osteogenic potency.

Compact bone is composed of concentric cylindrical **lamellae**, which form **Haversian systems** or **osteons** (Figure 3.24).

Each lamella is composed of ground substance and parallel collagen fibres; the direction of orientation of these fibres changes in adjacent lamellae. The lamellae are 3–7 µm thick and each osteon is made up of four to 20 lamellae, so that the diameters of individual osteons vary considerably. Some osteons are simple cylindrical structures, while others branch and anastomose with those nearby. The bone cells (**osteocytes**) lie in cavities (**lacunae**) in the matrix. Lacunae are connected to each other and with the **Haversian canal**, which lies at the centre of each osteon, by means of fine channels or **canaliculi**. Haversian canals are linked to each other by **Volkmann's canals**.

Between the osteons, there are lamellae filling in the spaces. These are called **interstitial systems** and on the surface of bones beneath the periosteum and endosteum there are usually a few circumferential lamellae, which extend around the periphery of the bone.

Cancellous bone also has a lamellar structure but does not have Haversian canals containing blood vessels, and the cells are connected to the blood vessels in the endosteum by the canaliculi.

Bone salt is mainly the complex molecule hydroxyapatite ($Ca_{10}(PO_4)_6(OH)_2$) and it is found on and within the collagen fibres. Other ions may either associate with the crystals of apatite (e.g. carbonate and citrate) or be substituted for ions within the molecule (e.g. fluoride (F^-) may substitute for the hydroxyl group OH^-). Na^+ and Mg^{2+} are also present. Some radioactive isotopes released in the fission of uranium and plutonium may become incorporated into the hydroxyapatite molecules. The most hazardous of these bone-seeking isotopes is strontium-90 (^{90}Sr).

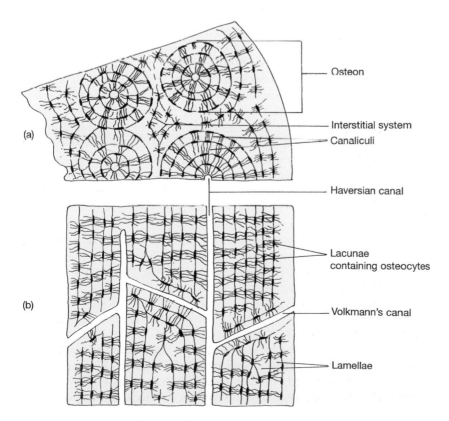

Figure 3.24 Diagrammatic **(a)** transverse and **(b)** longitudinal sections of compact bone.

Osteon

Interstitial system

Canaliculi

Haversian canal

Lacunae containing osteocytes

Volkmann's canal

Lamellae

(a)

(b)

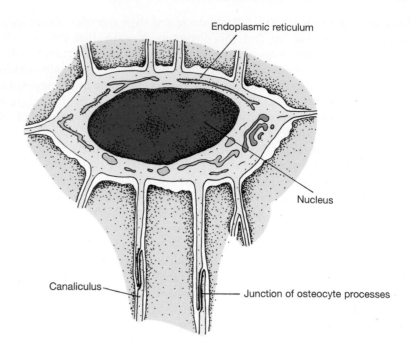

Endoplasmic reticulum

Nucleus

Canaliculus

Junction of osteocyte processes

Figure 3.25 Osteocyte within its lacuna. The cell's processes are in contact with those of adjacent cells.

BONE CELLS

Bone is laid down by cells called **osteoblasts**, which are present in the growing surfaces of bone. These are ovoid in shape with several cytoplasmic processes radiating outwards to connect with those of adjacent cells. As the bone matrix is laid down around the cells it leaves the lacunae and canaliculi surrounding the cells. The 'trapped' cells are the mature bone cells, the **osteocytes** (Figure 3.25), which maintain the matrix and also actively remove bone salts from the bone to the extracellular fluid filling the canaliculi and thence to the blood. The transfer of bone salt to blood by the osteocytes is called osteolysis and is stimulated by parathyroid hormone.

Bone surfaces that are undergoing resorption contain large, multinucleate cells called **osteoclasts**. These cells are often seen in shallow depressions in the bone surface called **Howship's lacunae.** The surface of the cell next to an area of bone undergoing resorption appears 'ruffled' because the cell membrane is deeply folded. The precise mechanisms of bone resorption are unknown, but it is probable that the osteoclasts secrete proteolytic enzymes into the matrix and then the digestion products are taken into the cells by pinocytosis. Parathyroid hormone stimulates osteoclast activity.

BLOOD SUPPLY

Bone, in contrast to other connective tissues, has an extensive blood supply. The hard nature of the matrix does not allow the bone cells to rely on diffusion for nutrition and removal of waste. The canaliculi in the matrix connect the bone cells to the blood vessels in the Haversian canals; each canal contains one or two blood vessels, usually capillaries.

The canaliculi are therefore effectively an extension of the circulatory system.

BONE MARROW

There are two types of bone marrow: red and yellow. Red marrow is found within most bones in newborn and young children. It contains haemopoietic cells and is a major source of blood cells in children.

After 4 or 5 years of age, blood-forming cells start to be replaced by adipose cells and the marrow changes from red to yellow. In adults, red marrow persists only in the proximal ends of the humerus and femur, and in the vertebrae, ribs, sternum and ilia of the pelvis. Yellow marrow can revert back to red marrow in response to a rise in body temperature or a fall in the blood cell count.

OSSIFICATION AND GROWTH OF LONG BONES

Bone is produced by osteoblasts and the events preceding its formation during development and growth are categorized as either intramembranous or endochondral ossification.

Most of the skull bones and the collar bones (clavicles) are formed by **intramembranous ossification**, that is, from primitive connective tissue (mesenchyme), which undergoes structural changes including vascularization and the development of osteoblasts from the connective tissue cells.

The first bone to be laid down is called woven bone and has collagen fibres running in all directions, rather than in regular lamellae, which are laid down subsequently. Woven bone has large channels containing blood vessels running through it.

Most bones, however, are formed by **endochondral ossification**. In this process, a template of cartilage is laid down which replaces the embryonic mesenchyme, and then the cartilage is, in turn, replaced by bone. The details of endochondral ossification are given here in connection with the ossification of a long bone (Figure 3.26).

The first, or primary, centre of ossification occurs in the diaphysis by the third month of foetal life. The chondrocytes enlarge and the matrix diminishes. Calcium phosphate crystals are deposited in the matrix,

Haemopoiesis is described in **Production of red blood cells (erythropoiesis)** (page 334) and **Production of white blood cells (leucopoiesis)** (page 345), in Ch. 11, Blood, Lymphoid Tissue and Immunity.

Figure 3.26 Growth of a long bone. **(a)** Cartilage template of a long bone in the fetus. **(b)** Primary centre of ossification and periosteal collar. **(c)** Invasion of the diaphysis by blood vessels and connective tissue. **(d)** Formation of trabeculae. **(e)** Postnatal formation of secondary centres of ossification. **(f)** Epiphyses completely ossified but cartilaginous epiphyseal plates still present. **(g)** Closure of epiphyses.

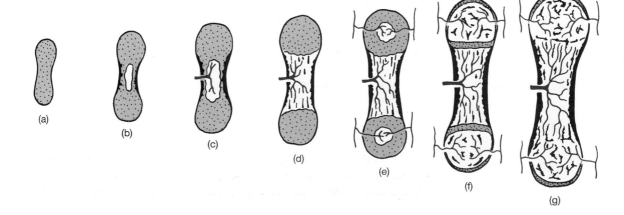

(a)   (b)   (c)   (d)   (e)   (f)   (g)

which causes the cells to die. Concurrently there are changes in the perichondrium resulting in the production of osteoblasts, which produce a periosteal band or collar of bone. Blood vessels grow into the diaphysis and carry with them, in the perivascular tissue, primitive connective tissue cells which subsequently develop into haemopoietic cells and osteoblasts. These osteoblasts congregate to form a layer on the spicules of calcified cartilage, which is disintegrating. The cells deposit bone matrix and form trabeculae.

Further increase in length occurs by interstitial growth of the cartilage, particularly at the junctions of the diaphysis and epiphyses of the bone. The diaphysis thickens by appositional growth, which increases the thickness of the periosteal band. Ossification progresses from the centre of the shaft towards the epiphyses, with cartilage being replaced by bone in the metaphyseal region. The bones are modelled as they grow by resorption by osteoclasts on the inner (endosteal) surface, which enlarges the marrow cavity, and also by osteoclasts on the periosteal surface, which shape the bone surface.

The primary bone is subsequently replaced by ordered secondary bone from about 1 year onwards and the replacement of bone continues throughout life. The primary bone is eroded by osteoclasts and then replaced by secondary bone arranged in osteons.

After birth, secondary centres of ossification occur in the epiphyses. In this case, there is no periosteal band and the ossification gradually replaces all but the articular cartilage and the cartilage between the epiphyses and the diaphysis. This cartilage becomes known as the epiphyseal plate and, because of its ability to divide, it is responsible for the increase in the length of long bones during childhood and adolescence. The thickness of the plate remains relatively constant, as ossification keeps pace with the additional cartilage produced. Eventually, the cartilage is completely replaced by bone, a process called **closure of the epiphyses**; this typically occurs around the age of 18 years in women and 21 years in men.

HORMONAL CONTROL OF BONE GROWTH

Bone growth in young children and adolescents is regulated primarily by **growth hormone**, which is produced by the adenohypophysis. Growth hormone promotes the synthesis and release of somatomedins, growth hormone-dependent peptides, by the liver. Somatomedin then stimulates division of chondrocytes and bone cells, which leads to bone growth.

Oestrogens in girls and androgens in boys promote the growth of long bones, thereby producing the growth spurt which occurs in puberty. The hormones also bring about closure of the epiphyses, which eventually stops further growth in length.

Thyroxine and tri-iodothyronine also promote the growth of bones, particularly in infancy and early childhood.

REPAIR OF FRACTURES

The breakage of bones is a relatively common occurrence but fortunately bone tissue has good powers of regeneration.

Somatomedins are discussed in **Growth promoting actions of growth hormone** (page 618), in Ch. 16, Endocrine Physiology.

The roles of the sex hormones in growth during puberty are described in **Female puberty** (page 660) and **Male puberty** (page 668), in Ch. 17, Sex and Reproduction.

The influences of T3 and T4 on bone growth are considered in **Metabolic actions of T3 and T4** (page 625), in Ch. 16, Endocrine Physiology.

A blood clot forms in the area of a break, and the matrix and bone cells in the vicinity die. There is intense proliferation of the periosteum and endosteum around the fracture and immature bone forms due to the endochondral ossification of small cartilaginous fragments in developing connective tissue. In addition, there is intramembranous ossification. Irregular trabeculae of immature bone temporarily unite the extremities of the fractured bone, forming a bone callus. Normal stress imposed on the bone leads to remodelling of this callus so that the latter is gradually replaced by lamellar bone.

SKELETON

Bones collectively form the skeleton, which is the primary supporting framework of the body (Figure 3.27).

It gives shape to the body and provides protection for internal organs such as the brain, heart and lungs. Muscles are attached to bone, enabling their movement, and the cells of the blood are produced in the marrow cavities of some bones. The tissue is a dynamic one in that it is constantly being renewed (**accretion**) and removed (**resorption**). Blood calcium concentration is kept relatively constant, in part by the maintenance of an equilibrium with calcium in the bone. If blood calcium levels fall, for example, then calcium is added from the bone.

The bones which make up the skeleton are divided into two groups. The **axial skeleton** includes those bones found in the skull, spine (vertebral column) and rib cage, while the **appendicular skeleton** includes the shoulder and pelvic girdles and the upper and lower limbs.

Lack of bone salt (osteoporosis and osteomalacia)

Osteoporosis is a decrease in total bone mass, which is found to a greater or lesser extent in most people over the age of 50. It is associated with low oestrogen levels and is therefore common in post-menopausal women.

Osteoporosis results from either excessive bone resorption, or decrease in new bone formation, or both. In addition, since bone remodelling occurs in response to external stress, the reduced physical activity of old age might be expected to lead to its reduction.

Osteoporosis affects all bones, but most commonly produces symptoms in those with a particular stress-bearing role. The bodies of vertebrae become compressed so that there may therefore be a reduction in overall height and altered curvatures of the spine (**kyphosis**). Bones are generally brittle and are therefore easily fractured.

Osteomalacia is a type of osteoporosis in adults that is caused by a lack of calcium salts in bone, usually due to a dietary deficiency of vitamin D.

As a result, the bones are soft and may become deformed or exhibit fine fractures; there is also pain. Since growth is complete, however, deformities are not extensive.

The low levels of blood Ca^{2+} which occur in osteomalacia may lead to increased secretion of parathyroid hormone and elevation of blood phosphate concentrations.

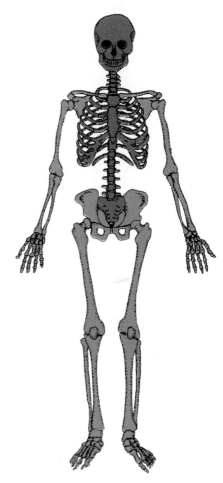

Figure 3.27 The skeleton – frontal view to show the axial skeleton [orange] and the appendicular skeleton [green].

Vitamin D deficiency is summarized in Table 15.2 (page 525), in Ch. 15, Digestion and Absorption of Food.

Regulation of PTH is described in **Parathyroid hormone (PTH)** (page 628), in Ch. 16, Endocrine Physiology.

Muscle tissue

Muscle tissue is capable of contraction and thereby cause movement of the whole body, or a part of it.

The cells are elongated in the direction of contraction and contain the proteins actin and myosin in much larger amounts than other types of cells. These proteins are arranged to form myofilaments in the cytoplasm (sarcoplasm) of the cells and it is these which cause contraction of the cell.

When viewed microscopically under polarized light or after staining, muscle cells appear either homogenous (**smooth**), or show alternate light and dark cross-banding (**striated**). The classification of muscle, together with its distribution, is given in Table 3.3.

Smooth muscle is also known as **involuntary muscle** as it is found in those structures not generally associated with voluntary activity, such as the walls of blood vessels and the gastrointestinal tract. Contraction is controlled by the autonomic nervous system.

There are two types of striated muscle: **skeletal** and **cardiac** (Figure 3.28). The former is usually, though not always, found in muscles attached to bone and is therefore responsible for such movements as walking and raising the rib cage during respiration. This tissue is also called **voluntary muscle**, although it can contract involuntarily by reflex action. Skeletal muscle is controlled by somatic motor neurones.

Cardiac muscle is found in the myocardium of the heart and is controlled by the autonomic nervous system.

Smooth muscle

Smooth muscle cells are long (15–500 µm) and spindle-shaped, with an ovoid central nucleus (Figure 3.28). Each smooth muscle cell is surrounded by a basal lamina (like that seen in epithelial tissues) and there are gap junctions linking the cells together. Cells are usually

Table 3.3 Classification and distribution of muscle	
Type	*Distribution*
Striated	
Cardiac	Heart
Skeletal	Attached to bones; wall of abdomen; diaphragm; extrinsic muscles of eye; facial muscles
Smooth	Iris, ciliary body of eye; respiratory tract; walls of arteries, veins and arterioles; walls of the larger lymphatic trunks; urinary, reproductive tract and alimentary canal; ducts of glands, arrector pili muscles of skin; subcutaneous tissue of scrotum; areolae of nipples

(a)

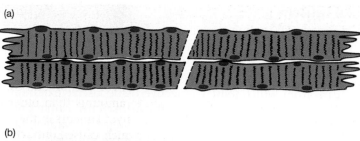

(b)

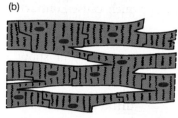

(c)

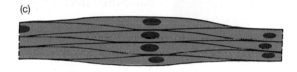

Figure 3.28 Types of muscle tissue. **(a)** Skeletal. **(b)** Cardiac. **(c)** Smooth.

arranged in small bundles or **fasciculi**, which are themselves arranged as sheets.

The orientation of the cells determines the type of movement effected, so that contraction of the cells in the circular muscle of the gastrointestinal tract causes constriction, while the longitudinal cells cause local shortening.

Connective tissue surrounds the fasciculi and carries blood and lymphatic vessels and nerves. The collagen, reticular and elastic fibres in the connective tissue are continuous with those forming a sheath around individual cells, so that when a cell contracts, the force is distributed via the fibres to the surrounding connective tissue.

Some smooth muscle appears to contract spontaneously, i.e. it is **myogenic**, or it is stimulated by stretching the muscle, as for example in the gastrointestinal tract, the uterus and ureters. In these cases the autonomic nervous system modifies the pre-existing rhythmic contraction. Smooth muscle also exhibits a sustained or **tonic contraction**.

Smooth muscle is found in the iris and ciliary body of the eye, in the walls of the respiratory tract, in the urinary and reproductive tracts, in the duct walls of glands, as arrector pili muscles attached to the hairs of the skin, as well as in blood vessels and the gastrointestinal tract.

REPAIR OF SMOOTH MUSCLE

Repair of damaged smooth muscle is thought to be achieved largely by the formation of scar tissue by the fibroblasts in the connective tissue, although some regeneration of muscle cells may also take place.

Skeletal muscle

There are some 600 whole muscles in the body composed of skeletal (voluntary) muscle tissue. They are mostly attached to the skeleton, usually by tendons.

Muscles are surrounded by a dense connective tissue sheath called **epimysium**, from which loose connective tissue fasciae extend into the muscle and divide it into primary bundles or **fasciculi**, containing 20–40 fibres (Figure 3.29). The fasciculi may be arranged in parallel, obliquely or spirally in relation to the direction of pull of the muscle.

Figure 3.29 Arrangement of connective tissue in muscle.

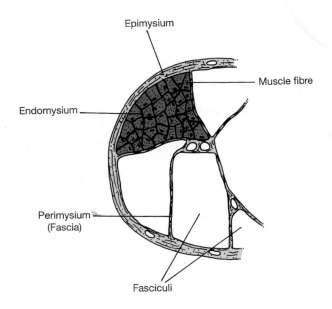

The connective tissue surrounding each fasciculus is known as the **perimysium**, and this in turn is continuous with the connective tissue surrounding each individual muscle fibre, the **endomysium**.

Arterial, venous and lymphatic vessels lie in the perimysium and epimysium, while the endomysium contains an extensive capillary network supplying each muscle fibre. The nerve supply (somatic motor neurones) to skeletal muscle cells is also distributed via the connective tissue network.

Skeletal muscle fibres are 10–100 µm in diameter and their length varies from a few millimetres to about 30 cm (in the sartorius muscle of the thigh). Usually, a fibre does not extend from one end of the muscle to the other, but is connected to a tendon at one end and to connective tissue within the muscle at the other.

Muscle fibres are cylindrical in shape and contain many hundreds of peripheral nuclei. Each fibre develops from a number of **myeloblasts**, which fuse to form **myotubules**, which then grow to become foetal muscle fibres. Under the light microscope, a characteristic banding pattern, consisting of alternating light and dark bands, can be seen across muscle cells.

Skeletal muscle structure and contraction are described in Ch. 9, Autonomic and Somatic Motor Activity.

REPAIR OF SKELETAL MUSCLE

Muscle cells have only a limited capacity for repair and, if cells are completely destroyed, new ones may not be formed and connective tissue accumulates instead. Regeneration of damaged fibres occurs when satellite cells, spindle-shaped cells associated with the muscle fibres, proliferate and fuse to form new cylinders of sarcoplasm, which then join with the undamaged portions. The nuclei of muscle fibres themselves are incapable of dividing.

Cardiac muscle

Cardiac muscle fibres are faintly striated, branched cylinders. The fibres consist of many individual cells about 80 μm in length and 15–20 μm in diameter, arranged end to end. The cell junctions stain darkly and are known as **intercalated discs** (Figure 3.30). Each cell has one or more centrally placed nuclei and one or two branches, so that adjacent fibres are joined.

The cells are surrounded by connective tissue endomysium (like the skeletal muscle cells), which contains lymphatic as well as blood capillaries and autonomic neurones. There are extensive nerve plexuses around the sinoatrial node and the conducting system of the heart.

In addition, the cardiac muscle is generally supplied with parasympathetic and sympathetic fibres, which have no specialized junctions with the muscle cells. The fibres are grouped in bundles of between a few hundred and a few thousand, surrounded by perimysium.

The striations of cardiac muscle arise from the same arrangement of myofilaments as in skeletal muscle. There are, however, several intracellular features that are different from skeletal muscle cells.

Cardiac muscle cells have an abundant sarcoplasm and larger, more numerous mitochondria (usually about the length of one sarcomere, but sometimes more) than those of skeletal muscle. The myofilaments are not grouped in regular myofibrils; instead the filaments form a continuous mass incompletely subdivided into fibrils.

Cardiac muscle cells have stores of glycogen and lipid and oxygen attached to myoglobin. Oxidative enzymes are abundant. The intercalated discs have various types of attachment joining adjacent cells

> See also **Conduction system and innervation of the heart wall** (page 377) and **Contraction of cardiac muscle cells** (page 382), in Ch. 12, Circulation of Blood and Lymph.

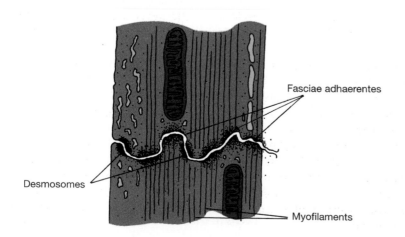

Figure 3.30 Intercalated disc of cardiac muscle.

Fasciae adhaerentes

Desmosomes

Myofilaments

together, maculae adhaerentes (desmosomes), gap junctions (like those in smooth muscle) and fascia adhaerentes. The cytoplasm immediately either side of the cell membranes serves as the attachment point for the thin myofilaments (Figure 3.30).

Although cardiac muscle cells are myogenic, the rate of contraction is dominated by the frequency of impulses arising from the sinoatrial node or pacemaker. The impulses are transmitted along the cell membranes of the branching fibres and through the gap junctions very rapidly, so the interconnected cells function as a unit or **functional syncytium**. There are two functional syncytia in the heart, the atrial and ventricular syncytia, separated by the fibrous connective tissue surrounding the heart valves.

REPAIR OF CARDIAC MUSCLE

Repair of cardiac muscle is effected by fibroblasts, which form scar tissue, rather than by regeneration of muscle cells.

Nervous tissue

Only 10% of the total number of cells comprising nervous tissue are nerve-cells or **neurones** (although they occupy 50% of the volume). These are cells which are capable of receiving, generating and transmitting impulses at great speed from one part of the body to another. The remaining 90% of cells are **neuroglia**, which have a secondary, supportive role to the neurones.

The nervous system can be divided into two primary sections, the **central nervous system** (CNS) which comprises the brain and spinal cord, and the **peripheral nerves** which connect the CNS with the tissues (see Figure 4.2). The latter are further subdivided into **sensory** (afferent) and **motor** (efferent) divisions. Sensory fibres carry information from the periphery to the brain and spinal cord while motor fibres carry information away from the CNS to effectors.

The nervous system is covered in Ch. 4, Cellular Mechanisms of Neural Control; Ch. 5, The Brain; Ch. 6, The Spinal Cord; Ch. 7, Sensory Processing; Ch. 8, The Special Senses and Ch. 9, Autonomic and Somatic Motor Activity.

Neurones

Neurones consist of a **cell body**, soma, or perikaryon, which is the nucleus and surrounding cytoplasm, and processes or **neurites**. The processes are of two kinds; one or more **dendrites**, which conduct impulses towards the cell body, and a single **axon**, which conducts impulses away from the cell body. Another, more recent, distinction is that axons generate action potentials, whereas dendrites generate graded potentials.

Neurones may be classified according to the number of processes joining the cell body (i.e. the number of poles) as multipolar, bipolar and unipolar (pseudounipolar) (Figure 3.31).

Multipolar cells have many dendrites and one axon connected to the cell body, which may have a variety of shapes. Cells in this category include somatic motor neurones, the Purkinje cells in the cerebellar cortices and the pyramidal cells in the motor cortices of the cerebrum.

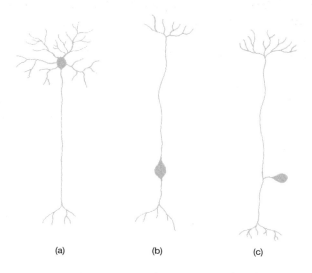

(a)   (b)   (c)

Figure 3.31 **(a)** Multipolar neurone. **(b)** Bipolar neurone. **(c)** Pseudounipolar neurone.

Bipolar cells have a spindle-shaped cell body with one axon and one dendrite. Most sensory cells pass through this stage during embryonic development before becoming pseudounipolar. Cells which remain bipolar include those in the retina, in the sensory ganglia of the cochlea and vestibular apparatus and cells in the olfactory epithelium.

Most sensory neurones are classified as **pseudounipolar**, because, after the embryonic bipolar stage, the two processes move together and combine, so that the cell has a single process attached to a pear-shaped cell body. The process divides into a dendrite and an axon (also called a peripheral process and a central process).

Another way of classifying neurones is by the length of the axon (Table 3.4). Short ones are classified as Golgi type II, and these are found in the retina and the cerebellar and cerebral cortices, whereas neurones with a long axon are Golgi type I neurones and they are found in peripheral nerves and fibre tracts in the CNS.

The cell body is concerned with the maintenance and repair of the cell and has the appropriate organelles present, including mitochondria, Golgi apparatus, lysosomes and yellow lipofuscin granules (which are probably a product of lysosomal activity and they accumulate with age), microfilaments, Nissl bodies (rough endoplasmic reticulum) and centrioles.

Dendrites are the receptive surfaces of the neurone. They are branched processes; the branches leave the cell body at an acute angle, and are covered by thorn-like spines or gemmules (Figure 3.32). In sensory neurones the dendritic tree is remote from the cell body and the peripheral process that connects this with the cell body is structurally identical to an axon, despite the fact that it transmits impulses towards the cell body. In other types of neurone, dendrites connect directly with the cell body.

Table 3.4 Classification of nervous tissue

1. Neurones

(a) Classified by number of processes

Number	Name	Example
Many	Multipolar	Somatic motor neurones
Two	Bipolar	Middle layer of retina
One	Pseudounipolar	Somatic sensory neurones

(b) Classified by length

Axon length	Name	Example
Long	Golgi type I	Peripheral neurones
Short	Golgi type II	Retina; cerebellar and cerebral cortices

(c) Classified by fibre diameter

Diameter	Name	Example
Large myelinated (3–20 μm) neurones	A fibres	Somatic motor neurones; sensory (touch, pressure, cold and sharp pain)
Small myelinated (1–3 μm)	B fibres	Autonomic preganglionic neurones
Small unmyelinated (less than 1 μm)	C fibres	Autonomic postganglionic neurones; sensory neurones (heat and dull pain)

2. Neuroglia

Name	Location
Microglia	Widespread within the CNS – equivalent to macrophages in other tissues
Macroglia	
Astrocytes	Widespread within the CNS, particularly in association with blood vessels and ependyma
Oligodendrocytes	White matter within the CNS

The axon usually arises from a conical extension of the cell body, the **axon hillock**. The first section is bare and is known as the **initial segment** of the axon. Branches along the axon are known as **collaterals**, and they leave at right angles. The terminal branches of the axon are known as **telodendria**.

Axons contain long, slender mitochondria, which are particularly abundant in the terminals. The cytoplasm within the axon is known as **axoplasm**. Thick and thin microfilaments run parallel to the long axis of the axon, although they interlace with each other. There are few microtubules present compared with dendrites. There is no endoplasmic reticulum present. Axons, in contrast to dendrites, may be surrounded by a myelin sheath.

Materials are moved from the nerve-cell body to the axon endings (**anterograde transport**) by two types of axonal transport, fast and slow. **Fast axonal transport** involves the microtubules, whereas slow

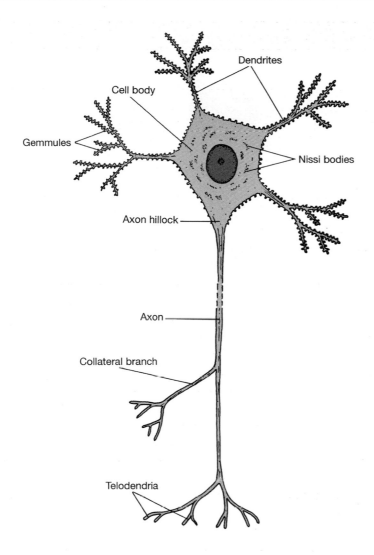

Figure 3.32 Structure of a multipolar neurone.

axonal transport operates by axoplasmic flow. Fast axonal transport (20–400 mm per day) moves membrane-bound organelles such as mitochondria and small vesicles. **Retrograde transport**, which is slower than anterograde transport, returns materials from the axon terminals for reuse or degradation within the nerve-cell body.

    Slow axonal transport (0.2–0.4 mm per day) moves individual molecules such as the protein components of neurofilaments and microtubules as well as enzymes. Proteins and small molecules picked up by the axon terminal are conveyed towards the cell body in vesicles that fuse with lysosomes when they reach the cell body.

Peripheral nerve fibres

The white colour of cranial and spinal nerves is due to the presence of myelin sheaths surrounding the axons of some of the neurones. An axon (or peripheral process of a sensory neurone), together with its myelin

Figure 3.33 Several unmyelinated peripheral nerve fibres embedded in a single Schwann cell.

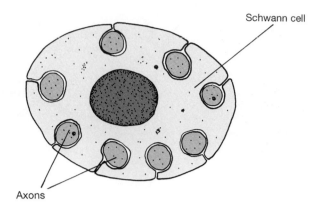

Figure 3.34 Electron micrograph of a Schwann cell (SC) in a peripheral nerve, showing several unmyelinated axons occupying deep recesses in its surface. Most are completely surrounded by Schwann cell cytoplasm, but one (A×2) is only partially enclosed. In such cases, the axon is covered only by the basal lamina (B). Another unmyelinated axon (Ax3) appears to be embedded in this Schwann cell, but is actually surrounded by a completely separate process which is probably an extension of the next Schwann cell in the row. (Reproduced with permission from Fawcett, D. W. (1993) *Bloom and Fawcett: A Textbook of Histology*, Chapman & Hall, London.)

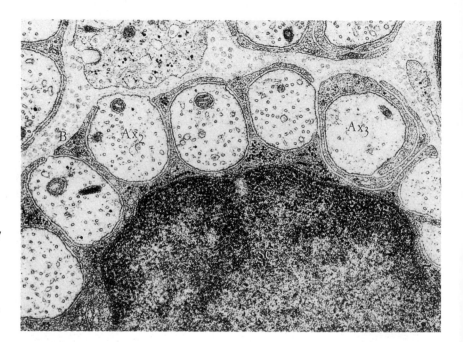

sheath, constitutes a **nerve fibre**. In peripheral nerves, neurites are associated with **Schwann cells** (similar to neuroglia). Several unmyelinated fibres share a single Schwann cell (Figures 3.33, 3.34) whereas myelinated fibres have a much more intimate association with Schwann cells.

The process of **myelination** starts before birth and is completed after birth at various times in different sites.

The Schwann cells develop alongside the neurites and each section of myelin is formed from a single Schwann cell wrapping itself around the neurite as many as 50 times, forming layer upon layer of Schwann cell membrane. The **myelin sheath** so formed appears striated; the major dense lines are due to the apposed inner surfaces of the membrane and these alternate with the dark intraperiod lines formed from the outer surfaces (Figures 3.35, 3.36).

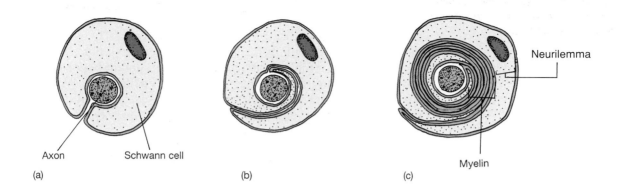

(a)   (b)   (c)

Neurilemma

Axon   Schwann cell   Myelin

Figure 3.35 Formation of a myelin sheath in a peripheral nerve. **(a)** Schwann cell wrapped around an axon. **(b)** Schwann cell overlaps itself around the axon. **(c)** Myelin formed by many layers of Schwann cell membrane.

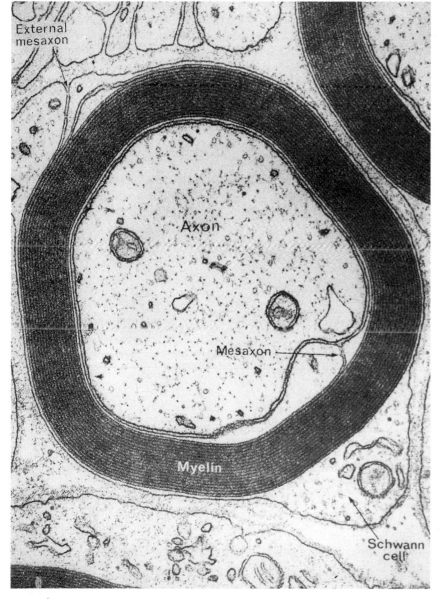

External mesaxon

Axon

Mesaxon

Myelin

Schwann cell

Figure 3.36 Electron micrograph of a large myelinated neurone. (Reproduced with permission from Fawcett, D. W. (1993) *Bloom and Fawcett: A Textbook of Histology*, Chapman & Hall, London.)

The section of myelin formed from a single Schwann cell is known as an **internode** and the junction between adjacent cells where the axon is partially uncovered is called the **node of Ranvier**. The length of the internode is 0.5–2.0 mm, being longer in thicker nerve fibres. The nuclei and most of the cytoplasm of Schwann cells are found peripheral to the myelin sheath and form a layer called the **neurilemma**. Within each internode there are several oblique structures called **Schmidt–Lantermann clefts**. These may act as channels to convey nutrients and metabolites to and from the axon (Figure 3.37).

The white matter in the CNS is due to myelin, but in this site, the myelin sheath is formed from a type of neuroglial cell, the oligodendrocyte (see Neuroglia, below). The Schmidt–Lantermann clefts are absent from myelin in the CNS.

Peripheral nerve fibres are classified according to their conduction velocities and fibre diameters. Erlanger and Gasser, in the 1930s, divided fibres into groups A, B or C. Group A are the largest-diameter myelinated fibres (up to 20 μm), with velocities between 15 and 120 m/s; group B are small-diameter myelinated fibres, with velocities between 3 and 15 m/s; group C are small-diameter unmyelinated fibres (less than 1.0 μm), with velocities of 0.5–2 m/s. Group A fibres may be further subdivided into Aα, Aβ, Aγ and Aδ, again according to conduction speed and fibre diameter (Aα being the largest-diameter fibres).

Nerves

A nerve (such as the vagus) consists of bundles of nerve fibres. Since both afferent and efferent fibres are present it is described as a 'mixed' nerve. All spinal nerves are mixed, but some cranial nerves, such as the vestibulocochlear nerves, are entirely sensory and others, such as the oculomotor, are entirely motor.

Figure 3.37 Longitudinal section through a myelinated axon as it would appear in **(a)** an electron micrograph; **(b)** a light micrograph.

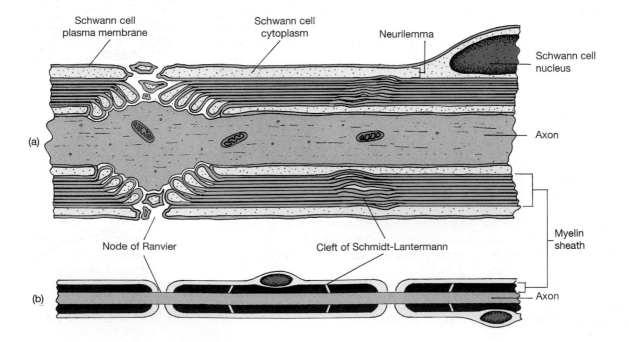

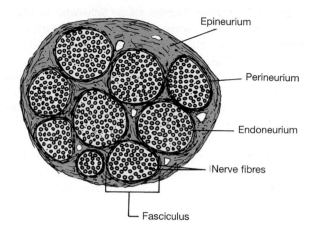

Epineurium

Perineurium

Endoneurium

Nerve fibres

Fasciculus

Figure 3.38 Arrangement of nerve fibres and connective tissue within a peripheral nerve.

The fibres within a nerve are grouped in bundles or **fasciculi**, containing a variable number of fibres (from a few to several hundreds) (Figure 3.38).

The arrangement of connective tissue is analogous to that in skeletal muscle. **Epineurium**, a dense, irregular connective tissue sheath, surrounds the whole nerve; **perineurium**, consisting of concentric rings of collagenous connective tissue, surrounds each fasciculus, and **endoneurium**, which is a loose, delicate connective tissue, surrounds each nerve fibre. In addition to providing support for the neural elements, the connective tissue framework is also the distribution route for blood and lymphatic vessels within the nerve.

Neuroglia

Collectively, neuroglia (literally, 'nerve glue') offer mechanical support and insulation to neurones within the CNS; they act as phagocytes and can form scar tissue. They play a regulatory role in neurone activity by affecting the ionic environment and also by taking up neurotransmitters released from synapses. They may play a role in providing nutrients to the neurones.

The principal types of neuroglia can be subdivided into **macroglia** and **microglia** (Table 3.4). The latter are found between neurones or outside capillaries in the CNS and they are now thought to be the same as connective tissue macrophages (that is, they start as monocytes in the blood). The macroglia comprise astrocytes and oligodendrocytes.

Astrocytes are cells with small bodies and cytoplasmic processes, like dendrites, which have leaf-like structures on them (Figure 3.39).

They are found in contact with blood vessels, the ependyma (lining the ventricles of the brain) and in the grey and white matter generally. They divide if brain tissue is damaged and phagocytose cell debris.

Oligodendrocytes are so named because they have a small number of processes (Figure 3.40).

They produce the myelin sheaths within the CNS and are therefore found in the white matter. A single oligodendrocyte can enclose several adjacent axons with separate myelin sheaths.

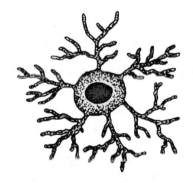

Figure 3.39 Astrocyte.

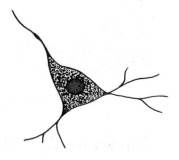

Figure 3.40 Oligodendrocyte.

Degeneration and regeneration of neurones

Neurones cannot divide and replace others that are destroyed or degenerate. Spontaneous degeneration of neurones begins during foetal development and continues throughout life, so that in old age the total number still in existence may only represent about 80% of those that were present originally.

If a neurone is damaged, its recovery is dependent upon an intact cell body. If this is destroyed, recovery cannot occur.

The essential requirement for the regeneration of a nerve pathway, assuming that the blood supply is adequate, is that the supporting framework remains more or less intact, i.e. Schwann cells and an endoneurial tube must be present. Regenerating axons grow into the tubes and are thereby guided to appropriate destinations. It should be noted that neither Schwann cells nor endoneurial tubes are present in the brain or spinal cord, so that regeneration in these locations is not possible.

The course and amount of time required for regeneration depends upon the degree of damage to the fibres and the surrounding tissues.

DEGENERATION OF NEURONES

A slightly damaged axon, due for example to compression of the nerve, will not conduct impulses and will lead to the condition known as **neuropraxia**. Recovery may occur within minutes but may take considerably longer.

An axon which is severed, but which remains enclosed within an intact supporting framework of connective will give rise to **axonotmesis**. In this case, the axon distal to the break will degenerate and the proximal axon will grow out along the original pathway. Recovery, although complete, will occur quite slowly.

If the whole or part of a nerve is severed so that not only the axons but also the endoneurial tubes are damaged, then **neurotmesis** is said to occur. In this case regeneration will be much more difficult and surgical intervention will be required to approximate the cut ends of the fibres as closely as possible.

The breakdown of tissues, **Wallerian degeneration**, starts to take place within 24 hours. The axon distal to the damaged area swells up and then fragments (Figure 3.41).

Later, but within about 4 days, myelin also breaks up into droplets. This breakdown of myelin is normally complete within 10 days and the debris is removed by phagocytosis. Retrograde degeneration of the axon proximal to the damaged area also occurs to an extent that is dependent upon the degree of damage. In some cases the cell body itself may start to degenerate and may subsequently die, or it may recover completely. Degeneration may also occur in cells to which it is linked synaptically.

REGENERATION OF NEURONES

Regeneration begins even before degeneration is complete. Schwann cells in the distal stump divide and, provided that the gap is small enough, grow proximally and bridge the damaged area. The proximal end of the axon puts out a number of processes, which grow down the endoneurial tube and cross the gap, which is already bridged by

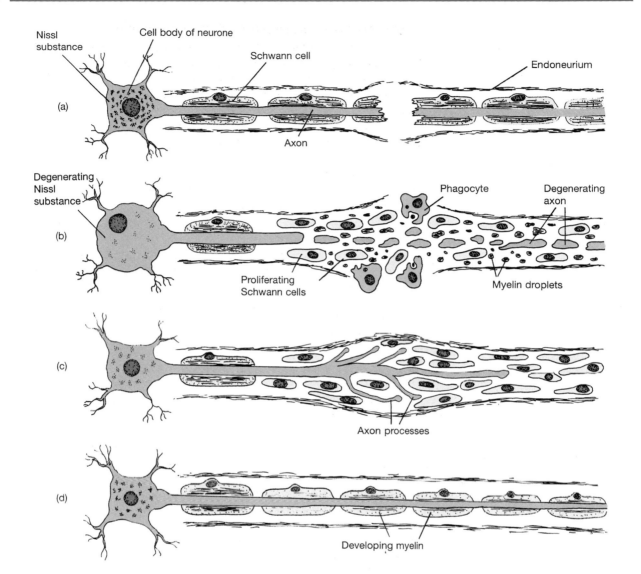

Figure 3.41 Degeneration and regeneration of a nerve fibre. **(a)** The axon has been severed. **(b)** Wallerian degeneration. The distal axon swells and fragments; myelin also breaks up and the fragments removed by invading phagocytes. **(c)** Distal Schwann cells divide and bridge the damaged area; proximal branches of the axon grow into the endoneurial tube **(d)** One branch only grows out and replaces the damaged fibre.

Schwann cells, before entering the distal part of the tube. Peripheral processes degenerate and only one finally grows out and becomes a new fibre. In axonotmesis fibres enter their own tubes and always end up in the 'right' place. In neurotmesis, however, axons may follow the 'wrong' route and so recovery will be variable. If sensory fibres enter motor tubes, or vice versa, then they will not function. If a sensory or a motor fibre links up with the wrong sensor or effector then its function can change to some extent. This phenomenon is known as **plasticity**. When regenerating, axons increase in diameter, but may not reach their original size; they do, however, become myelinated and nodes of Ranvier develop.

The initial bridging of the damaged area by Schwann cells occurs at a rate of about 1 mm/day. Fibres cross the gap at a similar rate but, once inside the distal endoneurial tube, growth of 3–4 mm/day may take place.

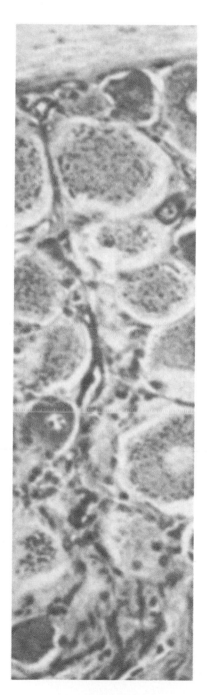

Cellular mechanisms of neural control

4

The nervous system is a rapid control system which operates by sending impulses (action potentials) from one part of the body to another at high speed. Although the nervous system exerts a continuous regulatory action, it can also bring about a rapid increase or decrease in the activity of the tissues it innervates (muscle and some secretory cells). This contrasts with the type of control effected by hormones, where again their action maintains basal levels of activity, but changes in tissue activity are generally slower in onset and longer in duration than those effected by neural regulation. Sites of hormone action are also much more widespread than those of neural action.

This chapter analyses the cellular events that bring about an action potential, its transmission or inhibition at junctions between neurones (synapses) and the mechanisms of stimulation or inhibition of the tissues innervated (effectors). The ways in which drugs interact with these physiological processes are also explored. The organization of the nervous system is outlined first, in order to place the cellular mechanisms into a broader context.

Organization of the nervous system

Structurally, the nervous system can be separated into two primary divisions, the **central nervous system** (**CNS**), which includes the brain and the spinal cord, and the **peripheral nervous system**, which consists of the nerves connecting the CNS with the tissues (Figure 4.1).

There are 12 pairs of cranial nerves and 31 pairs of spinal nerves. Within these nerves some neurones transmit impulses towards the CNS while others carry impulses away from it; such nerves are described as 'mixed'. **Sensory neurones** are also known as **afferent** neurones because they convey impulses towards the CNS from sensory receptors in the tissues. **Motor** (or **efferent**) **neurones** carry impulses from the CNS to muscles and some glands. Motor neurones can be subdivided, both structurally and functionally, into two parts, the **somatic nervous system** and the **autonomic nervous system** (ANS) (Figure 4.2).

The somatic nervous system connects the CNS with skeletal muscle by a single neurone pathway (Figure 4.3).

All voluntary muscular actions such as speaking, movement and the maintenance of posture, involve such pathways. Spinal reflexes, such as the withdrawal of a limb from the source of a painful stimulus, also use somatic motor pathways.

The autonomic nervous system connects the CNS with smooth muscle, cardiac muscle and glands. It controls involuntary activities such as the beating of the heart, the state of contraction of blood vessel walls, movements and secretions of the gut and the voiding of urine. In contrast to somatic motor pathways, autonomic pathways from the CNS to the effector organs generally comprise two successive neurones, with a junction (**synapse**) between them. A number of synapses are collected together in structures called **ganglia** (Figure 4.3).

The ANS is further subdivided into **sympathetic** and **parasympa-**

See also **Neurones** (page 100), in Ch. 3, Tissues.

thetic divisions. They operate continuously but with varying degrees of intensity in the maintenance of involuntary activities.

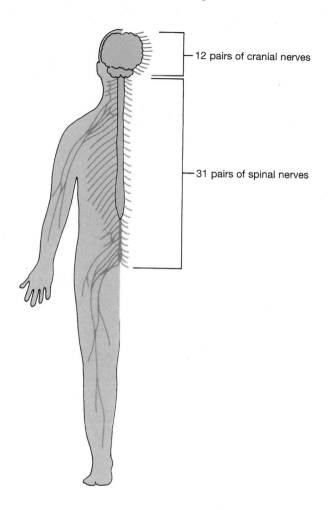

12 pairs of cranial nerves

31 pairs of spinal nerves

Figure 4.1   The central and peripheral nervous systems.

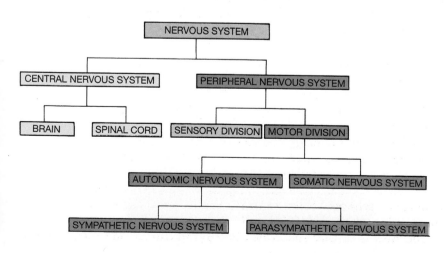

Figure 4.2   Organization of the nervous system.

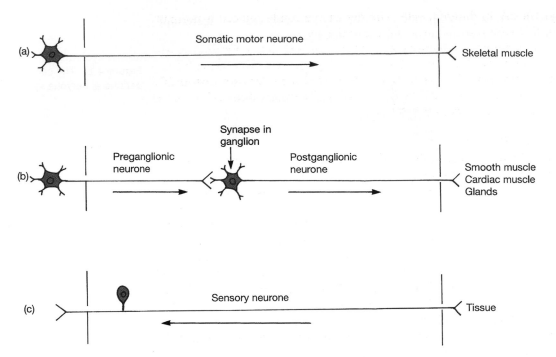

Figure 4.3 Nerve pathways.
(a) Somatic motor.   **(b)** Autonomic
motor.   **(c)** Sensory.

Cellular basis of the nerve impulse

Membrane potentials

If a microelectrode is inserted into a cell, connected to a voltmeter and to a second electrode placed outside the cell, then a voltage difference can be measured across the membrane (Figure 4.4).

This voltage, or potential difference, is very small, varying between 5

Figure 4.4 Measurement of the potential difference across the membrane of an axon.

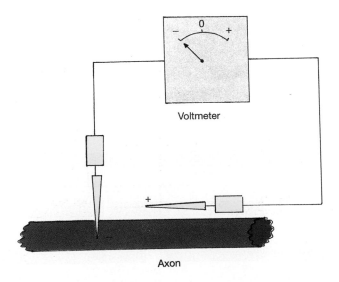

and 100 mV in different cells. The net charge inside the cell is normally negative with respect to the outside of the cell.

The membrane potential at a particular site on a neurone varies according to whether the cell is in a resting state (in which case it has a **resting potential**) or in an active, or excited, state (**action potential**). In the latter, the charge is reversed so that the inside of the cell becomes positive with respect to the outside.

THE RESTING POTENTIAL

Intracellular and extracellular fluids are very different in composition (see Table 2.1). Intracellular fluid has a relatively high concentration of K^+ and a relatively low concentration of Na^+, whereas extracellular fluid is rich in Na^+ and low in K^+; there are approximately 14 times more Na^+ ions outside the cell than inside and 35 times more K^+ inside than out. The unequal distribution of these ions depends upon the presence of an active transport system (the **sodium–potassium pump**) within the cell membrane which uses ATPase as a carrier to transport K^+ into the cell and Na^+ out of the cell (**Na^+–K^+–ATPase**). The exchange of ions is unequal so that, generally, three Na^+ are exchanged for two K^+. Such a pump is said to be **electrogenic** since it results in the separation of charge across the cell membrane, in this case a net negative charge inside the cell.

The concentration differences (gradients) between the inside and the outside of the cell act as a force promoting the diffusion of ions across the membrane. In the case of K^+, the concentration force acts outwards across the membrane, whereas that for Na^+ acts inwards (Figure 4.5).

The extent to which ions diffuse across the membrane is limited by the membrane permeability as well as the concentration gradient. The membrane is about 100 times more permeable to K^+ than to Na^+.

Potassium ions diffuse out of the cell down their concentration gradient, but movement is opposed by the build up of a positive charge on the outside which acts as a repellent force.

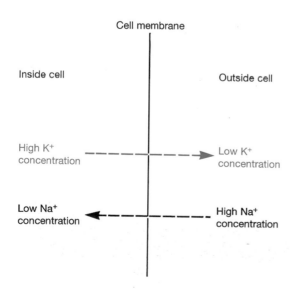

Figure 4.5 Concentration differences for Na^+ and K^+ across the nerve cell membrane.

If K$^+$ was the only cation present, an equilibrium would be established when the concentration force driving K$^+$ out of the cell was equalled by the electrical force repelling such movement. At this point there would be no net movement of K$^+$ and the membrane potential would be −94 mV (i.e. the inside of the cell is negatively charged with respect to the outside). This is known as the **equilibrium** (or **Nernst**) **potential** for K$^+$ (Figure 4.6). For Na$^+$ alone entering the cell the equivalent potential would be +61 mV.

Figure 4.6 Concentration and electrical forces for K$^+$ across the nerve cell membrane.

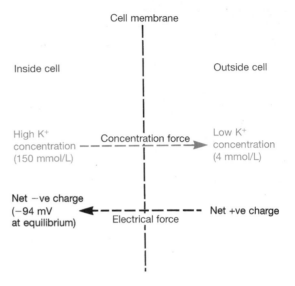

In cells, the movement of K$^+$ is also influenced by the activity of the Na$^+$–K$^+$ pump. This means that there are two forces promoting inward movement of K$^+$ (the Na$^+$–K$^+$ pump and the electrical gradient) which are balanced by a single force for outward movement (the concentration gradient) (Figure 4.7).

Figure 4.7 The forces influencing the distribution of K$^+$ across the nerve cell membrane.

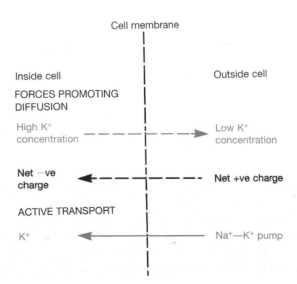

The movement of Na⁺ is similarly governed by the concentration gradient, the electrical gradient and the Na⁺–K⁺ pump. In this case, however, the concentration gradient and the electrical gradient (collectively known as the electrochemical gradient) both promote the diffusion of Na⁺ into the cell and the Na⁺–K⁺ pump actively extrudes Na⁺ from the cell (Figure 4.8).

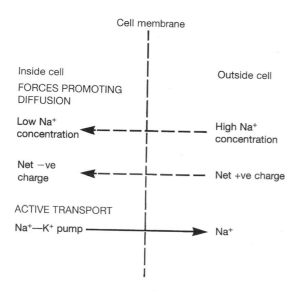

Figure 4.8 The forces influencing the distribution of Na⁺ across the nerve cell membrane.

The resting potential, which is typically about $-70\,\text{mV}$, represents an equilibrium point where there is no net movement of K⁺ or Na⁺. The number of Na⁺ ions diffusing down the electrochemical gradient into the cell is balanced by the number being pumped out, and the number of K⁺ ions diffusing out is balanced by the number being pumped in.

THE ACTION POTENTIAL

When a neurone is stimulated, the cell membrane becomes more permeable to Na⁺. For most neurones the stimulus is chemical, a neurotransmitter released from the previous neurone(s) in the nerve pathway. Sensory receptors, however, may be adapted to respond to other stimuli such as temperature, pressure, pain, or light.

The action potential, or nerve impulse, is the change in membrane potential from its resting value of around $-70\,\text{mV}$ to its peak of about $+30\,\text{mV}$ and back again, i.e. a total voltage change of about $100\,\text{mV}$ (Figure 4.9).

When the neurone is stimulated and becomes more permeable to Na⁺, the ions diffuse into the cell down their electrochemical gradient and thereby reduce the resting potential towards zero. This is known as **depolarization**. The equilibrium potential for Na⁺ alone is $+61\,\text{mV}$ so that the ions continue to diffuse in, changing the membrane potential to positive, thereby reversing the potential. The reversed potential does not, however, reach $61\,\text{mV}$ because Na⁺ permeability is not high enough. The

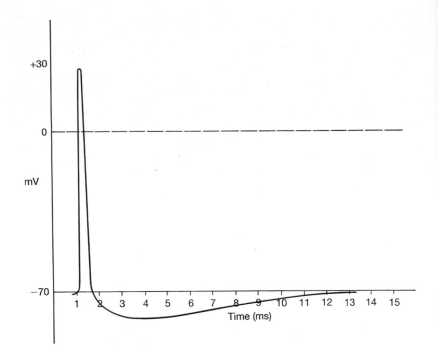

Figure 4.9 The action potential (AP) and afterpotential.

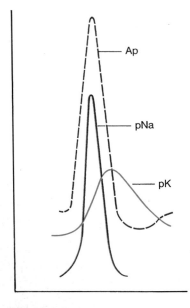

Figure 4.10 The changes in membrane permeability for Na⁺ (pNa), and K⁺ (pK) during the action potential (AP).

increased permeability only lasts for a fraction of a millisecond before being suddenly reduced again (Figure 4.10). At this point the cell membrane permeability to K⁺ increases and the downward phase of the action potential is caused by a loss of K⁺ from the cell by diffusion down its concentration gradient, the electrical gradient and enhanced by the increased permeability. This phase is called **repolarization**.

The membrane potential actually becomes more negative than the resting value (**hyperpolarization**) because the permeability to K⁺ remains higher than normal.

The original ionic distribution is finally restored by the **Na⁺–K⁺ pump**, which is stimulated to greater activity when the intracellular concentration of Na⁺ rises. This is the energy-requiring part of the action potential.

The action potential typically lasts for about 0.4 ms and the after-hyperpolarization for 10–15 ms.

Ion channels can be blocked by **local anaesthetics**; they therefore reduce conduction and induce local analgesia when applied to sensory fibres, and motor paralysis results from their action upon motor neurones.

Mechanism of membrane permeability changes

Sodium and K⁺ diffuse continuously through the cell membrane by means of protein **'leak' channels**; these channels are about 100 times more permeable to K⁺ than to Na⁺. However, in addition, there are also **'voltage-gated' channels** for Na⁺ and K⁺. These are protein channels with 'gates' that are able to open and close during the action potential, thereby altering the permeability of the membrane to the two ions.

There are two types of gate: **'activation gates'** and **'inactivation gates'**. Na⁺ channels have activation gates on the outer surface of the membrane and inactivation gates on the inner surface, whereas K⁺ channels have only activation gates, located on the inner membrane surface.

A fall in the potential difference between the inside of the cell and the surrounding fluid (i.e. as it approaches $-50\,mV$) leads to a sudden rearrangement of the Na⁺ activation gate protein molecules so that the gates open, increasing the permeability of the membrane to Na⁺ as much as 5000 times. As a result Na⁺ ions flood into the cell, further reducing the potential difference. This reduction brings about the opening of more channels which increases the rate of change; this is an example of a **'positive feedback'** mechanism (Figure 4.11).

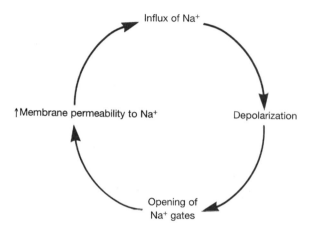

Figure 4.11   Positive feedback between membrane permeability to Na⁺ and depolarization during the generation of the action potential.

The Na⁺ channels are closed again by the inactivation gates, which operate more slowly than the activation gates. As the Na⁺ channels are closing, K⁺ channels are opened by the slow-acting K⁺ activation gates, so that K⁺ permeability increases, enabling K⁺ to flow into the cell and reverse the newly-established potential difference.

THRESHOLD POTENTIAL

There is a particular membrane potential ($5-15\,mV$ less negative than the resting potential) which, if reached, will result in the generation of an action potential: this is known as the **threshold potential**. At this point the positive feedback cycle between depolarization and increased membrane permeability to Na⁺ is initiated. A stimulus that is just strong enough to cause the membrane to depolarize to its threshold potential and hence initiate an action potential is known as a **threshold stimulus**. Weaker stimuli than this (**subthreshold stimuli**) elicit graded potentials (see *Graded potentials*, below), whereas stimuli greater than threshold (**suprathreshold stimuli**) result in action potentials, which are of constant size (Figure 4.12).

Thus, an action potential is either initiated (by a threshold or suprathreshold stimulus), or it fails to be initiated (by a subthreshold stimulus). This is known as the **'all-or-nothing'** principle.

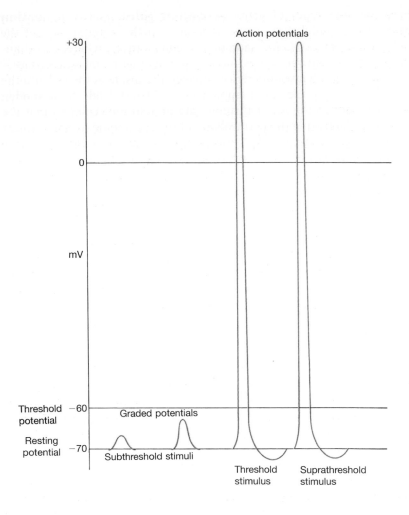

Figure 4.12 The effect of increasing stimulus strength on membrane potential. Subthreshold stimuli elicit graded potentials, which are not propagated along the neurone. Threshold and suprathreshold stimuli elicit action potentials of equal size, which are propagated along the neurone.

Different neurones have different thresholds but, in addition, thresholds also vary in different parts of the surface membrane of each individual neurone; the threshold is lowest at the initial segment of the axon.

REFRACTORY PERIODS

It is not possible to restimulate a neurone during the time when an action potential is still in progress, because the Na$^+$ inactivation gates remain closed until the resting membrane potential is restored. This is called the **absolute refractory period** and lasts for about 0.4 ms in type A fibres. During the hyperpolarization phase the neurone can be restimulated if a suprathreshold stimulation is applied so that the threshold potential is reached. This is the **relative refractory period** and lasts for 10–15 ms.

Clearly, the absolute refractory sets a limit upon the number of impulses that can be generated per unit of time. If each one lasts for 0.4 ms, then 2500 action potentials could theoretically be generated in 1 minute. The maximum frequency of impulses carried by any nerve fibre is actually far less than this.

GRADED POTENTIALS

In spite of the all-or-nothing principle, it is still possible for small changes in membrane potential to occur. They may be either depolarizations or hyperpolarizations, which vary in size according to the degree of stimulation; they are therefore described as 'graded potentials'. Such potentials occur at sensory receptors or at synapses; they are not action potentials because they vary in size and do not reach the threshold potential of the neurone.

When sensory receptors are activated, the stimulus (mechanical deformation, chemical, electrical, or heat) causes an increase in cell membrane permeability with the result that there is a net influx of Na^+, which diffuses down the electrochemical gradient into the cell and cause depolarization of the membrane. This is known as a **generator potential** and its size varies according to the strength of the stimulus. Graded potentials of this type can be transmitted by local current flow although they die out within a few millimetres.

If the generator potential reaches threshold, then action potentials are generated instead. The lowest threshold of a neurone is found at the beginning of the axon (the initial segment, or the first node of a myelinated fibre), so that is where the action potential first appears. Further increases in stimulation (suprathreshold stimuli) cause an increase in the frequency of the action potentials that are generated, but not an increase in their size (the all-or-nothing principle). In addition, with increasing levels of stimulation, adjacent neurones are also stimulated. Thus the **intensity of a stimulus** is conveyed to the central nervous system by the frequency of impulses travelling along a neurone, and by the number of neurones firing.

For details of graded potentials generated at synapses, see *Excitatory synapses* and *Inhibitory synapses*, below.

EFFECT OF ELECTROLYTE CHANGES ON EXCITABILITY

Because of the major role played by **K^+** in the generation of the resting potential, alterations to its concentration in body fluids also alter the membrane potential. Should K^+ concentration in ECF rise, its concentration gradient between intracellular and extracellular fluid is reduced, so that less K^+ diffuses out of the cell and the membrane potential rises (becomes less negative), nearer to the threshold value. The cell therefore becomes more excitable. Conversely, a fall in K^+ concentration in ECF results in a loss of K^+ from cells, hyperpolarization and less excitability.

Changes in **Na^+** in ECF are rare because, should there be a change in Na^+ a rapid movement of water by osmosis follows. If Na^+ rises, for example as a result of dehydration, renal adjustments rapidly correct the situation, principally by water retention and consequent dilution of ECF.

If the concentration of **Ca^{2+}** in ECF falls, cells become more excitable.

The explanation lies in the way that Ca^{2+} interacts with the outer surface of the cell membrane. Ca^{2+} ions are attracted to the negative surface charge on the cell membrane, thereby neutralizing it. In hypercalcaemia, fewer Ca^{2+} ions cover the outer aspect of the cell membrane, so that some areas remain negatively charged. The voltage across the membrane is therefore reduced, resulting in hyperexcitability. Measurement of the membrane potential by means of electrodes in the fluids does not show any change, because the voltage change is in the membrane itself.

Changes in electrolyte composition affect the excitability of muscle cells as well as neurones.

Propagation of action potentials

UNMYELINATED AXONS

In unmyelinated neurones the action potential is transmitted to adjacent sections of the cell membrane by local current flow. The active region of the neurone has the opposite charge inside and outside the membrane compared with adjacent areas (Figure 4.13).

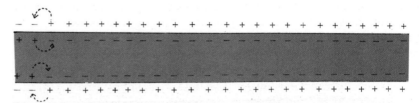

Figure 4.13 Local current flow in an unmyelinated fibre. Action potentials are generated in sequence along the fibre, from left to right of the diagram.

Ions are attracted to areas of opposite charge, so the positive ions on the inside of the cell therefore diffuse to the adjacent section, which has a resting negative charge, and depolarize the membrane to the threshold value. The positive feedback cycle between depolarization and Na^+ permeability is initiated and an action potential of the same value is thereby generated. The conduction of action potentials, in contrast to the conduction of graded potentials, is not decremental and can therefore cover large distances.

Action potentials can travel in either direction along a cell membrane; for example, they pass out along the sarcolemma towards both ends of a muscle fibre from a central motor end plate. However, since neurones normally come into contact with one another at synapses, when axon terminals link up with the dendrites and cell bodies of other neurones, nerve impulses normally only flow along dendrites towards the cell body and from there to the axon terminal.

The velocity of conduction of nerve impulses along axons depends upon their diameter: the larger the diameter, the greater their velocity. This is because an increase in the diameter of an axon is accompanied by a reduction of the resistance to the flow of ions through the membrane. The rate of conduction in the smallest-diameter non-myelinated axons is about 0.5 m/s.

MYELINATED AXONS

The rate of conduction of impulses in myelinated fibres is very much faster than in non-myelinated fibres (about 120 m/s in the most heavily myelinated). The myelin sheath acts as an insulator, offering an approximately 5000-fold increase in resistance to the flow of ions. The nodes of Ranvier that interrupt the myelin sheath, on the other hand, offer little resistance to the diffusion of ions. Action potentials can only be generated at sites where exchange of Na^+ and K^+ can take place between the cytoplasm and the surrounding fluid, and as a result can only be generated at the nodes of Ranvier. Since only a fraction of the total surface membrane of the axon is actually involved in the generation of action potentials, the fibre conducts impulses very rapidly. The impulse appears to jump from node to node; this is known as **saltatory conduction**. In fact, of course, each node generates a new impulse in rapid succession.

The presence of a net positive charge inside the axon at an active node repels adjacent positive ions in the axoplasm which, in turn, repel those adjacent to them. Effectively a column of positive ions drifts toward the next node, so that the ions that depolarize it are local ones. Ions do not jump from node to node! The mechanism can be likened to a tube filled with ball bearings. The net positive charge at one node is like an extra ball being pushed into one end of the tube, causing one at the other end to fall out; in this case, depolarizing the next node (Figure 4.14).

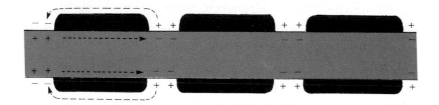

Figure 4.14 Saltatory conduction in a myelinated fibre. Action potentials are generated at successive nodes of Ranvier, from left to right of the diagram.

Demyelination

There are several conditions in which the myelin sheath degenerates, the most common of which is **multiple sclerosis**. The conduction of action potentials is impaired, which can affect a variety of functions, depending upon the location of the neurones involved. Clinical manifestations may include weak or poorly controlled muscles, urinary incontinence and visual disturbances. In **Guillain–Barré syndrome**, impaired function of the motor neurones to the respiratory muscles can be severe enough to cause respiratory failure.

Neurochemical transmission

Within the central nervous system, information is conducted along some 100 billion neurones by the propagation of action potentials. Neurones form part of neural networks or nerve pathways, which connect different parts of the CNS together and are also linked to peripheral structures that have sensory and motor functions.

The junctions between neurones in a nerve pathway (synapses) and between neurones and muscles or glands (neuroeffector junctions) always include a gap. Chemicals (neurotransmitters) released from the axon terminals diffuse across the gap, and become attached to 'receptors' on the postsynaptic or effector cell membrane.

This arrangement allows a number of neurones, secreting different neurotransmitters, to form junctions with the same postsynaptic neurone or effector cell. The latter can therefore be stimulated or inhibited depending upon the amount and type of neurotransmitter released and the types of receptor present on the postsynaptic cell surface.

So, although the nerve impulse itself does not vary in size, control of activity occurs by way of complex junctions between neurones in pathways involving many different chemicals and receptors.

Neurotransmitters

A large number of transmitter substances have been identified, at least tentatively, in the human nervous system. Chemically they are amino acids, amines or peptides. All of the boutons arising from the axon endings of a single neurone release the same neurotransmitter(s).

Neurones can be classified according to the neurotransmitters that they synthesize and release. The best known neurotransmitters are those operating in the peripheral nervous system. Neurones that use acetylcholine as a neurotransmitter are described as **cholinergic**, and those that use noradrenaline as **adrenergic** (although strictly the term '**noradrenergic**' should be used).

Functionally, neurotransmitters can be divided into two groups; those which are **fast-acting** (effects apparent in milliseconds) and a second group which are relatively **slow-acting** (effects apparent in seconds, minutes or even hours).

FAST-ACTING NEUROTRANSMITTERS

Fast-acting transmitters include amines, and amino acids (Table 4.1). They are synthesized in the boutons and stored in secretory vesicles. The enzymes required for this process are synthesized on ribosomes in the nerve-cell bodies, packaged by the Golgi apparatus into vesicles and transported from the cell body along the axon to its terminals. The neurotransmitter precursors are taken up into the vesicles containing the enzyme in the axon terminals, and synthesis occurs. The vesicles are recycled. After they have combined with the presynaptic membrane and released their contents, they reinvaginate, separate from the membrane and refill with neurotransmitter by active transport. These processes are driven by enzymes.

Acetylcholine is formed from acetyl-CoA under the influence of choline acetyltransferase. Having entered the synaptic cleft and stimulated the postsynaptic membrane it is then split into acetate and choline by the enzyme cholinesterase. Choline is actively transported back across the presynaptic membrane and used to resynthesize acetylcholine. Whether or not a particular neurotransmitter is excitatory or inhibitory depends upon the type of receptor proteins it combines with. Acetylcholine is, in most situations, excitatory. However, some postganglionic parasympathetic nerve endings exert an inhibitory influence; the vagus nerve, for example, reduces heart rate and the force of atrial contraction.

Table 4.1 The major neurotransmitters (from Kruk, Z. L. and Pycock, C. J. (1991) *Neurotransmitters and Drugs,* Chapman & Hall, London)

Chemical type	Mode of action	Name
Fast-acting neurotransmitters		
Amino acids	Excitatory	Glutamic acid
		Aspartic acid
	Inhibitory	Glycine
		Gamma-amino butyric acid
Amines	Excitatory	Acetylcholine (nicotinic)
		Serotonin
Slow-acting neurotransmitters		
Amines		Acetylcholine
		Dopamine
		Noradrenaline
		Histamine
		Serotonin
Peptides		Enkephalins
		Substance P
		Bradykinin

Gamma-amino butyric acid (GABA) is found in the brain and spinal cord and is always inhibitory in its action.

SLOW-ACTING NEUROTRANSMITTERS

Peptides (neuropeptides) are slow-acting neurotransmitters (Table 4.1). In contrast to other neurotransmitters, neuropeptides are synthesized in the ribosomes of the cell bodies of neurones and migrate to the axon tips by cytoplasmic streaming, at a rate of a few centimetres a day. Their release at a synapse is in response to the arrival of an action potential and is therefore identical to that of a fast-acting transmitter; slow-acting transmitters are not, however, reused.

The amine group of slow-acting neurotransmitters includes dopamine, noradrenaline, histamine and serotonin (5-hydroxytryptamine). Acetylcholine acting on non-nicotinic receptors also has a relatively slow transduction mechanism in contrast to its action on nicotinic receptors.

Noradrenaline is synthesized in the axon endings from the amine tyrosine.

Tyrosine $\longrightarrow$ L–DOPA $\longrightarrow$ Dopamine $\longrightarrow$ Noradrenaline.

It is secreted by many nerve endings both within the CNS and the periphery and is generally excitatory. Like acetylcholine, however, it exerts an inhibitory influence in some areas of the body.

The effects of these substances at synapses are extremely long-lasting, perhaps for years, and include changes in the metabolic activities of the postsynaptic cell and an alteration in the functions of some of its genes.

For actions of acetylcholine and noradrenaline in the tissues see **Neurotransmitters in the autonomic nervous system** (page 277), in Ch. 9, Autonomic and Somatic Motor Activity.

See also **Neurotransmitters in the brain** (page 178), in Ch. 5, The Brain, and **Neurotransmitters in the spinal cord** (page 199), in Ch. 6, The Spinal Cord.

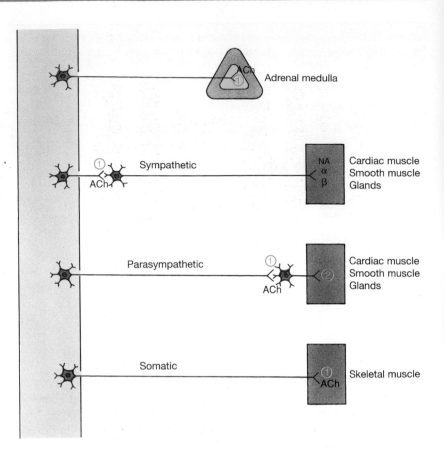

Figure 4.15 Neurotransmitters and receptors in motor pathways in the peripheral nervous system. Preganglionic autonomic neurones and somatic motor neurones secrete acetylcholine (ACh) which combines with nicotinic receptors (1) on the postsynaptic cell membrane. Postganglionic parasympathetic neurones secrete acetylcholine which combines with muscarinic receptors (2) on the effector cell membrane. Postganglionic sympathetic neurones release noradrenaline (NA) which combines with α-adrenoceptors and β-adrenoceptors on the effector cell membrane.

NEUROTRANSMITTERS IN THE PERIPHERAL NERVOUS SYSTEM

Acetylcholine is produced by preganglionic neurones in both sympathetic and parasympathetic pathways in the ANS. It is also produced by postganglionic parasympathetic neurones and by somatic motor neurones (Figure 4.15).

Noradrenaline is released by most postganglionic sympathetic neurones.

Receptors

The membranes of the postsynaptic cells contain receptor proteins, which have a binding component which projects into the synaptic cleft. The binding component is connected to either an ion channel (Figure 4.16(a)), or to a regulatory or G protein (Figure 4.16(b)), which is itself connected to an effector protein in the cell membrane.

Following release of neurotransmitter from the bouton, the chemical diffuses across the synaptic cleft and binds to the receptors on the postsynaptic or effector cell membrane. Depending upon the nature of the receptors present, one of three principal actions follows:

- opening of Na^+ channels;
- opening of K^+ and Cl^- channels;
- activation of an enzyme, which then catalyses specific chemical reactions within the cell.

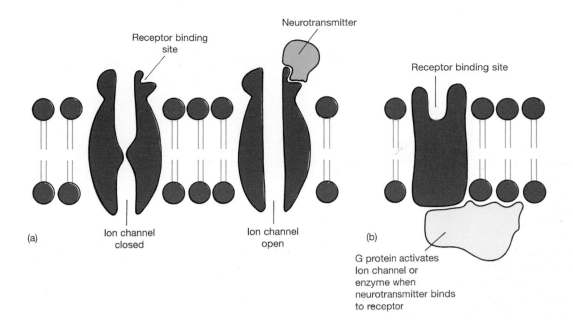

Figure 4.16 The two types of receptor to which neurotransmitters bind on postsynaptic or effector cell membranes. **(a)** Receptor linked to ion channel. **(b)** Receptor linked to G protein.

Fast-acting transmitters act by opening ion channels, whereas slow-acting transmitters stimulate effector proteins, which then either open ion channels or activate enzymes. Some of these enzymes promote the formation of cyclic-AMP, which facilitates other metabolic reactions; other enzymes activate genes within the nucleus of the postsynaptic cell; whereas some enzymes activate protein kinases, which decrease the number of neurochemical receptors. Thus neurotransmission can induce long-term changes in postsynaptic cells. Such mechanisms are thought to be involved in the storage of long-term memory.

Receptors may be classified according to their affinity for certain chemicals. Thus, acetylcholine receptors are classified into two types, named according to whether they bind with the drugs nicotine (from tobacco) or muscarine (from toadstools). Figure 4.15 shows the distribution of such receptors in the autonomic and somatic nervous systems. **Nicotinic receptors** are found in the autonomic ganglia and adrenal medullae as well as in skeletal muscle. **Muscarinic receptors** are found on the effector cells controlled by the parasympathetic nervous system.

There are also two main types of receptor that respond to adrenaline and noradrenaline found in the tissues: **alpha-adrenoceptors** (α-**adrenoceptors**) and **beta-adrenoceptors** (β-**adrenoceptors**).

See also **Neural mechanisms for storing long-term memory** (page 182), in Ch. 5, The Brain.

See also **Adrenergic receptors** (page 281), in Ch. 9, Autonomic and Somatic Motor Activity.

Synapses

Synapses are junctions between neurones and there are a variety of ways in which the neurones may be linked together. The commonest synapse is between an axon and a dendrite; the axon branch ending is a spherical structure known as a **bouton**. There may be one or many boutons at each axon ending and a single motor neurone may be in contact with 100 000 boutons. At least 80% of all boutons terminate on dendrites, the rest on cell bodies.

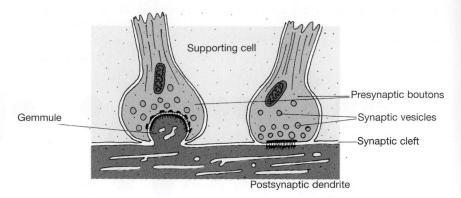

Figure 4.17 Presynaptic boutons associated with the postsynaptic membrane in an axodendritic synapse.

See also **Endocytosis and exocytosis** (page 51), in Ch. 2, Cells and the Internal Environment.

A synapse between an axon and a dendrite is known as an **axodendritic synapse**, while one between an axon and a soma is an **axosomatic synapse**. Other, less common, relationships exist, for example between two dendrites (dendrodendritic), two axons (axoaxonic), among others.

An axodendritic synapse consists of the boutons of the presynaptic cell(s), a 20 or 30 nm wide **synaptic cleft** and the postsynaptic membrane (Figure 4.17).

Boutons vary somewhat in size and shape, but usually contain numerous small synaptic vesicles containing neurotransmitter, mitochondria and networks of microtubules and filaments. Some filaments extend across the cleft. The postsynaptic side of the synapse has a filamentous mesh (subsynaptic web), which appears to support the synaptic structure. In addition, numerous glial cells wrap around the synaptic junction.

Presynaptic neurones exert their effects upon postsynaptic neurones by the release of **neurotransmitters**. These chemicals are contained within the **synaptic vesicles** in the presynaptic boutons; they are released into the synaptic cleft and combine with receptor sites on the postsynaptic cell membrane.

Action potentials arriving at a presynaptic bouton depolarize the membrane and increase its permeability to Ca^{2+} by opening voltage-gated Ca^{2+} channels. Ca^{2+} therefore enters the bouton down an electrochemical gradient and bind with proteins on the inside of the cell membrane. Synaptic vesicles nearby then fuse with the cell membrane and release their neurotransmitter into the synaptic cleft by **exocytosis**.

The neurotransmitter diffuses across the cleft and binds to receptors in the postsynaptic cell membrane.

EXCITATORY SYNAPSES

At these junctions, some neurotransmitter–receptor combinations open Na^+ channels in the postsynaptic cell membrane, thereby increasing its permeability to Na^+. Consequently there is an influx of Na^+ down its electrochemical gradient and the postsynaptic membrane becomes depolarized. A single presynaptic action potential will only cause slight depolarization of the postsynaptic cell. The difference in voltage between the resting and depolarized levels is called the **excitatory postsynaptic** potential (**EPSP**). This is a type of graded potential that does not necessarily lead to the development of an action potential in the postsynaptic neurone (see *Summation*, below).

In some cases, e.g. in response to acetylcholine, the depolarization is caused by a decrease in permeability of the postsynaptic neurone to K^+ and/or Cl^-.

A third mechanism of excitation across a synapse is mediated by enzymes. It may, for example, result in an increase in the number of excitatory receptors in the postsynaptic cell membrane.

INHIBITORY SYNAPSES

In contrast to excitatory synapses, the combination of neurotransmitter and receptor in inhibitory synapses has the effect of reducing transmission between neurones. This is achieved by the postsynaptic cell membrane becoming hyperpolarized and therefore refractory to stimulation by excitatory synapses; it is called postsynaptic inhibition.

In this case, instead of opening Na^+ channels in the postsynaptic membrane, there is an increase in the permeability to smaller ions (K^+ or Cl^-), so that they diffuse down their concentration gradients, thereby increasing the negativity of the membrane potential.

Some inhibitory neurotransmitters initiate metabolic changes in the postsynaptic cell, including the synthesis of more inhibitory receptors.

The difference between the hyperpolarized potential and the resting potential is known as the **inhibitory postsynaptic potential** (**IPSP**).

PRESYNAPTIC INHIBITION

Synaptic inhibition can also be brought about by neurones whose terminals lie upon the fibre immediately before the synapse (Figure 4.18).

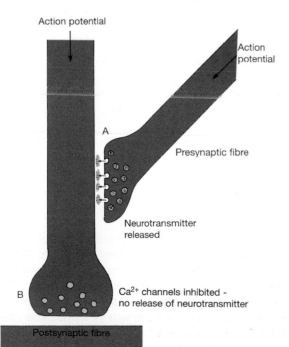

Action potential

Action potential

A

Presynaptic fibre

Neurotransmitter released

B

Ca^{2+} channels inhibited - no release of neurotransmitter

Postsynaptic fibre

Figure 4.18 Presynaptic inhibition. The neurotransmitter released by bouton A prevents the opening of Ca^{2+} channels in bouton B and inhibits its activity.

In this case, release of the presynaptic neurotransmitter prevents the opening of Ca^{2+} channels in the synaptic bouton, which will therefore become refractory to stimulation. Such inhibition occurs in many sensory pathways and prevents impulses from spreading laterally. The effect is slow to develop, but may persist for minutes, or even hours.

SUMMATION

A single EPSP or IPSP has little influence over the activity of a post-synaptic neurone but, given that each postsynaptic neurone has many, in some cases thousands, of synaptic connections, each of which is capable of firing repeatedly, the effects of individual PSPs can be added together by the process of summation. There are two types of summation: temporal and spatial.

Temporal summation of PSPs is achieved by the repeated firing of a synapse and is dependent upon the relatively long duration of PSPs (up to 15 ms). While the postsynaptic membrane is still depolarized, additional impulses may travel down the presynaptic fibre and cause further release of neurotransmitter. In the case of an excitatory synapse, this increases the size of the EPSP. The result of several impulses arriving at the same bouton in rapid succession is that the potential of the postsynaptic membrane will reach its threshold value and an action potential will be generated. Summation at an inhibitory synapse results in a larger IPSP.

Spatial summation of PSPs occurs when more than one presynaptic neurone fires simultaneously, thereby increasing the total amount of neurotransmitter released.

Individual PSPs travel to the initial segment of the axon, where summation occurs. This is because the initial segment contains more voltage-gated Na^+ channels than either the soma or the dendrites of the neurone, and therefore the threshold potential of the initial segment is lower than that of nearby sections and it fires.

A postsynaptic neurone that is in contact with several excitatory and inhibitory fibres may be influenced in a number of ways depending on the number and type of active synapses. If the excitatory effect dominates and there is net depolarization, then the postsynaptic neurone is said to be **facilitated**, as it is nearer to the threshold potential. Once the threshold potential of the initial segment is reached, then an action potential will be generated. If the inhibitory effect dominates, then the neurone becomes hyperpolarized and an action potential will not be generated. If the postsynaptic fibre is already firing, inhibitory synapses can switch it off.

SYNAPTIC DELAY

Even in non-myelinated fibres nerve impulses travel very quickly, at a rate of at least 0.5 m/s. At the synapse, however, neurotransmitter release, its passage to the postsynaptic membrane and its combination with receptors, the subsequent increase in membrane permeability and the generation of an action potential takes a relatively long time. The sum total of these processes gives rise to a synaptic delay of about 0.5 ms. Clearly, the more synapses there are in a neural pathway the slower impulses will travel.

SYNAPTIC FATIGUE

Repeated stimulation of a postsynaptic neurone results in a progressive reduction in the number of action potentials that are generated. This is due to fatigue of synaptic transmission. Such fatigue is caused mainly by exhaustion of neurotransmitter substance in the presynaptic endings, even though it is estimated that enough is stored for about 10 000 transmissions. Other contributing factors include inactivation of postsynaptic receptors and build up of Ca^{2+} in the postsynaptic neurone.

Synaptic fatigue is a common occurrence and helps to explain how nerve impulses die out in reverberating neuronal circuits.

See also **Circuits in the interneurone pool** (page 198), in Ch. 6, The Spinal Cord.

Neuroeffector junctions

In addition to the synaptic junctions between pre- and postsynaptic fibres, similar junctions are found between neurones and other structures. Such neuroeffector junctions include those between neurones and smooth, cardiac and skeletal muscle cells (**myoneural junctions**), and those between neurones and glands, which are found typically associated with the ANS. Of these, the myoneural junctions of skeletal muscle are the most complex and their structures are considered separately in Chapter 9.

Smooth muscle cells are innervated by unmyelinated neurones of the ANS. Axons pass between muscle cells; generally, those associated with slow-acting muscles branch extensively, while those which innervate fast-acting muscles, such as those of the iris, exhibit much less branching. The axon terminals lie parallel to, and usually some distance away (15–50 nm or more) from the muscle cell surfaces. Neurotransmitter is released from synaptic vesicles within multiple 'varicosities' along the axon branches. Schwann cells cover the axons between, but not over, the varicosities (Figure 4.19).

The heart is innervated by both divisions of the ANS. Unmyelinated fibres end close to the SA and AV nodes and also to the cardiac muscle cells of the atria. Sympathetic fibres also innervate the ventricles (the

See also **Conduction system and innervation of the heart wall** (page 377), in Ch. 12, Circulation of Blood and Lymph.

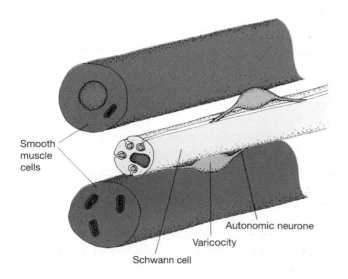

Figure 4.19 Autonomic neuroeffector junction. Unmyelinated fibres, supported by Schwann cells, run parallel to smooth muscle fibres. Neurotransmitter is released from the uncovered varicosities along the axon branches.

Smooth muscle cells

Autonomic neurone

Varicocity

Schwann cell

PNS does not innervate the ventricles). Although such nerve endings contain synaptic vesicles, in neither case is there a well-developed myoneural junction.

The junctions between autonomic neurones and glandular cells are also simple, with varying distances between the elements. In the islets of Langerhans the axon terminals are in close contact with hormone-secreting cells and the presence of an electrical rather than a chemical neuroeffector junction has been postulated.

The mechanism of transmission between neurones and the effector cells is essentially the same as that operating at synapses. The arrival of an action potential causes the opening of Ca^{2+} channels and the subsequent entry of Ca^{2+} into the axon terminal. The Ca^{2+} ions cause a number of vesicles of neurotransmitter to move to the cell membrane and the neurotransmitter is released into the cleft between the axon terminal and the effector cell. The neurotransmitter then binds to receptors on the effector cell.

There is an important difference between the innervation of skeletal muscle (by somatic motor neurones), and that of smooth muscle, cardiac muscle and glands (by autonomic motor neurones). The somatic motor neurones that innervate skeletal muscle are all cholinergic and stimulate the cells to contract. Relaxation of skeletal muscle is brought about by central inhibition of the somatic motor neurones. In contrast, most of the tissues innervated by the autonomic nervous system have dual innervation by sympathetic (adrenergic) and parasympathetic (cholinergic) motor neurones, in which case one chemical stimulates the effector and the other inhibits it. Inhibitory activity in the autonomic nervous system, therefore, occurs at the tissue site, as well as at the level of the central nervous system.

See also **Neurotransmitters in the autonomic nervous system** (page 277) and **Neuromuscular junction** (page 293), in Ch. 9, Autonomic and Somatic Motor Activity.

Inactivation of neurotransmitters

Neurotransmitters are inactivated by two principal mechanisms: enzyme inactivation in the synaptic cleft or reuptake of the neurotransmitter into the bouton.

In the case of **acetylcholine**, the enzyme **cholinesterase** in the postsynaptic cell membrane splits the molecule into choline and acetate. The choline is actively transported into the nerve terminal and reutilized by the cell.

The **catecholamines**, adrenaline, noradrenaline and dopamine are broken down in the synapse by the enzyme **catechol-O-methyl transferase** (**COMT**) or removed by reuptake into the axon terminal where they may be recycled or broken down by another enzyme, **monoamine oxidase** (**MAO**), in the mitochondria (Figure 4.20).

Actions of drugs on neurochemical transmission

Drugs are known that stimulate or inhibit neurotransmission at each stage of the process: synthesis, storage, release, receptor binding and inactivation of neurotransmitter. One example of a drug that acts at each of these stages is given here.

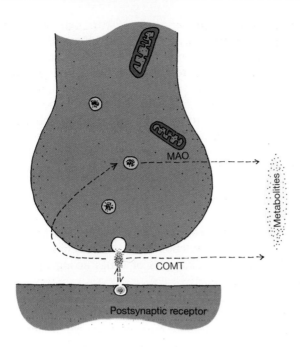

Figure 4.20 Inactivation of noradrenaline. Noradrenaline is metabolized by the enzymes monoamine oxidase (MAO) in the mitochondria and catechol-O-methyl transferase (COMT) in the synapse. Alternatively, the neurotransmitter may be taken back into the bouton.

SYNTHESIS

Laevodopa (**L-dopa**) is a drug which stimulates neurotransmitter synthesis. It is taken up by neurones that synthesize dopamine, resulting in an increase in the amount of stored neurotransmitter. L-dopa is used in the treatment of dopamine deficiency, which occurs in Parkinson's disease. **Disulfiram**, on the other hand, inhibits noradrenaline synthesis and is used in the treatment of alcoholism.

STORAGE

Amphetamines displace noradrenaline from its storage vesicles and therefore effectively increase the release of noradrenaline, resulting in an increase in the level of activity of the sympathetic nervous system.

RELEASE

Histamine release is prevented by **disodium cromoglycate (DSCG)**, which is used to prevent the inflammatory effects of histamine in conditions such as asthma and hayfever.

RECEPTOR BINDING

Drugs that act on receptors may be classified according to their mode of action.

Agonists or stimulants

Molecules of the drugs combine with receptors and mimic the effects of the neurotransmitter. **Carbachol** combines with muscarinic receptors and mimics the effects of acetylcholine. It is used in the treatment of glaucoma to reduce the size of the pupil, thereby relieving any obstruction to the flow of aqueous humour.

See also **Enzyme inhibition** (page 25), in Ch. 1, Molecules, Ions and Units.

Antagonists or blockers

These combine with receptors and block the effects of neurotransmitter. **Propranolol** blocks beta-adrenoceptors in cardiac muscle and is used to reduce cardiac activity in the treatment of angina pectoris.

Competitive antagonists

These compete with neurotransmitter molecules for the receptor sites, they therefore only block neurotransmission when they are present in a higher concentration than the neurotransmitter. **Tubocurarine** is a competitive blocker for acetylcholine at nicotinic receptors in skeletal muscle; it is used as a muscle relaxant.

Physiological antagonists

These are substances that act upon different receptors and have different actions on effectors, e.g. acetylcholine and noradrenaline.

Tables 9.2 and 9.4 give examples of drugs acting upon the different receptors.

INACTIVATION OF NEUROTRANSMITTERS

For more examples of drugs acting on neurotransmission see **Neurotransmitters in the Brain** (page 178), in Ch. 5, The Brain.

GABA is inactivated by reuptake into the presynaptic terminal followed by catabolism by the mitochondrial enzyme GABA-T. The drug **vigabatrin** inhibits the action of GABA-T and therefore increases the amount of GABA in the CNS. This has a tranquillizing action and vigabatrin is used in the treatment of epilepsy.

The brain

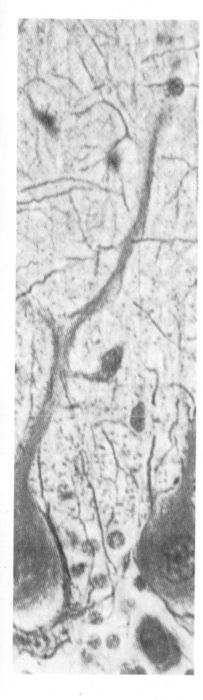

Approaches to brain research

Traditionally, neuroanatomists and neurophysiologists have studied the brain with a view to locating specific functions in particular 'centres' or anatomical regions. The identification of such functional regions derives from animal experiments in which parts of the brain were either stimulated electrically, isolated, or removed and the resulting physiological or behavioural changes were recorded. Data from human subjects was relatively sparse, involving observations of the effects of damage from either physical trauma (such as a cerebrovascular or road accident), tumours or congenital malformations.

The relative crudity of animal experiments and the paucity of data on humans indicates the need for caution in order to avoid a somewhat simplistic view of brain function. The remarkable recovery made by some individuals following a cerebrovascular accident or other trauma, in which relatively large sections of brain tissue have been destroyed, suggests that other parts of the brain are able to take over the functions of the damaged areas. This refutes the concept of discrete localization of brain functions. The ability of neurones to change their functions is known as **plasticity**.

New imaging techniques introduced in the 1970s have enabled non-invasive and much more sophisticated studies of the brain to be undertaken both for research and as clinical investigations. The techniques or 'scans' include computed tomography (CT), magnetic resonance imaging (MRI) and positron emission tomography (PET) (Figure 5.1).

CT scans use X-rays which rotate around the body and produce a series of images that are combined by computer to produce a 'slice' through the body.

MRI uses magnetic fields and radio waves to energize hydrogen atoms in the body. Three-dimensional colour images are produced of tissues (soft and hard), comparative metabolic activity and blood flow.

PET scans are taken following the injection of a radioactive molecule such as glucose into the bloodstream. More glucose is taken up by the more active areas of the brain and, since it is radioactive, the glucose gives off positrons. The computer analyses the gamma-rays (formed when positrons hit electrons) and produces a colour map reflecting different levels of metabolic activity. By such means, particular areas of the brain can be 'seen' to be associated with specific functions e.g. the occipital lobes are more active when the eyes are open; the hippocampus is active in memory tasks.

More recently, techniques derived from information technology have been adopted, which create a mathematical 'model' of brain activity. Brain 'systems' have been devised that involve sensory inputs from somatic and special sensory pathways, neural connections between different parts of the brain, and the initiation and coordination of motor responses. Such systems have been used, for example, to produce a 'robot' that can perform mechanical tasks such as picking up objects and respond to sensory inputs such as sight, touch or even smell.

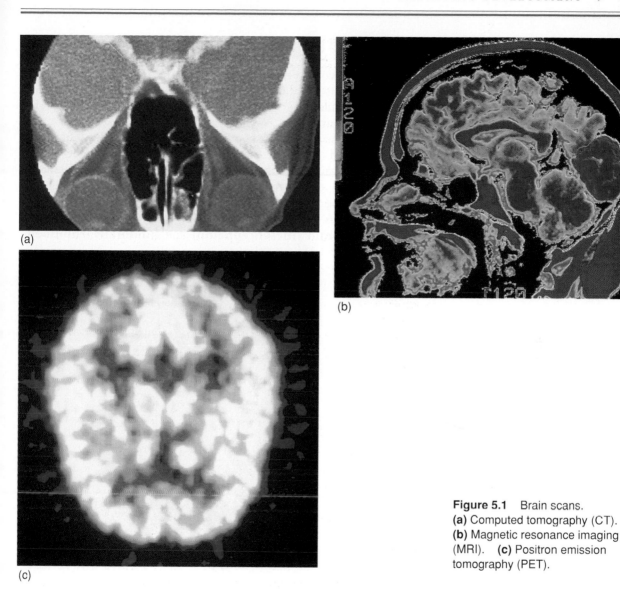

Figure 5.1 Brain scans.
(a) Computed tomography (CT).
(b) Magnetic resonance imaging
(MRI). **(c)** Positron emission
tomography (PET).

The approach to brain research, therefore, has shifted from the search for discrete 'centres' to multisite systems. When analysing the particular functions of the parts of the brain, therefore, students should view them not as isolated structures but as areas that have neural links with each other as well with other parts of the body.

Embryonic development

In order to understand the anatomical relationships between the various parts of the adult brain it is useful to study its early development first, because the rather complex structures comprising the adult brain are present in a simpler form in the embryo. When each brain structure is introduced in the text, the reader is recommended to locate the structure on the diagrams of the embryonic brain before referring to diagrams of the adult brain.

The central nervous system develops from the neural plate, a strip of tissue lying in the top surface (ectoderm) of the embryo. This strip thickens and its sides rise up to form neural folds on either side of a neural groove (Figure 5.2).

By the end of the third week of embryonic life the folds have begun to fuse together and form the **neural tube**. This simple tube is the precursor of the brain and spinal cord. At the head end the folds enlarge before fusing and two transverse constrictions develop, dividing the newly-formed tube into three sections (**cerebral vesicles**). These are the main divisions of the primitive brain; the **forebrain (prosencephalon)**, **midbrain (mesencephalon)** and **hindbrain (rhombencephalon)** (Figure 5.3).

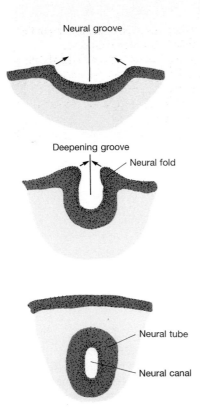

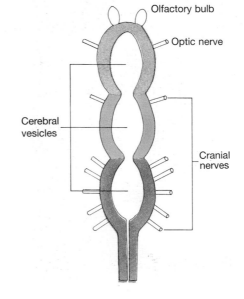

Figure 5.2 Development of the neural tube in the first few weeks of embryonic life.

Figure 5.3 The brain at around 1 month of embryonic life showing the three main areas and associated cranial nerves. Forebrain [pink], midbrain [green], hindbrain [purple].

The cavity of the neural tube persists within each division of the brain, becoming the fluid-filled **ventricles**, which are continuous with the much narrower spinal canal that runs the length of the spinal cord.

The cerebral vesicles enlarge and change shape, the forebrain incompletely dividing into two large hemispheres; as a result, there are four, rather than three ventricles, since each hemisphere contains a lateral ventricle.

The forebrain develops two vesicles: the **telencephalon** (endbrain) and the **diencephalon** (interbrain). The midbrain develops four protrusions on its posterior surface (the corpora quadrigemina) and two vertical pillars on its anterior surface (the cerebral peduncles). The hindbrain gives rise to three areas: the cerebellum, the pons varolii and the medulla oblongata. By about the fourth month of development, most of the major brain structures have been established (Figure 5.4). The forebrain then develops at a faster rate than the other areas and curls over anteriorly towards the hindbrain. Figure 5.5 summarizes the major parts of each region of the brain.

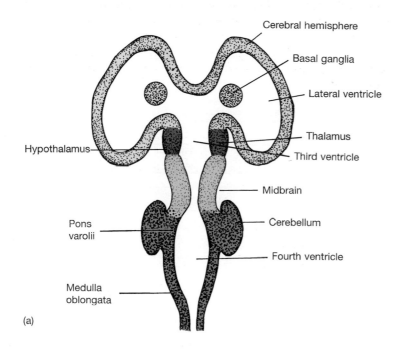

(a)

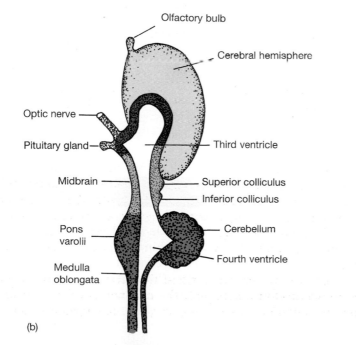

(b)

Figure 5.4 The major areas of the brain in a 4-month embryo.
(a) Horizontal section. **(b)** Midline section. Forebrain: telencephalon [light pink], diencephalon [dark pink]; midbrain [green]; hindbrain [purple].

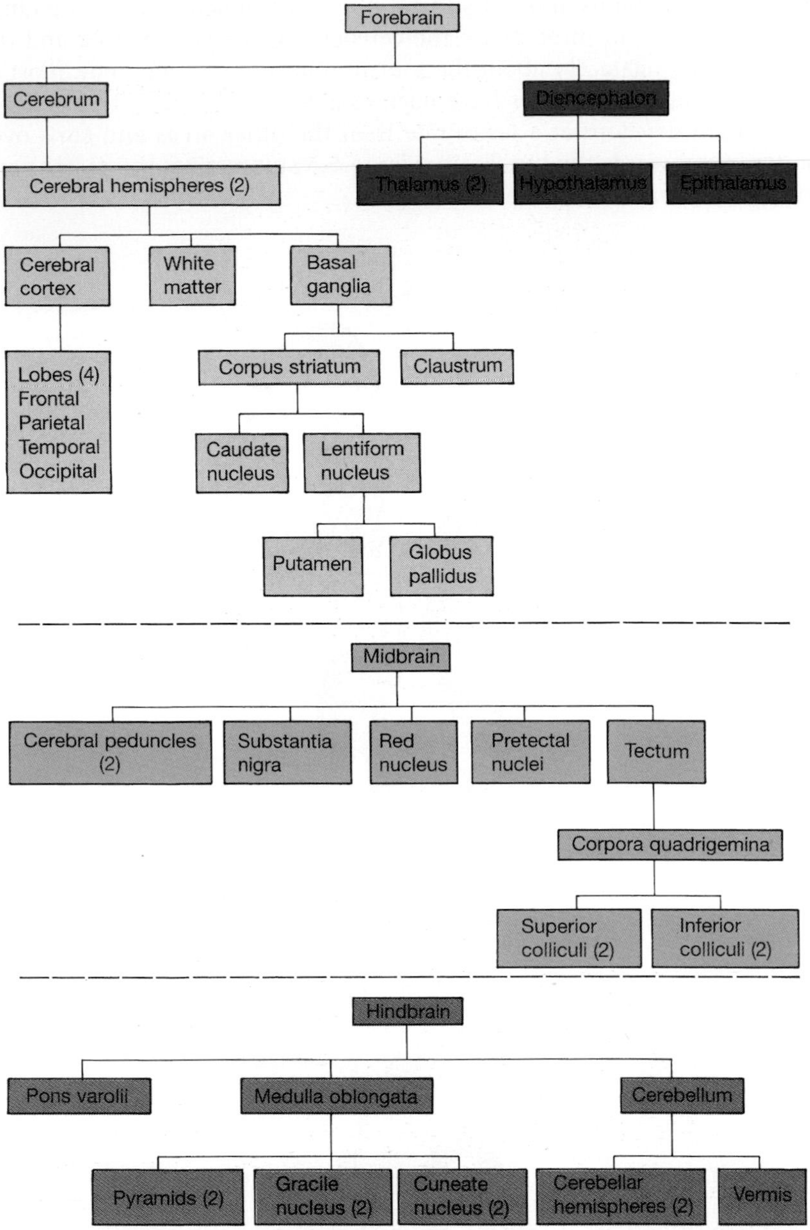

Figure 5.5 The major structures of the forebrain [pink], midbrain [green] and hindbrain [purple]. The locations of the cranial nerve nuclei are shown in Figure 5.17 and listed in Table 5.1.

Major regions of the brain

The brain typically weighs about 1.4 kg in an adult man, usually slightly less in women. It is held in position within the skull by tough, protective membranes, the meninges. The brain is ovoid in shape, being slightly wider posteriorly than it is anteriorly. The largest part of the brain is the cerebrum, which comprises the right and left cerebral hemispheres (Figure 5.6).

Anterior

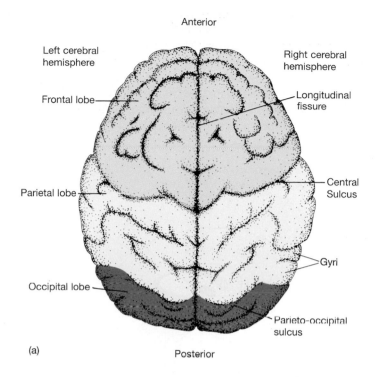

Left cerebral hemisphere

Right cerebral hemisphere

Frontal lobe

Longitudinal fissure

Central Sulcus

Parietal lobe

Gyri

Occipital lobe

Parieto-occipital sulcus

(a)

Posterior

Anterior

Longitudinal fissure

Olfactory bulb

Frontal lobe of cerebrum

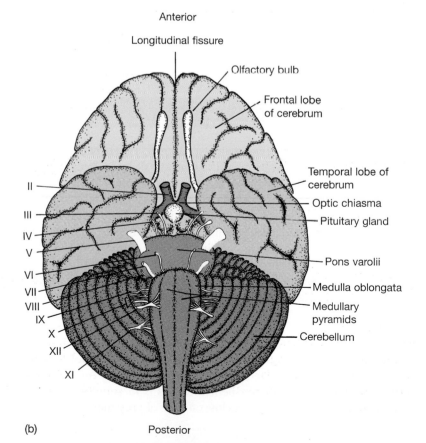

II

Temporal lobe of cerebrum

III

Optic chiasma

IV

Pituitary gland

V

VI

Pons varolii

VII

Medulla oblongata

VIII

IX

Medullary pyramids

X

Cerebellum

XII

XI

Figure 5.6 The brain.
(a) Viewed from above.
(b) Viewed from below. The cranial nerves are numbered. Frontal lobe [blue], parietal lobe [yellow], occipital lobe [pink], temporal lobe [orange].

(b)

Posterior

Viewed from below, the base of the brain reveals the hindbrain, comprising the medulla, pons and cerebellum, and the midbrain as well as the lower surface of the cerebrum. The origins of 11 of the 12 cranial nerves are also visible (Figure 5.6(b)).

Although the brain is divided anatomically into three regions, the forebrain, midbrain and hindbrain, the additional term **brain stem** is used to identify the stalk-like section (consisting of the medulla, pons and midbrain) that is connected to the spinal cord (Figure 5.7).

Figure 5.7 Midline section of the brain. Forebrain: telencephalon [light pink], diencephalon [dark pink], midbrain [green], hindbrain [purple], brain stem [blue].

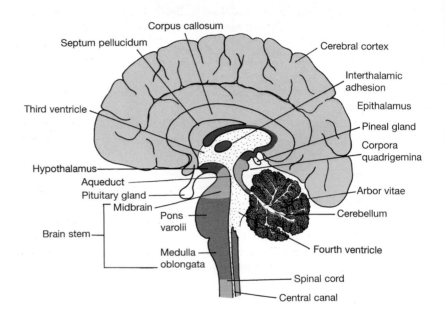

Forebrain

The forebrain comprises two major structures, the **cerebrum** and the **diencephalon**. The diencephalon, which is situated deep within the cerebrum consists principally of the **thalami** (joined by the interthalamic adhesion) and the **hypothalamus** below (Figure 5.7).

In animals, the term **rhinencephalon** is used to describe those parts of the brain concerned with smell (olfaction). In many animals it is a dominant feature of the brain, and in the early human embryo the two **olfactory bulbs** are prominent (Figure 5.3). In the adult human brain, however, the olfactory bulbs are disproportionately small (Figure 5.6(b)), reflecting the relative unimportance of the sense of smell.

Cerebrum

The cerebrum consists of the two **cerebral hemispheres** containing the lateral ventricles, incompletely separated by the **septum pellucidum**.

Each cerebral hemisphere has a surface layer of grey matter, the cerebral cortex, with white matter beneath. This is in contrast to the spinal cord, where the white matter encloses a core of grey matter.

CEREBRAL CORTEX

The cerebral cortex contains the cell bodies of the cerebral neurones; they are arranged in vertical columns 0.5–1.0 mm in diameter, in six layers (with a variable depth of 1.5–4.5 mm). Layers I and II have neuronal links from lower brain areas; II and III have extensive neural links with adjacent areas of the cerebral cortex. Sensory pathways terminate mainly in layer IV, whereas layers V and VI contain the cell bodies of neurones in outgoing pathways. The thickness of each layer varies in different regions of the cortex.

In addition to the numerous neuroglia, there are two principal types of neurone in the cortex: **pyramidal** and **stellate cells** (Figure 5.8).

Each pyramidal cell has a pyramidal cell body with a long apical dendrite orientated towards the brain surface. A number of short dendrites radiate from the base of the cone and from its centre an axon passes down to the underlying white matter. The axon sends collateral branches to adjacent regions. Pyramidal cells are particularly abundant in layers IV and V, from where they send axons to other areas of the cortex (association fibres) as well as down the spinal cord as the cortico-spinal tracts.

Stellate (star-shaped) cells have small round cell bodies with short, highly branched dendrites, and a short axon. Stellate cells are found in all layers of the cortex, except for layer I, with layers II and IV having particularly high densities. In contrast to pyramidal cells, stellate cells operate entirely within the cerebral cortex. The human cortex has a higher density of stellate cells than other species, suggesting a correlation with intelligence.

> See also **Neuroglia** (page 107), in Ch. 3, Tissues.

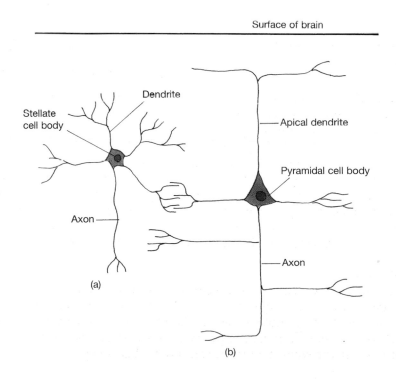

Figure 5.8 Cells in the cerebral cortex. **(a)** Stellate cell. **(b)** Pyramidal cell.

While 99% of cortical cells send axons only to other cortical areas, only 1% send them to subcortical areas.

The surface of the cerebrum is covered with ridges (**gyri**), which are separated by shallow grooves (**sulci**). This folding of the surface of the cerebrum increases its surface area to approximately 2500 cm². The two cerebral hemispheres are incompletely separated by a deep groove, the **longitudinal fissure** (Figure 5.6(a)). In the middle section this fissure extends down to the **corpus callosum**, a wide band of white matter that links the two hemispheres (Figure 5.7). The **transverse fissure** separates each cerebral hemisphere from the cerebellum beneath.

Each cerebral cortex is divided into four primary areas, the **frontal, parietal, occipital** and **temporal lobes** (see Figure 5.10). The boundaries of the lobes are demarcated by the **lateral, parieto-occipital** and **central sulci**.

WHITE MATTER OF THE CEREBRUM

The white matter of the cerebrum contains tracts of fibres which are orientated in three principal directions: they connect lower and upper parts of the brain (**projection fibres**), different parts of the same hemisphere (**association fibres**) and the right and left hemispheres (**commissural fibres**) (Figure 5.9).

The largest structure containing commissural fibres is the **corpus callosum**, which lies below the longitudinal fissure and above the lateral ventricles (Figure 5.7). It is usually larger in women than in men.

TELENCEPHALIZATION AND THE NEOCORTEX

As the telencephalon has evolved it has enlarged and developed disproportionately compared with other areas of the brain, a process known as

Figure 5.9 **(a)** Frontal section of the cerebrum showing the orientation of the projection fibres and the commissural fibres.
(b) Midline section showing the association fibres that connect different parts of the same hemisphere.

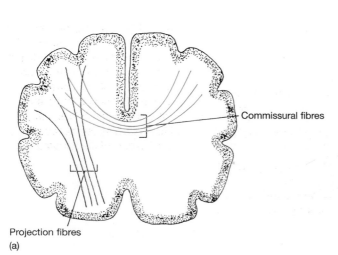

Commissural fibres

Projection fibres

(a)

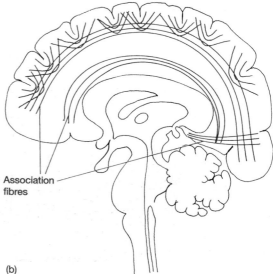

Association fibres

(b)

telencephalization. As a result, humans have a proportionally larger telencephalon than other animals.

During evolution, the sense of smell has become progressively less dominant over the other senses. The cortex of the 'older' brain, which is primarily concerned with smell, is known as the **palaeocortex**. The newer parts of the cortex are identified as the **neocortex**.

The neocortex is associated with 'higher' mental functions such as reasoning, intelligence, memory, many aspects of personality, interpretation of sensations, initiation of voluntary movement and the moderation of reflex movements. Physiologists often use the rather vague term **'higher centres'** when referring to areas of the neocortex.

FRONTAL LOBES

Each frontal lobe lies anterior to the central sulcus and above the lateral sulcus. The frontal lobes have nerve connections with the hypothalamus, thalamus, brain stem and spinal cord. Much of the activity of the frontal lobes is concerned with the control of voluntary movements, including speech.

Primary motor cortex (precentral gyrus)

Immediately in front of the central sulcus is the precentral gyrus, which is the location of the primary motor cortex of the cerebrum (Figure 5.10).

Each motor cortex controls voluntary movements of the opposite side of the body, with the individual parts of the body being controlled by groups of nerve cells along the gyrus (somatotopic organization). These cell groups are arranged with approximately the same relationships as the parts of the body they control, although they are inverted and differ markedly in their proportions. Those parts of the body that are capable of fine, complex movements, such as the face and hands, are represented by a relatively large area of the motor cortex, whereas those with only limited capability for subtle movement, such as the trunk, arms and legs, are controlled by much smaller areas of cortex. A representation of the

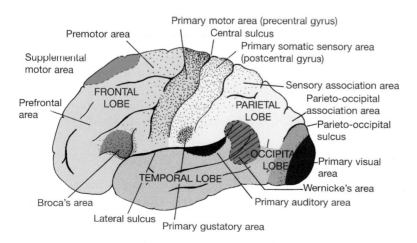

Anterior   Posterior

Figure 5.10 The lateral surface of the left cerebral cortex showing the four lobes and the major functional areas. Special sensory areas not visible: the vestibular cortex lies near the primary auditory area, deep in the lateral sulcus; the primary olfactory cortex lies on the medial aspect of the temporal lobe.

body with its parts in the same proportion as the regulatory areas of the motor cortex is known as a **motor homunculus**. Detailed mapping of the cortex was carried out by the Canadian surgeon Wilder Penfield, who stimulated exposed areas of the cerebral cortex on conscious patients (Figure 5.11).

Although Penfield's concept of spatial representation of the body along the motor cortex is still supported in general terms, research published in the 1990s suggests more complex maps within the head, arm, torso and leg areas. Individual cortical neurones appear to control *groups* rather than *individual* muscles so that, for example, areas controlling hand movements are interspersed with and overlap areas involved in upper arm movements. A mosaic arrangement of cortical areas which control muscles that work together to produce a movement (synergystic muscles) is emerging.

Figure 5.11 Penfield's motor homunculus. (Reproduced with permission from Penfield, W. and Rasmussen, T. (1950) *The Cerebral Cortex of Man*, Macmillan, London.)

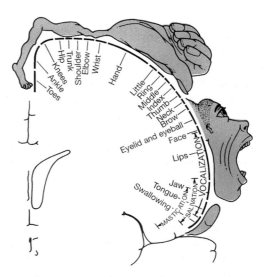

The principal nerve pathways controlling voluntary movements are the **corticospinal tracts**, as many as 80% of which are thought to arise in the motor cortex.

Some tracts start in the cortex and then synapse in other areas of the brain before passing down the spinal cord and innervating skeletal muscle.

Should the primary motor cortex be damaged, there is a loss of voluntary control of discrete movements of the limbs, particularly of the hands and fingers. In addition, since the motor cortex exerts a tonic stimulatory influence upon skeletal muscles, damage leads to a loss of muscle tone (hypotonia).

See also **Lateral and anterior corticospinal (pyramidal) tracts** (page 196), in Ch. 6, The Spinal Cord, and **Neural control of voluntary movement** (page 299), in Ch. 9, Autonomic and Somatic Motor Activity.

Premotor area

Anterior and parallel to the primary motor cortex is the premotor area (Figure 5.10), which controls learned complex movements such as typing or riding a bicycle, by sending impulses into other motor areas. Loss of function in this area, therefore, results in the loss of ability to perform these activities skilfully.

Some 15% of the corticospinal tract neurones, which control voluntary movement, originate in this area.

Supplemental motor area

The supplemental motor area lies above and in front of the premotor area (Figure 5.10). Most of it lies within the tissue lining the longitudinal fissure, with a centimetre or so extending on to the upper surface of the cortex. As its name suggests, the supplemental motor area works with the other motor areas, providing background movements that support the fine control exerted by the premotor and primary motor cortices. Some of the fibres in the corticospinal tracts arise in the supplemental motor area. It is also involved in the planning of complex movements and damage to this area results in an inability to carry them out, leaving simple movements unaffected.

Broca's area

Anterior to the primary motor cortex, just above the lateral sulcus, lies Broca's area (Figure 5.10), which is responsible for the initiation of word formation and grammatical construction in **speech**. In right-handed people it is found in the left inferior frontal gyrus, whereas in left-handed people it is in the corresponding position in the right cerebral hemisphere. Broca's area lies close to that part of the motor cortex which controls the movements of the jaws and the tongue and another which initiates the short inspirations and long, controlled expirations required for speech. Damage to Broca's area leads to **motor aphasia**, in which the ability to form words is lost.

Prefrontal area

Anterior to the motor area of each frontal lobe lies the prefrontal area (Figure 5.10). Isolation of this area by **prefrontal lobotomy** was frequently carried out, between the 1930s and the early 1960s, on patients with extreme anxiety. The operation did not impair intelligence, but social behaviour was often severely affected and there was frequently a complete loss of inhibitions. Clearly the area is associated with personality, but it is not the seat of intelligence, as was once thought, even though damage to the area reduces both problem-solving ability and attention span.

PARIETAL LOBES

The parietal lobes lie behind the central sulcus and above the lateral sulcus on each side. Their functions are predominantly sensory in nature.

Primary somatic sensory area (postcentral gyrus)

The postcentral gyrus on each side is known as the primary somatic sensory (somaesthetic) cortex and is concerned with the perception of somatic sensations such as touch, pressure, temperature and pain. Like the motor cortex, the sensory cortex can be mapped out and represented by a **sensory homunculus** (Figure 5.12), which is very similar in appearance to the motor homunculus. The representation of the body is

> Somatic senses are covered in Ch. 7, Sensory Processing.

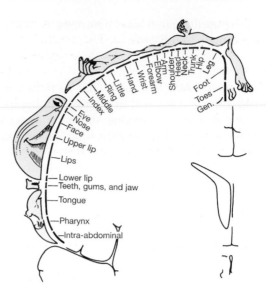

Figure 5.12   Penfield's sensory homunculus. (Reproduced with permission from Penfield, W. and Rasmussen, T. (1950) *The Cerebral Cortex of Man*, Macmillan, London.)

Taste is covered in Ch. 8, The Special Senses.

upside down and the left hemisphere receives impulses from the right side of the body and *vice versa*. Just at the bottom of the somatic sensory area lies the primary gustatory area, which is responsible for the perception of taste.

Loss of function of this area leads to an inability to localize sensations in different parts of the body; crude localization may still be possible, however, due to the activities of the thalamus and other parts of the cortex. The ability to judge the degree of pressure against the body, the weight and form of objects and texture are also lost. Pain and temperature sensations become poorly localized.

Sensory association area

Behind the primary sensory area is a sensory association area (Figure 5.10) where somatic sensations are interpreted, for example by comparing them with a memory of a similar sensation or contrasting them with different sensations. Damage to this area causes problems of interpreting sensations, so that the ability to recognize complex objects by touch is lost. Since information is being relayed from the opposite side of the body, damage to the sensory association area can result in the affected person forgetting that the other side of the body exists at all, so that there is a loss of a sense of form of the body as a whole. Motor function is, as a result, also abandoned on the affected side.

Parieto-occipitotemporal association area (posterior parietal cortex)

Posterior to the somatic sensory association area is the much larger parieto-occipitotemporal association area (Figure 5.10). It receives visual signals from the posterior occipital cortex and somatic sensory information from the postcentral gyrus. This enables the brain to place the body's position relative to its surroundings and the relative positions of the parts of the body. All of this information is required in order to coordinate movement.

Output from the posterior parietal cortex goes to motor areas of the brain: the premotor cortex, cerebellum and basal ganglia.

Damage to the parieto-occipitotemporal association area on one side results in a lack of awareness of the body and its surroundings on the opposite side. The coordination of movements consequently fails to take account of half of the body.

See also **Neural control of voluntary movement** (page 299), in Ch. 9, Autonomic and Somatic Motor Activity.

OCCIPITAL LOBES

Each occipital lobe lies behind the parieto-occipital sulcus and contains the visual areas.

Visual areas

The **primary visual cortex** lies at the back of the occipital lobe (Figure 5.10). The sensory pathways ending here form the optic radiation from the lateral geniculate body on each side. There is spatial separation of parts of the retina in the visual cortex and images are represented upside down. Interpretation of the stimulus is aided by the **visual association area** found adjacent to the primary area.

See also **Visual pathways** (page 243), in Ch. 8, The Special Senses.

Damage to one visual cortex results in an inability to see objects on the opposite side of the visual field. The condition can also be caused by damage to the optic tract or of the optic radiation on one side. The visual cortex may be destroyed by infarction of the posterior cerebral artery, due to thrombosis; although the foveal area may be spared, so that central vision is relatively unimpaired.

TEMPORAL LOBES

Each temporal lobe lies below the lateral sulcus and contains areas concerned with the perception of auditory, vestibular and olfactory sensations as well as the interpretation of language.

Auditory areas

Most of the **primary auditory area** lies on the superior temporal gyrus (Figure 5.10). It receives the auditory radiations from the medial geniculate body, perceives sound and depends on the adjacent association or auditopsychic area for interpretation. The auditory cortex has been mapped with regard to the separation of sounds with differing frequencies (tonotopic maps). Impulses from the vestibular apparatus are conveyed to areas that lie adjacent to those dealing with auditory information.

Auditory and vestibular functions are covered in Ch. 8, The Special Senses.

Total destruction of both auditory cortices reduces hearing sensitivity, but may not lead to total deafness. The many cross-connections between the cortices of the two sides mean that destruction of one cortex alone has little effect upon hearing itself, although the ability to detect the direction of sounds is lost.

Vestibular area

Information from the vestibular apparatus of the ear concerning the position and movements of the head is thought to be perceived in an area of the temporal lobe close to the primary auditory area, deep in the lateral sulcus.

Smell (olfaction) is covered in Ch. 8, The Special Senses.

Olfactory areas

The **primary olfactory cortex** lies in the uncus, on the medial aspect of the temporal lobe. The surrounding area is also involved in the conscious perception of smell.

Wernicke's area

Wernicke's area lies behind the primary auditory cortex in the temporal lobe (Figure 5.10). This is a **language** interpretative area and is therefore particularly important in intellectual functions. The nearby visual and auditory areas feed word information into Wernicke's area. In right-handed people, Wernicke's area in the left cerebral cortex is dominant.

Damage to Wernicke's area can result in **sensory aphasia**, in which understanding of both written and spoken language is impaired. Speech production, on the other hand, is unaffected, although the sequence of words spoken often makes little sense.

CEREBRAL ASYMMETRY

Although the right and left cerebral hemispheres are structurally similar overall, detailed studies have shown some anatomical differences. Generally, in right-handed people the left occipital and parietal lobes are wider than the right, whereas the right frontal lobe is usually wider than the left.

Functionally too, there tend to be differences between the two hemispheres. In most people, the left hemisphere is associated particularly with language, both spoken and written, mathematical skills and reasoning. Damage to the left hemisphere usually causes psychological disturbance and depression. The right hemisphere is generally associated with non-verbal skills such as musical and artistic awareness, the perception of space and patterns and imagination. Damage to the right hemisphere often does not cause the emotional disturbances that are seen in left-sided damage.

BASAL GANGLIA

The basal ganglia, or nuclei, are areas of grey matter embedded within the white matter of each cerebral hemisphere, near to the thalamus (Figure 5.13).

The basal ganglia include the **corpus striatum**, which consists of the **caudate** and **lentiform** (Latin, 'lens-shaped') **nuclei**, the latter being divided into the **putamen** (Latin, 'pod') and the **globus pallidus** or **palaeostriatum** ('old striatum'). The putamen and the caudate nucleus together constitute the **neostriatum** ('new striatum'). The **claustrum** (Latin, 'barrier') is another nearby basal nucleus. These nuclei are surrounded or separated by broad bands of white matter, the **internal capsule**, formed by projection fibres (Figure 5.13(a)). These fibres comprise ascending pathways from the thalamus to the cerebral cortex and descending pathways from the cerebral cortex to the thalamus, brain stem and spinal cord. The internal capsule is a common site for a stroke (see *Cerebrovascular accident (stroke)*, below).

The **subthalamic nucleus** in the diencephalon and the **substantia**

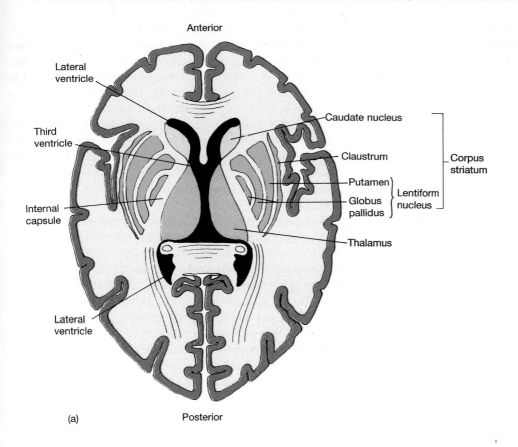

(a)

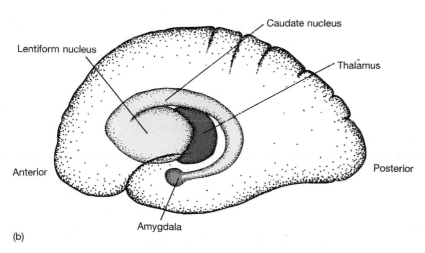

(b)

Figure 5.13 **(a)** Horizontal section through the cerebral hemispheres, showing the positions of the basal ganglia and thalami. **(b)** Three-dimensional representation of the basal ganglia.

nigra in the midbrain (see Figure 5.23) are also functionally part of the basal ganglia.

The amygdaloid nucleus or **amygdala** (Latin, 'almond') is connected to the other basal ganglia, although it is functionally part of the limbic system.

The basal ganglia form part of a neural circuit, receiving input from large parts of the cerebral cortex and sending output mainly to the motor

See also **Neural control of voluntary movement** (page 299), in Ch. 9, Autonomic and Somatic Motor Activity.

areas of the cerebral cortex, via the thalamus, which also relays information from the cerebellum to the cortical motor areas.

As the motor areas of the brain are interdependent and modify the activities of the other areas, it is difficult to ascribe specific functions to each component of the motor system. The basal ganglia do, however, appear to exert a generally inhibitory influence on muscle tone via the nerve connections with the motor cortex and lower brain stem. The corpus striatum has a role in the initiation of gross voluntary movements which are normally refined by the motor cortex. A range of specific activities are dependent upon the integrity of the basal ganglia. They include all those activities that require a particular skill, such as writing and throwing a netball through a hoop.

Damage to the basal ganglia gives rise to a range of involuntary movements depending upon the location of the damage. Destruction of the globus pallidus leads to writhing movements of the hands, face and tongue in the condition known as **athetosis**. Damage to the subthalamic nuclei initiates violent movements of one side of the body (**hemiballismus**, from the Greek meaning 'half jumping'). **Huntington's chorea**, which is characterized by flicking movements of the hands and face, is caused by degeneration of the neostriatum.

Parkinson's disease is a relatively common condition in people over 70 years of age. Two of the principal symptoms, muscle rigidity and tremor, are associated with degeneration of inhibitory dopaminergic neurones that connect the substantia nigra in the midbrain with the neostriatum. The resultant lack of inhibition of the neostriatum leaves the excitatory cholinergic neurones in the neostriatum unopposed, and this causes muscle rigidity and tremor (see also *Acetylcholine and Dopamine*, in *Neurotransmitters in the brain*, below). Another symptom, disinclination to voluntary movement (**akinesia**) is due to lack of stimulation of motor areas of the cerebral cortex from the basal ganglia.

Diencephalon

The diencephalon comprises the two thalami, the hypothalamus and the epithalamus which forms the roof of the IIIrd ventricle and contains a choroid plexus. The pineal gland is attached to the posterior surface of the epithalamus (Figure 5.7).

THALAMI

The thalami (Greek, 'inner chambers') are two oval masses of grey matter that form the lateral walls of the IIIrd ventricle (see Figures 5.4, 5.13 and 5.15). Each **thalamus** is subdivided into a number of **nuclei** which are arranged in four major groups, anterior, medial, lateral and ventral (Figure 5.14). In addition, the **medial** and **lateral geniculate** ('knee-shaped') **bodies** are usually classified as part of the thalamus (Figures 5.14 and 5.17).

All areas of the cerebral cortex have both afferent and efferent connections with the thalamus. All sensory pathways (except smell) synapse in the thalamus and then project to the sensory cortex. The auditory pathways relay in the medial geniculate bodies, the visual pathways relay in the lateral geniculate bodies and the general somatic

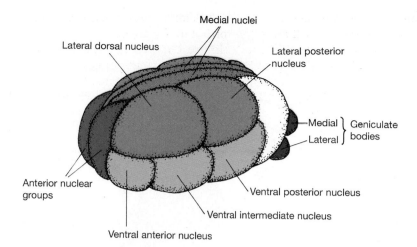

Figure 5.14 The thalamic nuclei. Anterior group [orange], medial group [purple], lateral group [light orange], ventral group [green] and geniculate bodies [red].

senses, and taste, relay in the ventral posterior nuclei (Figure 5.14). Some sensations, such as pain, may reach consciousness at the thalamic level.

The thalamus also plays a role in the control of voluntary movements and has nerve connections with the other motor areas, the motor cortex, cerebellum and basal ganglia.

The thalamus receives afferent neurones from the hypothalamus and brain stem nuclei, as well as the spinal cord, basal ganglia, cerebellum and cerebral cortex. The anterior thalamic nucleus is associated with memory and emotions.

Blockage of the posterolateral branch of the posterior cerebral artery (see Figure 5.26) by a thrombus leads to destruction of the nuclei in the ventral posterior region of the thalamus (Fig. 5.14). The resultant '**thalamic syndrome**' comprises a loss of sensation (**parasthaesia**) from the opposite side of the body and, because of the loss of proprioceptive input, the ability to control movements precisely is also lost (**ataxia**).

After a few weeks or months, some sensation is restored, but it is usually poorly localized and almost always painful. The medial nuclei of the thalamus are not affected by the thrombus and are believed to facilitate pain sensations.

HYPOTHALAMUS

The hypothalamus, as its name suggests lies beneath the thalamus, in the wall of the IIIrd ventricle (Figure 5.15).

The **pituitary gland** is connected to the hypothalamus and indeed is sometimes regarded as a part of it (certainly the neurohypophysis is embryologically derived from the hypothalamus). The **mammillary bodies** are two small round structures that project from the anterior surface of the hypothalamus.

The nerve connections between the cerebral cortex and the hypothalamus provide a 'psychosomatic' link whereby emotional feelings may result in diverse bodily changes such as a rise in blood pressure, urgent defaecation and micturition and the release of adrenaline.

Figure 5.15 Midline section through the brain in the region of the IIIrd ventricle. The surfaces of the thalamus and hypothalamus can be seen in the wall of the IIIrd ventricle.

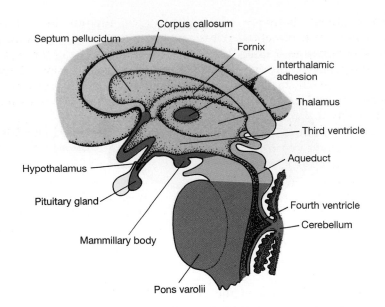

The autonomic nervous system is covered in Ch. 9, Autonomic and Somatic Motor Activity.

See also **Regulation of osmotic pressure by antidiuretic hormone** (page 503), in Ch. 14, Renal Control of Body Fluid Volume and Composition; **Hypothalamic control of body temperature** (page 318), in Ch. 10, The Skin and the Regulation of Body Temperature, and **Insulin** (page 633), in Ch. 16, Endocrine Physiology.

See also **Cardiovascular centre** (page 387), in Ch. 12, Circulation of Blood and Lymph.

See also **Regulation of water balance** (page 501), in Ch. 14, Renal Control of Body Fluid Volume and Composition, and **Neurohypophysis** (page 621), in Ch. 16, Endocrine Physiology.

See also **Oxytocin** (page 676), in Ch. 17, Sex and Reproduction.

The hypothalamus controls all the functions of the autonomic nervous system. The latter controls the activities of a number of glands, the heart and structures containing smooth muscle, e.g. the walls of blood vessels, gastrointestinal tract and urinary tract. The hypothalamus contains various sensory receptors including osmoreceptors, temperature receptors and glucoreceptors. The hypothalamus also receives sensory inputs from the viscera and initiates motor responses by means of its nerve connections with the sympathetic and parasympathetic nervous systems.

Body temperature is regulated by the hypothalamus. Warm blood flowing into the hypothalamus stimulates heat-losing reflexes, while cold blood initiates heat-gaining reflexes.

In many cases the pathways between the hypothalamus and its effectors include secondary integrating 'centres' in the brain stem or spinal cord; for example, stimulation of the hypothalamus increases heart rate and raises blood pressure. These effects are mediated through the 'cardiovascular centre' in the medulla. Digestive activity is mediated in the medulla oblongata and defaecation and micturition reflexes involve the sacral regions of the spinal cord.

The hypothalamus contains areas that promote eating and drinking and satiety and consequently controls the intake of food and drink.

Water output in the urine is regulated by the action of the hormone ADH on the kidneys. ADH is synthesized in the supraoptic nucleus of the hypothalamus and is released into the blood from the neurohypophysis.

The hormone oxytocin is synthesized in the paraventricular nucleus of the hypothalamus. Oxytocin, like ADH, is released from the neurohypophysis; it stimulates the ejection of milk in lactation and contraction of uterine muscle during labour.

The hypothalamus produces a number of releasing hormones that promote the release of other hormones from the adenohypophysis. They include growth hormone releasing hormone; thyrotrophin releasing hormone; corticotrophin releasing hormone and gonadotrophin releasing hormone. Through these releasing hormones and through the adenohypophysis, the hypothalamus regulates the secretion of many hormones, including those from the thyroid, adrenal cortices and gonads, as well as growth hormone and prolactin from the adenohypophysis itself.

In addition, the hypothalamus also appears to house a pacemaker, or biological clock, which generates circadian rhythms such as variations in hormone levels (e.g. cortisol) and body temperature at different times of day. Functionally linked to this 'clock' is a sleep-inducing 'centre'.

The hypothalamus, as well as several other brain areas, distinguishes between pleasant and unpleasant sensations (see *Limbic system*, below).

Damage to the hypothalamus results in a wide range of effects, including altered autonomic functions, obesity, ADH deficiency (diabetes insipidus), sleepiness and memory loss.

Limbic system

Behavioural manifestations of emotional states such as pleasure, pain, rage, docility, affection and sexual arousal have been elicited in many animals by stimulating parts of the hypothalamus and adjacent structures, which are collectively called the limbic (Latin, 'border') system or 'emotional brain'. It includes the cingulate gyrus, the parahippocampal gyrus, the hippocampus, the amygdala, the septal nuclei, the anterior thalamic nuclei and the mammillary bodies. The parts of the limbic system are linked together by a nerve fibre tract, the fornix (Figure 5.16).

The major motor output from the limbic system is via the **hypothalamus**. As a result of electrical stimulation of specific areas in the hypothalamus of animal brains, it has been suggested that there are 'centres' for reward and punishment. Strong stimulation of the punishment centres in animals results in a rage response, whereas stimulation of the reward centres causes placid, tame behaviour. It is further suggested that these centres are important in the process of learning, since if something

See also **Hypothalamic regulation of adenohypophysial hormone secretion** (page 617), in Ch. 16, Endocrine Physiology.

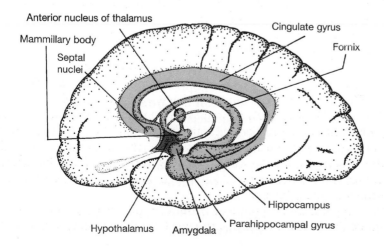

Figure 5.16 The components of the limbic system.

is rewarding, it continues to be carried out, whereas if punishment is involved, the activity is stopped (see also *Learning and memory*).

The **hippocampus** (Greek, 'sea horse') plays a particular role in learning and memory. Destruction of the hippocampi leads to an inability to learn or remember anything new for more than a few minutes. This is **anterograde amnesia**. In addition, there may be some deficit in previously learned memories. The hippocampus receives somatic and special sensory information from the sensory cortices and learns information about the body's position in the environment.

The **amygdala** is thought to act as a 'window' into the limbic system, through which information about an individual's state of mind is fed in; the amygdala may then coordinate behavioural responses. Stimulation of different parts of the amygdala causes a large range of effects including stimulation or inhibition of the autonomic nervous system mediated via the hypothalamus. Additional responses include involuntary movements of skeletal muscle, rage, pleasure and sexual activity.

The **mammillary bodies** control several reflexes involved in feeding, e.g. swallowing and licking the lips (see also *Learning and memory*).

Midbrain

The midbrain is about 2.5 cm long and forms the connection between the pons and the diencephalon (see Figures 5.4, 5.7 and 5.17); it contains the **cerebral aqueduct**, which links the IIIrd and IVth ventricles (Figure 5.15). It is essentially tubular, with two anterior elevations, the **cerebral peduncle**s, and four posterior elevations comprising the **tectum**.

The cerebral peduncles contain ascending and descending fibre tracts, the red nucleus and the substantia nigra. Each red nucleus receives descending fibres from the motor cortex and ascending fibres from the cerebellum, and projects to the cerebellum, reticular formation, thalamus, and olive, as well as the spinal cord in the rubrospinal tract. Of these, the largest number of fibres connect to the olive in the medulla oblongata, which they inhibit. The olives are thought to be involved in the acquisition of motor skills.

The substantia nigra contains melanin and synthesizes the neurotransmitter dopamine. It works with the basal ganglia and the thalamus in the control of motor functions (see *Basal ganglia*)

The tectum (Latin, 'roof') comprises the **corpora quadrigemina** which are made up of the **superior** and **inferior colliculi** (Figure 5.17).

The **optic nerves** (cranial nerve **II**) terminate in the **pretectal nuclei**. The two superior colliculi contain reflex pathways for eyeball movements as well as pupillary reflexes and accommodation. They have neural connections with the pretectal nuclei, and contain the origin of the **oculomotor** (**III**) and the **trochlear** (**IV**) nerves. Table 5.1 summarizes the locations of the cranial nerves and their principal functions. Figure 5.18 shows the locations of the cranial nerve nuclei within the brain. The ascending **spinotectal** and spinothalamic tracts from the

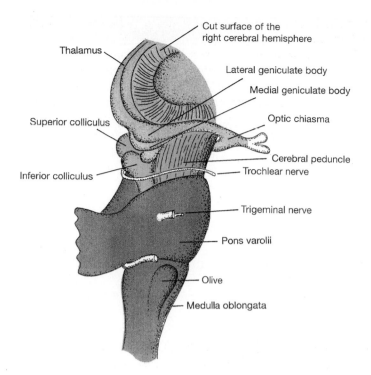

Figure 5.17 Surface view of the midbrain and surrounding structures.

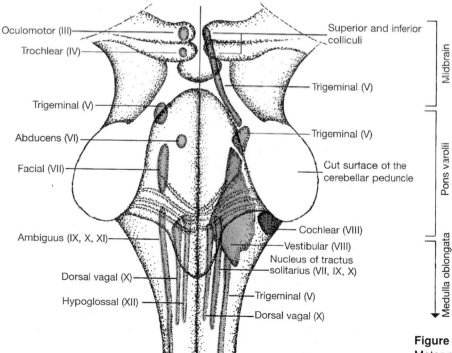

Figure 5.18 Cranial nerve nuclei. Motor nuclei are shown only on the left and sensory nuclei only on the right. The vestibular nuclei are further subdivided into four groups: superior, inferior, lateral and medial.

Table 5.1 Origins and functions of the sensory and motor neurones in the cranial nerves

No. Nerve	Origin	Termination	Actions
I Olfactory	Olfactory mucosa	Olfactory cortex	Sensory – smell
II Optic	Retina	Visual cortex	Sensory – vision
III Oculomotor	Midbrain	Upper eyelid muscle	Motor – raises upper eyelid
		Extrinsic eye muscles (superior, medial, inferior recti; inferior oblique)	– eyeball movement
		Ciliary muscles	– accommodation of lens
		Sphincter muscle of iris	– pupillary constriction
	Proprioceptors in extrinsic eye muscles	Midbrain	Sensory – proprioception
IV Trochlear	Midbrain	Extrinsic eye muscle (superior oblique)	Motor – eyeball movement
	Proprioceptors in extrinsic eye muscle (superior oblique)	Midbrain	Sensory – proprioception
V Trigeminal	Pons varolii	Muscles of mastication	Motor – chewing
	Ophthalmic branch – skin of upper eyelid, eyeball, lacrimal glands, nasal cavity, side of nose, forehead, anterior half of scalp	Midbrain, pons varolii and medulla oblongata	Sensory – touch, pain, temperature proprioception
	Maxillary branch – nasal mucosa, palate, pharynx, upper teeth and lip, cheek, lower eyelid		
	Mandibular branch – anterior two-thirds of tongue, lower teeth, skin over mandible and side of head in front of ear		
VI Abducens	Pons varolii	Extrinsic eye muscle (lateral rectus)	Motor – eyeball movement
	Proprioceptors in lateral rectus	Pons varolii	Sensory – proprioception
VII Facial	Pons varolii	Face, scalp, neck muscles. Lacrimal glands, salivary glands (sublingual, submandibular)	Motor – facial expression, lacrimation, salivation, lowers upper eye lid
	Taste buds on anterior two-thirds of tongue	Gustatory cortex	Sensory – taste
	Proprioceptors in muscles of face and scalp	Pons varolii	– proprioception

Table 5.1 continued

No. Nerve	Origin	Termination	Actions	
VIII Vestibulocochlear	Ear – cochlea, vestibule	Pons varolii – cochlear nuclei Medulla oblongata– vestibular nuclei	Sensory – hearing – equilibrium	
IX Glossopharyngeal	Medulla oblongata	Pharynx – swallowing muscles Parotid gland	Motor – swallowing – salivation	
	Taste buds on posterior one-third of tongue	Gustatory cortex	Sensory – taste	
	Carotid sinus	Medulla oblongata		– monitoring arterial blood pressure
	Carotid body	Medulla oblongata		– monitoring arterial O_2, CO_2, H^+
	Proprioceptors in swallowing muscles	Medulla oblongata		– proprioception
X Vagus	Medulla oblongata	Visceral muscles – (pharynx, larynx, respiratory tract, oesophagus, heart, stomach, small intestine, proximal large intestine, gall bladder, liver, pancreas)	Motor – swallowing, digestive movements and secretions	
	Receptors in visceral muscles (pharynx, larynx, respiratory tract, oesophagus, heart, stomach, small intestine, proximal large intestine, gallbladder, liver, pancreas)	Medulla oblongata and pons varolii	Sensory – Sensory inputs from organs supplied and muscle proprioception	
	Carotid sinus, aortic arch and carotid and aortic bodies	Medulla oblongata and pons varolii	Sensory – monitoring arterial blood pressure and O_2, CO_2, H^+	
XI Accessory	Medulla oblongata – cranial root	Muscles of pharynx, larynx, soft palate	Motor – swallowing	
	Cervical spinal cord – spinal root	Sternocleidomastoid and trapezius muscles		– head movements
	Proprioceptors in muscles supplied by motor fibres	Medulla oblongata	Sensory – proprioception	
XII Hypoglossal	Medulla oblongata	Muscles of tongue	Motor – tongue movements	
	Tongue proprioceptors	Medulla oblongata	Sensory – proprioception	

spinal cord terminate in, and pass through, respectively, the superior colliculi. The **tectospinal** tract originates in the midbrain.

The two inferior colliculi receive auditory stimuli and initiate head and trunk movements. They also receive vestibular stimuli which initiate head and postural movements. See *Brain stem reflexes*, below, for clinical tests of midbrain function.

The **medial lemniscus** is a band of white fibres, found in the medulla and pons as well as the midbrain, that carries sensory fibres concerned with touch, proprioception and vibrations to the thalamus.

See also **Posterior column – lemniscal system** (page 194), in Ch. 6, The Spinal Cord.

Hindbrain

The hindbrain comprises the **pons varolii**, the **medulla oblongata** and the **cerebellum**.

Pons varolii

The pons (Latin, 'bridge') is about 2.5 cm long and lies anterior to the cerebellum and above the medulla (Figure 5.7). It contains large numbers of fibres orientated both transversely and longitudinally. The transverse fibres connect the pons with the cerebellum (**pontocere-bellar fibres**), while the longitudinal fibres consist of sensory and motor tracts between the spinal cord and the higher parts of the brain. The **corticopontine** tracts originate in the association areas of each cerebral cortex, cross over to the opposite side of the pons and then relay with the pontocerebellar fibres. These neural pathways convey information about intentional movements to the contralateral cerebellar hemisphere.

The **cranial nerve nuclei** in the pons include: **V**, which is associated with chewing and various sensations from the face; **VI**, concerned with movement of the eyeballs; and **VII**, facial expression, salivation, lacrimation and taste (Figure 5.18). The cochlear nuclei (**VIII**), part of the auditory pathway, are also found in the pons; from here fibres travel to the medial geniculate bodies and the inferior colliculi, and thence to the temporal cortex.

See also **The respiratory centres** (page 457), in Ch. 13, Respiration.

One of the respiratory centres, the **pneumotaxic centre**, is found in the pons. This modifies the activities of the medullary respiratory centres.

Pain pathways (page 219), in Ch. 7, Sensory Processing.

The central aqueduct is surrounded by periaqueductal grey matter, which is involved in pain control, next to which is the locus coeruleus on each side. The locus coeruleus (see Figure 5.22) contains the cell bodies of noradrenergic neurones (see *Neurotransmitters in the brain*, below).

Medulla oblongata

The medulla (Latin, 'middle') is 2.5–3 cm long and widens as it approaches the pons. The central canal of the spinal cord is continuous with a canal in the medulla and this in turn connects with the IVth ventricle (Figure 5.7).

The medulla coordinates many autonomic activities and is said to contain a number of specialized 'centres' which, in turn, are controlled by the hypothalamus. These include the **cardiovascular, inspiratory** and **expiratory, swallowing, vomiting, coughing** and **sneezing** centres; each contains the nerve-cell bodies of motor neurones that initiate their respective activities.

The **nuclei of cranial nerves IX–XII** are found in the medulla (Figure 5.18); IX is associated with swallowing, salivation and taste; X contains sensory and motor fibres from and to the thoracic and abdominal viscera; XI controls head and shoulder girdle movements and XII tongue movements. The vestibular nuclei of cranial nerve VIII, the lateral, medial and inferior, are also found in the medulla (Table 5.1). Vestibular nuclei receive input from the vestibular apparatus in the ears and send efferents to the vestibulospinal tract, which helps maintain the upright position by causing extensor muscle contraction.

On each upper lateral surface there is an oval structure, the **olive** (Figure 5.17), which contains several olivary nuclei having nerve connections with the cerebellum and is involved in motor control, particularly the acquisition of motor skills.

Anteriorly, on either side of the anterior median fissure, there are two rounded columns, the **pyramids** (Figure 5.6(b)). These contain the **pyramidal (corticospinal)** tract fibres, which control voluntary movement. Most of these fibres cross over in the medulla, the decussation of the pyramids. Fibres then descend in the lateral corticospinal tracts of the spinal cord. Fibres in the lateral part of each pyramid, however, remain uncrossed and travel in the anterior corticospinal tracts of the spinal cord.

The **fasciculus gracilis** and **fasciculus cuneatus** on each side of the spinal cord contain ascending fibres that convey proprioception and fine touch. The fibres terminate at the bottom of the IVth ventricle as the **gracile nucleus** and **cuneate nucleus** on each side. Neurones arising from these nuclei cross over in the medulla and ascend in the medial lemniscus to the thalamus.

There are many other fibre tracts passing through the medulla, including the anterior and posterior spinocerebellar, the anterior and lateral spinothalamic, spinotectal and tectospinal, vestibulospinal and rubrospinal.

See also **Pathways and neuronal circuits in the spinal cord** (page 192), in Ch. 6, The Spinal Cord.

The death of tissue following a lack of blood supply (**infarction**) in the medulla caused, for example, by a thrombus, results in a variety of changes, depending on which pathways and nuclei are affected. Damage to the spinocerebellar tracts causes cerebellar ataxia (see *Cerebellum,* below) on the same side. Damage to the lateral spinothalamic tract results in a loss of pain and temperature sensation from the contralateral side. Damage to the vestibular nucleus causes vertigo, and to the nucleus ambiguus causes hoarseness and sometimes difficulty in swallowing. Interruption of sympathetic pathways to the spinal cord results in **Horner's syndrome**, which is characterized by a constricted pupil, drooping upper eyelid and lack of sweating.

Cerebellum

The cerebellum lies behind the pons and medulla and below the occipital

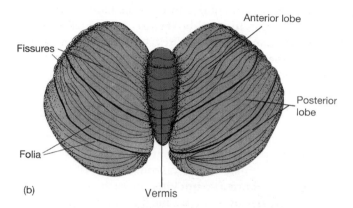

Figure 5.19 The cerebellum.
(a) Inferior surface.   **(b)** Superior surface.

lobes of the cerebrum. The two **cerebellar hemispheres** are joined by a smaller **vermis** (Latin, 'worm'). The whole structure is divided into three lobes: the **anterior**, **posterior** and **flocculonodular lobes** (Figure 5.19).

Inferiorly, the vermis is divided into the **uvula** (Latin, 'little grape') and the **pyramid**. Also inferiorly there is a lobule of each cerebellar hemisphere known as the **tonsil**. The cerebellar tonsils lie near to the uvula (as indeed do the palatine tonsils in the pharynx).

The surface of the cerebellum is composed of grey matter, like the cerebrum, with parallel curved **fissures** separating narrow **folia**. These are analogous to the sulci and gyri of the cerebrum.

The deeper white matter contains fibre tracts orientated like those in the cerebrum: there are commissural and projection fibres, although association fibres connecting different parts of the cerebellum are lacking. The projection fibres are arranged in three bundles on each side, forming the superior, middle and inferior **cerebellar peduncles**. The white matter projects into the grey as fine laminae to form a structure known as the **arbor vitae** (Latin, 'tree of life', Figure 5.7).

The cerebellum functions principally in the control of rapid muscular movements such as running. Whereas other parts of the brain and spinal cord may initiate muscle contraction, the cerebellum serves to monitor and make appropriate adjustments to the timing and strength of contractions of groups of muscles. It can be regarded as comparing intended with actual movements.

The cerebellum receives sensory input from virtually all types of mechanoreceptor, including muscle spindles, Golgi tendon organs, touch receptors in the skin and joint receptors, as well as the special sense organs.

Each half of the cerebellum controls the movement of its own side of the body, and the efferent connections influencing its activity generally reflect this. Somatic sensory information is conveyed along the **spino-cerebellar tracts** to the cerebellum on the same side (ipsilaterally). Visual and vestibular afferent pathways also connect to the cerebellum ipsilaterally, as do the **reticulocerebellar** fibres.

Connections from the pons and the olive via the **pontocerebellar** and **olivocerebellar** tracts arise from the opposite (contralateral) side.

There is **somatotopic organization** in the cerebellum whereby impulses conveying a particular sensory modality from a specific part of the body are conveyed to different parts of the cerebellar cortex. The face, arm and leg are represented ipsilaterally in the anterior lobe and bilaterally in the posterior lobe (Figure 5.20). The maps for movement correspond with the sensory maps.

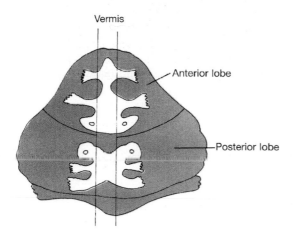

Vermis

Anterior lobe

Posterior lobe

Figure 5.20 Somatotopic organization in the sensorimotor cortex of the cerebellum.

Outflow from the cerebellum via the **vestibulocerebellar** tract is projected to both sides, controlling eye movements (via the midbrain) and balance (via the vestibulospinal tract). Connections with the reticular formation and thereafter to the reticulospinal tracts control posture and locomotion.

Cerebellar connections to the red nuclei and thence to the olivary nuclei form a neural circuit responsible for motor learning.

The cerebellum also has neural connections with the thalamus and the motor cortex. These inter-relationships are explored further in Chapter 9.

The cerebellum has motor connections with other parts of the brain.

See also **Neural control of voluntary movement** (page 299), in Ch. 9, Autonomic and Somatic Motor Activity.

The pathways arise in the deep **cerebellar nuclei**, including the dentate and fastigial (see Figure 8.32). Voluntary motor activity is coordinated via motor pathways to the motor cortex and the coordination of conscious control from the motor cortex with subconscious body postural control involves nerve connections between the cerebellum, thalamus and motor cortex as well as the basal ganglia and reticular formation.

Damage to the cerebellum, particularly if it involves the deeper nuclei, leads to a number of conditions characterized by disturbances of complex motor control. The ability to predict the extent of a movement is lost (**dysmetria**) and movements become uncoordinated (**ataxia**). Attempting to perform a voluntary act leads to an 'intention tremor' as the body (or part thereof) tries to hit a specific mark. In complex movements the point at which one element ends and another begins is also lost, so that movements do not progress in the normal sequence (**dysdiadochokinesia**). This lack of coordination also extends to vocalization and leads to speech that is unintelligible (**dysarthria**).

Reticular formation

The reticular formation is a core of grey matter that extends from the spinal cord through the medulla, pons and midbrain to the hypothalamus and medial thalamus. It is analogous to the central grey matter in the spinal cord and contains a number of nuclei with indistinct boundaries. The reticular formation can be divided into two parts, **excitatory** and **inhibitory**. The excitatory portion extends along the whole length of the reticular formation, whereas the inhibitory reticular formation lies mainly in the lower medulla (Figure 5.21).

Figure 5.21 The location of the excitatory and inhibitory portions of the reticular formation.

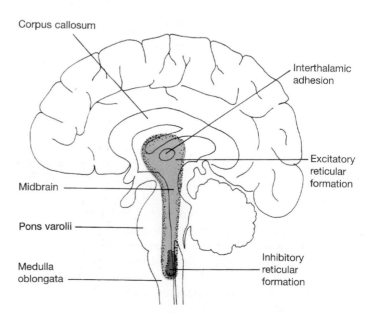

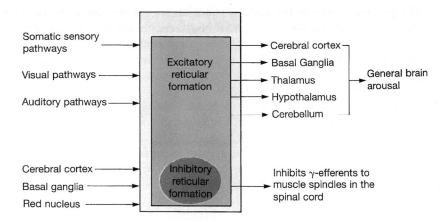

Figure 5.22 Major neural connections of the reticular formation.

One of the main functions of the reticular formation is determining the level of wakefulness or alertness in the brain as a whole. The reticular formation receives collaterals from all the sensory pathways, including those conveying proprioceptive information from joints and muscles, those conveying pain and touch from the skin, and visual and auditory pathways. Such sensory input stimulates the excitatory reticular formation, which in turn produces general arousal in the brain via nerve pathways to the thalamus, hypothalamus, basal ganglia, cerebellum and cerebrum (Figure 5.22). The **reticular activating system** is the name given to the stimulating action of the excitatory reticular formation.

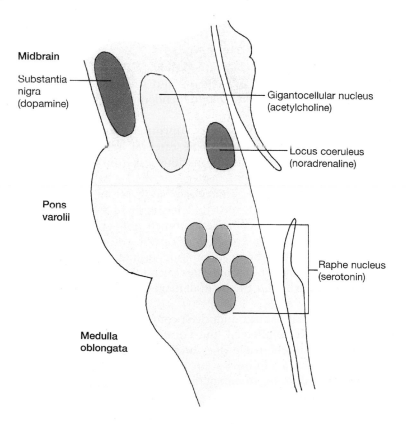

Figure 5.23 Brain stem nuclei containing the cell bodies of neurones that synthesize acetylcholine, dopamine, noradrenaline and serotonin.

Two neurotransmitters particularly associated with the reticular activating system are **noradrenaline** and **acetylcholine**. Noradrenergic neurones are concentrated in the **locus coeruleus** (Latin, 'dark blue place'), a bilateral area located at the junction of the midbrain and the pons. Acetylcholine is produced by **gigantocellular neurones** in the pons and the midbrain (Figure 5.23).

The lateral vestibular nuclei, together with the reticular formation control the muscles that support the body against the effects of gravity, e.g. the extensor muscles of the limbs. The lateral vestibular nuclei stimulate both alpha and gamma motor neurones continuously. The inhibitory reticular formation balances this by exerting an inhibitory influence on the gamma motor neurones. If the body's posture changes, sensory stimuli from the vestibular apparatus to the vestibular nuclei can result in changes in the degree of contraction, thereby maintaining equilibrium.

If the inhibitory reticular formation is stimulated, it causes general inhibition of brain activity. The principal action of the area, however, is moderating spinal cord activity. Several areas of the brain connect to the inhibitory reticular formation, including the cerebral cortex, the basal ganglia and the red nucleus (Figure 5.22). **Muscle tone** is controlled from the reticular formation by means of the sensitivity of the spindles which, in turn, is regulated by gamma-efferents. The reticular formation alters the level of activity of these gamma-efferents. Transection of the brain at midbrain level results in **decerebrate rigidity**, which is caused by overactive stretch reflexes affecting the extensor muscles. The transection blocks the connections between the red nucleus and the inhibitory reticular formation.

> See also **Muscle tone** (page 204), in Ch. 6, The Spinal Cord.

Consciousness and unconsciousness

Consciousness, the state of wakefulness that enables the perception of sensations, the initiation of movements and thinking to take place, is manifested by the cerebral cortex but dependent on input from the excitatory reticular formation.

The transient lack of consciousness (unconsciousness) which accompanies fainting (**syncope**) is caused by cerebral ischaemia due to low arterial blood pressure. **Sleep** is unconsciousness from which one can be awakened.

Coma, on the other hand, is unconsciousness for an extended period from which one cannot be aroused. The depth of unconsciousness is assessed using the Glasgow coma scale, which tests opening of the eyes and motor and verbal responses. Coma can be caused by a variety of things, including blows to the head, tumours or infections, anoxia, hypoglycaemia and high doses of barbiturates, alcohol or opiates. The type of coma is affected by whether the brain damage is to the cerebral cortex or to the brain stem.

Widespread cortical damage induces a coma in which respiratory and cardiac functions are unaffected, the vocal cords can move and make noises, albeit incomprehensible ones and reflex swallowing can occur. Periods of apparent wakefulness occur in which the eyes are open and move, but not in response to commands. The individual is in a **persistent vegetative state**.

Severe brain stem damage causes unconsciousness in which respiration only occurs with the help of a ventilator; the heart stops after a few days (despite the myogenic nature of its contraction); there is no vocalization or swallowing; the eyes are fixed.

Brain stem reflexes

Several reflex pathways pass through the brain stem, and these can be tested clinically. Absence of reflex responses would indicate brain stem death.

Direct light and consensual light reflexes

If a bright light is shone into one eye, both pupils constrict. Sensory neurones in the optic nerve of the eye are stimulated and convey impulses to the pretectal nucleus in the midbrain. Motor neurones in cranial nerve III (oculomotor) cause contraction of the radial muscles in the irises of both eyes.

See also **Visual pathways** (page 243), in Ch. 8, The Special Senses.

Vestibulo-ocular reflexes

In a conscious person, when the head is turned suddenly, signals from the semicircular canals in the ear initiate reflex movements of the eyes whereby the gaze moves slowly in a direction opposite to the direction of movement. In an unconscious person, either the head can be turned passively or ice-cold water can be introduced into the external auditory meatus, which sets up convection currents in the nearby semicircular canal, simulating head rotation. The eyes move towards the cooled side in a person lying face upwards (supine). The sensory neurones are in the vestibular nerve (VIII), which relays to the vestibular nucleus in the medulla, the medial longitudinal fasciculus to the ocular nuclei in the midbrain. Motor neurones stimulate movement in the extrinsic muscles of the eyes.

See also **Vestibular pathways** (page 264), in Ch. 8, The Special Senses.

Facial nerve reflex

Pressure on the supra-orbital notch produces reflex grimacing. The sensory neurones are in the ophthalmic branch of cranial nerve V (trigeminal) which relays with cranial nerve VII (facial) in the pons.

Corneal reflex

If the cornea is touched with a wisp of cotton wool, reflex blinking occurs. The sensory neurones are in the ophthalmic branch of cranial nerve V (trigeminal), which relays with cranial nerve VII (facial) in the pons.

Gag reflex

Touching the back of the pharynx causes gagging, muscular movements that occur during vomiting. The sensory neurones are in cranial nerve X (vagus), which relays with several motor neurones in the medulla and pons.

Cerebral meninges

The brain is surrounded by three membranes collectively known as the cerebral meninges (*sing*. meninx). They are: the dura mater, which is attached to the inside of the skull; the arachnoid mater; and the pia mater, which covers the surface of the brain (Figure 5.24).

Figure 5.24 The cerebral and spinal meninges and the approximate locations of the choroid plexuses which produce CSF. The fluid fills the ventricles of the brain, the central canal of the spinal cord and the subarachnoid space. **Inset:** junction between the brain and spinal cord, showing the single layer of dura mater and the epidural space around the spinal cord, and the double layer of dura mater around the brain.

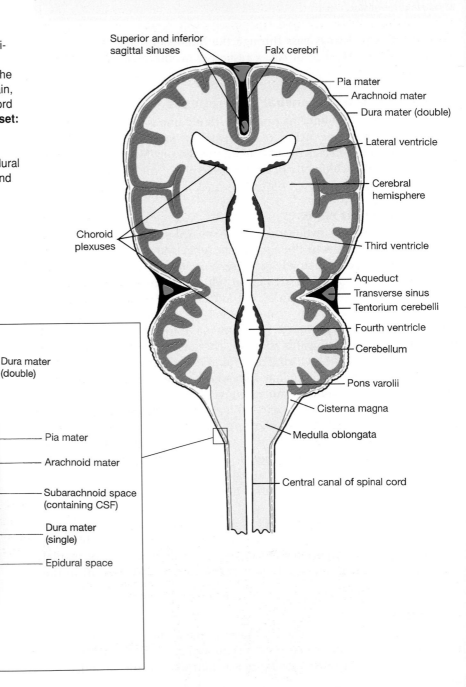

Superior and inferior sagittal sinuses

Falx cerebri

Pia mater

Arachnoid mater

Dura mater (double)

Lateral ventricle

Cerebral hemisphere

Choroid plexuses

Third ventricle

Aqueduct

Transverse sinus

Tentorium cerebelli

Fourth ventricle

Cerebellum

Pons varolii

Cisterna magna

Medulla oblongata

Central canal of spinal cord

Brain

Dura mater (double)

Skull

Periosteum

Vertebra

Pia mater

Arachnoid mater

Subarachnoid space (containing CSF)

Dura mater (single)

Epidural space

The main function of the meninges is protection of the brain. The dura mater (Latin, 'hard mother'), as its name implies, is a tough outer layer. The pia mater (Latin, 'tender mother') and the arachnoid mater (Greek, 'like a spider's web') form and reabsorb, respectively, the cerebrospinal fluid that surrounds and nourishes the brain and cushions it against blows.

The **dura mater** is a double layer of dense fibrous tissue. The outermost layer is attached to the skull, forming an endosteum, so that there is no epidural space like that surrounding the spinal cord, where the dura mater is a single layer only. Epidural injections into the spine, therefore, do not reach the brain because the outer layer of dura mater is attached to the skull and therefore prevents the injection from entering the cranial vault.

The two layers of dura mater separate at certain points, where they contain venous sinuses. One such structure is the **falx cerebri**, which runs along the longitudinal fissure between the two cerebral hemispheres and contains the superior and inferior sagittal sinuses (Figure 5.24). An equivalent structure, the **tentorium cerebelli**, lies between the cerebellum and the cerebrum and contains the transverse and superior petrosal sinuses on each side.

The **arachnoid mater** is a delicate, fibrous membrane covered by mesothelium on both surfaces. It lines the dura mater and is separated from it by a potential **subdural space** containing a very small amount of serous fluid, which acts as a lubricant. The arachnoid mater is separated from the pia mater by the **subarachnoid space** which contains cerebrospinal fluid (CSF). Connective tissue strands cross the space, linking the two membranes. The arachnoid mater projects into several of the venous sinuses as finger-like **arachnoid villi** or as larger **arachnoid granulations** (Figure 5.25). CSF passes through these projections into the blood in the sinuses (see Cerebrospinal fluid, below). The cavity of the hindbrain, the IVth ventricle, has both median and lateral connections with the subarachnoid space.

In a number of places the arachnoid mater is less closely applied to the brain surface. Between the cerebellum and the medulla, for example, the arachnoid mater bridges the space between the two structures, giving rise to the **cisterna magna** (cerebello-medullary cistern) (Figure 5.24).

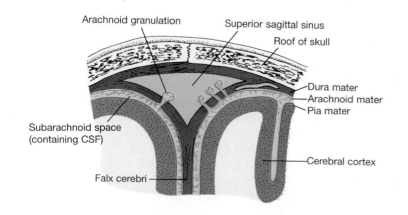

Arachnoid granulation
Superior sagittal sinus
Roof of skull
Dura mater
Arachnoid mater
Pia mater
Subarachnoid space (containing CSF)
Cerebral cortex
Falx cerebri

Figure 5.25 Frontal section through the falx cerebri showing the arachnoid granulations projecting into the superior sagittal sinus.

The **pia mater** is a delicate, highly vascular membrane, which is closely applied to the surface of the brain. The membrane invaginates the brain at certain points and joins the lining of the ventricles, forming fringe-like structures that project into the ventricles. These are the **choroid plexuses**, highly vascular structures which give rise to CSF.

Inflammation of the meninges (meningitis)

The meninges are susceptible to infection by a variety of organisms, including those populating the skin, intestine and respiratory tract. The organisms travel in the bloodstream and cause inflammation of the pia mater and arachnoid mater (meningitis). This irritates the underlying nerve tissues and leads to headaches, vomiting and reflex spasm of spinal muscles. The manifestations of infection include a rash, high temperature and septicaemia, which can lead to shock. Chronic meningitis may lead to destruction of neural tissue, causing permanent brain damage.

Cerebrospinal fluid

Cerebrospinal fluid (CSF) surrounds the brain and spinal cord, as well as filling the central ventricles and canals. It performs a protective function in that the brain floats in the CSF within the skull, thereby providing a cushion against a blow to the head.

CSF is formed from the blood and is returned to it and so is analogous to lymph or interstitial fluid. The composition is similar, but not identical to plasma (Table 5.2).

CSF contains more Na^+ and Cl^- than plasma and less K^+, glucose and protein. It is more acid and contains more dissolved CO_2 and less HCO_3^- than plasma. CSF is produced by a combination of filtration and active secretory processes by the choroid plexuses found in the inferior horns of the lateral ventricles, the posterior part of the third ventricle and the roof of the fourth ventricle (Figure 5.24). Some CSF is also produced through the ependymal lining of the ventricles.

The total volume of fluid present is about 150 mL and it is produced at a rate of about 600–700 mL/day (0.5 mL/min). The fluid is filtered and secreted into the ventricles, most of it being produced in the lateral ventricles. Fluid then flows through the interventricular foramina into the third ventricle and thence to the fourth. There are two lateral apertures and one median aperture through which the fluid can pass out of the fourth ventricle. CSF flows from the fourth ventricle into a large space, the cisterna magna, which lies behind the medulla and beneath the cerebellum. From here the fluid fills the subarachnoid space; the main direction of flow is upwards towards and around the cerebrum. The fluid also fills the central canal and surrounds the spinal cord.

The return of CSF to the blood takes place through the arachnoid villi and granulations, which project through the walls of the venous sinuses (Figure 5.25). The pressure of the CSF is slightly (about 10 mmHg when the body is horizontal) higher than that of the venous blood in the head and the arachnoid villi act as one-way valves, allowing CSF to pass only

Table 5.2 The compositions of plasma and cerebrospinal fluid

	CSF	Plasma
Na^+ (mmol/L)	148.0	142.0
K^+ (mmol/L)	2.9	4.0
HCO_3^- (mmol/L)	22.0	27.0
Cl^- (mmol/L)	125.0	100.0
Glucose (mmol/L)	4.5	5.0
Urea (mmol/L)	5.0	5.0
P_{CO_2} (kPA)	6.6	5.3
PH	7.3	7.4
Protein (mg/dL)	30.0	7000.0

into the blood in the sinus. The mechanism is similar to that operating in lymphatic capillaries.

Excess cerebrospinal fluid (hydrocephalus)

Excessive production of CSF, reduction in its absorption or obstruction to its flow leads to hydrocephalus, in which the ventricles become dilated and the brain is flattened against the skull. In a young child hydrocephalus causes the pliable skull to enlarge, but in an older child or an adult there is compression of the brain within the rigid skull. Sites of obstruction include the aqueduct of Silvius (between the third and fourth ventricles), the subarachnoid space at the base of the brain, or the arachnoid villi. The extent and type of damage is variable. Blindness may result, for example, due to a rise in pressure in the sheath that surrounds the optic nerve.

Contrecoup

If the head is struck hard, then any damage to the brain occurs on the side opposite the blow. The brain floats in CSF, so that the blow pushes the fluid and the brain away from it. The skull has more inertia than the floating brain, so it only moves slightly and consequently the brain strikes the inner surface of the skull on the opposite side from the blow (contrecoup).

Cerebral circulation

Blood enters the skull through the left and right **internal carotid arteries** and, to a lesser extent, through the two **vertebral arteries**.

The carotid arteries give off a number of branches that are applied to the underside of the brain. Two **anterior cerebral arteries** link together through an **anterior communicating artery**. Other branches enable them to communicate with the **middle cerebral arteries**, the largest branches of the carotid arteries (Figure 5.26).

The right and left vertebral arteries fuse, giving rise to the **basilar artery**. From the latter arise the two **posterior cerebral arteries**, which communicate with the middle cerebral arteries through **posterior communicating arteries**. The extensive anastomoses between the carotid and vertebral arteries create the **circulus arteriosus**, or **circle of Willis**. There are considerable variations in the extent to which the circle is developed and it may be absent in up to a third of the population.

The entire supply of the cerebral cortex is derived from cortical branches of the anterior, middle and posterior cerebral arteries. They pass to the cortex in the pia mater and give off branches that penetrate the grey matter; some of them reach the underlying white matter.

The choroid plexuses of both the lateral and the third ventricles are supplied by branches of the internal and posterior cerebral arteries; that of the fourth ventricle receives its blood supply from the posterior cerebral artery.

Blood is drained from the substance of the brain by cerebral and cere-

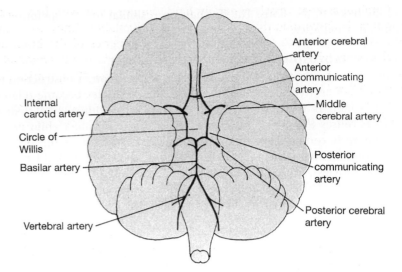

Figure 5.26 Arteries at the base of the brain. The brain is supplied by the anterior, middle and posterior cerebral arteries which arise from the circle of Willis.

bellar veins and a number in the brain stem. Blood flows into the **dural sinuses**, channels between the two layers of dura mater. The venous sinuses are devoid of muscle and are composed entirely of endothelium. The falx cerebri contains the superior and inferior **sagittal sinuses** which drain into the **transverse sinus** in the tentorium cerebelli on each side (Figures 5.24 and 5.27). Blood from each transverse sinus joins blood draining the eye orbit and part of the face via the **cavernous sinus** before flowing into the **internal jugular vein** (Figure 5.27).

Figure 5.27 The major dural sinuses taking venous blood from the brain to the internal jugular vein.

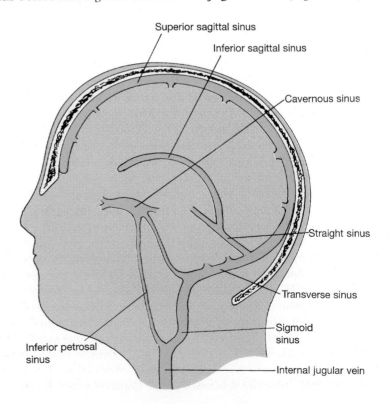

Cerebral arterial vessels generally have thinner walls with less elastic and muscle tissue than those of the systemic circulation. They are therefore capable of much less constriction. The capillaries of the brain are supported by glial cells and have tight junctions between the endothelial cells. They are consequently less permeable than typical capillaries (see *Blood–CSF and blood–brain barrier*, below).

Blood flow through the brain normally remains constant at a rate of about 55 mL/100 g/min (750 mL/min) and only when cardiac output drops below 3 L/min does cerebral circulation become deficient. The constant nature of this circulation is very important since the tissues of the brain are very delicate and sensitive to hypoxia (see *Brain metabolism*, below). The brain is housed within a rigid membrane, the dura mater, inside a rigid shell, the skull. The incompressibility of the brain tissue is one of the factors that actually helps to maintain a constant blood flow, i.e. the vessels can only dilate very slowly because of the tissues around them. Although cerebral vessels are innervated by both sympathetic and parasympathetic fibres, neural control appears to be of only minor importance, compared with chemical factors.

If arterial pressure rises, for example during heavy exercise, the arteries supplying the brain constrict, thereby preventing the high pressure from being transmitted onwards into the brain. Strong arterial constriction can also occur if the brain is damaged, for example by a cardiovascular accident, or by a subdural haemorrhage or tumour.

Cerebral blood flow is regulated by the levels of carbon dioxide and H^+ in arterial blood. Should the levels of carbon dioxide or H^+ in arterial blood rise, and/or the level of oxygen fall, vasodilation occurs, thereby increasing blood flow and reversing the stimuli. Usually, of course, arterial concentration of oxygen, carbon dioxide and H^+ remain relatively constant.

Although the total rate of cerebral blood flow is constant, the distribution of the blood to different parts of the brain is constantly being adjusted in accordance with the prevailing levels of activity; the greater the level, the higher the blood flow. In physical exercise, for example, the motor areas of the brain receive an increased blood flow at the expense of other areas. The redistribution of blood to active areas of the brain is brought about by the local changes that accompany an increase in activity, i.e. a rise in carbon dioxide and H^+ levels and a fall in the level of oxygen. As in other tissues, these changes cause local vasodilation and a consequent increase in blood flow.

Central nervous system ischaemic response

If blood flow to the brain falls considerably i.e. if the pressure drops to around 50 mmHg or less, then an 'emergency' reflex is initiated; this is known as the central nervous system ischaemic response.

Ischaemia raises tissue carbon dioxide concentration (because of reduced blood flow away from the tissue) and, if this happens in the brain, the carbon dioxide is thought to stimulate the pressor area of the vasomotor centre in the medulla. This initiates a massive sympathetic discharge, which brings about intense arteriolar constriction and a rise in arterial blood pressure, which in turn improves cerebral blood flow.

An example of this response can be seen in someone who has **raised intracranial pressure** due to a head injury, and the pressure of fluid compresses the cerebral arteries and reduces blood flow. This, in turn, elicits the CNS ischaemic response and thereby raises arterial pressure. If the response is caused by raised intracranial pressure it is known as the **Cushing reaction**. Usually, it is accompanied by a reduction in heart rate due to the secondary action of the baroreceptor reflex initiated by the rise in blood pressure.

Cerebrovascular accident (stroke)

The term 'stroke' is used to describe the sudden seizure that results from an interruption in the flow of blood to the brain, followed by the death of brain tissue. A cerebrovascular accident (CVA) is analogous to a heart attack (myocardial infarction). The cessation of blood flow to an area of brain is caused, in the vast majority of cases, by blockage of an artery by a thrombus or atheromatous plaque. Alternatively a haemorrhage, which then compresses brain tissue, can also cause cerebral ischaemia. The nature and severity of the consequences depend upon the precise location of the accident and how large an area of brain is supplied by the affected vessel.

Frequently, a CVA results in paralysis of one side of the body, as well as sensory and speech disturbances. The precise consequences clearly depend on which areas of the brain have been affected. Coverage of the individual brain areas in this chapter includes the consequences that could result from damage.

Transient ischaemic attacks (**TIA**) constitute a milder and reversible form of cerebral ischaemia than that which follows a CVA. The attacks last from a few minutes to an hour and involve similar symptoms to those experienced in a CVA. TIA is most often due to emboli that have become detached from atherosclerotic plaques in feed arteries such as the carotid.

Brain oedema

See also **Physiological causes of oedema** (page 412), in Ch. 12, Circulation of Blood and Lymph.

Oedema is excess interstitial fluid, which has a variety of causes, including injury. An accumulation of fluid in the brain is potentially much more serious than in other organs because the brain is encased in the rigid skull and so oedema leads to the compression of blood vessels, with resultant cerebral ischaemia. This, in turn, leads to a rise in the concentration of CO_2, H^+ and other metabolites and a fall in O_2 concentration. These changes cause arteriolar dilation, which increases the blood flow and capillary hydrostatic pressure and therefore further increases the oedema. The hypoxia also increases capillary permeability, further exacerbating the oedema. A positive feedback cycle has, therefore, been elicited (Figure 5.28).

Medical intervention could involve the withdrawal of CSF from the lateral ventricles or infusing a solution of a substance such as mannitol into the blood, thereby drawing water out of the CSF by osmosis.

Blood–cerebrospinal fluid and blood–brain barriers

With the exception of the hypothalamus, the capillaries supplying the

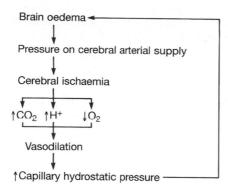

Figure 5.28 Positive feedback between brain oedema and raised capillary hydrostatic pressure.

brain, including those in the choroid plexuses, are composed of endothelial cells with very tight junctions and therefore very low permeability. As a consequence some substances are either partially or completely prevented from gaining access to brain tissue. These blood–brain and blood–CSF barriers enable the local environment of the brain (CSF and interstitial fluid) to be maintained at a level which is more constant than that of the rest of the body. Thus, bilirubin and circulating neurotransmitters, for example, are unable to gain access; K^+ levels are kept relatively low, which favours optimal resting and action potential function; H^+ ions are also largely excluded from crossing the blood–brain and blood–CSF barriers.

The hypothalamus contains capillaries that do allow the passage of materials from the blood to the tissue of the brain, thereby allowing them to gain access to the chemoreceptors and osmoreceptors.

Water, carbon dioxide, alcohol and anaesthetics can, however, gain access to the brain via the bloodstream, but non-lipid-soluble drugs and antibodies do not. However, drugs administered into the CSF can readily gain access through the ependymal cells lining the ventricles, or through the pia mater covering the brain, as these are both highly permeable membranes.

Hypothalamic chemoreceptors are discussed in **Neural control of eating** (page 535), in Ch. 15, Digestion and Absorption of Food, and **Regulation of blood glucose concentration** (page 645), in Ch. 16, Endocrine Physiology. Hypothalamic osmoreceptors are discussed in **Regulation of water balance** (page 501), in Ch. 14, Renal Control of Body Fluid Volume and Composition.

Brain metabolism

The brain has a relatively high metabolic rate compared with other tissues and, although it constitutes only about 2% of body mass, it receives approximately 15% of cardiac output. The energy is used mainly for the active transport of ions in the generation of action potentials.

The major nutrient oxidized by the brain is glucose. This diffuses into the brain cells by an insulin-independent mechanism; consequently, its uptake does not fluctuate during absorptive and postabsorptive states.

The stores of oxygen and glycogen within neurones are minimal and therefore the cells depend upon a constant blood flow to maintain their metabolism. If cerebral blood flow ceases, then unconsciousness follows within 5–10 seconds.

See also **Regulation of blood glucose concentration** (page 645), in Ch. 16, Endocrine Physiology.

Electroencephalogram

If electrodes are placed on the scalp and connected up to an instrument that measures voltage differences between the electrodes, the record of the resultant electrical activity is known as an electroencephalogram (**EEG**).

In contrast to the ECG, brain waves are frequently irregular and lack a discernible pattern. However, if neurones from a particular region of the brain fire synchronously, then brain waves are recorded. They are classified as delta, theta, alpha and beta waves according to their frequency (Figure 5.29).

Figure 5.29   The four different brain waves that can be recorded as an electroencephalogram. Alpha waves are recorded from the occipital region when a person is awake, calm and relaxed. Beta waves are recorded from the parietal or frontal regions when a person is awake and mentally alert. Delta waves occur in very deep sleep. Theta waves are recorded from the parietal and temporal lobes in children.

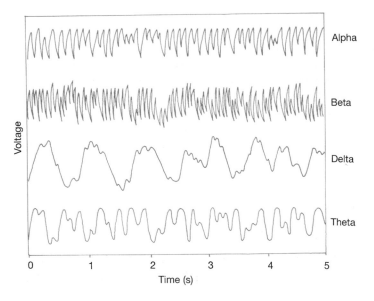

Delta waves have a frequency lower than 4 Hz and a high amplitude. They occur in very deep sleep, in anaesthesia, in infancy and in some organic brain diseases.

Theta waves are somewhat irregular and have a frequency range of 4–7 Hz. They emanate from the parietal and temporal lobes in children, but are normally absent from adults except in the early stages of sleep, in emotional stress or in some brain disorders.

Alpha waves have a frequency range of 8–13 Hz, and a low amplitude. They are most intense in the occipital region of the brain when a person is awake, calm and relaxed. If attention is drawn to something they are replaced by beta waves.

Beta waves have the highest frequency of the brain waves (14–25 Hz). They are more irregular than alpha waves and emanate from the parietal or frontal regions of the brain when a person is awake and mentally alert.

The frequency of brain waves is reduced by drugs that depress brain activity, and in coma. A flat EEG is evidence of cortical brain death. An increase in frequency may be caused by fear, drug intoxication or epilepsy.

Excess activity within the CNS (epilepsy)

Epilepsy results from uncontrolled excess activity of all or a part of the CNS. In the form of epilepsy known as **grand mal**, all areas of the brain are involved, probably stimulated by excess activity in the reticular activating system. The person loses consciousness and uncontrolled jerky movements (**convulsions**) occur. Loss of bowel and bladder control can occur and the violence of the convulsions can cause bones to break and the tongue to be bitten. The seizure or 'fit' lasts from a few seconds up to a few minutes. A predisposition to epilepsy is usually genetic, with episodes being triggered by flashing lights, loud noises, emotional states, drugs, fever or alkalosis due to hyperventilation. Blows to the head, stroke, infections and tumours can also cause epilepsy.

A sensory hallucination (**aura**) such as a taste, smell or flashes of light often precedes a seizure.

Focal epilepsy involves excess activity in one part of the brain, which may then spread, causing muscular contraction in the opposite side of the body, often starting at the mouth and progressing down to the legs (**Jacksonian epilepsy**). A **psychomotor seizure** is a type of focal epilepsy that does not spread and that often involves the limbic system. The consequences are variable and include amnesia, incoherent speech and attacks of rage or anxiety.

A much milder form of epilepsy, known as **petit mal**, involves loss of consciousness for up to 30 seconds, with some muscle twitches, usually of the face.

Sleep

Sleep is a form of unconsciousness from which a person can be roused (in contrast to a coma, from which a person cannot be roused). Sleep generally follows a circadian rhythm controlled by the hypothalamus, although some control can be exerted over when and how much sleep is taken. The need for sleep is variable, with a tendency for the amount to reduce with age. In the middle years, some individuals may require only 3–4 hours per 24 hours, but most people seem to need 7–8 hours. The nature of the restorative role of sleep is not clear, but periods of enforced wakefulness result in increased sluggishness, irritability and even psychotic behaviour.

There are two principal types of sleep: **orthodox**, slow-wave or non-rapid-eye-movement sleep; and **paradoxical**, **rapid eye movement** (**REM**) sleep.

Sleep typically consists of alternating periods of orthodox and REM sleep every 90 minutes, with the latter occupying progressively more of the cycle. The first 90 minutes of sleep is orthodox, followed by 5–10 minutes of REM sleep, back to orthodox sleep, followed by REM sleep, but lasting longer each time, up to about 50 minutes. REM sleep occupies 20–25% of the total (night's) sleep.

Orthodox sleep involves a fall in arterial blood pressure, respiration and metabolic rate. Serotonin released from the midline raphe nuclei in the reticular formation is thought to generate orthodox sleep by opposing the actions of the reticular activating system (cholinergic), thereby reducing cortical activity. Orthodox sleep is relatively light sleep, from which one is easily aroused.

REM sleep is also known as paradoxical sleep because, although this is deep sleep from which one is not easily aroused, the brain is highly active and the brain waves are more like those recorded when the person is awake. Arterial blood pressure and respiration rise. The eyes move rapidly under the lids and most **dreaming** occurs during this type of sleep. It has been suggested that dreaming is a process whereby the neural network is cleared of meaningless or accidental thoughts by a process of reverse learning. The Freudian view of dreams suggests that they express frustrated desires. Alcohol and sleeping pills generally suppress REM sleep. The noradrenaline released from the locus coeruleus may generate REM sleep. **Narcolepsy** is uncontrolled lapses into REM sleep during waking hours.

Neurotransmitters in the brain

The large number of chemicals in the brain and their relative inaccessibility has made the search for definitive neurotransmitters and their actions very difficult. They are often described as 'putative', to convey the uncertainty that still exists about them. Table 4.1 lists the major neurotransmitters for which there is a moderate degree of consensus. Their cellular modes of action are covered in Chapter 4.

This section describes the following neurotransmitters: acetylcholine, gamma-aminobutyric acid (GABA), dopamine, aspartic acid, glutamic acid, noradrenaline, opioid peptides and serotonin. Their major sites of origin, actions and relationship to illness and drugs are reviewed.

Acetylcholine

There are many pathways in the brain that use acetylcholine as a neurotransmitter. A major source of acetylcholine is the neurones of the gigantocellular nucleus in the excitatory reticular formation (Figure 5.23) which send fibres up to higher levels of the brain and down into the spinal cord.

The effects of acetylcholine in the brain are generally excitatory. It mediates the arousal and wakefulness functions of the reticular formation and is thought to activate mechanisms for storing and recalling memories. Drugs that mimic the actions of acetylcholine induce nausea, vomiting and vertigo. It is deduced, therefore, that acetylcholine is involved in these conditions.

The resting tremor and rigidity that occur in **Parkinson's disease** are attributed to excess production of acetylcholine. Patients with presenile dementia (**Alzheimer's disease**), on the other hand, have been found to have reduced acetylcholine-synthesizing capacity, especially in the hippocampus.

Agonists and antagonists to acetylcholine are covered in Table 9.2.

Gamma-aminobutyric acid (GABA)

The amino acid GABA has a widespread distribution in the brain and is the principal inhibitory neurotransmitter in the higher centres.

GABA deficiency results in a decrease in central inhibitory mechanisms, which leads to convulsive, tetanic and spastic conditions. Loss of GABA in the basal ganglia occurs in both **Huntington's chorea** and **Parkinson's disease**, in which there are impaired voluntary movements (**dyskinesia**). GABA deficiency may be a cause of **epilepsy**, **schizophrenia** and **anxiety states**. Low concentrations of GABA have been measured in the **dementias**.

The effects of GABA are enhanced by the **benzodiazepine** group of drugs which are used as anxiolytics, hypnotics, muscle relaxants, anticonvulsants and sedatives.

Dopamine

Dopamine is a catecholamine, a precursor of adrenaline and noradrenaline as well as acting as a neurotransmitter in its own right. It is excitatory in some areas, inhibitory in others.

Dopamine is also one of the hypothalamic regulatory hormones, prolactin inhibitory hormone.

Schizophrenia is associated with increased activity of dopaminergic neurones in the anterior tegmentum of midbrain. Fibres project into medial and anterior portions of the limbic system, the emotional brain. This psychotic condition is manifested in a variety of ways, including delusions of grandeur, hearing voices, paranoia or incoherent speech. Antipsychotic drugs (also known as neuroleptics or major tranquillizers) such as chlorpromazine act by blocking dopamine receptors.

Parkinson's disease is associated with degeneration of dopaminergic neurones in the substantia nigra (see Figure 5.23) causing tremor and rigidity (see *Basal ganglia*). The precursor of dopamine, **L-dopa**, is given to relieve the rigidity. It crosses the blood–brain barrier (unlike dopamine itself), and is subsequently taken up by dopaminergic neurones, which then synthesize dopamine. Some people with Parkinson's disease develop symptoms of schizophrenia when treated with L-dopa.

> See also **Prolactin** (page 675), in Ch. 17, Sex and Reproduction.

Excitatory amino acids (aspartic and glutamic acids)

The excitatory amino acids aspartic and glutamic acid are found in the brain and spinal cord.

At least half of the synapses in the mammalian CNS are glutaminergic.

The role of the hippocampus in memory storage is thought to be associated with its high concentration of one type of excitatory amino acid receptor, the *N*-methyl-D-aspartate (**NMDA**) **receptor**. Synaptic activity can be enhanced for hours, days or weeks by a mechanism known as long-term potentiation (see *Learning and memory*, below).

High local concentrations of the excitatory amino acid neurotransmitters have a toxic action (**excitotoxic**) within the CNS and are thought to play a role in the aetiology of Alzheimer's disease and other dementias, Huntington's chorea, olivopontino-cerebellar degeneration and brain damage associated with anoxia/ischaemia, hypoglycaemia, stroke and epilepsy.

Excess of excitatory amino acids may cause epilepsy.

Noradrenaline

Noradrenaline (NA) is a catecholamine. The greatest accumulation of noradrenergic nerve-cell bodies is in the brain stem. In the medulla oblongata, the noradrenergic neurones are believed to control peripheral sympathetic tone. In the pons varolii, the locus coeruleus (Figure 5.23) contains nerve-cell bodies from which axons ascend to many parts of the brain. There are also three descending spinal noradrenergic pathways in the posterior, anterior and lateral grey matter, which influence vaso-motor activity and muscle flexion.

NA reaches virtually every area of the brain, where it generally has a stimulating action. The amounts of NA present affect mood and behaviour and vary with the sleep–waking cycle. NA in the locus coeruleus is thought to prevent motor activity during REM sleep (see also *Sleep*, above). NA is also associated with the reward–recognition system (see also *Hypothalamus*, above).

In **endogenous depression**, there is a deficit of stimulation of adrenergic and serotonin receptors in the CNS. Symptoms include grief, unhappiness, despair and misery, loss of appetite, lack of sex drive, insomnia and psychomotor agitation. Antidepressant drugs inhibit the breakdown of NA, thereby returning the level of receptor stimulation to that which is closer to the non-depressed level.

Electroconvulsive therapy (**ECT**), which causes a generalized seizure, like an epileptic attack, has been used to treat depression. One of its effects is to enhance the efficiency of transmission of NA.

Agonists and antagonists to NA are covered in Table 9.4.

Opioid peptides

Opioid peptides have morphine-like actions in the brain – they promote: a fall in heart rate; shallow, slow respiration; cough suppression; analgesia, drowsiness, sleep and euphoria; nausea and vomiting; pupil constriction; and increased release of ADH. There are at least 10 endogenous opioids, which fall into three groups: **enkephalins, endorphins** and **dynorphins**. The principal compounds are leucine-enkephalin (**leu-enkephalin**), methionine-enkephalin (**met-enkephalin**) and **beta-endorphin**.

High concentrations of opiate receptors are found in the posterior horn of spinal cord, the periaqueductal grey matter and medial parts of the thalamus. These regions contain the pain pathways of the anterolateral system, which conducts dull diffuse pain. Exogenous opiate analgesics decrease pain by acting on receptors in these regions.

High concentrations of enkephalins and opiate receptors are found in

See also **Pain pathways** (page 219), in Ch. 7, Sensory Processing.

parts of the limbic system (the amygdala, frontal cortex and hypothalamus). It is probable that this area mediates the analgesic, euphoric and dependency-inducing actions of opiates.

High concentrations of enkephalins and opiate receptors are also found in the brain stem, where opiates cause respiratory depression, nausea, vomiting and cough suppression.

Within the CNS, there are three major opioid receptors: mu, delta and kappa. Mu-receptors, which bind more strongly to beta-endorphin than to the enkephalins, are widely distributed in both the peripheral and central nervous systems, particularly in the brain stem, the trigeminal nucleus, the periaqueductal grey, the neostriatum, the amygdala and the cerebral cortex. Mu-receptors induce hyperpolarization and are therefore generally inhibitory, although in the hippocampus they inhibit the release of GABA presynaptically. Since GABA is an inhibitor, the action here of mu-receptors is excitatory. The centrally induced effects of morphine are mediated by mu-receptors.

Drugs that bind to opiate receptors and act as agonists include morphine, heroin, pethidine, methadone and codeine. The drug naloxone blocks all the opioid receptors, but mu-receptors most strongly.

Serotonin (5-hydroxytryptamine)

Serotonin is a monoamine, is usually inhibitory and is involved in the control of mood and behaviour, including hunger, feeding, sleep and motor activity. Serotonin has an analgesic role in the posterior horn of the spinal cord.

A major collection of serotoninergic nerve-cell bodies is located in the midline raphe nuclei in the pons (Figure 5.23). From here, ascending pathways connect to many areas of the brain and serotoninergic neurones and descending pathways connect with the posterior horn of the spinal cord.

Reduced formation of serotonin, along with noradrenaline, is associated with depression (see *Noradrenaline*, above).

Monoamine oxidase inhibitors block the breakdown of serotonin and **tricyclic antidepressants** block its reuptake by axon endings. These drugs, therefore, increase the amount of serotonin present.

See also **Analgesia in the substantia gelatinosa** (page 220), in Ch. 7, Sensory Processing.

Learning and memory

Memory can be defined as the stored form of learned information which is manifested by the ability to recall it.

There appear to be three different types of memory: **short-term** or **immediate memory** (seconds to minutes); **working memory** (days to weeks); and **long-term memory** (years).

Short-term memory is a temporary store of quite limited capacity, such as a telephone number, which is held in the cerebral cortex. It may become transferred into a longer-term form.

Memory areas in the brain

It is predictable that the neocortex, the area that has evolved into the largest area of the brain, should be associated with its most sophisticated functions, including learning and memory.

The **frontal lobes** are particularly concerned with working memory, which processes and stores information. The information processing involves systems that (1) focus attention on a specific object, (2) receive the language-based or visual information emanating from the object and (3) retrieve the long-term stored information which enables sense to be made of the object. For example, (1) could be a memorandum about equal opportunities policy, (2) would be reading the written words and (3) would be retrieval of the memory of the meaning of the words and related information such as where information about equal opportunities might be found in the filing cabinet or computer.

Working memory may be interrupted by a blow to the head, so that events prior to the accident are not remembered. A similar type of memory loss (**retrograde amnesia**) is induced by deep anaesthesia, coma, brain ischaemia and ECT.

Memory consolidation consists of the transfer of working memories to the long-term memory. The **hippocampus** seems to be central in the organization of long-term memory. It receives stored information from the visual, auditory and vestibular and somatic sensory association areas of the cerebral cortex. The **amygdala** is, like the hippocampus, part of the limbic system, and also functions to receive information. Other areas of the limbic system are also involved, since amnesia follows destruction of the mamillary bodies or bilateral interruption of the fornix.

Damage to the hippocampus results in an inability to store new memories (**anterograde amnesia**) and an inability to remember the position of things (**spatial memory**).

Damage to the amygdala affects the memory of highly pleasurable or highly fearful events.

The processed information is despatched to various parts of the brain for storage including the diencephalon, basal cortex and prefrontal cortex.

Damage to some areas in the thalamus can result in retrograde amnesia.

In Alzheimer's disease, a principal characteristic of which is memory loss, there is loss and disorganization of neurones in the cortical cell layers; the cortical gyri become narrower and the sulci become wider, thereby 'smoothing out' the cerebral cortex.

Neural mechanisms for storing long-term memory

Long-term memory storage is associated with both anatomical and functional changes in the brain as a result of neural pathways being activated. The ability of neurones to change in this way is known as **plasticity**.

Anatomical changes, particularly in the cerebral cortex, hippocampus and cerebellum, have been correlated with increased learning and memory in experimental animals. These changes include an increase in numbers of neuroglia, more dendritic branching, more spines and an increase in the total area from which neurotransmitters are released.

A phenomenon known as **long-term potentiation** (**LTP**) has been suggested as the basis of 'memory traces' or neural pathways used in the storage and retrieval of long-term memories.

Information which is 'meaningful' to the individual appears to involve neural pathways in which synaptic transmission is facilitated. The excitatory amino acid glutamic acid and the NMDA receptors (see *Excitatory amino acids,* above) are thought to be major mediators of LTP. The hippocampus has the highest number of NMDA receptors in the brain. Pharmacological blocking of these receptors results in impaired spatial memory. Normally the NMDA receptor–channel complex is blocked by Mg^{2+}. If the glutaminergic neurones are stimulated strongly (by meaningful information), then sufficient glutamate is released to unblock the NMDA channel and Ca^{2+} enters the postsynaptic cell and activates the intracellular biochemical processes that cause LTP.

6

The spinal cord

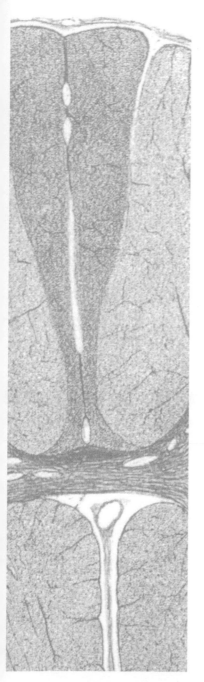

Gross structure and location of the spinal cord

The spinal cord lies within the vertebral canal; its average length is 45 cm in adult European men. It extends from the opening on the underside of the skull (the foramen magnum) to the level of the first or second lumbar vertebrae. Damage to the vertebral column below L2 does not, therefore, damage the spinal cord. Below this the vertebral canal is occu-

Figure 6.1 Longitudinal section of the vertebral column, showing the segmentation of the spinal cord and the origins of the spinal nerves.

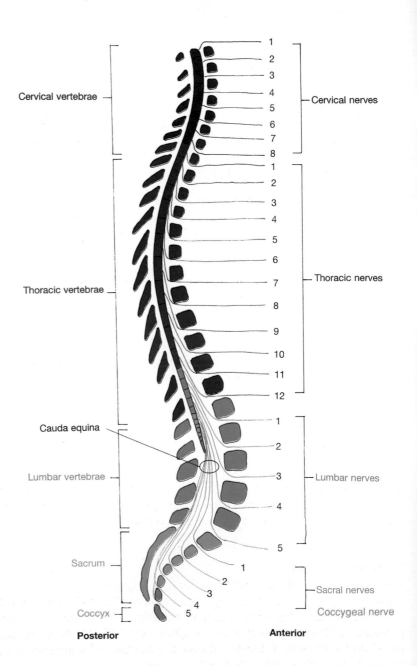

Cervical vertebrae

Cervical nerves

Thoracic vertebrae

Thoracic nerves

Cauda equina

Lumbar vertebrae

Lumbar nerves

Sacrum

Sacral nerves

Coccyx

Coccygeal nerve

Posterior

Anterior

pied by nerve roots from the lumbar and sacral segments of the cord which exit well below their points of origin (Figure 6.1). These nerve roots constitute the **cauda equina**, or 'horse's tail'.

The diameter of the cord narrows from the top to the bottom with enlargements in the cervical and lumbar regions. These enlargements correspond with the origins of the nerves to the upper and lower limbs.

The cord is incompletely divided into right and left halves along the whole of its length by a deep anterior median fissure and a shallow posterior median sulcus (Figure 6.2).

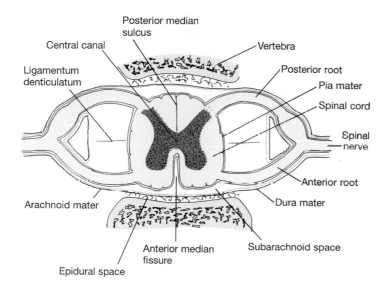

Figure 6.2 Transverse section of the spinal cord and the surrounding meninges.

A central canal filled with CSF runs down the whole length of the cord from the fourth ventricle of the brain.

Lumbar puncture

CSF can be sampled by inserting a needle between the lower lumbar vertebrae, through the dura and arachnoid maters, below the level at which the spinal cord ends. This procedure is known as a lumbar puncture. The nerve roots move aside from the needle. A pressure-measuring manometer attached to the needle measures the pressure of CSF, a sample of which can be withdrawn into a syringe.

Spinal segments

The spinal cord is divided functionally into segments, each of which is connected to one left and one right spinal nerve. These emerge from the vertebral column between adjacent vertebrae. There are 31 spinal segments distributed among five regions; cervical, thoracic, lumbar, sacral and coccygeal. Table 6.1 shows the number of segments, spinal nerves and vertebrae associated with each region.

Table 6.1 Comparison of the numbers of vertebrae and spinal cord segments of each region. Each spinal cord segment is connected to one pair of spinal nerves. With the exception of the first pair of cervical nerves, each pair of spinal nerves emerges below the corresponding vertebra.

Region	Vertebrae	Spinal cord segments and pairs of spinal nerves
Cervical	C1–C7	C1–C8
Thoracic	T1–T12	T1–T12
Lumbar	L1–L5	L1–L5
Sacral	Five fused	S1–S5
Coccygeal	Four or five fused	$C_0 1$

Spinal nerves

The first seven pairs of cervical nerves lie above the equivalent cervical vertebrae, and the eighth pair lies below vertebra C7. Thereafter, each pair of spinal nerves lies below the equivalent vertebra, so that there are 12 pairs of thoracic nerves, five pairs of lumbar nerves, and five pairs of sacral nerves. Although the coccyx comprises four fused vertebrae, there is only one pair of coccygeal nerves (Table 6.1, Figure 6.1)

Each spinal nerve has a **posterior (dorsal) root** and an **anterior (ventral) root**. The posterior roots contain sensory nerve fibres which carry impulses from the periphery to the cord. These neurones are pseudounipolar and have their cell bodies in **posterior root ganglia**, small swellings on the posterior roots. The anterior roots contain fibres of multipolar motor neurones which carry impulses away from the cord.

With the exception of the cervical nerves, all spinal nerve roots travel at least a short distance within the vertebral canal before exiting between the vertebrae.

After only 1–2 cm, each spinal nerve branches into an **anterior** and a **posterior ramus** (and a small meningeal branch, which innervates the blood vessels in the spinal cord meninges). The anterior ramus is connected to the sympathetic chain of ganglia by a **grey** and a **white ramus communicans** (see Figure 9.2).

The posterior and anterior rami, like the short spinal nerves, are mixed. The posterior ramus supplies the skeletal muscles and skin of the posterior trunk, whereas the anterior rami supply the muscles and skin of the rest of the body.

The posterior trunk is innervated in a segmental pattern that corresponds to the points of emergence of the spinal nerves from the spinal cord (Figure 6.3).

With the exception of nerves T2–T12, all anterior rami join interconnecting nerve networks called **nerve plexuses** (Figure 6.4).

As a result of the cross connections made in the plexuses, limb muscles are innervated by neurones from several spinal nerves. This means that damage to one spinal segment or root does not result in complete paralysis of a particular muscle.

Table 6.2 summarizes the distribution of the spinal nerves.

NERVE DAMAGE

Nerve damage is most commonly due to accidents, although compression or stretching of an individual peripheral nerve can lead to damage followed by demyelination. Such mechanically induced lesions typically recover within a few weeks. During the period of hypofunction, the innervated areas have sensory loss and the muscles become wasted and weak.

Compression of the radial nerve against the humerus can occur by adopting an awkward sleeping position, particularly when drunk. The resultant dropped wrist has been termed '**Saturday night palsy**'. Another vulnerable site is the elbow, where prolonged pressure can

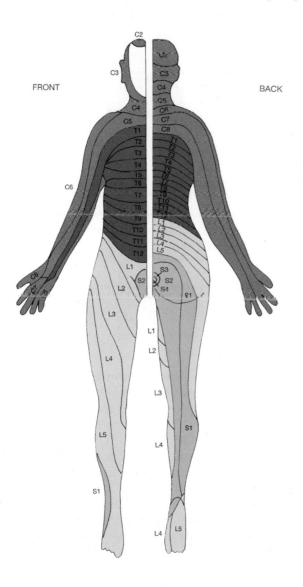

Figure 6.3 Map of the skin dermatomes supplied by spinal nerves. C= cervical; T = thoracic; L = lumbar; S = sacral. (Modified from Williams, P. L., Warwick, R., Dyson, M. and Bannister, L. H. (1989) *Gray's Anatomy*, 37th edn, Churchill Livingstone, Edinburgh).

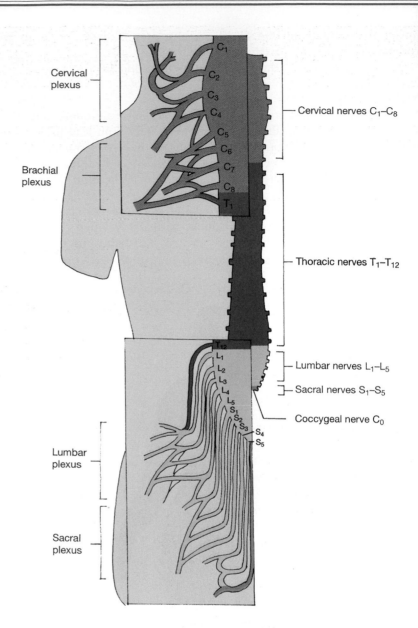

Figure 6.4 Distribution of anterior rami of spinal nerves, most of which connect to nerve plexuses (**inset, enlarged**). Note that there is no thoracic plexus.

cause an ulnar nerve lesion. **Carpal tunnel syndrome** is another example of a compressive neuropathy, in this case due to compression of the median nerve as it passes through the carpal tunnel in the wrist.

NEUROPATHIES

Polyneuropathy affects peripheral nerves in general; paraesthesia and motor weakness usually starts distally and progresses proximally. The causes of polyneuropathy are many and varied including nutritional deficiency (e.g. beriberi), chemical poisoning (e.g. lead and mercury), metabolic (e.g. diabetes mellitus, renal and liver failure), infection (e.g. diphtheria), vascular (e.g. polyarteritis) and malignancy (e.g. carcinoma of the lung).

Table 6.2 Summary of the distribution of the anterior rami of the spinal nerves. All spinal nerves, except T2–T12, form interconnecting plexuses lateral to the vertebral column. The names of the *major nerves* and **areas innervated** are given. The nerves contain sensory and motor neurones.

Ventral rami of spinal nerves	Plexus	Innervation
C1–C4	Cervical	*Nerves from the cervical plexus* innervate skin and muscles of **neck and anterior chest** *Phrenic nerve* innervates **diaphragm**
C5–C8, T1	Brachial	*Axillary, musculocutaneous, median, ulnar and radial nerves* innervate **upper limb**
T2–T12	None	*Intercostal (T2–T12) and subcostal (T12) nerves* innervate **intercostal muscles** and **skin of anterolateral chest wall, subcostal and abdominal muscles**
L1–L4	Lumbar	*Femoral and obdurator nerves* innervate **anterior and medial thigh**
L4–S4	Sacral	*Sciatic nerve* innervates **posterior thigh** *Tibial* and *common peroneal nerves* innervate **leg** *Superior* and *inferior gluteal nerves* innervate **buttocks** *Pudendal nerve* innervates **perineum**

Discrete lesions in several peripheral nerves can occur simultaneously, for example in diabetes mellitus and leprosy.

Blood supply of the spinal cord

Blood enters the cord from a series of anastomotic channels derived from branches of the intercostal, vertebral, deep cervical and lumbar arteries and the anterior and posterior spinal arteries (Figure 6.5).

Blood drains out of the cord into six vessels which form a tortuous plexus in the pia mater. They drain into the intervertebral veins.

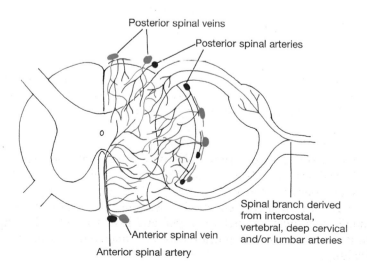

Posterior spinal veins
Posterior spinal arteries
Anterior spinal vein
Anterior spinal artery
Spinal branch derived from intercostal, vertebral, deep cervical and/or lumbar arteries

Figure 6.5 Arterial supply and venous drainage of the spinal cord (left side only).

Spinal meninges

The spinal cord is surrounded and protected by the same three meninges that cover the brain. The innermost meninx, the **pia mater**, is closely attached to the surface of the cord and is separated from the **arachnoid mater** by the subarachnoid space, which contains CSF. The arachnoid mater is separated by a potential space, the subdural space, from the tough, outer **dura mater** (Figure 6.2). In contrast to the dura mater surrounding the brain and lining the skull, the dura mater around the spinal cord is a single layer only.

Outside the dura is the **epidural (extradural) space**, which is filled with fatty tissue and which contains the epidural veins. These tissues separate the dura from the wall of the vertebral canal.

An injection given into the epidural space, such as anaesthetic given during childbirth, can spread for a short distance upwards, downwards or laterally to adjacent areas. Fluid, such as a dye, injected under pressure into the sacral hiatus can reach the base of the skull in the epidural space. As the brain, in contrast to the spinal cord, is surrounded by a double layer of dura mater, epidural injections do not affect the brain (see Figure 5.24).

The pia mater is connected to the dura mater at each thoracic and cervical segment by means of a **ligamentum denticulatum** on each side. These anchor the cord to the dura. The lower end of the cord is anchored to the lower end of the vertebral column by an extension of the pia mater, the filum terminale.

Pathways and neuronal circuits in the spinal cord

In transverse section, the spinal cord consists of two distinct regions (Figure 6.6).

In the centre is an H-shaped mass of grey matter which is embedded

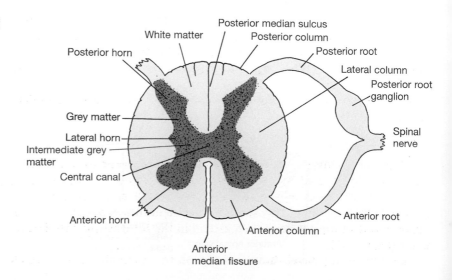

Figure 6.6 Transverse section of the spinal cord showing the principal regions of grey and white matter.

in the surrounding **white matter**. The posterior (dorsal) and anterior (ventral) projections of the grey matter are known as the **posterior** and **anterior horns**, with **intermediate grey matter** in between the two. Additionally, in the thoracic, upper lumbar and sacral regions there are short **lateral horns** or **columns**. The white matter may be separated into three regions on each side of the cord: the **posterior**, **anterior** and **lateral columns**. The grey matter consists of large numbers of nerve cell bodies, their processes (mostly unmyelinated) and neuroglia. The colour of the white matter is due to the presence of large numbers of myelinated axons.

White matter

The white matter of the spinal cord consists mainly of nerve axons which are grouped together to form tracts. These are usually named according to their position in the white matter and their points of origin and termination. The lateral corticospinal tract, for example, is found in the lateral column of the white matter, and it contains neurones that connect the motor cortex with the spinal cord. Within each tract, information being transmitted to or from a specific part of the body travels along neurones that occupy a particular position. This is described as **somatotopic organization**.

Ascending tracts carry sensory information to the brain, and different sensory modalities are conveyed by separate tracts. Descending tracts transmit motor information to all levels of the cord. Since the two sides of the cord are mirror images, each tract is duplicated on the opposite side.

ASCENDING (SENSORY) PATHWAYS

Sensory pathways in the spinal cord fall into two groups: the anterolateral system and the posterior column–lemniscal system.

The anterolateral system includes sensory pathways in the lateral and the anterior areas of white matter. The pathways convey the modalities of pain, temperature, crude touch, pressure, tickle, itch and sexual sensations.

The posterior column–lemniscal system includes those sensory pathways that travel in the posterior white matter of the spinal cord to the medulla, cross over and then ascend in the medial lemniscus to the thalamus. The pathways convey the modalities of fine touch, vibration and proprioception.

Sensory pathways comprise three consecutive neurones: first-order, second-order and third-order neurones (see Figures 7.5 and 7.6).

Anterolateral system

The first-order sensory neurones of **pain** and **temperature pathways** enter the spinal cord and then ascend or descend for one or two segments before entering the posterior grey matter and synapsing with second-order neurones. The second-order neurones cross over to the opposite side of the cord and then ascend in the **lateral spinothalamic tract** (Figure 6.7).

These neurones travel through the pons and midbrain in the medial

See also **Somatic sensory pathways** (page 217), in Ch. 7, Sensory Processing.

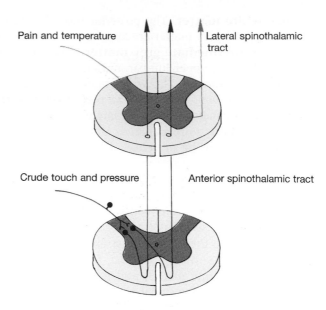

Figure 6.7 The anterolateral system. **Pain and temperature:** second-order neurones cross over and ascend in the lateral spinothalamic tract. **Crude touch and pressure:** some second-order neurones cross over and ascend in the anterior spinothalamic tract, others ascend in the corresponding tract on the same side.

lemniscus. They synapse with third-order neurones in the thalamus. The third-order neurones pass through the internal capsule to the somatic sensory cortex in the postcentral gyrus of the parietal lobe of the cerebrum.

Crude touch and **pressure pathways** travel a similar route to those for pain and temperature, but in the **anterior spinothalamic tracts** on either side of the cord (Figure 6.7). There is a difference, however, in that some of the fibres do not cross over in the spinal cord but ascend on the same side to the medulla, cross over and ascend to the thalamus.

Posterior column–lemniscal system

The first-order sensory neurones of pathways involving conscious proprioception, fine touch and vibration ascend in two tracts in the posterior white matter, the **fasciculus gracilis** and **fasciculus cuneatus**, (Figure 6.8) before synapsing in the medulla oblongata.

The fasciculus gracilis runs the whole length of the cord and contains fibres from the lower part of the body up to the midthorax. As additional fibres are added at each higher level, the existing ones are displaced medially (Figure 6.8). The fasciculus cuneatus arises in the thoracic region and contains fibres that derive from the upper thoracic and cervical nerves. These first-order neurones also have collateral branches in the grey matter, which relay with reflex spinal pathways as well as to the spinocerebellar tracts.

A third group of fibres in the posterior column, the **posterior spinocerebellar tract** (Figure 6.9), conveys proprioceptive information, mainly arising in muscle spindles, from the trunk and lower limbs to the cerebellum on the same side.

The **anterior spinocerebellar tract** (Figure 6.9) also conveys proprioceptive information, although less than the posterior spinocerebellar tract, from the trunk and lower limbs to the cerebellum on the same

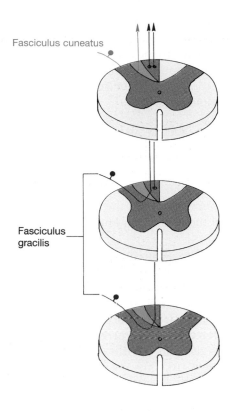

Figure 6.8 The posterior column–lemniscal system (fine touch, vibration and proprioception). The fasciculus gracilis contains fibres from midthorax downwards. The fasciculus cuneatus contains fibres from midthorax upwards. As additional fibres are added at each higher level, the existing ones are displaced medially.

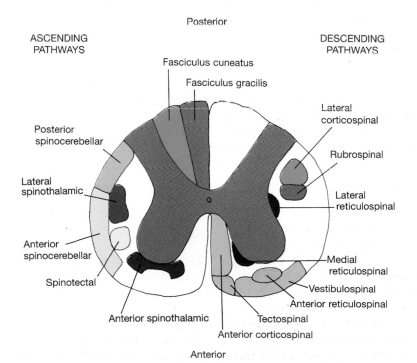

Figure 6.9 Pathways in the white matter of the spinal cord. For clarity ascending and descending pathways are shown on one side only.

side. The anterior spinocerebellar tract is stimulated by motor signals from the corticospinal and rubrospinal tracts, thereby conveying feedback on muscle movements to the cerebellum.

As the spinocerebellar tracts terminate in the cerebellum rather than the somatic sensory cortex, the impulses propagated along these tracts do not result in conscious sensation.

DESCENDING (MOTOR) PATHWAYS

Lateral and anterior corticospinal (pyramidal) tracts

The corticospinal tracts connect the motor cortex, and other parts of the cerebral cortex, with lower motor neurones that innervate skeletal muscle. They are concerned with the regulation of voluntary movements, particularly of the most distal muscles such as those in the fingers and toes.

The axons of neurones from the cerebral cortex, known as upper motor neurones, pass through the internal capsule, the cerebral peduncle and pons before reaching the medulla oblongata. About 80% of the fibres cross over in the medullary pyramids and enter the white matter of the cord in the lateral corticospinal tract (Figure 6.10). About 5% of the fibres enter the lateral corticospinal tract on the same side. The remaining fibres descend on the same side in the anterior corticospinal tract (Figure 6.10), crossing over in the spinal cord at the cervical and upper thoracic levels. The name 'pyramidal tract' refers to the pyramids in the medulla oblongata. The name 'corticospinal tract' is, however, more meaningful in that it conveys that the tract starts in the motor cortex and travels in the spinal cord. If 'lateral' or 'anterior' are added to 'corticospinal', then this specifies which region of the white matter in the spinal cord contains the tract.

Figure 6.10 The anterior and lateral corticospinal (pyramidal) tracts. About 80% of the upper motor neurones cross over in the medulla oblongata and descend in the lateral corticospinal tract; 15% of the upper motor neurones descend on the same side in the anterior corticospinal tract until they reach the cervical and upper thoracic levels, where they cross over. The upper motor neurones relay with interneurones and then with lower motor neurones, which innervate skeletal muscles.

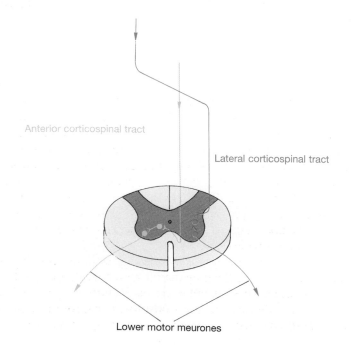

Anterior corticospinal tract

Lateral corticospinal tract

Lower motor meurones

Most corticospinal neurones terminate on interneurones in the intermediate grey matter, although those that control the limb muscles terminate directly on the cell bodies of lower motor neurones lying in the lateral region of each anterior horn. The anterior tract is present only in the cervical and upper thoracic levels, because its fibres supply motor neurones to the neck muscles, whereas the lateral tract extends the whole length of the cord.

See also **Neural control of voluntary movement** (page 299), in Ch. 9, Autonomic and Somatic Motor Activity.

Subcorticospinal (extrapyramidal) tracts

The term **extrapyramidal pathways** has traditionally been used to describe pathways other than those originating in the cerebral cortex and passing through the medullary pyramids to the spinal cord. The term is now seldom used, mainly because it covers such a diversity of pathways that a particular function cannot be ascribed to it. Also, since the medullary pyramids contain some extrapyramidal fibres, the nomenclature is confusing.

There are several motor pathways to skeletal muscle arising in the brain stem which can be called 'subcorticospinal' pathways, thereby distinguishing them from corticospinal pathways.

The **vestibulospinal tract** (Figure 6.9) arises from cells in the vestibular nucleus of the pons. Fibres descend uncrossed and terminate around motor cells in the anterior grey matter. The tract conveys impulses that affect posture and balance.

The **rubrospinal tract** (Figure 6.9) originates from nerve cells in the red nucleus of the midbrain. Fibres cross over and then descend on the opposite side and terminate in the anterior grey matter. The tract controls movements of the limbs and contributes to the maintenance of muscle tone.

Other subcorticospinal tracts include the **lateral**, **medial** and **anterior reticulospinal** (from the reticular formation) and the **tectospinal** (from the tectum in the midbrain).

Grey matter

The colour of grey matter is due to the presence of large numbers of nerve cell bodies that contain dark-staining nuclei. These cell bodies are grouped according to function. The cell bodies of somatic motor neurones are found in the anterior horns of the grey matter, whereas autonomic preganglionic neurones are found in the lateral horns. The posterior horns contain the cell bodies of the first interneurones in pathways which connect: 1) the posterior and anterior horns, 2) one side of the cord to the other, and 3) one segment of the cord to another. Interneurones are approximately 30 times more numerous than other neurones; they are found in all parts of the grey matter and are collectively called the **interneurone pool**.

The grey matter can be subdivided into nine, roughly parallel **laminae** on each side of the grey matter with a tenth around the central canal (Figure 6.11). These laminae are distinguished by the appearance, size, shape and density of the constituent neurones. Functionally, laminae I–VI receive first-order sensory neurones, VII–VIII contain much

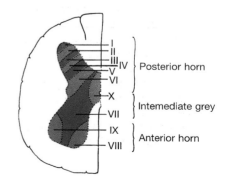

Figure 6.11 Transverse section of half of the spinal cord, showing the laminae in the grey matter.

of the interneurone pool, and IX contains the cell bodies of somatic motor neurones (both alpha and gamma, see *Stretch reflex*, below).

First-order neurones conveying pain and temperature terminate in laminae I, II and III. Laminae II and III are collectively known as the **substantia gelatinosa**. Laminae I, IV, V and VI contain the cell bodies of second-order neurones of the anterolateral system; their fibres cross to the other side of the cord in the anterior commissure.

CIRCUITS IN THE INTERNEURONE POOL

The CNS contains a very large number of collections of interconnecting groups of neurones described as neuronal pools. Impulses are trans-

Figure 6.12 Neuronal pools in the spinal cord. Input neurones on the left; output neurones on the right.
(a) Converging pathway.
(b) Diverging pathway.
(c) Reciprocal innervation circuit.
(d) Parallel circuits.
(e) Reverberating circuit.

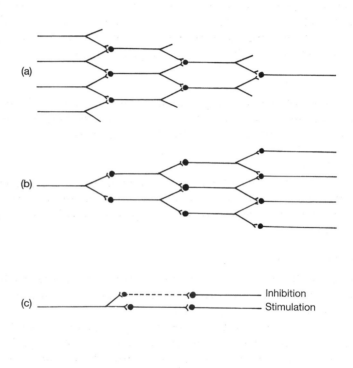

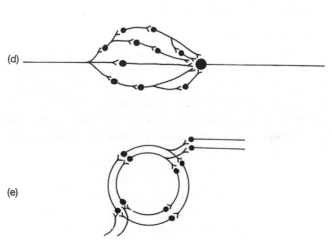

mitted into the interneurone pool through afferent (input) fibres and leave via efferent (output) fibres. The interneurone pools described here (Figure 6.12) enable impulses to:

- converge upon a final common pathway;
- diverge along a number of different routes;
- bring about reciprocal inhibition;
- prolong neural activity.

Convergence

Impulses may enter the pool along several afferent fibres to stimulate a smaller number of efferent fibres. The impulses entering the pool may come from a single source or from a number of sources. Interneurones in the grey matter of the spinal cord receive inputs from a number of sources, so that first-order sensory neurones, other interneurones and neurones in descending pathways all converge upon them.

Divergence

A small number of afferent fibres stimulate a larger number of efferent fibres. This is found in corticospinal pathways: a single pyramidal cell in the cerebral cortex may excite up to 10 000 muscle fibres.

Reciprocal inhibition

Afferent impulses may cause excitation of some neurones and inhibition of others in the pool. This type of arrangement is found in the reciprocal inhibition circuits that regulate antagonistic pairs of muscles (see *Spinal reflexes*, below).

Circuits that prolong neural activity

Figure 6.12(d) shows a parallel circuit in which the pathways have different numbers of synapses. As a result, impulses arrive sequentially at the output fibre and prolong neural activity.

The neurones in reverberatory or oscillatory circuits (Figure 6.12(e)) are arranged so that their output re-stimulates the same pathway. Impulses may therefore continue to pass around the circuit for up to several hours following a single stimulation.

NEUROTRANSMITTERS IN THE SPINAL CORD

Many of the neurotransmitters that are found in the spinal cord are also found in the brain (see *Neurotransmitters in the brain*, Ch. 5, for details).

There are differences in distribution of the neurotransmitters in the two sites. The major inhibitory amino acid neurotransmitter in the brain is GABA, whereas in the spinal cord it is glycine. Table 6.3 summarizes the location and functions of the major neurotransmitters in the spinal cord.

Table 6.3 Major neurotransmitters in the spinal cord

Name	Location	Functions
Acetylcholine	Anterior horns	Regulates motor activity
Aspartic acid	Posterior and anterior horns	Regulates motor activity Spinal reflexes
Enkephalins	Posterior horn	Analgesia
GABA	Posterior horn	Spinal reflexes Pain modulation
Glutamic acid	Posterior horn	Relays sensory and regulates motor activity
Glycine	Anterior horn	Regulates motor activity Spinal reflexes
Noradrenaline	Lateral grey	Vasomotor tone
Serotonin	Posterior horn	Pain modulation
Substance P	Posterior horn	Pain Weal of axon reflex

Spinal reflexes

Autonomic reflexes: **Vascular reflexes** (page 407), in Ch. 12, Circulation of Blood and Lymph. **Reflex sweating induced by a local rise in skin temperature** (page 319), in Ch. 10, The Skin and the Regulation of Body Temperature. **Reflex secretion and movements in the gut** are covered in Chapter 15, Digestion and Absorption of Food. **Micturition** (page 478), in Ch. 14, Renal Control of Body Fluid Volume and Composition.

In addition to its role in the transmission of information to and from the brain, the spinal cord also has an integrative function, particularly with respect to reflexes. A reflex is a rapid, automatic response to a stimulus, a particular stimulus always causing the same response. Tapping the knee, for example, causes the leg to jerk forwards; stepping on a drawing pin results in withdrawal of the foot by bending the leg.

This section covers reflex activity involving skeletal muscle, innervated by somatic motor neurones, i.e. somatic reflexes. In addition to these, there are a large number of reflexes involving the autonomic nervous system that are mediated through pathways in the spinal cord.

Reflex arc

The components of a reflex pathway or arc are: 1) a sensory receptor; 2) a sensory neurone; 3) an integrating 'centre', usually within the CNS; 4) a motor neurone; and 5) an effector (skeletal muscle in the case of a somatic reflex, Figure 6.13).

The stimulus activates a sensory receptor, which is connected to a sensory neurone. All first-order sensory neurones enter the spinal cord through the posterior roots, with their cell bodies lying within the posterior root ganglia. Once inside the spinal cord, the sensory neurones branch, one or more branches serving the reflex pathways covering a few (in some cases many) segments of the cord, and another branch conveying sensory information to the brain.

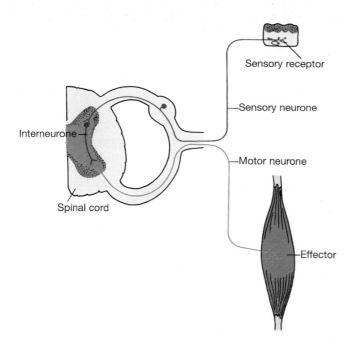

Figure 6.13 The components of a polysynaptic reflex arc.

Most reflexes are **polysynaptic**, i.e. there is at least one interneurone and therefore at least two synapses in the pathway between the sensory neurone and the motor neurone. The stretch reflex, however, has no such interneurone, and is therefore designated as **monosynaptic**. Synaptic transmission is relatively slow compared with the propagation of impulses along neurones, so that the more synapses a nerve pathway has, the longer it takes for impulses to be propagated along it.

Stretch reflex

A sharp tap on the patellar tendon leads to a contraction of the quadriceps femoris muscle, which raises the leg. This is a demonstration of the **knee-jerk reflex**, a type of stretch reflex. Tapping the tendon stretches the muscle, and receptors within it initiate impulses along the sensory neurones to the spinal cord (Figure 6.14).

The sensory neurones synapse directly with somatic motor neurones which are thereby stimulated and cause muscle contraction. Stretching a muscle, therefore, initiates a reflex which tends to counteract the change. Stretch reflexes can be initiated by stretching any muscle. They are the only monosynaptic reflexes in the body.

MUSCLE SPINDLE

Muscle spindles contain the sensory nerve endings that are stimulated by stretch. Each muscle spindle contains up to 14 small fibres, 1–5 mm long, which lack the striations caused by the regular arrangement of myofilaments in their central regions. Spindle fibres are known as **intrafusal fibres** to distinguish them from ordinary muscle or **extrafusal fibres**. The intrafusal fibres are enclosed in a connective tissue capsule and

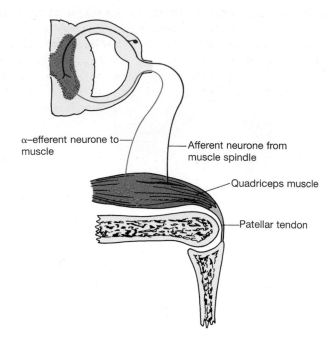

Figure 6.14 The monosynaptic nerve pathway of the stretch reflex.

α–efferent neurone to muscle

Afferent neurone from muscle spindle

Quadriceps muscle

Patellar tendon

Figure 6.15 A muscle spindle.

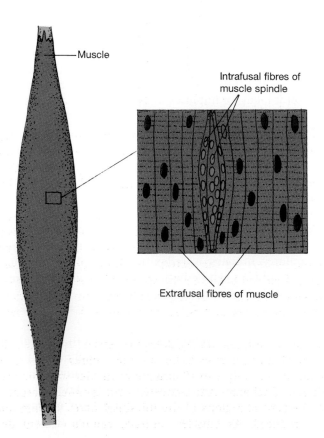

Muscle

Intrafusal fibres of muscle spindle

Extrafusal fibres of muscle

attached to the connective tissue sheaths of the surrounding extrafusal fibres and are orientated parallel to them (Figure 6.15).

There are two types of intrafusal fibre: nuclear bag and nuclear chain fibres. **Nuclear bag fibres** are larger, with a swollen central region containing many nuclei. **Nuclear chain fibres** are narrower and their nuclei are arranged in a row in the central region (Figure 6.16).

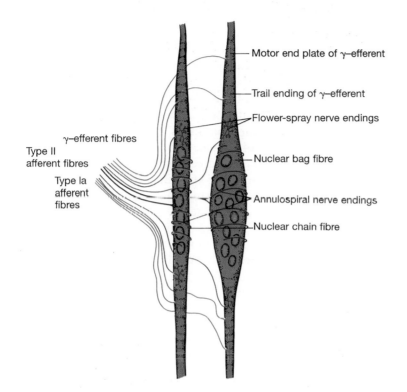

Motor end plate of γ–efferent

Trail ending of γ–efferent

Flower-spray nerve endings

γ–efferent fibres

Type II afferent fibres

Type Ia afferent fibres

Nuclear bag fibre

Annulospiral nerve endings

Nuclear chain fibre

Figure 6.16 The intrafusal fibres of a muscle spindle and their innervation.

Both types of fibre are innervated by large myelinated (type Ia) sensory neurones. Annulospiral nerve endings wrap around the non-contractile central regions of the fibres. A second type of smaller sensory neurone (type II) has flower-spray terminals on either side of the type I junctions, mainly on the nuclear chain fibres.

Motor innervation of the intrafusal fibres is by small-diameter neurones, known as **gamma-efferents** (γ-efferents), to distinguish them from the larger somatic motor neurones or **alpha-efferents** (α-efferents), that innervate the extrafusal fibres. Both types of motor neurone have their cell bodies in the anterior horns of the grey matter. The gamma-efferents can be further subdivided into those that end in typical motor end-plates and those that end in less specialized trail-endings.

Gamma-efferent stimulation regulates the sensitivity of the spindle by causing contraction of the ends of the intrafusal fibres. This stretches the central region so that only a small amount of further stretching will lead to rapid afferent discharge. Alternatively, if the gamma-efferent activity is reduced, the central regions of the intrafusal fibres slacken and their sensitivity is reduced. As muscles contract, gamma-efferent discharge

See also **Reticular formation** (page 164), in Ch. 5, The Brain.

causes concomitant shortening of the intrafusal fibres so that they maintain their sensitivity. The activity of these gamma-efferents is regulated by descending spinal pathways which originate in the reticular formation in the brain stem.

Muscle spindles are a type of proprioceptor that play an important role in the maintenance of **posture** since they provide constant feedback to the cerebellum through the posterior spinocerebellar tracts. The cerebellum, in turn, controls gamma-efferent activity via the brain stem.

DYNAMIC AND STATIC STRETCH REFLEXES

The knee-jerk reflex is an example of a **dynamic stretch reflex**. The actual stimulus, induced by a tap on the knee, is the increasing length of the intrafusal fibres, primarily the nuclear bag fibres.

A stretched muscle stimulates both type Ia and type II sensory nerve endings, mainly in the nuclear chain fibres. The frequency of discharge is proportional to the degree of stretch. The resulting muscle contraction will also be in proportion to the degree of stretch and lasts as long as the muscle is stretched; this is the **static stretch reflex**.

Reciprocal inhibition of the opposing muscle during the stretch reflex is brought about by a pathway that includes a collateral branch from the Ia sensory neurone, which synapses with an inhibitory interneurone. The latter then synapses with a motor neurone to the antagonistic muscle. In the knee-jerk reflex, when the stretch reflex causes the quadriceps muscle to contract, the antagonistic (hamstring) muscle is inhibited. Reciprocal inhibition is illustrated in Figures 6.12 and 6.18.

MUSCLE TONE

Since muscle spindles are stimulated when muscles are stretched and their action is to oppose that stretch, then they have a damping function i.e. they help to smooth out contractions that would otherwise be very jerky.

Passive stretching of a muscle induces the stretch reflex which opposes the stretch. This constitutes **muscle tone**, which exerts a slight inhibitory influence upon passive movements of the limbs. Excessive tone results in a **spastic** muscle in which passive stretching is very difficult, and very low tone results in floppy or **flaccid** muscles.

Golgi tendon reflexes

There are two reflexes initiated by Golgi tendon organs: the inverse stretch reflex and the tendon reflex. In both cases, increased tension in a tendon results in reflex muscle relaxation. Tendon tension is increased by both muscle relaxation and contraction.

GOLGI TENDON ORGAN

Golgi tendon organs are found in tendons, near the junction with the muscle. Each organ is 500–700 µm long and consists of an encapsulated bundle of tendon fibres, which are innervated by Ib sensory fibres with spray-type endings (Figure 6.17).

Impulses from the Golgi tendon organs ascend to the cerebellum and to the cerebral cortex, conveying proprioceptive information.

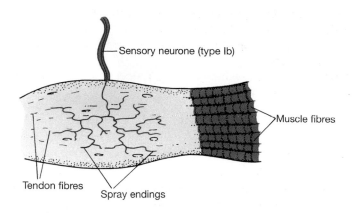

Figure 6.17 Golgi tendon organ.

INVERSE STRETCH REFLEX

Passive stretch of a muscle will only increase the tension in the tendon slightly and the Golgi tendon organs are unaffected. If, however, a muscle is stretched a lot, the stretch reflex initiated by the muscle spindles is suddenly replaced by relaxation, the inverse stretch reflex, initiated by stimulation of the Golgi tendon organs.

DYNAMIC AND STATIC TENDON REFLEXES

The tendon reflexes are the converse of the stretch reflexes. While a muscle is contracting, a burst of impulses is generated from the Golgi tendon organ. The sensory neurones transmit the impulses to the spinal cord where they are relayed to interneurones, which inhibit activity in the somatic motor neurones to the muscle, thereby causing muscle relaxation. During muscle contraction, therefore, the tendon organs elicit a dynamic tendon reflex.

As long as the muscle contracts and exerts tension on the tendon, the Golgi tendon organs are stimulated proportionally and cause reflex muscle relaxation (static tendon reflex), which has a damping function in the control of muscle movement.

Flexor (withdrawal) reflex

A painful stimulus to the hand or foot initiates reflex contraction of the flexor muscles, which causes withdrawal of the arm or leg, respectively, from the source of the pain. Reciprocal innervation causes simultaneous inhibition of the extensor muscles (Figure 6.18), which facilitates the bending action of the limb.

Diverging pathways (Figure 6.12(b)) cause accessory muscles (e.g. trunk and shoulder muscles) to be stimulated, aiding movement of the limb. Pathways that prolong neural activity are also involved (Figure 6.12(d) and (e)), so that the muscular responses can last as long as a few seconds.

Crossed extensor reflex

A strong painful stimulus will not only induce withdrawal of the affected limb, but also extension of the other limb (Figure 6.18). Afferent

Figure 6.18 Nerve pathways of the flexor and crossed extensor reflexes. In the **flexor reflex**, a painful stimulus is applied to the right hand (left-hand side of the diagram). The sensory neurone transmits the impulses into the interneurone pool of the grey matter. A minimum number of interneurones is shown here for the motor neurone to the flexor muscle to be stimulated by one interneurone [purple] and the motor neurone to the extensor muscle to be inhibited by a different interneurone [broken line]. The arm consequently flexes, moving the hand away from the source of the pain. In the **crossed extensor reflex**, a collateral from the interneurone in the flexor reflex pathway is shown crossing over to the other side of the cord and synapsing with one interneurone [purple], which stimulates extension of the opposite limb, and a second interneurone [broken line], which causes relaxation of the flexor muscle by inhibiting the motor neurone to it. The opposite arm therefore straightens, pushing the body away from the source of the pain.

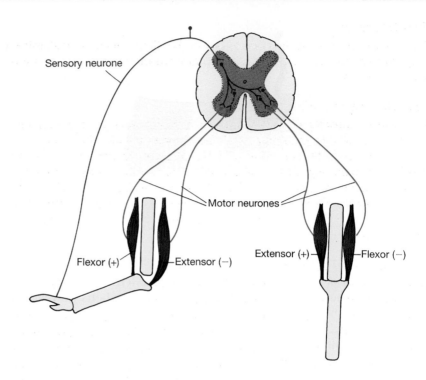

impulses to the cord pass through a series of interneurones to the opposite side. Here, the synapses are so arranged that stimulation of the extensor muscle and inhibition of the flexor muscle occur. The presence of a number of synapses in the pathway causes a delay of up to 0.5 s in the crossed extensor reaction.

The action of the crossed extensor reflex can be illustrated by the example of stepping on a drawing pin with the left foot. The flexor response causes the leg to bend, lifting the foot off the floor. The crossed extensor reflex causes the right leg to straighten, providing support to the body.

Standing and walking

Pressure on the underside of the foot causes the limb to extend against the pressure. This is called the **positive supportive reaction**, a spinal reflex.

Although walking is a voluntary activity controlled by the motor areas of the brain, the rhythmic movements, particularly of the legs but also of the arms, shoulders, trunk and hips, are mediated by central pattern generators in the spinal cord.

Stepping movements comprise repeated cycles of forward flexion followed by backward extension of each limb. Reciprocal inhibition circuits in the spinal cord 1) inhibit extensor muscles during flexion of a limb and vice versa and 2) cause one limb to move back when the other moves forwards.

Sensory signals from the feet and limb proprioceptors influence the amount of foot pressure and the rate of walking.

Scratch reflex

The sensation of a tickle or itch caused by light touch or histamine, respectively, initiates scratching, a two and fro movement akin to stepping movements.

Muscle spasm induced by pain

Pain causes muscles in the vicinity to contract, so that, for example, contraction of the abdominal wall accompanies abdominal pain and muscles around a broken bone contract. **Muscle 'cramp'** is thought to result from pain, e.g. to be due to ischaemia causing reflex contraction which, in turn, increases the ischaemia, a positive feedback cycle. If the antagonistic muscle is voluntarily contracted, it is possible to stimulate the reciprocal inhibition circuits and thereby reduce the contraction in the affected muscle.

Plantar reflex and the Babinski sign

If a blunt object is drawn along the lateral sole of the foot, the usual response is that the toes bend downwards towards the floor, as in walking. This response is not, however, the reflex response, but is controlled by the corticospinal tract. Should there be any damage to the foot area of the primary motor cortex or the corticospinal tract, then the stimulus results in dorsiflexion of the big toe and a fanning out of the other toes. This response is known as the Babinski sign and demonstrates the spinal reflex without the influence of the voluntary motor pathway from the brain. The Babinski sign is also present in babies one year old, before myelination of the corticospinal tract is complete.

Effects of damage to the spinal cord

Damage to a specific part of the spinal cord that transects the whole cord results in loss of motor function in muscles (**paralysis**) and loss of sensation (**paraesthesia**) from all parts of the body innervated from below the lesion. This is because the descending motor and ascending sensory pathways have been interrupted.

Spinal shock

The short term effect of spinal cord damage (3–14 days) is known as spinal shock and is due to the lack of neural input from the brain. Skeletal muscles are completely relaxed (flaccid) and spinal reflexes are temporarily lost, including the micturition reflex and maintenance of vasomotor tone. Reflex activity recovers in stages, flexor reflexes return first followed by extensor ones, which become exaggerated.

If the spinal cord injury is above T6, episodes of **mass reflex** activity involving both autonomic and somatic motor neurones can occur in response to hitherto trivial stimuli. There are flexor spasms, and autonomic actions such as excess sweating, evacuation of the bladder and colon and very high arterial blood pressure. The mass reflex has been described as epilepsy of the spinal cord.

See also **Excess activity within the CNS (epilepsy)** (page 177), in Ch. 5, The Brain.

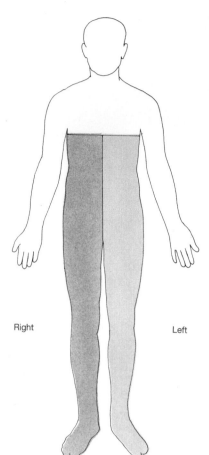

Right   Left

Figure 6.19 Effects of right hemisection of the spinal cord in the mid-thoracic region: the Brown–Séquard syndrome. Pain and temperature [green] is lost on the opposite side below the lesion, because the pathways cross over in the spinal cord. Fine touch, proprioception and vibration is lost and muscles are paralysed [orange] on the same side below the lesion, because the pathways cross over in the brain.

Hemisection of the spinal cord (Brown–Séquard syndrome)

If the damage is confined to one side of the spinal cord, then paralysis of the same side (**ipsilateral**) below the damage occurs (Figure 6.19).

This is because most motor fibres are carried in the corticospinal tract, which crosses over in the brain. Pain and temperature sensations are lost from the opposite (**contralateral**) side below the lesion, because the lateral spinothalamic pathways cross over in the spinal cord. Crude touch and pressure, however, are transmitted in the anterior spinothalamic tracts both on the ipsilateral side as well as contralaterally, so that some sensation from each side is maintained. The perception of proprioception, fine touch and vibration is lost ipsilaterally, however, as these modalities are conveyed in the posterior column–lemniscal system, which does not cross over in the spinal cord.

Destruction of motor neurones in the anterior horns (poliomyelitis)

The poliovirus causes inflammation and destruction of the motor neurones in the anterior horns of the grey matter. Loss of reflex or voluntary muscle movement can result, in a limb or other muscle groups such as the respiratory muscles. Paralysed muscles atrophy rapidly.

Incomplete closure of the neural plate (spina bifida)

Sometimes during development, the neural plate fails to close. This occurs most often in the lumbosacral region and gives rise to the condition known as spina bifida. In its mildest form (**spina bifida occulta**) only the vertebrae do not close up, but the structures are covered by skin. In its most severe form (**spina bifida aperta**), the neural plate does not close at all and the spinal cord is laid open. This leads to impaired neural control of the legs, rectum and bladder, as well as a predisposition to infection.

7

Sensory processing

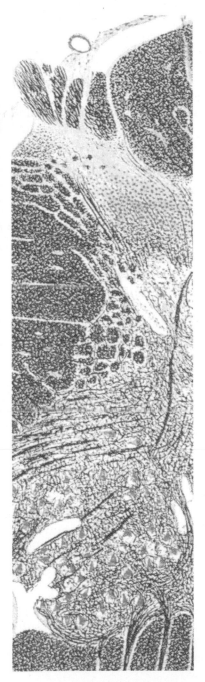

Overview of sensory processing

The conscious experience of a sensation involves the generation of action potentials along sensory pathways, beginning with a sensory receptor in the tissues and ending in the cerebral cortex of the brain. Depending upon the area of the cortex where the pathways terminate, sensations of a particular type are experienced. Stimulation of the eyes by light, for example, results in the passage of impulses to the visual cortex at the back of the brain and an image is 'seen'; impulses generated by sound in the ears are propagated along auditory pathways to the auditory areas of the cerebral cortices and sound is 'heard'.

The ability to discriminate one sensation from another also depends on the specificity of sensory receptors to particular stimuli. Touch receptors are only stimulated by touch, cold receptors by cold and so on.

For the general body (**somatic**) **senses** of touch, pressure, cold and heat, the stimulus that initiates activity in specific sensory pathways and elicits a particular sensation is known as its **modality**. The sensation of pain is different from the other sensations because it is elicited by a variety of different stimuli, mechanical, chemical and thermal.

Sensory receptors convert stimuli into action potentials, which are then propagated along sensory pathways which terminate in the cerebral cortex. The somatic senses terminate in the primary somatic sensory (somaesthetic) cortex; the special senses of taste, smell, sight and hearing and balance have separate sensory areas in the cerebral cortex.

The stimulation of all sensory receptors does not give rise to a conscious sensory experience. Many of the deep-lying receptors such as baroreceptors, arterial chemoreceptors and osmoreceptors are vital parts of the regulation of the internal environment but, because the sensory pathways do not reach the sensory cortex, no conscious sensation is perceived.

The labelled line principle

The all or nothing principle is described in **Threshold potential** (page 119), in Ch. 4, Cellular Mechanisms of Neural Control.

Action potentials are all the same size, and so cannot distinguish between different sensations. It is the spatial separation of the neural pathways that determines the nature and perceived location of sensations. A particular modality activates a specific sensory receptor which, in turn, activates a specific sensory pathway, which terminates in a particular part of the sensory cortex. This is known as the labelled line principle. For example, the sensation of light touch to the back of the left hand is initiated by touch receptors and conveyed by touch pathways to a specific spot on the primary somatic sensory cortex. This pathway is unique for the sensation of touch in the left hand and is, in effect, 'labelled' for this activity.

Perception of stimulus strength

Despite the constant size of action potentials, differing intensities of a particular stimulus can be conveyed to the brain in two ways: by changing impulse frequency or by changing the number of neurones firing. The greater the frequency of impulses propagated along a nerve pathway and/or the greater the number of neurones firing, the more intense the sensation.

Sensory receptors

The brain is informed of events occurring both within and outside the body by nerve impulses, which originate in various different sensory receptors. Somatic sensory receptors are nerve endings (the tips of dendrites), either free or encapsulated. The receptors of the special senses (except smell) are non-neural cells, which communicate with sensory neurones by means of neurotransmitters.

Sensory receptors are attached to sensory neurones, which typically have a branched dendrite, with the end of each branch either acting as the receptor or connecting with it (Figure 7.1). As all the branches of the dendrite converge to a single fibre, all the sensory receptors convey impulses along the same pathway. The sensory receptors associated with a single sensory neurone are known as a **sensory unit**. The area of tissue in which the sensory unit is located is called the **receptive field**.

Classification of sensory receptors

There are several different ways of classifying sensory receptors. A simple division is into **exteroceptors** in the skin, which respond to stimuli originating in the external environment, and **interoceptors**, which monitor the internal environment. Receptors that give information about the relative position of parts of the body are known as

Figure 7.1 A sensory unit.

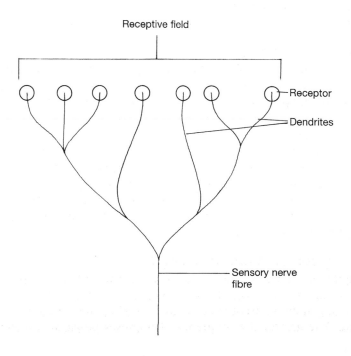

Receptive field

Receptor

Dendrites

Sensory nerve fibre

Table 7.1 Classification of sensory receptors (P) = also classified as proprioceptors

Receptors	Location	Stimuli
Mechanoreceptors		
Free nerve endings	Skin	Light touch, light pressure
Free nerve endings	Skin hairs	Bending of hair
Free nerve endings	Skin	Tickle, itch
Merkel's discs	Skin	Light pressure
Meissner's corpuscles	Glabrous skin	Light touch, low-frequency vibration
Krause's end bulbs	Mouth, conjunctiva, tongue, external genitalia	Light touch, low-frequency vibration
Ruffini's end organs (P)	Skin and hypodermis, joints	Deep pressure and stretch
Pacinian corpuscles (P)	Skin and hypodermis, tendons, ligaments, joints, periostea, mesentery	Deep pressure and stretch, high-frequency vibration
Muscle spindles (P)	Skeletal muscles	Muscle stretch
Golgi tendon organs (P)	Tendons	Tendon stretch
Baroreceptors (free nerve endings)		
High pressure	Carotid sinus, aortic arch, left atrium	↑arterial blood pressure
Low pressure	Right atrium	↑venous blood pressure
Hair cells	Ear (cochlea)	Sound waves
Hair cells	Ear (saccule and utricle)	Linear acceleration
Hair cells	Ear (semicircular canals)	Rotational acceleration
Chemoreceptors		
Gustatory cells	Taste buds of the tongue	Chemicals in mouth
Olfactory receptors	Olfactory epithelium in nasal cavity	Air-borne chemicals
Arterial chemoreceptors (free nerve endings)	Aortic and carotid bodies	↑CO_2 and H^+ ↓O_2
Medullary chemoreceptors	Medulla oblongata	↑H^+
Hypothalamic chemoreceptors	Hypothalamus	↑or ↓Amino acids ↑or ↓Fatty acids ↑or ↓Glucose
Osmoreceptors	Hypothalamus	↑Osmotic pressure
Thermoreceptors		
Cold receptors (free nerve endings)	Skin	Cold
Heat receptors (free nerve endings)	Skin	Heat
Hypothalamic cold receptors	Hypothalamus	Cold
Hypothalamic heat receptors	Hypothalamus	Heat
Photoreceptors		
Rods	Retina of eye	Low-intensity light
Cones	Retina of eye	High-intensity light
Blue		Blue light
Green		Green light
Red		Red light
Nociceptors		
Free nerve endings	Most tissues	Strong heat and cold, mechanical stimuli, various chemicals

proprioceptors. They are stimulated by movement of joints, tendons and muscles (Table 7.1).

A more detailed classification system separates receptors according to the type of stimuli involved: **mechanoreceptors**, which respond to mechanical stimuli; **chemoreceptors**, which respond to chemicals; **thermoreceptors**, which detect heat or cold; **photoreceptors**, which respond to light; and **nociceptors**, which do not quite fit this scheme, because they respond to a variety of stimuli all of which, however, elicit the sensation of pain (Table 7.1).

Mechanoreceptors

Touch is detected by superficial skin receptors, pressure by deep-lying receptors and vibration by touch and pressure receptors.

Free nerve endings of Aβ fibres are found everywhere in the skin and detect light touch and pressure (Figure 7.2). Similar endings are wrapped around the hair follicles and are stimulated when the hairs are disturbed, and so they convey the sensation of light touch. Some free

Fibre types are classified in **Peripheral nerve fibres** (page 103), in Ch. 3, Tissues.

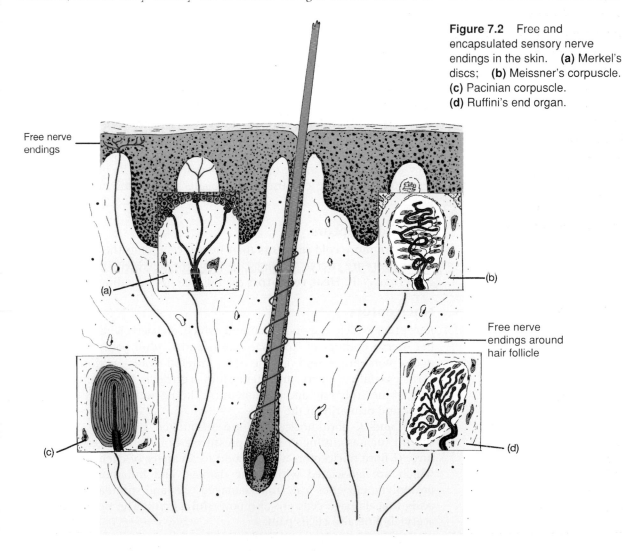

Figure 7.2 Free and encapsulated sensory nerve endings in the skin. **(a)** Merkel's discs; **(b)** Meissner's corpuscle. **(c)** Pacinian corpuscle. **(d)** Ruffini's end organ.

Free nerve endings

Free nerve endings around hair follicle

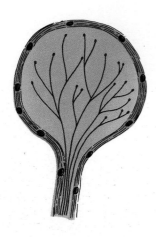

Figure 7.3 Krause's end bulb.

Other specialized receptors include muscle spindles and Golgi tendon organs, which are covered in **Spinal reflexes** (page 200), in Ch. 6, The Spinal Cord.

nerve endings in the skin elicit the sensation of tickle and itch. These fibres are the slow-conducting type C fibres, the same as those that mediate dull pain.

Merkel's discs are the expanded ends of sensory nerve fibres closely applied to Merkel cells in the epidermis of the skin. Collections of Merkel's discs are grouped in the skin to form the Iggo dome receptor. They are stimulated by touch and give continuous signals along Aβ fibres.

Meissner's corpuscles are elongated, encapsulated receptors found in the dermal papillae of hairless skin, including the lips, fingertips, nipples, palms, soles and external genitalia. They are rapidly adapting and give information about light touch and low frequency vibration along Aβ fibres.

Krause's end bulbs (Figure 7.3) are roughly spherical structures found in the dermal papillae of the skin in the mouth, the tongue and external genitalia.

Ruffini's end organs are spindle-shaped, branched encapsulated receptors found deep in the dermis and underlying tissue, particularly on the plantar surface of the foot. They are stimulated continuously by crude touch and pressure. They are also found in the joints and provide proprioceptive information during movement, which is conveyed along Aβ fibres.

Pacinian corpuscles lie in and immediately below the skin, in the mesentery and in the periosteum around bones. A central axon is surrounded by 20–60 concentric lamellae, separated by a gel. The receptors respond to deformation of the tissues as well as to high-frequency vibration. They are also found in tendons, ligaments and joints, where they are stimulated at the onset of movement. Like the other specialized receptors, Pacinian corpuscles propagate action potentials along Aβ fibres.

Thermoreceptors

There are more cold receptors than heat receptors in the skin. The **cold receptors** are nerve endings of Aδ fibres which innervate basal epidermal cells. **Heat receptors** are the free nerve endings of C fibres.

Nociceptors

Receptors which respond to stimuli which are perceived as painful are free nerve endings of Aδ (sharp pain) and C (dull pain) fibres. C-fibre nociceptors are found in the skin, arterial walls, periosteum, joint surfaces, falx cerebri and tentorium cerebelli and parietal serous membranes (pleurae and peritoneum). The nociceptors of the Aδ fibres are found primarily in the skin.

Aδ and C-fibre nociceptors are stimulated by strong mechanical stimuli such as cutting or strong pressure and large changes in temperature. C-fibre nociceptors also respond to a variety of chemicals, many of which are associated with tissue damage and inflammation. K^+ and proteolytic enzymes leak from damaged cells and stimulate nociceptors; acids that damage cells are also powerful stimuli. The neurotransmitter acetylcholine also elicits pain.

Histamine, serotonin and bradykinin concentrations in interstitial fluid all rise during inflammation and all stimulate nociceptors. Prostaglandins potentiate the effects of the chemicals produced in inflamed tissue, which thereby becomes very painful, a state of hyperalgesia.

ISCHAEMIC PAIN

If the blood supply to a tissue is interrupted, pain is experienced. One probable stimulus is lactic acid, which accumulates in hypoxic conditions. If the ischaemia is sufficient to cause cell damage, then the inflammatory responses are stimulated and chemicals such as bradykinin increase in concentration and stimulate the nociceptors.

PAIN OF MUSCLE SPASM

Muscle spasm is a strong, involuntary contraction which causes pain: colic, for example, is severe abdominal pain that accompanies spasm of the colon. The mechanical tissue deformation stimulates nociceptors and, if the muscle spasm impedes the blood flow, the resultant ischaemia will exacerbate the pain.

Receptor potentials

Sensory receptors act as transducers, converting the energy of the stimulus into receptor potentials. Despite the diversity of both stimuli and receptors, the effect of stimulating a receptor is remarkably constant. That is, the permeability of the receptor's cell membrane to ions increases. The principal consequence of this is that the diffusion of Na^+ into the cell increases and the membrane potential is therefore reduced. Subthreshold stimuli generate graded potentials, known in this site as receptor potentials.

For an action potential to be generated in a sensory neurone, summation of receptor potentials has to occur; in myelinated sensory neurones, this takes place at the first node of Ranvier. Each receptor potential depolarizes the node and, when the threshold potential is reached, sufficient voltage-gated Na^+ channels are open to generate an action potential, which is then propagated along the sensory fibre.

Adaptation of receptors

If a receptor is stimulated continuously for a period of time, the frequency of impulses in the sensory nerve fibre reduces and they may cease completely. The process is known as **adaptation**. The mechanism can be due to changes in the receptor itself. In the photoreceptive cells of the retina, for example, prolonged exposure to light reduces the concentration of photosensitive chemicals. Stimulation of a Pacinian corpuscle occurs by compression, which disturbs the fluid within the receptor. This fluid rapidly redistributes itself, however, even though the compression is still present, and so the nerve fibre in the centre of the corpuscle is no longer stimulated.

Another mechanism of adaptation is when sensory nerve fibres lose their responsiveness as they accommodate to continuous stimulation. The Na^+ channels open less in response to the stimulus. This occurs in

Chemoreceptors are described in **Chemoreceptor reflexes** (page 459), in Ch. 13, Respiration; **Regulation of water balance** (page 501), in Ch. 14, Renal Control of Body Fluid Volume and Composition; **Neural control of eating** (page 535), in Ch. 15, Digestion and Absorption of Food; **Hypothalamus** (page 153), in Ch. 5, The Brain.

Summation is explained in **Synapses** (page 127), in Ch. 4, Cellular Mechanisms of Neural Control.

Pacinian corpuscles, in addition to the redistribution of fluid.

Different receptors adapt at different rates and this is the basis of subdividing them into two functional groups: **tonic receptors**, which adapt slowly, and **rate receptors**, which adapt rapidly. Figure 7.4 illustrates cutaneous sensory receptors, their nerve fibres and adaptation rates.

TONIC RECEPTORS

Tonic receptors are able to respond continuously to their stimuli and send impulses into the central nervous system. They probably would

Figure 7.4 Sensory receptors in the skin, their nerve fibres and adaptation rates.

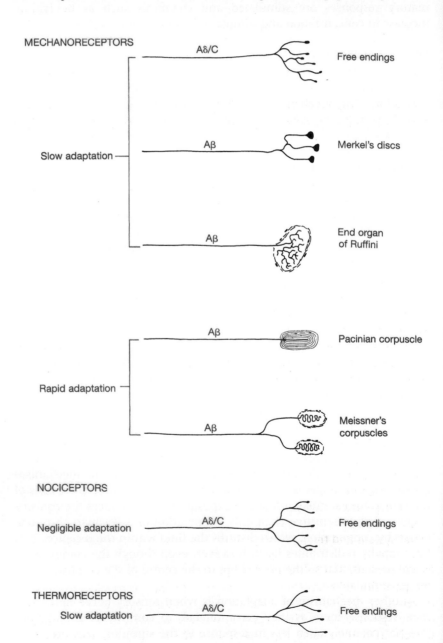

cease firing eventually if their stimuli remained constant, but this does not happen in the case of receptors stimulated by movement (muscle spindles, Golgi tendon organs and hair cells in the utricle and saccule), potential or actual damage (nociceptors), changes in blood pressure (baroreceptors) or blood chemistry (chemoreceptors), touch (Ruffini's end organs and Merkel's discs) or temperature (cold and heat receptors in the skin).

RATE RECEPTORS

Rate receptors respond to sudden changes. Pacinian corpuscles respond to sudden pressure to the skin; limb proprioceptors and hair cells in the semicircular canals respond to movement while it is changing. During actions such as running, proprioceptive information to the brain enables the coordination of many different muscles to take place.

Somatic sensory pathways

Sensory pathways between somatic receptors and the cerebral cortex of the brain (somatic sensory pathways) all have a minimum of three consecutive neurones. These are identified as first order, second-order and third-order sensory neurones. This provides a general framework for somatic sensory pathways, upon which specific variations can be overlaid.

First-order neurones connect the tissues with the spinal cord. They are pseudounipolar neurones whose cell bodies lie within the posterior root ganglia. **Second-order neurones** ascend to the thalamus; some cross over in the spinal cord, others in the medulla oblongata. **Third-order neurones** project from the thalamus to the primary somatic sensory cortex.

Fibres conveying sensory information from different receptive fields in the body are relayed systematically through the thalamus to the primary somatic sensory cortex, where the body surface is represented by the homunculus (see Figure 5.12). This is known as **somatotopic organization**. The thalamus and the primary sensory cortex, therefore, both contribute to the ability to distinguish different sensory modalities and their points of origin in the body.

The primary somatic sensory cortex plays the major role in determining the location of body sensations in general, and in the perception of fine touch in particular. The thalamus is able to discriminate between pain, temperature and crude touch.

Sensory pathways in the spinal cord fall into two groups: the anterolateral system and the posterior column–lemniscal system (Table 7.2).

See also **Thalami** (page 152) and **Primary somatic sensory area** (page 147), in Ch. 5, The Brain.

Posterior column–lemniscal system

The posterior column–lemniscal system refers to sensory pathways that travel in the fasciculi gracilis and cuneatus in the posterior white matter of the spinal cord to the medulla, synapse in the gracile or cuneate nuclei, cross over, and then ascend in the medial lemniscus to the

---

Table 7.2   General features of somatic sensory pathways

Anterolateral system (pain, temperature, crude touch, pressure, tickle, itch, sexual sensation)

First-order neurones	– Tissues to spinal cord
Second-order neurones	– Cross over in spinal cord, ascend to thalamus (some terminate in reticular formation)
Third-order neurones	– Project from thalamus to primary somatic sensory cortex

Posterior column–lemniscal system (proprioception, kinaesthesia fine touch, vibration)

First-order neurones	– Tissues to medulla
Second-order neurones	– Cross over in medulla, ascend to thalamus
Third-order neurones	– Project from thalamus to primary somatic sensory cortex

---

See also **Posterior column – lemniscal system** (page 194), in Ch. 6, The Spinal Cord.

thalamus. The pathways convey the modalities of **fine touch**, including **vibration**, proprioception and **kinaesthesia**. Proprioception is the sense of movement and position of body parts in relation to each other; kinaesthesia is the sense of movement and position of joints. The first-order neurones have large-diameter Aβ fibres and conduct impulses relatively fast (30–100 m/s). The second-order neurones cross over in the medulla oblongata and ascend to the thalamus in the medial lemniscal tract. This contrasts with the anterolateral system in which the second-order neurones cross over in the spinal cord. The third-order neurones connect the thalamus with the primary somatic sensory cortex (Figure 7.5).

Anterolateral system

See also **Anterolateral system** (page 193), in Ch. 6, The Spinal Cord.

The anterolateral system includes sensory pathways in the lateral and anterior areas of white matter. The pathways convey the modalities of **pain**, **temperature**, **crude touch** and **pressure**, **tickle**, **itch** and **sexual sensations**.

The first-order neurones are typically Aδ and conduct impulses relatively slowly at velocities between 8 and 40 m/s. The second-order neurones cross over in the spinal cord and ascend to the thalamus in the lateral spinothalamic tract (pain and temperature) or the anterior spinothalamic tract (crude touch and pressure). Some second-order neurones terminate in the reticular formation. The third-order neurones connect the thalamus with the primary somatic sensory cortex (Figure 7.6).

Spatial localization of sensory modalities conveyed by pathways in the anterolateral system is poorer than those in the posterior column–lemniscal system, because a smaller number of third-order neurones reach the primary somatic sensory cortex (see, for example, the pathways conveying dull pain).

PAIN PATHWAYS

There are two pathways that convey the sensation of pain following the stimulation of nociceptors. One pathway conveys sharp pricking pain rapidly, the other conveys dull, aching pain more slowly. A sharp blow to the thumb can stimulate both pathways, so that firstly a sharp pain and secondly a dull, persistent ache is experienced.

The pathway conveying sharp, pricking pain conforms to the general features of the anterolateral system. The first-order neurones, which have Aδ fibres, synapse in lamina I of the posterior horn of the spinal cord (see Figure 6.11); the second-order neurones cross over and ascend in the lateral spinothalamic tract to the thalamus; and the third-order neurones project from the thalamus to the primary sensory cortex (Figure 7.7). The source of this type of pain is thereby located accurately.

The first-order neurones conveying dull, burning or aching pain have C fibres, and therefore transmit action potentials more slowly than the

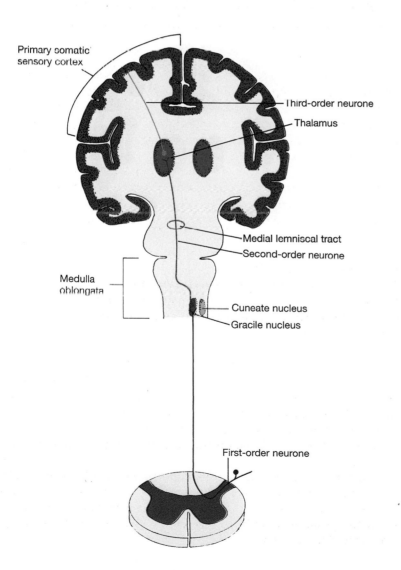

Figure 7.5 Posterior column–lemniscal system pathways: fine touch, vibration proprioception and kinaesthesia.

Primary somatic sensory cortex

Third-order neurone

Thalamus

Medial lemniscal tract

Second-order neurone

Medulla oblongata

Cuneate nucleus

Gracile nucleus

First-order neurone

Aδ fibres of the sharp pain pathway. The first-order neurones relay with one or more short neurones in laminae II and III (the substantia gelatinosa) of the posterior horn of the spinal cord. The final neurone in the circuit has its cell body in lamina V; the axon crosses over to the anterolateral pathway in the lateral white matter of the spinal cord. Most of the fibres ascend and terminate in various parts of the reticular formation in the brain stem. From here, several short neurones relay to various other parts of the brain, including the thalamus. The C pathway is therefore relatively diffuse compared with the Aδ pathway, and localization of this type of pain is much poorer than for sharp pain, because of the relatively few fibres relaying impulses to the primary somatic sensory cortex.

Analgesia in the substantia gelatinosa

Ronald Melzack and Patrick Wall, in the 1960s, proposed a model of how the flow of impulses along pain pathways, particularly the C

Figure 7.6 Anterolateral system pathways: pain and temperature [orange] and crude touch and pressure [red].

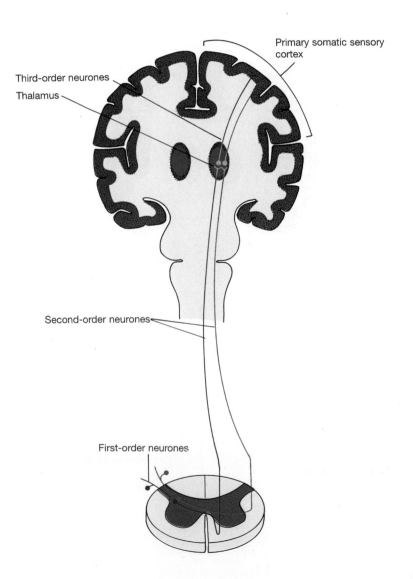

Primary somatic sensory cortex

Third-order neurones

Thalamus

Second-order neurones

First-order neurones

pathway, could be increased or decreased. They likened the situation to a gate opening and closing, thereby allowing more or fewer impulses through. Their **gate theory of pain**, although subject to considerable modification over the years, still provides a model for the integration of different pathways influencing pain, as well as understanding how various methods of pain relief work.

Attempts to determine which neurotransmitters are associated with particular pathways within the CNS is clearly much more difficult than studying neurotransmitters in the periphery. That is one reason why such transmitters are frequently described as 'putative'. The interconnections within the CNS are so many and varied, that one simple story may never emerge!

One peptide that has been proposed as the neurotransmitter released by the C fibres is **substance P** (see Table 6.3).

The Aδ neurones synapse with short neurones in the substantia

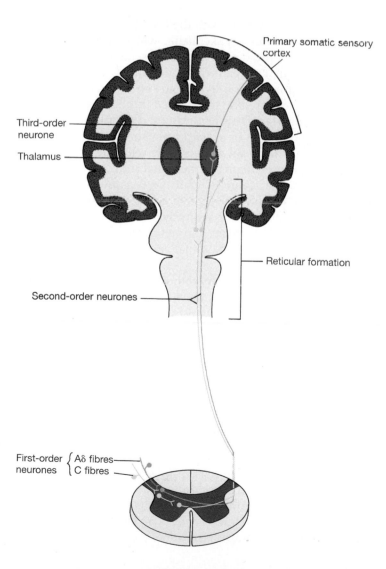

Primary somatic sensory cortex

Third-order neurone

Thalamus

Reticular formation

Second-order neurones

First-order neurones { Aδ fibres / C fibres

Figure 7.7 Pathways conveying sharp pain [orange] and dull pain [green]. Sharp pain is well localized because the majority of fibres project to the primary somatic sensory cortex. Dull pain is poorly localized as the majority of fibres terminate in the reticular formation.

Figure 7.8 Schematic diagram of pain pathways and their control in the substantia gelatinosa. C: Dull pain pathway. Aδ: Sharp pain (e.g. acupuncture) and temperature pathways (e.g. ice packs) inhibit dull and sharp pain via interneurones in the substantia gelatinosa, which release enkephalin. Enkephalin causes presynaptic inhibition of both C and Aδ pathways. Aβ: Fine touch, vibration pathway (e.g. TENS) inhibits dull pain via interneurones in the substantia gelatinosa, which release GABA. Descending pathways from the raphe magnus nucleus in the brain stem terminate in the substantia gelatinosa and release the neurotransmitter serotonin which stimulates the release of enkephalin.

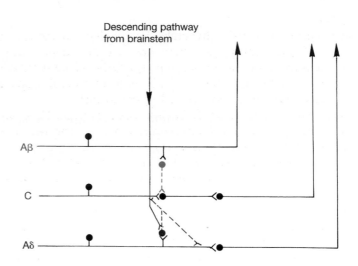

Descending pathway
from brainstem

Aβ

C

Aδ

> **Presynaptic inhibition** (page 129), in Ch. 4, Cellular Mechanisms of Neural Control.

gelatinosa that are inhibitory to both the C and the Aδ pathways (Figure 7.8). The neurotransmitter is enkephalin, which reduces the release of neurotransmitter from the C-fibre and Aδ-fibre neurones, an example of presynaptic inhibition. This pathway is dominant, therefore, it inhibits the C and the Aδ pathways, 'closes the gate' and reduces the sensation of pain. Sensations of cold are also transmitted through Aδ pathways to the lateral spinothalamic tract. This pathway then affords an explanation of how the application of cold or a sharp pain, such as that experienced in **acupuncture**, could act as an analgesic, by releasing enkephalin in the posterior horn of the grey matter of the spinal cord.

Another pathway that connects with the C pathway carries impulses along Aβ fibres from mechanoreceptors and conveys sensations of fine touch and proprioception. This pathway is in the posterior column–lemniscal system. The first-order neurones ascend in the posterior white matter, without synapsing in the spinal cord and without crossing over to the other side of it.

The Aβ fibres synapse with short neurones in the substantia gelatinosa which, like those connecting with the Aδ pathway, are inhibitory to the C pathway. A putative neurotransmitter in this case is **GABA**. **Transcutaneous electric nerve stimulation** (**TENS**) is a form of pain relief afforded by applying an electric current to electrodes placed on the skin. This procedure is thought to stimulate the Aβ fibres which, via their collaterals which synapse in the substantia gelatinosa, are able to reduce the flow of impulses along the dull pain pathway.

Descending pathways from the periaqueductal grey matter and the raphe magnus nucleus in the brain stem also end in the substantia gelatinosa, release **serotonin**, stimulate the enkephalinergic neurones and 'close the gates'. It may be that these descending pathways act as a negative feedback loop back to the substantia gelatinosa, initiated by action potentials reaching the brain stem in the pain pathways. The perception of pain by the brain, therefore, initiates analgesic activity. This pathway could be elicited by acupuncture or indeed by stimulation from the cerebral cortex effecting psychological control of pain.

> Areas in the brain associated with analgesia are described in **Opioid peptides** (page 180) and **Serotonin** (page 181), in Ch. 5, The Brain.

Hyperalgesia

Excessive sensitivity to pain (hyperalgesia) involves an increase in the excitability of pain pathways. There are two functional causes: 1) increased sensitivity of the nociceptors (**peripheral sensitization** or **primary hyperalgesia**); and 2) facilitation of neural transmission (**central sensitization** or **secondary hyperalgesia**).

Primary hyperalgesia occurs following tissue damage, for example a burn. It is thought that the increased sensitivity of the nociceptors is mediated by serotonin and bradykinin, whose concentrations rise during inflammation. Chemicals that lower the threshold of stimulation of nociceptors and therefore increase their sensitivity are termed **algogens**. Prostaglandins potentiate the effects of algogens.

Secondary hyperalgesia is found in an area surrounding the tissue damage. Here, the threshold stimulus is unchanged, but the intensity of the pain experienced is enhanced. This effect is due to facilitation of pathways in the spinal cord or the brain which are stimulated by neural inputs from nociceptors in the damaged area.

Phantom limb pain

Following the amputation of part or all of a limb, pain can be experienced as if the limb were still intact. The probable mechanism is a combination of three things.

1. The 'labelled line' pathway proximal to the amputated limb is still intact and therefore able to transmit information to the brain.
2. Damaged neurones become hypersensitive to excitatory neurotransmitters, so that small amounts released at neighbouring synapses could stimulate the pain pathway from the limb.
3. Sensory inputs along temperature and touch pathways, which would normally act to reduce pain sensation, are missing.

Referred pain

Pain caused by stimulation of nociceptors in the viscera is usually 'felt' in a different place, somewhere on the body's surface. Such pain is known as **referred pain**. The explanation of this phenomenon is largely anatomical. Branches of visceral pain fibres synapse in the spinal cord with some of the same second-order neurones that convey nociceptive information from the skin (Figure 7.9). A common pathway for both skin surface and visceral pain therefore conveys impulses to the primary somatic sensory cortex. The source of the pain is perceived to be from the skin surface rather than the viscera because the skin has more nociceptors, and the brain has therefore 'learned' to interpret impulses arriving via the common pathway as pain from the skin.

Pain resulting from damage to part of the thalamus is described in **Thalami** (page 152), in Ch. 5, The Brain.

Table 7.3 gives some examples of referred pain and the nerve pathways involved.

Pain from many abdominal organs (e.g. pancreas, kidney, bladder) is referred to the skin in front of or behind the organ.

Headache

Head pain can originate from structures superficial to the cranium or

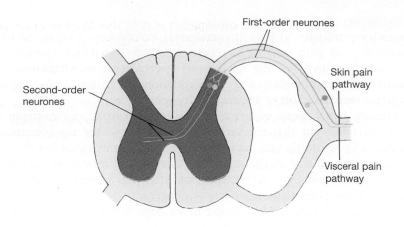

Figure 7.9 Referred pain. Branches of first-order visceral pain fibres [green] synapse with some second-order neurones receiving pain fibres from the skin [orange]. There is therefore a common pathway from the two locations and the brain interprets impulses from either route as pain in the skin.

Table 7.3 Referred pain		
Source of pain	*Referred site*	*Nerve pathway*
Upper part of cranial vault	Anterior half of scalp	Cranial nerve V
Lower part of cranial vault	Posterior half of scalp	Cranial nerve II
Diaphragm	Shoulder	C4 and C5
Gall bladder	Right shoulder	C5
Heart	Left arm	T1

from intracranial blood vessels, the falx cerebri or the tentorium cerebelli.

Headache of extracranial origin can be caused by stress, eye strain or a head cold. Stress or tension headache can be caused by strong contraction of muscles which are attached to the scalp (see *Pain of muscle spasm*, above). Eye strain headache is caused by strong contraction of the ciliary muscles, which are used in changing the shape of the lens during focusing. A head cold can inflame the nasal and sinus mucosae, thereby causing pain.

The brain itself does not generate the sensation of pain. If the pain areas of the primary sensory cortex are stimulated electrically then the pain sensation is 'felt' in the parts of the body represented, not in the brain itself.

Stimulation of nociceptors in blood vessels in the dura mater, or in the falx cerebri or tentorium cerebelli causes headache. The stimulus might be 1) mechanical, for example due to a head injury or surgery or withdrawal of cerebrospinal fluid, or 2) part of the inflammatory response, for example in meningitis. Stimulation of nociceptors above the tentorium causes headache in the front half of the head, whereas stimulation below the tentorium results in pain at the back of the head (Table 7.3).

The headache of a 'hangover' probably results from excess alcohol stimulating nociceptors in the dura mater.

Headache that accompanies constipation may be due to a rise in toxins absorbed from the large intestine stimulating intracranial nociceptors.

Lateral inhibition

Sensory pathways can involve thousands of fibres lying very close together. Different fibres relay information that distinguishes between different sensory modalities, parts of the body or, in the case of auditory pathways, sound frequencies. Should excitation spread laterally along sensory pathways, the information would become very confused.

The mechanism of lateral inhibition, which takes place at the synapse points in sensory pathways, prevents the spread of excitation. Collateral fibres branch off from one sensory pathway and inhibit adjacent pathways either by presynaptic inhibition or by relaying with another neurone, which releases an inhibitory neurotransmitter.

Presynaptic inhibition (page 129), in Ch. 4, Cellular Mechanisms of Neural Control.

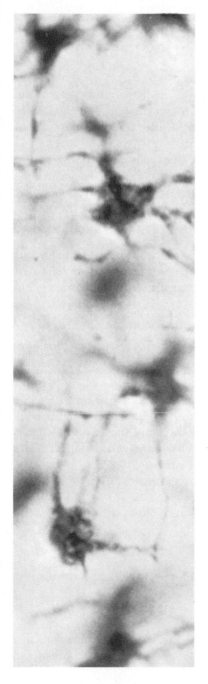

The special senses

8

The **special senses** – vision, hearing, balance, taste and smell – are designated as 'special' because they derive from the stimulation of specialized receptor cells, all of which are located in sense organs or tissues in the head. This is in contrast to somatic senses which derive from sensory neurone endings which have a wide distribution in the body.

VISION

The process by which images are 'seen' by the brain involves quite a long sequence of events.

1. The eyes look towards the object.
2. Adjustments are made to the shape of the lens and the size of the pupil so that the light that passes through the lens and the refractive media within the eye is focused on the retina at the back of each eye.
3. The light stimulates receptor cells (the rods and cones) in the retina.
4. Action potentials are propagated along neural pathways, beginning with the optic nerves and ending in the visual cortex at the back of the brain.

Images are received by the retina and the visual cortex upside down, but are interpreted as being the right way up. Neural pathways mediated through the midbrain stimulate reflex changes in pupil diameter and lens shape.

The eyes

The two eyes are located within the orbits of the skull, one on either side of the nose, facing forwards. Each eyeball is roughly spherical and averages 2.4 cm in diameter. It is protected by the bony socket in which it is located, by the ridge of the eyebrow and by the eyelid, anteriorly. The eyeball is cushioned by fat, which lines the orbit.

Movements of the eyes are achieved by extrinsic muscles that attach the socket to the outer surface of each eye.

Lacrimal glands produce fluid that constantly flows over the surface of the eyes, lubricating and cleansing them.

Layers of the eye

The eye contains three principal layers: the outer sclera and cornea, the middle uvea and the inner retina (Figure 8.1).

SCLERA AND CORNEA

About five-sixths of the outer surface of the eyeball is made up of a tough, white fibrous layer, the **sclera**. The anterior one-sixth consists of

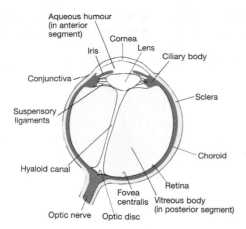

Aqueous humour
(in anterior
segment)
Cornea
Iris
Lens
Ciliary body
Conjunctiva
Sclera
Suspensory
ligaments
Hyaloid canal
Choroid
Retina
Fovea
centralis
Vitreous body
(in posterior segment)
Optic nerve
Optic disc

Figure 8.1 Horizontal section through the right eyeball viewed from above.

the **cornea**, a transparent structure that is continuous with the sclera. Both sclera and cornea consist mainly of collagen fibres. The transparency of the cornea is due to the even size and regular arrangement of the collagen fibres, together with the lack of blood vessels. The frontal surface of the cornea is covered by stratified squamous non-keratinized epithelium, which is continuous with the **conjunctiva**, the mucous membrane that covers the sclera and is reflected back to line the eyelids. The conjunctiva secretes mucus, which lubricates the surface of the eye. Vitamin A is necessary for this process, so that deficiency causes the layer to become dry, scaly and opaque, which impedes vision. Inflammation of the conjunctiva is called **conjunctivitis**.

Within the sclera, near its junction with the cornea, an oval canal passes around the circumference of the eyeball. This is the **canal of Schlemm** (sinus venosus sclerae), which drains aqueous humour from the anterior chamber. Posteriorly, the sclera is pierced by the optic nerve, which contains the sensory nerve fibres of cells that have their cell bodies in the retina.

UVEA

The middle layer of the eyeball, the uvea, comprises three parts: the choroid, which lines the sclera; the ciliary body, which supports the lens; and the iris in front of the lens (Figure 8.2).

The **choroid** is a thin, highly vascular, pigmented layer, which supplies the retina with oxygen and nutrients. The dark brown pigment absorbs light and prevents it from being reflected back through the retina.

The **ciliary body** contains smooth muscle fibres arranged in three directions: longitudinal (meridional fibres), oblique (radial fibres) and circular. The lens is suspended from the ciliary body by fine suspensory ligaments, so that changes in contraction of the smooth muscle fibres alter the shape and therefore the focusing properties of the lens.

The surface of the ciliary body is folded into **ciliary processes**, which contain the capillaries from which aqueous humour is secreted.

The **iris** varies in colour from pale blue to dark brown and separates the **anterior** and **posterior chambers** of the **anterior segment** of the

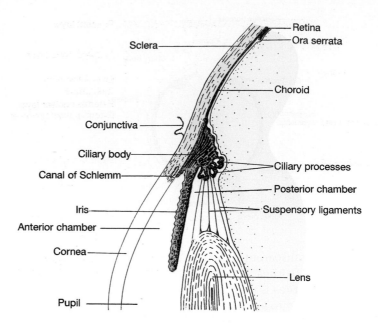

Figure 8.2 Section through the ciliary body and part of the lens.

eye. The **pupil** is a hole in the middle of the iris through which light passes to the posterior parts of the eye, and the aqueous humour flows forwards into the anterior chamber. The iris has two layers of smooth muscle: circular fibres (sphincter pupillae) and radial muscle fibres (dilatator pupillae). Contraction of the circular fibres causes constriction of the pupil (meiosis), whereas contraction of the radial fibres brings about pupillary dilatation (mydriasis). By these means, pupil size can vary from about 1 mm to 8 mm in diameter.

RETINA

The retina is the innermost layer of the eyeball, lining the whole of the posterior segment and terminating in a ragged line (**ora serrata**) behind the ciliary body (Figure 8.2). The retina contains the rods and cones (photoreceptors) and other short neurones, which connect the photoreceptors with each other and with the neurones whose axons lie in the optic nerve.

The microscopic appearance of the retina has given rise to 10 smaller layers, which are illustrated in Figure 8.3. Note that the photoreceptors face away from the light, which has to pass through several layers of neural tissue before reaching them.

The cells in the outermost layer of the retina, the **pigment layer**, which lies next to the choroid, contain the pigment melanin. The **pigment cells** absorb light and prevent it scattering, store vitamin A, synthesize the photoreceptor pigments and are phagocytic. Their microvilli extend between the outer segments of the rods in the next layer, thereby lending them support.

The photoreceptors and the ganglion cells are connected by **bipolar cells**.

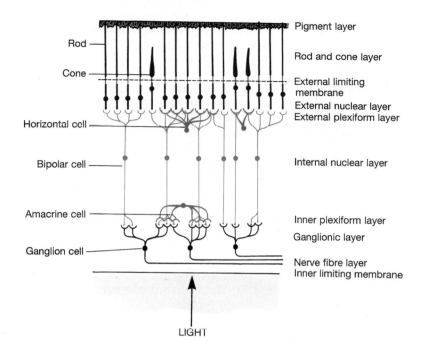

Rod

Cone

Horizontal cell

Bipolar cell

Amacrine cell

Ganglion cell

Pigment layer

Rod and cone layer

External limiting membrane

External nuclear layer
External plexiform layer

Internal nuclear layer

Inner plexiform layer

Ganglionic layer

Nerve fibre layer
Inner limiting membrane

LIGHT

Figure 8.3 Schematic diagram of the layers of the retina.

Ganglion cells are neurones whose cell bodies lie in the retina and whose axons form the optic nerve.

Lateral connections in the retina are made by **horizontal cells** and **amacrine cells**. Horizontal cells lie close to the basal regions of the rods and cones; their action is always inhibitory. Amacrine cells lie horizontally at the level of the junctions of the bipolar and deep ganglion cells. There are a great many different types of amacrine cells and their actions, when elucidated, may well be as varied.

Blind spot

The layer of rods and cones is present throughout the retina, except at the point where the optic nerve joins the eyeball (Figure 8.1). This area, the **optic disc**, is about 1.5 mm in diameter. Since it lacks photoreceptors, it is also known as the 'blind spot'.

Fovea centralis

In the centre of the retina, lateral to the blind spot, is an oval, yellow area, the **macula lutea**. This area has a small depression in its centre, the **fovea centralis** (Figure 8.1). In this region, the neurones in the retina are displaced and, as a result, the photoreceptors, which in this region are exclusively cones, are exposed directly to light (Figure 8.4). Visual resolution at the fovea, therefore, is the highest in the retina.

At the fovea, cone density is about 150 000/mm², compared with about 5000/mm² in the rest of the retina. Rods are absent from the fovea.

Figure 8.4 Photomicrograph of the fovea of a retina showing the reduced thickness in this area of maximal visual acuity. (Reproduced with permission from Fawcett, D. W. (1993) *Bloom and Fawcett: A Textbook of Histology*, Chapman & Hall, London.)

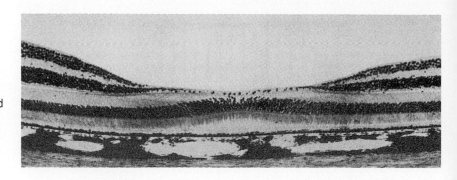

Blood supply of the eyeball

The eyeball is supplied with blood from the **ophthalmic artery**, which enters the orbital cavity through the optic canal next to the optic nerve. Branches of the ophthalmic artery – the long and short posterior ciliary arteries, the anterior **ciliary arteries** and the **central retinal artery** – supply the eyeball (Figure 8.5). The **ophthalmic vein** drains into the cavernous sinus.

The cornea contains no blood vessels; the sclera has very few. The choroid and ciliary body receive arterial blood from the seven short posterior ciliary arteries, which divide into 15–20 branches and pierce the sclera in a circle around the optic nerve.

The iris contains two vascular circles, the major one near to the attached margin, the other near to the free margin. The blood vessels are supplied by two long posterior ciliary arteries, which pierce the sclera near to the optic nerve, and anterior ciliary arteries, which pierce the sclera near the sclerocorneal junction.

The outer third of the retina is supplied by the blood vessels in the choroid, the inner third by the central retinal artery, which runs along

Figure 8.5 Branches of the ophthalmic artery supply the eyeball: the long and short posterior ciliary arteries, the anterior ciliary arteries and the central retinal artery.

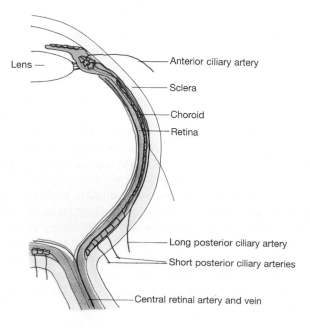

the centre of the optic nerve to the optic disc or papilla. This can be seen by ophthalmoscopy. Oedema of the disc (**papilloedema**) may indicate raised intracranial pressure, which compresses the central retinal vein, thereby raising capillary hydrostatic pressure in the tissues draining into it.

Rotational movements of the eyeballs

The rotational movements of the eyeballs are brought about by the **extrinsic muscles**, comprising two pairs of **rectus muscles** (superior and inferior, medial and lateral) and one pair of **oblique muscles** (superior and inferior) (Figure 8.6).

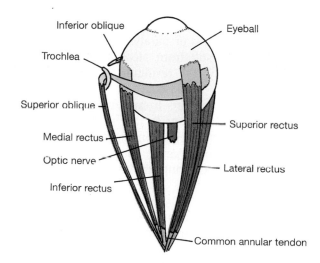

Figure 8.6 Extrinsic muscles of the right eye viewed from above.

The four recti insert into the sclera posterior to the corneal margin and originate in a fibrous ring (common annular tendon) which surrounds the exit point of the optic nerve from the orbit. The superior, inferior, medial and lateral recti move the eyes upwards, downwards, medially and laterally, respectively.

The oblique muscles are arranged such that, for part of their length at least, they lie around the circumference of the eyeball. The superior oblique lies above the eyeball and originates in the common annular tendon. Near the front of the orbit it passes through a fibrocartilage loop (**trochlea**) and the tendon of the muscle then inserts into the superolateral aspect of the eyeball behind its equator. Thus the superior oblique turns at an angle of more than 90° between its origin and insertion: contraction moves the eye downwards and outwards. The inferior oblique muscle originates from the medial surface of the orbit, runs around beneath the eyeball and inserts into the inferolateral surface of the sclera. Its contraction moves the eyeball upwards and outwards.

The lateral rectus is innervated by cranial nerve VI; the superior oblique by cranial nerve IV, and the remaining extrinsic muscles are all innervated by cranial nerve III (see Table 5.1). Each pair of muscles is innervated reciprocally, so that when one muscle of a pair is active the other is inhibited.

Reciprocal inhibition (page 199), in Ch. 6, The Spinal Cord.

Eye movements are of two types – quick, jerky (**saccadic**) movements, and slow, scanning movements. Saccadic movements direct the eyes from one point in the visual field to another, e.g. when reading, whereas **scanning** movements enable the gaze to be maintained on one moving object, e.g. when looking out of a train window.

A sudden visual disturbance at the edge of the visual field initiates reflex movements of the eyes (and the head) towards the source of the disturbance. The neural pathway is mediated through the superior colliculi in the midbrain.

Focusing upon distant objects requires that the optical axes are parallel to each other and that the corresponding muscles of the two eyes work in concert. This is known as **conjugate movement**. If movements of the two eyes are not synchronized, there is double vision (**diplopia**) in which two images are seen rather than one. This can be caused by congenital weakness or paralysis of an extrinsic eye muscle. Temporary diplopia can result from alcohol intoxication. If one eye rotates medially or laterally, the resultant 'squint' is known as **strabismus**.

When the focus of the eye shifts from a distant to a near object, the two eyes move within their sockets so that their optical axes converge. In this way, images can be formed upon the corresponding areas of the retinas of the two eyes. In convergence, the medial recti of the two eyes contract simultaneously, which brings the two optical axes together.

Blinking

Each eyelid (**palpebra**) comprises a flat sheet of connective tissue (tarsal plate), which contains **tarsal glands** and is covered by muscles and skin. The tarsal glands are modified sebaceous glands that secrete a lubricating fluid into ducts that open behind the eyelashes. Inflammation of the tarsal glands results in a cyst, known as a **chalazion**. There are sebaceous glands and modified sweat glands (**ciliary glands**) between the hair follicles of the eyelashes. Inflammation of any of the small glands results in a '**stye**'.

A detached portion of the lower eyelid (**caruncle**) is found at the medial angle (canthus) of the eye. The secretion from sebaceous and sweat glands in the caruncle often collects at the medial canthus during sleep.

The **levator palpebrae superioris** muscle lies above the eye and inserts into the upper eyelid: contraction raises the upper eyelid and 'opens' the eye (Figure 8.7).

The **orbicularis oculi** muscle runs around the eye, and its contraction 'closes' the eye. Reflex blinking occurs every 3–7 s, spreading lacrimal fluid across the surface of the eye. The follicles of the eyelashes are extensively innervated by hair root plexuses and stimulation of these by very light touch initiates blinking. The sensory neurones are in the ophthalmic branch of cranial nerve V (trigeminal) which relays with cranial nerve VII (facial) in the pons and causes contraction of the orbicularis oculi, closing the eye, and with cranial nerve III in the midbrain, which causes contraction of the levator palpebrae, opening the eye.

Sebaceous glands (page 313) and **sweat glands** (page 313), in Ch. 10, The Skin and the Regulation of Body Temperature.

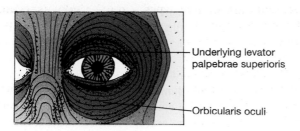

Underlying levator palpebrae superioris

Orbicularis oculi

Figure 8.7 The muscles of blinking. Somatic motor neurones in cranial nerve III cause contraction of the levator palpebrae superioris which raises the upper eyelid. Contraction of the orbicularis oculi lowers the upper eyelid, stimulated by somatic motor neurones in cranial nerve VII.

Focusing the image

The parts of the eye that enable light to be focussed on to the retina are the cornea, the lens and the refractive media – the vitreous humour and the aqueous humour. Changes in the size of the pupil also affect image formation.

When light enters the eye it is bent (refracted) by a constant and relatively large amount by the cornea and refractive media and by a variable and much smaller amount by the lens.

LENS

The lens is a transparent, biconvex, encapsulated structure suspended from ligaments attached to the ciliary body, posterior to the iris. The lens divides the eye into anterior and posterior segments (Figure 8.1). If removed from the eye, the lens is almost spherical, but in position in the eye it is flattened by the **suspensory ligaments**. The front surface of the lens consists of a layer of cuboidal epithelial cells, and at the equator the cells become elongated, lose their nuclei and become fibres, which make up the bulk of the lens. Although the lens does not contain blood vessels, it receives nutrients from the aqueous humour, which bathes it and contains transparent proteins (crystallins) that act as glucose-oxidizing enzymes. The lens is elastic and changes its shape when the eye is focused. This is brought about by contraction of the muscles in the ciliary body, which alters the tension in the suspensory ligaments.

The lens may become cloudy (**cataract**) and eventually cause blindness if it is not removed.

Accommodation

The eye is able to focus light from objects at different distances by altering the curvature of the lens in a process known as accommodation (Figure 8.8). As an object moves closer to the eye, the curvature of the lens is increased, so that the image remains in focus upon the retina.

When the eye is at rest, the ligaments supporting the lens are under tension, which flattens the lens; it is therefore focused on distant objects. As the eye focuses on closer objects, the ciliary muscles contract, causing the ciliary body to decrease in diameter and thereby reduce the tension in the ciliary ligaments. As a consequence, the lens is less restrained and its elasticity causes it to adopt a more spherical shape. The lens steadily flattens and loses elasticity with age, so that its ability to accommodate is reduced.

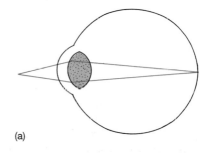

(a)

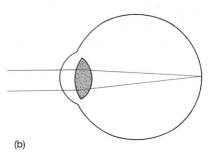

(b)

Figure 8.8 Accommodation. **(a)** Light from a source close to the eye is focused by a rounded lens. **(b)** Light from a distant source is focused by a flattened lens.

There is a limit to how close an object may be to the eye and remain in focus. The closest point is called the 'near' point and it increases with age (**presbyopia**) so that at 20 years it is about 10 cm and at 60 years it averages 83 cm.

The ciliary body is innervated by parasympathetic pathways from the oculomotor nucleus in the midbrain, through the third cranial nerve to the ciliary ganglion behind the eye. Parasympathetic stimulation causes contraction of the ciliary muscles and the lens becomes more convex.

Sympathetic fibres originate at the first thoracic segment of the spinal cord and pass up to the superior cervical ganglion. They then follow a number of arteries to the eyeball where they innervate the ciliary body. Sympathetic stimulation causes relaxation of the ciliary muscles, and the lens flattens.

A blurred image on the retina is relayed to the midbrain, which then increases or decreases activity in the parasympathetic pathways to the ciliary body, resulting in compression or stretching of the lens until a sharp image is formed.

AQUEOUS HUMOUR

The aqueous humour is a clear, watery fluid that fills the cavities around the lens (anterior and posterior chambers). It nourishes the cornea and the lens. The fluid, which contains less protein than plasma, is produced by a combination of active secretion and diffusion from the capillaries in the ciliary processes. It passes through the surface epithelium into the posterior chamber, and then forwards through the pupil to the anterior chamber where it is absorbed into the ciliary veins and the canal of Schlemm. If drainage of the aqueous humour becomes impaired, the fluid may accumulate and compress the retina and optic nerve, a condition called glaucoma.

VITREOUS BODY

The vitreous body occupies the bulk of the eyeball cavity behind the lens and the ciliary body. It consists of a transparent gel composed mostly of water with some electrolytes, mucoprotein (vitrein), hyaluronic acid and some collagen fibres. The gel is condensed at its edges into a membrane. The pressure exerted by the vitreous body supports the lens, presses against the retina and resists the forces generated by the extrinsic eye muscles. The vitreous body is doughnut-shaped because it contains the **hyaloid canal**, which passes from the optic disc to the posterior surface of the lens (Figure 8.1). In the foetus, the canal contains the hyaloid artery, which nourishes the anterior structure of the eye until about 6 weeks before birth, when it atrophies.

CHANGES IN PUPIL SIZE

If the pupil is constricted, then less light can enter the eye. As a result, light only passes through the central part of the lens, which reduces the chromatic and spherical aberrations that tend to occur at its edges. Secondly, the depth of focus of the eye also improves, since with a narrow pupil the beams of light entering the eye are themselves very

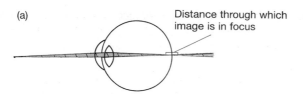

(a)

Distance through which image is in focus

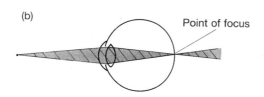

(b)

Point of focus

Figure 8.9 The effect of changes in pupil diameter upon image formation. **(a)** A constricted pupil produces a narrow cone of light that is in focus over a short distance. **(b)** A dilated pupil produces a wide cone focused at a single point.

narrow and remain in focus over a short distance rather than at a specific point (Figure 8.9).

Pupillary reflexes

The iris responds reflexly to changes in ambient light intensity. An increase in light intensity initiates pupillary constriction whereas a decrease in light intensity causes pupillary dilation. If only one eye is illuminated, then that eye shows a direct effect in response to the light change (**direct light reflex**). The other eye, however, also shows an identical response (**consensual light reflex**).

Alterations in the size of the pupil depend upon light hitting the retina. This then passes impulses to the midbrain, which then either sends impulses along parasympathetic pathways to bring about contraction of the circular muscles of the iris (pupillary constriction) or along sympathetic pathways to bring about contraction of the radial muscles of the iris (pupillary dilatation). Pupillary reflexes are used as a clinical test of brain stem function.

The pupil is capable of about a five-fold change in area, although light intensities with a million-fold variation may be experienced. Generally, pupil diameter changes rapidly in response to changes in light intensity, but longer-term adaptation depends upon photochemical changes in the retina.

Brain stem reflexes (page 167), in Ch. 5, The Brain.

Long- and short-sightedness and astigmatism

If the eyeball is short in the anteroposterior dimension, images are formed at a point beyond the retina. This is **long-sightedness (hyperopia)** and may be compensated by the use of convex lenses which refract the light to a nearer point (Figure 8.10).

If the eyeball is long in the anterior posterior dimension, an image is formed in front of the retina and the person is said to be **short-sighted (myopic)**. This is compensated by the use of biconcave lenses.

Astigmatism describes a condition where the cornea is not uniformly curved. This leads to distortion of the image formed on the retina, since light in different planes is focussed in front of or behind the retina. The use of cylindrical lenses can compensate for astigmatism.

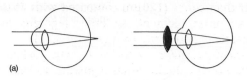

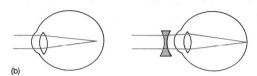

Figure 8.10 (a) Long-sightedness due to a short eyeball, corrected with a convex lens. **(b)** Short-sightedness due to a long eyeball, corrected with a biconcave lens.

Photoreceptors

STRUCTURES OF RODS AND CONES

Retinal photoreceptors are of two types, rods and cones. Rods give rise to black and white vision, cones to colour vision. The total number of rods in each retina is estimated to be around 120 million, and the number of cones about 6.5 million. Rod density is typically $160\,000/mm^2$ falling to $30\,000/mm^2$ at the ora serrata. Cone density is about $5\,000/mm^2$, except at the fovea, where it is about $150\,000/mm^2$.

Figure 8.11 Structure of a rod and cone, supported by Müller cells, and their positions in the layers of the retina.

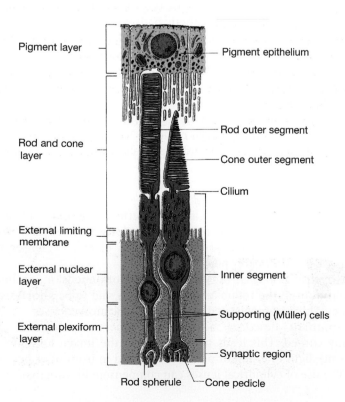

Rods are longer than cones (120 µm compared with 75 µm). Both cell types consist of an outer segment, an inner segment containing the nucleus and a synaptic region at the base (Figure 8.11).

The outer segments contain stacks of closely packed, membrane-bound sacs (discs), which contain visual pigments. In rods, the discs are totally separate from the cell membrane, but in cones they are infoldings of it. Rod outer segments are generally longer than those of cones, although at the fovea cones are also quite long and very narrow.

In rods, new discs arise at the basal end of the outer segment and are lost at the apex and phagocytosed by cells of the pigment layer. The turnover of discs can be as high as 100 per day from a single outer segment.

In cones, new visual pigment moves along existing discs from the base to the apex of the cell.

The inner segments of both rods and cones are longer and wider than the outer segments. At the apex of the inner segment of each cell type there is a projection, which has an internal structure characteristic of a cilium, from which the outer segment (appears to) develop. This cilium links the inner and outer segments.

The synaptic regions of the photoreceptors terminate in bulbous extensions called **rod spherules** and **cone pedicles**, which synapse with the neurones in the internal nuclear layer.

PHOTORECEPTOR PIGMENTS

Both rods and cones contain pigments that alter physically and chemically as a result of the effect of light. This is the first process in the sequence of events that results in action potentials being propagated along the optic nerve from the retina.

The rod pigment is known as **rhodopsin** and is incorporated into the disc membranes of the outer segments. Rhodopsin is a complex of vitamin A aldehyde, **retinal** (also known as retinene) and a protein, **scotopsin** (an opsin). The colour of rhodopsin gives it its alternative name of **visual purple**.

In the intact rhodopsin molecule, retinal is in the folded form (11-cis isomer), which fits into a 'pocket' on the surface of the much larger scotopsin molecule (Figure 8.12). Light energy causes the retinal to alter

Figure 8.12 The effect of light on rhodopsin. Light causes the 11-cis retinal to be converted into the all-trans form. The change in the molecular configuration of retinal means that it will no longer fit into its slot on the scotopsin molecule. As a result, the retinal is released from the scotopsin. The scotopsin also changes its shape slightly.

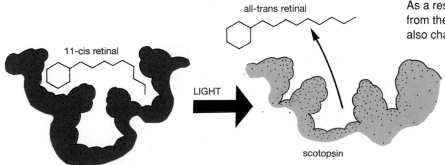

its configuration to the straight (all-trans) form, which no longer fits into the scotopsin. As a result, the retinal and the scotopsin separate and the visual purple becomes colourless or 'bleached'. Rhodopsin is extremely sensitive to even poor levels of illumination.

Rhodopsin is regenerated with the aid of the enzyme **retinal isomerase**, which is present in the epithelial cells of the pigment layer. All-trans retinal migrates into the pigment layer where it is converted into the 11-cis form before passing back to the rods, where it recombines with scotopsin.

There are three types of cone, each with a different pigment, each of which has a different spectral sensitivity (Figure 8.13).

Figure 8.13 Spectral sensitivities of the cone pigments.

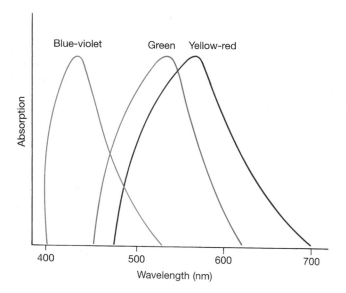

See also **Electromagnetic radiation** (page 30), in Ch. 1, Molecules, Ions and Units.

One pigment absorbs light maximally in the blue–violet portion of the spectrum, one in the green portion and one in the yellow–red portion. These are normally referred to as blue, green and red cones, although this is somewhat misleading, as it refers to the colour of light to which each responds maximally and not to the actual colour of the cones. The action of light on cone pigments is thought to be comparable to its action on rhodopsin.

For a particular colour of light, the pattern of response from the three types of cone forms a code which the brain interprets as that particular colour. Since blue, green and red are the primary colours, then stimulation of the different cones to different levels of excitation allows the brain to 'see' any colour. For example, if the red cones are excited to 83% of their maximum, green cones to 83% and blue cones not at all, the brain 'sees' the colour yellow. If all three cone types are excited equally, white light is perceived.

The eye reacts in the same way to a monochromatic light source such as yellow, as it does to an appropriate mixture of light (in this case red and green light). In both cases the brain receives an impression of yellow light. Stage lighting takes advantage of this process and can therefore create all manner of colours from various combinations of blue, red and green lights.

The three cone pigments are formed by a combination of retinal (as in rods) and one of three opsins, collectively called **photopsins**. Cone pigments are much less sensitive to light than rhodopsin, and there are fewer molecules of pigment in each cone compared with rods. Rods, therefore, are much more sensitive to light than cones.

Colour blindness

If one or more types of cone are congenitally absent from the retina, the person (usually male) will be 'colour blind'. Most commonly, lack of red- or green-sensitive cells is found and in either case the person will not be able to discriminate colour changes over the red–green portion of the spectrum. He will therefore be **red–green colour blind**.

Light and dark adaptation

The sensitivity of the retina is dependent upon the amount of pigments in the rods and cones. If the eye is exposed to bright light for a long period, then the total amount of pigment is greatly reduced. As a result the eye is **light-adapted** and its overall sensitivity is reduced.

If, conversely, the eye is kept in darkness for a long time, then the photopigments are synthesized to their maximum concentration, which is determined by the number of opsin molecules present. In this case the eye is **dark-adapted** and it is maximally sensitive.

The rods adapt more slowly than the cones, but they eventually reach a higher level of sensitivity. This means that the rods are used more than the cones in poor lighting conditions, in which case one can only discriminate between shades of black and white (**scotopic vision**). In bright light, however, when the cones are operating, different colours can be discriminated (**photopic vision**).

The absence of rods in the fovea means that focusing light on to this area in dim lighting conditions results in an inability to see detail. Consequently, whereas distant and peripheral objects can be detected quite readily, close work such as reading a book is very difficult.

Light and dark adaptation enable the eyes to function over a wide range of levels of illumination, despite the fact that pupil size and there-fore the amount of light entering the eyes can only be varied by rela-tively small amounts.

Night blindness

Night blindness (**nyctalopia**) is impaired rod function, usually due to vitamin A deficiency. The reduced amount of rhodopsin results in inade-quate bleaching of the pigment, resulting in poor vision, particularly in dim light.

Convergence and visual acuity

There are much larger numbers of rods and cones than of bipolar cells and ganglion cells. An average of 60 rods and two cones converge, via bipolar cells, on to each ganglion cell. In the periphery, some 200 rods may converge on to a single ganglion cell, whereas in the fovea, which contains only cones, each photoreceptor is connected to one ganglion cell.

The lack of converging pathways from the fovea facilitates maximal discrimination by the visual cortex. **Visual acuity**, the smallest distance between two points which can be seen, is therefore highest at the fovea.

Ganglion cell receptive fields

A ganglion cell has a receptive field consisting of the area of retina containing all the photoreceptors connected to it. The photoreceptors in the centre of the receptive field are linked to the ganglion cells via the bipolar cells, whereas those in the periphery are linked to bipolar cells via horizontal cells. The size of receptive fields, therefore, varies in different parts of the retina depending upon the degree of convergence.

Retinal processing

Ganglion cells generate action potentials continuously. The stimulation of photoreceptors in the retina results in a change in the frequency of impulses propagated along the optic nerve fibres from the ganglion cells.

In dark-adapted rods and cones there is a steady flow of Na^+ from the inner segment of the photoreceptor to the outer segment (Figure 8.14).

This flow relies upon a Na^+ pump in the surface membrane of the inner segment which removes Na^+ from the cell continuously and creates a negative membrane potential (about $-40\,mV$). The membranes of the outer segments are highly permeable to Na^+ and therefore Na^+ re-enters the cell down its electrochemical gradient.

Under the influence of light, the photochemical changes that take place in the outer segment reduce its permeability to Na^+ so that fewer ions re-enter the cell. This results in an increase in the negative charge

Figure 8.14 Effect of light on a photoreceptor. In the dark, the Na^+ pump generates a negative membrane potential and the photoreceptor releases the excitatory neurotransmitter glutamic acid. In the light, the photochemical changes reduce Na^+ permeability so that less Na^+ enters the cell, which thus becomes hyperpolarized. Neurotransmitter release is inhibited.

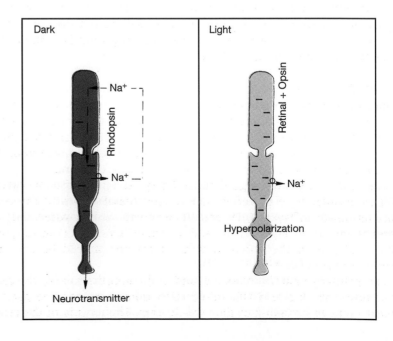

within the cell, i.e. it becomes hyperpolarized (−70 to −80 mV). The receptor potential of photoreceptors is therefore more negative than the resting potential. This is very unusual, as receptors usually become depolarized when stimulated.

Cones respond to light with rapid hyperpolarization, which dies away quickly (fast onset and fast offset). Rods, on the other hand, respond rapidly but the hyperpolarization dies away more slowly (fast onset and slow offset).

In the dark, the photoreceptor releases the excitatory neurotransmitter **glutamic acid**. Light hyperpolarizes the cell, which inhibits the release of neurotransmitter.

The change in frequency of impulses from the ganglion cells is mediated by two types of bipolar cell, one of which stimulates the ganglion cells, the other which inhibits them. The glutamic acid released by the photoreceptors stimulates one type of bipolar cell and inhibits the other type.

Horizontal cells and amacrine cells modify the information passing to the ganglion cells, principally by lateral inhibition.

Neither the photoreceptors nor the neural elements in the pathway between the photoreceptors and the ganglion cells operate by the usual action potentials, however. The cells communicate by direct current flow (**electrotonic conduction**).

Many of the ganglion cells produce a burst of impulses when a field is illuminated and a second burst when the illumination is switched off. Stimulation of the photoreceptors and the subsequent activities of bipolar, horizontal and amacrine cells therefore bring about an increase or decrease in the number of impulses travelling along the optic nerve fibres.

Information from the retina is perceived by the brain in terms of colour, shape and movement. These different aspects of vision appear to be processed separately, in parallel with each other, because some individuals have impairment of one of these functions, but not the others. For example, the perception of movement of images can be lost, but the ability to see colour and static shape retained.

Visual pathways

Figure 8.15 shows the nerve pathways from each retina to the lateral geniculate body in the thalamus and thence to the visual cortex. It can be seen that fibres from the lateral retina travel to the lateral geniculate body and to the visual cortex of the same side, whereas fibres from the nasal retina cross over, forming the X-shaped **optic chiasma**.

The cells of the **lateral geniculate body** are arranged in six layers, I–VI from anterior to posterior. The crossed (nasal) fibres of the optic tract terminate in layers I, IV and VI, whereas the uncrossed (lateral) fibres terminate in layers II, III and V. There is precise point-to-point transmission from the retina to these layers and indeed beyond this point to the visual cortex.

The **primary visual cortex** is found in the occipital lobe of the cerebral cortex (see Figure 5.10). Information from corresponding parts of the two retinae juxtapose in the visual cortex. The macula of the retina

See also **Receptor potentials** (page 215), in Ch. 7, Sensory Processing.

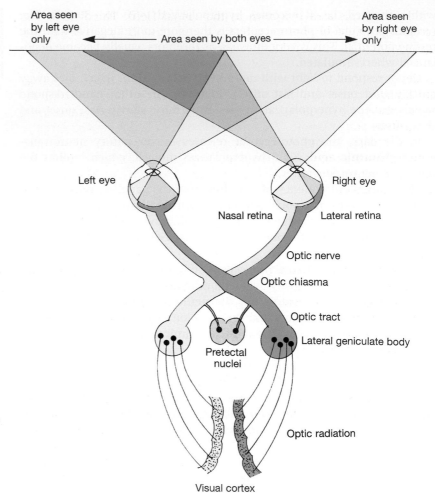

Area seen
by left eye
only

←——— Area seen by both eyes ———→

Area seen
by right eye
only

Left eye

Right eye

Nasal retina

Lateral retina

Optic nerve

Optic chiasma

Optic tract

Lateral geniculate body

Pretectal
nuclei

Optic radiation

Visual cortex

Figure 8.15 Visual pathways. Nerve impulses travel from the retina along the optic nerve to the optic chiasma. Fibres from the lateral retina of each eye travel in the optic tract on the same side to the lateral geniculate body in the thalamus. Fibres from the nasal retina of each eye cross over and travel to the lateral geniculate body of the opposite side. The neurones synapse in the geniculate bodies with neurones that travel in the optic radiation to the visual cortex.

See also **Direct light and consensual light reflexes** (page 167), in Ch. 5, The Brain.

is represented at the occipital pole, with other areas of the retina arranged in concentric circles around it. Superior regions of the retina are relayed to inferior positions on the cortex and vice versa. The fovea is represented by an area several hundred times greater than a simple projection of the retina on to the visual cortex would produce.

Impulses from the visual cortex pass to other areas of the brain, including the **visual association areas** which lie inferior, superior and anterior to the primary visual cortex. The association areas relate the image to memories, which give it meaning.

Some of the fibres of each optic nerve leave the optic tract and terminate in the **pretectal nuclei** in the midbrain. Reflex pathways connect the pretectal nuclei with the oculomotor and trochlear nuclei in the midbrain and the abducens nuclei in the pons varolii which regulate lens shape, pupil size and eye movements (see *Accommodation, Pupillary reflexes* and *Rotational movements of the eyeballs, above*).

BINOCULAR VISION

Each eye, when facing directly forwards, is capable of 'seeing' over quite a wide area; this area is known as the **visual field**. This field is not circular, as might be expected, because it is cut off by the nose and orbital ridge. The visual fields of the two eyes overlap for the most part, with smaller lateral areas that can only be seen by one eye (Figure 8.15). Images generated at corresponding points on the two retinae are fused into a single image within the visual cortex. The two images, however, are not absolutely identical, rather they are two views of the same object obtained at points about 10 cm apart (the distance between the two foveae). Images formed on the nasal and central parts of the retinae result in binocular images which give an appreciation of depth. Impulses generated within the lateral parts of each retina obviously cannot be fused in this way, and they give rise to flat monocular images in the brain.

LOSS OF VISION

Damage to one eye or one optic nerve results in the loss of three-dimensional vision, and the loss of the visual field of one eye. If however, the damage (such as that caused by a cerebrovascular accident) is beyond the optic chiasma (the cross-over point), in one optic tract, thalamus or visual cortex, then part or all of the opposite half of the visual field is lost. As the intact visual pathway takes information from both eyes to the visual cortex, three-dimensional vision is retained.

> See also **Cerebrovascular accident (stroke)** (page 174), in Ch. 5, The Brain.

Glaucoma

Glaucoma is characterized by a raised intraocular pressure, usually caused by impaired drainage into the canal of Schlemm (see *Aqueous humour*, above). The raised pressure causes indentation (cupping) of the optic disc with damage to or death of the neurones, exacerbated by ischaemia due to compression of the retinal artery (Figure 8.5). Chronic simple glaucoma is hereditary, progresses slowly and leads to enlargement of the blind spot and a reduction in peripheral vision. Without treatment with drugs (e.g. pilocarpine, which increases pupil size and therefore promotes drainage of aqueous humour) or the formation of a new drainage channel by surgery, blindness results.

Detached retina

A part of the retina may become detached from the pigment epithelial lining for a variety of reasons, including degenerative changes in the vitreous body or trauma. The retina becomes torn and vitreous humour leaks into the space between the pigment epithelium (which is attached to the choroid) and the inner layer of the retina. The retina thereby becomes deprived of its blood supply from the choroid, causing deterioration and loss of vision in the corresponding area of the visual field.

Lacrimation

Each of the two **lacrimal glands** comprises an orbital and a palpebral part. The former is the larger of the two parts and lies in a depression in the frontal bone above the eyeball and towards its lateral margin (Figure 8.16).

The gland has a lobular tubulo-acinar structure which secretes a clear

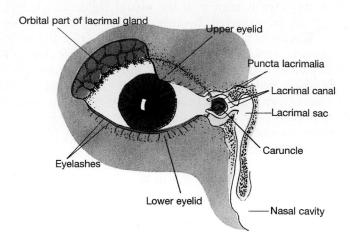

Figure 8.16 The lacrimal apparatus of the right eye.

dilute fluid containing Na$^+$ and Cl$^-$ over the front of the eyeball through several small ducts.

Two small openings (**puncta lacrimalia**) at the medial canthus of each eye lead into the **lacrimal canals**, which drain into the **lacrimal sac**. This is the upper, blind end of the nasolacrimal duct which, carries the lacrimal secretions (tears) down to the nasal cavity, where it terminates in the anterior part of the inferior meatus. Infection causing inflammation in the nasal cavity can easily spread to the ducts which drain lacrimal fluid, thereby blocking them and causing the eyes to 'water'.

Lacrimal fluid is secreted continuously on to the frontal surface of the eyeball and is spread over it by blinking. Excess fluid then drains down into the nasal cavity. Apart from keeping the eye moist, lubricated with mucus, it contains an enzyme, **lysozyme**, which is bactericidal.

The lacrimal glands are stimulated by parasympathetic fibres in response to chemical and mechanical irritants, so producing **tears**, which may wash away the irritants. Pain and emotion can also cause '**crying**', accompanied by a copious secretion of tears, stimulated by parasympathetic neurone activity.

HEARING AND BALANCE

Sound

Sound is generated by the vibration of an object such as a violin string. As the string moves forwards it causes compression of the air in front of it; as it moves backwards the molecules of gas in the air move further apart creating an area of expansion (Figure 8.17). Sound waves, therefore, are regions of alternate compression and expansion of molecules, their **frequency** being the number of compressions or expansions

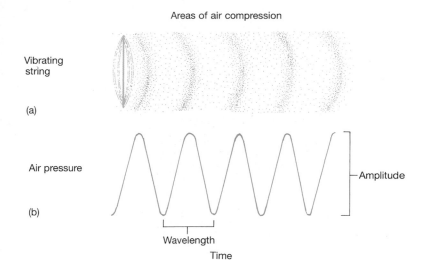

Areas of air compression

Vibrating string

(a)

Air pressure

Amplitude

(b)

Wavelength

Time

Figure 8.17   Sound waves.
(a) When a violin string vibrates, as it moves to the right it compresses the air molecules in front of it. When the string moves in the opposite direction, the air molecules to its right move further apart.
(b) Sound waves consist of alternating regions of compression and expansion of air (or water) molecules.

passing a fixed point per second, measured in hertz (Hz). The amount of energy in a wave is reflected in its height, or **amplitude**.

The ears

The ears play an important role in both hearing and balance. They convert the pressure changes generated by sound waves into electrical potentials which are then transmitted to the auditory areas of the brain. The ears also provide information about the position and movements of the head and initiate reflex postural adjustments that maintain balance.

The externally visible part of each of the two ears, the auricle or pinna, is located on the lateral surface of the head. The remaining parts of each ear are embedded in the bone of the skull beneath.

Each ear is subdivided into three parts, the outer, middle and inner ears (Figure 8.18).

Outer ear

The outer ear comprises the **auricle** and the **external auditory meatus** or canal.

Each auricle consists of a piece of elastic cartilage covered with skin. The rim (**helix**) is thicker than the rest. The earlobe (**lobule**) does not contain cartilage, but is composed of fibrous and adipose tissue, which makes it softer than the rest of the auricle, and easier to pierce.

The external auditory meatus is an S-shaped tube, oval in cross-section and about 2.5 cm long. The outer (distal) third of its length channels through cartilage, the inner (proximal) two-thirds through bone. The skin lining the meatus contains **ceruminous glands**; these produce wax (**cerumen**), which repels both water and insects. The cerumen traps particles and usually falls out of the meatus after it has dried. It

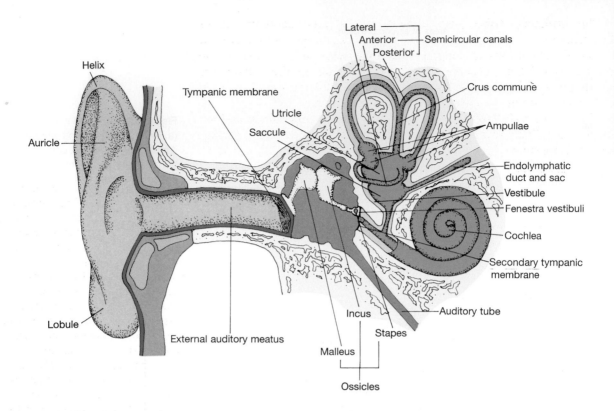

Figure 8.18 Schematic diagram of parts of the ear: outer ear [pink], middle ear [dark pink] and inner ear: osseus labyrinth [light green] and membranous labyrinth [dark green].

can, however, accumulate and become compacted and impair hearing if it is not removed. Coarse hairs project into the outer third of the meatus; these provide additional protection against the entry of small organisms. The external auditory meatus resonates at high frequencies (generated by some speech sounds) and therefore boosts them. A canal 2.5 cm long resonates at a frequency of 3440 Hz; shorter canals resonate at correspondingly higher frequencies.

The eardrum (**tympanic membrane**), which lies at the end of the external auditory meatus, is semi-transparent, cone-shaped and oval, with a longest diameter of about 10 mm. It has a three-layered structure: the outermost layer is skin, the middle layer is connective tissue containing collagen and elastic fibres, and the innermost layer is mucous membrane, continuous with that lining the middle ear.

Middle ear

The air-filled middle ear contains the three smallest bones in the body (the **ossicles**), which transmit sound from the outer to the inner ear.

The middle ear is very irregular in shape and measures some 15 mm both vertically and from front to back. It is bounded laterally by the tympanic membrane and medially by the inner ear; posteriorly it connects with air-filled cavities within the mastoid part of the temporal bone in the skull and anteriorly it connects with the auditory tube.

The **auditory tube** (also known as the pharyngotympanic or Eustachian tube) connects the middle ear with air in the nasopharynx. It is usually about 40 mm long and is lined with mucous membrane containing ciliated, columnar epithelium. The air in the middle ear slowly dissolves in its moist lining. It is topped up when the pharyngeal orifice of the auditory tube opens during swallowing.

The three ossicles are shaped like a mallet, anvil and stirrup and are named accordingly (**malleus, incus** and **stapes**). Further details of their structure are shown in Figure 8.19.

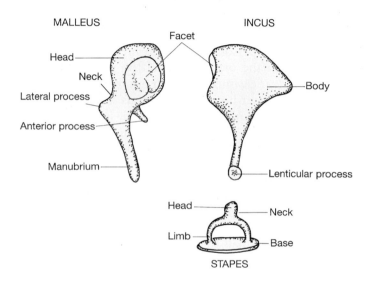

Figure 8.19 The three ossicles from the middle ear. The **malleus** (8–9 mm long) consists of a head, neck and three processes: handle (manubrium), anterior process and lateral process. The head articulates with the incus at the facet. The manubrium lies on the tympanic membrane. The **incus** has a body and two processes. The body articulates with the malleus. The longer of the two processes has a rounded end, the lenticular process, which articulates with the head of the stapes. The **stapes** consists of a head, neck, two limbs and a footplate or base. The head articulates with the incus and the base is held in the fenestra vestibuli by an annular ligament.

The malleus is attached to the tympanic membrane, the stapes is attached to the circumference of the fenestra vestibuli and the incus articulates with the other two ossicles by means of synovial joints. The ossicles are attached to the wall of the middle ear by ligaments.

The **tensor tympani** muscle lies in a canal above and parallel to the auditory tube and has its origin on the cartilaginous wall of the tube. The muscle inserts into the neck of the malleus and pulls it inwards. The **stapedius** muscle arises from the posterior wall of the middle ear and inserts into the neck of the stapes. Contraction of the stapedius pulls the stapes away from the fenestra vestibuli (see *Attenuation reflex*, below).

TRANSMISSION OF SOUND IN THE MIDDLE EAR

Sound waves hitting the tympanic membrane cause it to vibrate. These vibrations are then transmitted directly to the malleus, then to the incus and finally to the stapes, each bone moving against the next at its joint. The footplate of the stapes moves in and out of the fenestra vestibuli in a rocking motion. The force of the sound waves increases by about a third as they pass through the middle ear, because the ossicles act as levers. Furthermore, the tympanic membrane is some 17 times larger than the footplate of the stapes and therefore the force is transmitted to a smaller surface area. Overall, the pressure (force per unit area) of the sound waves is increased some 20 times as they pass through the middle ear.

The tympanic membrane and the ossicles are most responsive to sound waves with frequencies in the range generated by speech.

MAINTENANCE OF EQUAL PRESSURES ON EITHER SIDE OF THE TYMPANIC MEMBRANE

The molecules of gas in the air within the middle ear slowly dissolve in the mucous membrane, and consequently the pressure tends to fall. When swallowing, the pharyngeal end of the auditory tube is opened and air flows from the higher pressure in the pharynx into the lower pressure in the middle ear until the two pressures are equal.

The auditory tube can also be opened by a technique known as the **Valsalva manoeuvre**. The nose is pinched between the fingers, the mouth closed and the person attempts to breathe out forcefully. This raises the pressure in the oral cavity and the pharynx and opens the auditory tube. This 'ear clearing' is carried out repeatedly by divers using self-contained underwater breathing apparatus (scuba) as they descend underwater. The opening of the tube admits air into the middle ear and raises its pressure to that of the water pressure outside the tympanic membrane. Failure to do this results in a **burst eardrum**. This can occur even in the deep end of a swimming pool.

Another example of a situation in which the pressures either side of the eardrum are not equal is when flying in an aeroplane. In this case, on ascent, the atmospheric pressure falls below that at ground level, and therefore also below that in the middle ear. The auditory tube usually opens on its own and a small amount of air escapes from the middle ear until its pressure equals that of the air pressure outside the tympanic membrane. When the aircraft descends, atmospheric pressure rises and air is admitted into the middle ear until the two pressures are equal.

If the auditory tube becomes blocked with mucus, for example during a head cold, then ear clearing is impaired and the eardrum becomes displaced or ruptured. Either of these conditions are very painful and sound transmission into the middle ear is impaired.

ATTENUATION REFLEX

A sudden loud noise stimulates the sensory neurones in the cochlear nerve and causes reflex contraction of the tensor tympani and stapedius muscles in the middle ear, mediated by somatic motor neurones in cranial nerves V and VII respectively. The ossicles move closer together and become more rigid, thereby reducing their ability to transmit sound waves, particularly those of low frequency.

This reflex is a protective mechanism which prevents excessive vibrations from being transmitted to the internal ear. The reflex does not, however, prevent damage to sensory cells in the internal ear caused by prolonged excessive noise, such as from rock concerts or loud machinery.

Inner ear

The inner ear is composed of several interconnecting fluid-filled sacs and tubes (**membranous labyrinth**) suspended in fluid within a bony cavity (**osseous labyrinth**) within the temporal bone of the skull (Figure 8.18).

OSSEOUS LABYRINTH

The osseous labyrinth, the bony cavity within the temporal bone, is composed of three parts: the vestibule, the cochlea and the semicircular canals.

The **vestibule** lies medial to the tympanic cavity and measures about 5 mm from front to back and 3 mm across. The cochlea extends from the vestibule anteriorly and the semicircular canals arise posteriorly.

The **cochlea** is a helical cavity, like the inside of a snail's shell, consisting of a canal in the bone winding around a central cone-shaped piece of bone (**modiolus**) for two and three-quarter turns. The cochlea is some 35 mm long and its diameter is about 3 mm at its base, reducing towards the apex. A shelf of bone (**osseous spiral lamina**) projects from the modiolus like the thread of a screw (Figure 8.20).

At the base of the cochlea there are three openings in the bone, the oval window (**fenestra vestibuli**), which is closed by the base of the stapes; the round window (**fenestra cochleae**), which lies below the

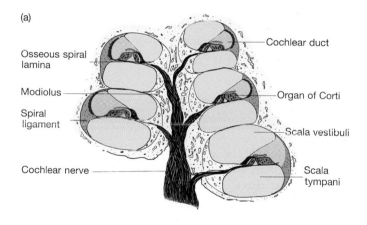

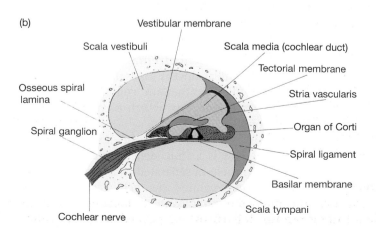

Figure 8.20 **(a)** Cross-section through the cochlea, a helical canal that winds around a central cone-shaped piece of bone (modiolus). A shelf of bone (osseous spiral lamina) projects from the modiolus like the thread on a screw. The cochlea contains three channels: the scala vestibuli and the scala tympani contain perilymph and the cochlear duct contains endolymph. **(b)** Detail: the sense organ of hearing (organ of Corti) lies in the cochlear duct and is innervated by sensory neurones which lie in the cochlear nerve.

fenestra vestibuli and which is closed by the **secondary tympanic membrane**; and the aperture of a tube (**cochlear canaliculus**), which opens out on the inferior surface of the temporal bone, thereby connecting the subarachnoid space with the cochlea.

Each ear contains three **semicircular canals**, orientated approximately perpendicular to each other; the **anterior** or **superior canal**, the **posterior canal** and the **lateral canal**.

The anterior canal is orientated vertically when the head is bent forward at an angle of about 30°. Posteriorly it joins the posterior canal, which is also vertical at right angles to the anterior canal, to form a common limb, the **crus commune**. The lateral canal is orientated in the horizontal plane.

MEMBRANOUS LABYRINTH

The membranous labyrinth comprises: 1) the **cochlear duct**, which is concerned with hearing, and 2) the **vestibular apparatus**, which is concerned with proprioceptive information about head position and rotation.

The membranous labyrinth lies within the osseous labyrinth, to which it is attached at certain points. It contains fluid (**endolymph**) and is surrounded by fluid of a different composition (**perilymph**) (see below).

The membrane has three layers. The outermost layer consists of fibrous tissue with blood vessels, the middle layer is loose, vascular connective tissue, whereas the inner layer is simple epithelium, variously squamous, cuboidal or polygonal.

The cochlea and hearing

A cross-section through the cochlea shows a kidney-shaped structure comprising three canals (scalae) (Figure 8.20). The middle canal (**scala media**, or **cochlear duct**) is part of the membranous labyrinth and is filled with endolymph, which is continuous with that in the vestibular apparatus.

On either side of the middle canal there are two canals filled with perilymph (Figure 8.20). The **scala vestibuli** contains fluid that is continuous with that in the vestibule: the fluid in the **scala tympani** bathes the secondary tympanic membrane. The two canals communicate at the apex of the cochlea at the **helicotrema**.

The outer wall of the cochlear duct is known as the **stria vascularis** and is composed of stratified epithelium containing capillaries. This structure overlies the **spiral ligament**, which is composed of thickened endosteum lining the bone.

The cochlear duct is separated from the scala vestibuli by the **vestibular membrane**. This is a thin, delicate structure composed of two layers of squamous epithelium separated by a basal lamina.

The **basilar membrane** separates the cochlear duct from the scala tympani. It is attached to the spiral ligament along its outer edge, and to the osseous spiral lamina along its inner edge. The basilar membrane is

much stronger than the vestibular membrane and contains protein filaments lying across it.

The structure and physical properties of the basilar membrane vary
along its length. At the basal end the membrane is narrow (0.21 mm),
the fibres short and the membrane stiff; towards the apex the membrane
is much wider (0.36 mm) and more flexible.

Organ of Corti

The sensory receptors associated with hearing are found in the organ of
Corti, which lies along the length of the basilar membrane (Figure 8.20).
The receptors are **hair cells** that are arranged in two groups (outer and
inner) and surrounded by a variety of packing cells. The most distinctive
of these supporting cells are the rod cells of Corti, which separate the
two groups of hair cells. The rod cells have expanded bases resting on
the basilar membrane. They are orientated in such a way as to create a
triangular-shaped tunnel (Figures 8.21, 8.22).

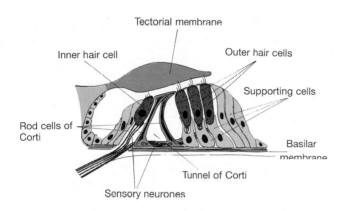

Figure 8.21 The organ of Corti. The hair cells are the sensory receptors which are stimulated when the basilar membrane vibrates and the cilia are bent and stretched. The hair cells are innervated by bipolar sensory neurones whose cell bodies lie in the spiral ganglion.

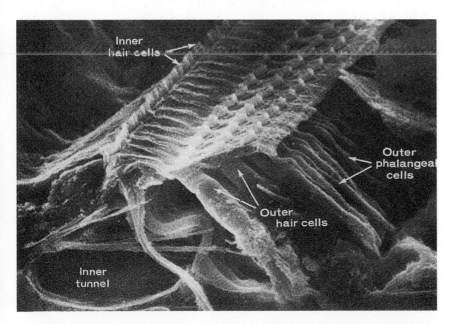

Figure 8.22 Scanning electron micrograph of guinea pig organ of Corti, cut transversely and viewed longitudinally. Note the rows of 'hairs' (stereocilia) and the outer phalangeal (supporting) cells. (Reproduced with permission from Fawcett, D. W. (1993) *Bloom and Fawcett: A Textbook of Histology*, Chapman & Hall, London.)

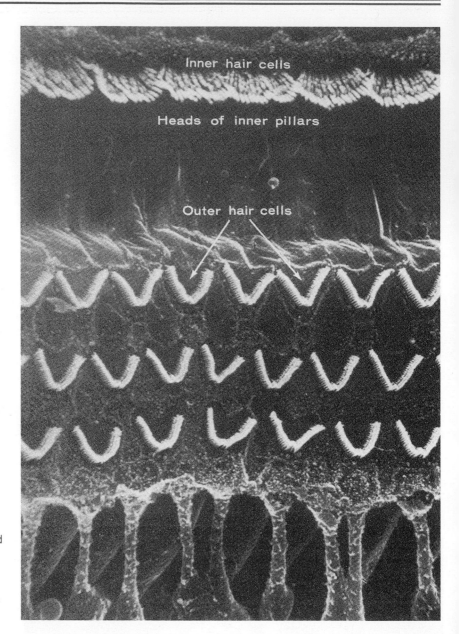

Inner hair cells

Heads of inner pillars

Outer hair cells

Figure 8.23 Scanning electron micrograph of guinea pig organ of Corti showing the rows of inner and outer hair cells. (Reproduced with permission from Fawcett, D. W. (1993) *Bloom and Fawcett: A Textbook of Histology*, Chapman & Hall, London.)

The outer hair cells are arranged in three rows, Each cell has some 50–100 **stereocilia** projecting from its apex in either a V- or W-shaped pattern (Figure 8.23).

The tallest of these cilia are embedded in the overlying **tectorial membrane**. This is a gelatinous structure, containing fibres, which is attached to the periosteum covering the osseous spiral lamina. The cells comprising the single row of inner hair cells have 50–60 stereocilia arranged in a shallow U-shaped pattern. These stereocilia do not embed in the tectorial membrane.

Both types of hair cell are innervated by **bipolar sensory neurones**, whose cell bodies lie in the spiral ganglion. The inner hair cells are supplied by many more sensory neurones than those in the outer group. The sensory fibres form the **cochlear nerve** (a branch of cranial nerve VIII) which lies in the modiolus.

Resonance of the basilar membrane

The movement of the stapes in and out of the oval window sets up pressure waves in the perilymph within the vestibule. The waves are then transmitted through the perilymph into the scala vestibuli and from there into the cochlear duct across the flexible vestibular membrane (Figure 8.24). The basilar membrane then vibrates and the sound waves are transmitted across into the scala tympani, where they are dissipated as the secondary tympanic membrane bulges from the round window.

High notes have a high frequency of vibration compared with low notes. The flexibility of the basilar membrane varies along its length, with the result that it is maximally displaced (resonates) by high-frequency notes at positions relatively near to the base of the cochlea, where it is stiff. Low-frequency sound waves, on the other hand, travel further towards the apex of the cochlea, where the membrane is much more flexible, before causing it to resonate (Figure 8.25).

Another factor affecting the position of resonance of a particular note along the basilar membrane is the mass of fluid involved in the vibration. Vibrations near the base of the cochlea involve a smaller mass of fluid than vibrations travelling further along the cochlea. This means that the basilar membrane has a smaller fluid 'loading' nearer to its base than its apex.

Figure 8.24 Transmission of sound through the ear. Perilymph [green]; endolymph [pink].

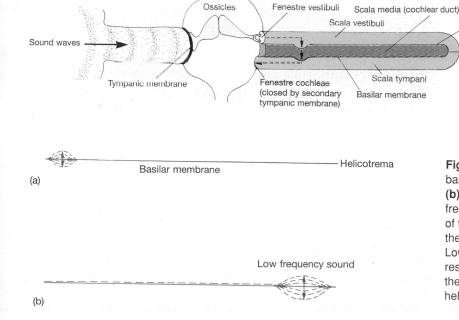

Figure 8.25 Response of the basilar membrane to **(a)** high- and **(b)** low-frequency sounds. High-frequency sounds cause resonance of the basilar membrane close to the secondary tympanic membrane. Low-frequency sounds initiate resonance over a longer length of the membrane closer to the helicotrema.

Stimulation of the hair cells in the organ of Corti

Displacement of the basilar membrane brings about movement of the organ of Corti, which lies upon it. The cilia of the outer hair cells, which are embedded in the tectorial membrane, are alternately bent and stretched as they move against this stationary membrane. As the cilia bend and stretch they are alternately depolarized and hyperpolarized, which leads to the development of alternating receptor potentials in the hair cells. Depolarization releases a neurotransmitter (probably glutamic acid), which stimulates the 20 or so sensory neurones which innervate them. Alongside the potential changes occurring within the hair cells, there are complementary changes in the fluid bathing them. These electrical potentials have the same frequency as the sound waves which stimulate them and are termed 'cochlear microphonics'. The cilia of the inner hair cells, which are not embedded in the tectorial membrane, are thought to be stimulated by movements of the endolymph.

Perilymph, endolymph and the endocochlear potential

Perilymph has a very similar composition to CSF, and indeed is connected to the subarachnoid space surrounding the brain through the cochlear canaliculus.

Endolymph is produced by blood vessels lining the membranous labyrinth, both from the stria vascularis in the cochlear duct and by blood vessels in the vestibular apparatus. After circulating through the membranous labyrinth, endolymph is returned to the blood in vessels surrounding the **endolymphatic sac** (Figure 8.18).

Endolymph has a high K^+ concentration and a low Na^+ concentration, which results in a potential difference (**endocochlear potential**) between it and the perilymph of some +80 mV with respect to endolymph. The hair cells have a resting potential of −60 mV. The total potential difference, therefore, between the endolymph and the hair cells is about −140 mV with respect to the hair cells. It is likely that this relatively large membrane potential sensitizes the hair cells to respond to slight movements of the stereocilia.

Pitch discrimination and the place principle

The **frequency** of a note is the number of sound waves passing a fixed point per second. **Pitch** is the subjective sensation of sound frequency, which involves sensory processing from the inner ear to the auditory cortex. The process of pitch discrimination begins in the organ of Corti. A high-frequency note stimulates hair cells near the base of the cochlea and stimulates the sensory neurones supplying them. Low frequency notes, on the other hand, stimulate neurones nearer the apex of the cochlea (Figure 8.25). As the nerve pathways from the different positions along the organ of Corti are kept separate right up to the auditory cortex in the brain, the same principle is also used in the cortex. It is called the **place principle for the discrimination of pitch**. Typically, humans can distinguish pitch over a frequency range of about 20–20 000 Hz, being most sensitive to tones from 1000–3000 Hz, which are in the middle of the frequency range of human speech.

Loudness

The detection of the loudness of a note is achieved in several ways. A louder note causes a greater amplitude of vibration of the basilar membrane and therefore a greater stimulus to the hair cells. This results in an increased frequency of action potentials from the sensory neurones innervating them.

The greater amplitude of vibration of the basilar membrane also means that more neurones on the edges of the vibrating area are stimulated. Thirdly, some sensory neurones have a higher threshold than others and therefore are stimulated only by a louder note.

Loudness is measured in **decibels** (dB). A barely audible sound, the threshold for hearing, is 0 dB. The decibel scale is non-linear, so that every increase of 10 dB represents a tenfold increase in loudness or intensity. Normal conversation at 1 m is about 60 dB, damage to hearing occurs after prolonged exposure to noise around 100 dB, and the threshold of pain is reached at about 120 dB.

An **audiometer** is an instrument that generates and measures the intensity of sound, and is used to measure hearing ability. The instrument also has an inbuilt electronic vibrator to test bone conduction from the mastoid process into the cochlea (see *Deafness*, below).

Auditory pathways

As impulses are relayed along the nerve pathways in the brain, successive neurones in the pathway respond to a narrower frequency band. It is likely that this is brought about by the mechanism of lateral inhibition.

Figure 8.26 shows the major routes between the sensory neurones from the cochlea to the brain stem and cerebral cortex. Impulses from each ear travel to both sides of the cerebral cortex, i.e. some pathways cross over from one side to the other whereas others do not. This contrasts with sensory pathways in general, where sensory information from the left side of the body is relayed to the right cerebral cortex, and vice versa.

The auditory pathways between the cochlea and the auditory cortex consist of several neurones. Synapses occur in the medulla (in the **cochlear nuclei**), the midbrain (in the **superior olivary nuclei**, the nuclei of the **lateral lemniscus** and the **inferior colliculi**) and the thalamus (in the medial geniculate bodies).

There are several points at which crossing over from one side of the brain to the other occurs: 1) between the superior olivary nuclei; 2) between the nuclei of the lateral lemniscus; and 3) between the inferior colliculi. The inferior colliculi mediate pathways that cause reflex head and trunk movements that turn the upper body towards the source of a sudden sound (the **auditory** or **startle reflex**).

There are also pathways to the reticular activating system, which has a general alerting effect on the nervous system, and to the cerebellum which is also activated by sound.

Lateral inhibition (page 225), in Ch. 7, Sensory Processing.

Figure 8.26 Auditory pathways. Sensory neurones from the cochlea have their cell bodies in the spiral ganglion and enter the upper medulla of the brain and synapse in the posterior and anterior cochlear nuclei. The second-order neurones mostly cross over to the superior olivary nucleus where most of them synapse. The third-order neurones ascend through the lateral lemniscus; some of them synapse in the nucleus of the lateral lemniscus, others terminate in the inferior colliculus in the midbrain. Some fibres cross over at the level of the nuclei of the lateral lemniscus, others cross over between the inferior colliculi. Neurones ascend and synapse in the medial geniculate nucleus in the thalamus and from there the final neurones in the pathway run to the auditory cortex in the auditory radiation.

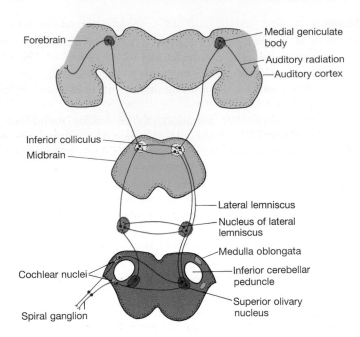

See also **Auditory areas** (page 149), in Ch. 5, The Brain.

Localization of a sound source

If the source of a sound is not exactly equidistant from the two ears, then the sound waves arrive at the two ears 1) at slightly different times and 2) with different intensities.

The localization of low-frequency sounds below 3000 Hz is determined principally by a comparison of the different times at which the two ears are stimulated by the sound. The information from the two ears is first compared in the medial area of the superior olivary nuclei and then despatched to the auditory cortices.

Higher-frequency sounds, on the other hand, are localized mainly by the difference in intensity of the sound arriving in each ear. Neurones in the lateral part of the superior olivary nuclei compare this information from each ear.

In both of these mechanisms of sound localization, turning the head changes the pattern of response and gives additional information about the direction of the sound.

Deafness

Partial or complete hearing loss can be one of two principal types: nerve deafness or conduction deafness.

NERVE DEAFNESS

The causes of nerve deafness can arise in the cochlea, the cochlear nerve, the auditory pathways or the auditory areas of the brain.

The sensory receptor cells in the organ of Corti are gradually lost as people age. Exposure to loud noise (which is usually of low frequency) can damage and even cause degeneration of the hair cells. The organ of Corti can also be damaged by some drugs, for example the antibiotic streptomycin.

Cochlear nerve degeneration can be a cause of deafness, and may cause a clicking or ringing sound in the ears in the absence of an external stimulus (**tinnitus**). Tinnitus can also be caused by inflammation in the middle or inner ear, or by aspirin.

Brain tumours or cerebrovascular accidents can damage the auditory pathways or the auditory cortices and cause deafness. Unilateral damage to auditory pathways below the level of the cochlear nuclei does not, however, result in deafness. This is because of the many points along the auditory pathway where the fibres cross over from one side of the brain to the other.

CONDUCTION DEAFNESS

Conduction deafness can be caused by impaired vibration of the tympanic membrane or of the ossicles.

Vibration of the tympanic membrane can be impaired by impacted cerumen, or by blockage of the auditory tube with mucus (due to a cold), which results in uneven pressures either side of the ear drum. A ruptured ear drum will not transmit sound from the outer to the middle ear very effectively.

Inflammation in the middle ear (otitis media) or fusion of the ossicles (otosclerosis, hardening of the ear) can impair their vibration.

A limited amount of sound is transmitted from the mastoid process (part of the temporal bone lying behind and below the external auditory meatus), through the skull bones into the cochlea. This is not affected in conduction deafness.

The vestibular apparatus, head movements and balance

The sense organs in the ear, which generate information about the position and movements of the head, are located in the parts of the inner ear collectively called the **vestibular apparatus**. This information leads to postural adjustments which maintain equilibrium and provide a sense of balance.

The vestibular apparatus (Figure 8.27) comprises the membranous **semicircular ducts**, each one having an enlarged section at one end, the **ampulla**, which houses a sense organ (**crista ampullaris**); the **utricle**, which is a sac connecting with the semicircular ducts and with a second sac, the **saccule**.

The utricle and the saccule each contain a sense organ (**macula** or **otolith organ**). Arising posteriorly from the saccule is the **endolymphatic duct**, which ends in a blind expansion, the **endolymphatic sac**, from where endolymph is returned to the blood.

The semicircular ducts are only about a quarter of the diameter of the bony semicircular canals and are attached to the wall by fibrous strands (Figure 8.28).

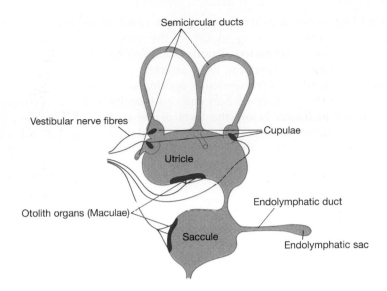

Figure 8.27   The vestibular apparatus.

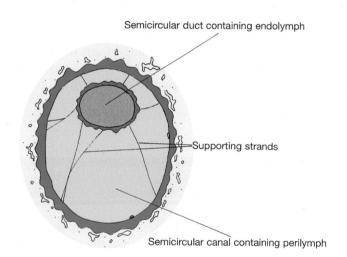

Figure 8.28   Section through a semicircular canal.

Crista ampullaris

The sense organs in the semicircular canals, the cristae ampullares, give information about the direction and rate of change (both acceleration or deceleration) of **rotational head movements**.

Within each ampulla, the membrane is thickened and projects into the cavity as a ridge called the ampullary crest (Figure 8.29).

On the surface of the crest are two types of **hair cell**, together with supporting cells. The type I hair cells are surrounded by a goblet-shaped nerve terminal, the calix, which is very close to, but does not actually touch the hair cell (Figure 8.29). Type II cells, on the other hand, are not surrounded with a calix but by a number of boutons, Some of these are sensory terminals, whereas others are motor and may be involved in altering the threshold of the type II cells.

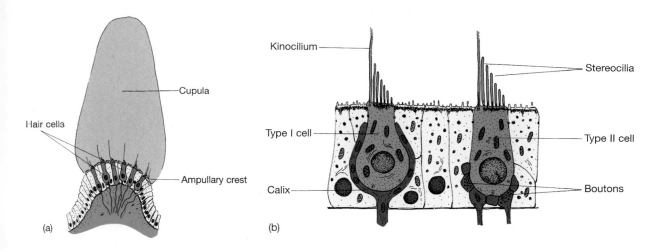

Figure 8.29 Structure of a crista ampullaris in the semicircular canals. **(a)** Ampullary crest and cupula. **(b)** Type I and type II hair cells on the ampullary crest.

Each sensory fibre innervating the type I cells innervates only a few such cells which are located near to each other. In contrast, type II cells are innervated by a number of different neurones, which themselves innervate a large number of type II cells spread over a large area. This pattern of innervation results in the type I cells being more discriminating.

The hairs of type I and type II cells are in fact **stereocilia**, or modified microvilli. There are between 40 and 100 stereocilia per cell, arranged into a hexagonal group. In addition, one border of the cell has a **kinocilium**, which has the usual nine doublets of microtubules around the periphery, but the central pair are normally poorly developed or may be absent.

Within each ampulla, the hair cell processes project into a jelly-like dome-shaped structure, the **cupula**, which projects across the ampulla and can be deformed by endolymph swirling within the semicircular duct when the head starts, or stops, turning. The jelly is composed of a protein–polysaccharide complex.

The way that the receptors are stimulated explains why they function only when the speed of rotation is changing and not if it is constant.

At the onset of rotation, the semicircular canals move as the head moves, but the endolymph within them lags behind. Therefore, inside those canals that lie in the plane of rotation, the cupula is dragged in a direction opposite to that of the movement. Since the canals in each ear are mirror images of each other, the two corresponding cupulae are dragged in opposite directions.

There is a resting discharge of impulses from the sensory neurones supplying the cristae, and as a cupula is moved it pulls the stereocilia either towards or away from the kinocilium. Movement of the stereocilia towards the kinocilium depolarizes the hair cells and increases the rate of firing of the sensory neurones, whereas movement away from the kinocilium leads to hyperpolarization and a decreased firing frequency (Figure 8.30).

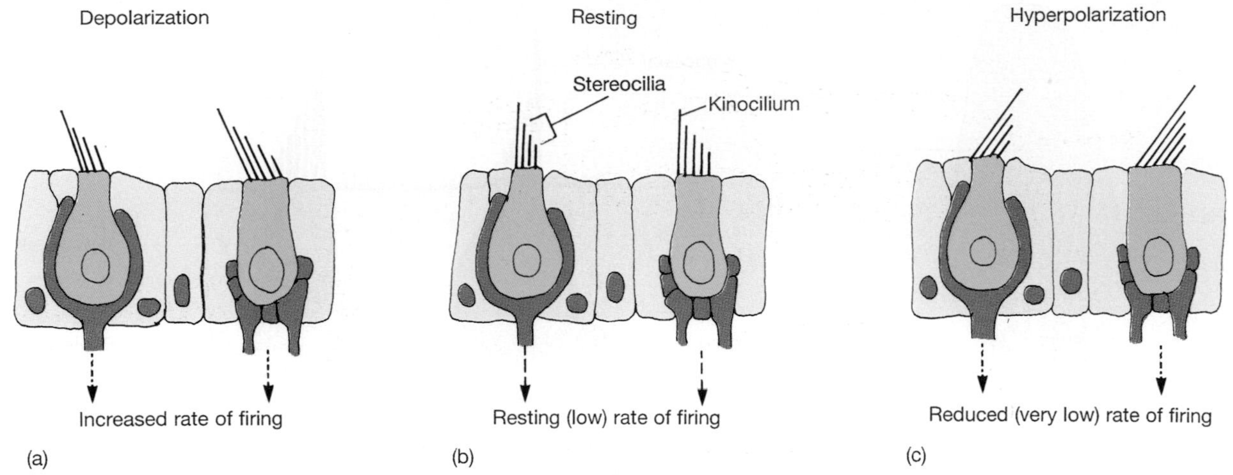

Figure 8.30 Relationship between the position of stereocilia and activity in sensory neurones in the sense organs of the vestibular apparatus. **(a)** Movement of the stereocilia towards the kinocilium increases the rate of firing. **(b)** Resting activity. **(c)** Movement of the stereocilia away from the kinocilium decreases the rate of firing.

At the onset of a rotational movement of the head, one cupula will generate an increased frequency of impulses, the corresponding one in the other ear a decreased frequency. A similar effect occurs if the head, already turning, suddenly moves faster. If, however, the movement is at a steady speed, then the endolymph catches up with the semicircular canal, the cupula recovers its resting position and the basal discharge rate is resumed.

At the end of the movement, the endolymph continues to flow and drags the cupula in the direction of the movement. The stereocilia bend in the opposite direction from that at the onset of movement, so that the rate of discharge changes in the opposite direction.

For a particular head movement, impulses from the six cristae are conveyed to the sensory cortex and the pattern of change at the onset or the end of the movement forms a code, which is interpreted as the movement in question.

Such information is particularly useful when a person is carrying out fast, intricate movements. If, for example a person is running and suddenly veers off in a different direction, then the change in firing patterns from the cristae lead to reflex **postural adjustments**, maintaining balance. Because the firing patterns from the cristae alter at the start of a movement, the information they generate rapidly becomes sufficient to initiate the appropriate postural changes, so that the new position is anticipated, and equilibrium maintained by the end of the turn.

Macula (otolith organ)

Within the utricle and the saccule is a sense organ 2–3 mm in diameter, known as a macula or otolith organ (Figures 8.27, 8.31). The four maculae (two in each ear) appraise the brain of the **static position of the head** and also of **linear**, but not **rotational,** acceleration.

In the utricle the macula is orientated horizontally on the floor, whereas in the saccule the macula is orientated vertically on the anterior wall, at right angles to the utricular macula.

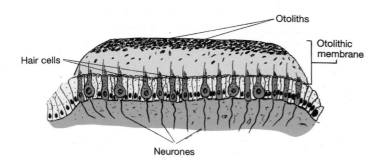

Figure 8.31 Macula or otolith organ from the utricle and saccule.

The hair cells and supporting cells of the maculae are similar to those on the ampullary crests but they project into an **otolithic membrane** composed of a glycoprotein jelly, containing particles of calcium carbonate and protein, called **otoliths** or **otoconia**. The otolithic membrane is flat and kidney-shaped, in the case of the utricle, and hook-shaped in the saccule.

The maculae emit a basal frequency of impulses. As the head is tipped, the otolithic membrane containing the heavy otoliths moves, causing some of the embedded stereocilia to be bent. When the hairs move towards the kinocilium, the frequency of action potentials increases; when the hairs move away from the kinocilium, the frequency reduces (Figure 8.30). The utricular macula responds mostly to horizontal movements because the hair cells are orientated vertically, whereas the saccular macula responds to vertical movements. Each head movement results in a different pattern of response from the four maculae.

If there is a sudden movement forwards, such as a car accelerating suddenly, the otolithic membrane, which has a greater inertia than the endolymph, tends to drag backwards. The stereocilia which bend are those which are also moved when falling backwards. This explains why suddenly moving forward elicits the sensation of falling backwards. The discharge pattern from the otolith organs initiates reflex postural changes which result in the body leaning forwards.

Nystagmus

If the head is turned suddenly, signals from the semicircular ducts initiate reflex movements of the eyes whereby the gaze moves slowly in a direction opposite to the direction of movement. If the head continues to turn, the eyes 'jump' forwards and fix on an object in view. With further movement of the head the eyes continue their backward gaze remaining fixed upon the object, before jumping forwards again to focus upon a new object.

Nystagmus consists of a slow component (the backward gaze) and a fast component (the jump forward). The effect of these movements is that the eyes have a better chance of focusing on an object if the gaze is maintained upon it. If the eyes always looked forwards, everything would be out of focus all the time as the head is turned.

See also **Brain stem reflexes** (page 167), in Ch. 5, The Brain.

In an unconscious person, semicircular canals can be stimulated artificially by introducing ice-cold water into the external auditory meatus. If the reflex pathway is intact, the eyes move towards the cooled side when the person is supine.

Vestibular pathways

The information from the vestibular sense organs is transmitted to the **vestibular nuclei** in the brain stem, where it is integrated with information from somatic proprioceptors and the eyes and initiates reflex postural adjustments that maintain balance as well as eye movements that maintain the gaze on particular objects. The vestibular nuclei have neural connections with the cerebellum, which coordinates muscle activity, and the reticular formation, which controls muscle tone. Neural pathways to the cerebral cortex mediate conscious awareness of the position and movement of the head.

Sensory neurones from the maculae and the cristae travel in the vestibular branch of the **vestibulocochlear nerve**. Figure 8.32 shows the nerve connections made by the vestibular nerves with the brain.

Figure 8.32 Vestibular pathways. Most vestibular nerve fibres synapse in the vestibular nuclei at the medullary/pontine junction. From here, second order neurones travel to various parts of the cerebellum; to the vestibulospinal tract; into the medial longitudinal fasciculus to the midbrain; and to the reticular formation in the brain stem.

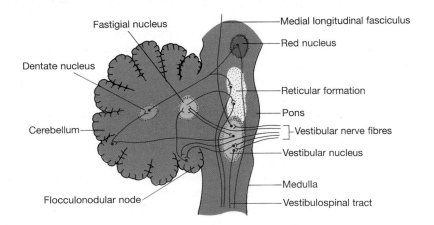

The main pathway for reflexes maintaining balance is via the vestibular nuclei, the cerebellum, the reticular formation and thence down the spinal cord to the muscles.

Eye movements are mediated via pathways from the vestibular nerves to the vestibular nuclei that then pass into the medial longitudinal fasciculus and on to the ocular nuclei in the midbrain.

Perception of the position and movement of the head involves pathways from the vestibular nerves to the vestibular areas in the temporal lobes of the cerebral cortex.

Impaired vestibular function (Ménière's syndrome)

The vestibular sense organs are distorted by an accumulation of endolymph within the membranous labyrinth and consequently give confused information to the brain in a condition called Ménière's syndrome. Balance can be so severely affected that standing upright is impossible. The person feels dizzy and this leads to nausea and vomiting.

The cochlea is also affected and may lead to tinnitus and hearing loss.

See also **Vomiting** (page 558), in Ch. 15, Digestion and Absorption of Food.

Vertigo

Vertigo is a sensation of falling, accompanied by dizziness and nausea, often induced by looking down from high places. It seems to be caused by an unexpected combination of vestibular and other, particularly visual, sensory inputs.

Motion sickness

The causes of motion sickness and vertigo are similar: a mismatch between sensory signals, particularly visual and vestibular ones. In the case of motion sickness, the body is moved about in an unpredictable way, stimulating the vestibular organs. The visual signals are also confusing in that the immediate environment of boat or plane moves with the person, but objects beyond this do not! The principal symptoms are typical of those resulting from upset balance: dizziness, nausea and vomiting.

TASTE (GUSTATION)

The organs of taste, the **taste buds**, are found in the epithelial coverings of the tongue, soft palate, posterior wall of the pharynx, and the epiglottis. There are typically about 3000 taste buds on the tongue and a further 7000 in the other areas. Recent work has demonstrated, however, that there is a very great variation in the number of taste buds on the tongue, with a correspondingly variable degree of sensitivity to taste. The taste buds contain **chemoreceptors** that respond to chemicals in the diet and generate patterns of impulses, which are transmitted to the gustatory cortex in the parietal lobes of the cerebral cortex. It is here that the sensation of taste is perceived. Reflex stimulation of salivary and gastric secretion is mediated by neural pathways through the brain stem.

The ability to detect different flavours is particularly important in achieving a **balanced diet**. It has been demonstrated, for example, that sodium-deficient laboratory rats selected a salt-rich diet; hypoglycaemic animals selected sweet foods; whereas hypocalcaemic ones chose calcium chloride solution to drink.

Animals and humans avoid bitter substances, many of which are poisonous, thus demonstrating the protective role of taste.

Taste buds

Taste buds are most numerous on the upper and lateral surfaces of the tongue. They are found on the surfaces of the circumvallate and fungiform papillae that cover the palatine surface of the tongue (Figure 8.33).

Circumvallate papillae (seven to 12) lie immediately anterior to the sulcus terminalis, each comprises a short cylinder sunk into the surface of the tongue. The taste buds are found on their side walls.

Fungiform papillae are mushroom-shaped, smaller than the

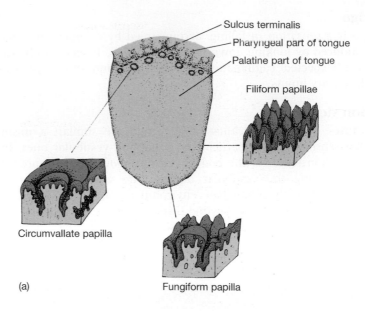

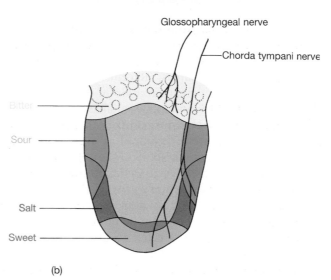

Figure 8.33 The dorsal surface of the tongue. **(a)** The different types of papillae (only the circumvallate and the fungiform papillae contain taste buds). **(b)** The areas most sensitive to particular tastes.

circumvallate papillae and found mainly on the tip and margins of the tongue, as well as being scattered over the entire dorsum. Taste buds are present on their upper surfaces.

The numerous filiform papillae that cover all of the palatine surface and margins of the tongue do not contain taste buds.

Each taste bud consists of about 50–90 cells arranged to form an ovoid structure lying deep within the epithelium and opening on to the surface through a small **gustatory pore** (Figure 8.34). There are three types of cell: sensory, supporting and basal cells.

Both the **sensory cells** and the **supporting cells** have microvilli (**gustatory hairs**) projecting from their apical surfaces. The sensory cells synapse with unmyelinated sensory nerve fibres.

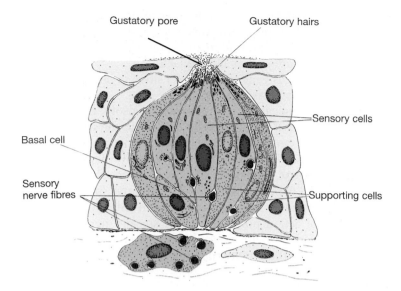

Gustatory pore

Gustatory hairs

Sensory cells

Basal cell

Sensory nerve fibres

Supporting cells

Figure 8.34 A taste bud. Chemicals attach to the surface membrane of the gustatory hairs (microvilli). The sensory cells become depolarized and stimulate action potentials in the unmyelinated sensory nerve fibres. The basal cells divide and replenish the supporting cells and the sensory cells.

The supporting cells insulate the sensory cells and the sensory fibres from one another, as well as forming the outer layer of the taste bud.

The basal cells renew the other cells of the taste bud by cell division, on average every 10 days.

Stimulation of taste receptors

There are four primary tastes: sweet, sour, salt and bitter.

Sweet substances include the organic molecules – carbohydrates, alcohols, aldehydes, ketones, esters and amino acids – and the inorganic salts of lead and beryllium. The non-carbohydrate sweetener saccharin is some 600 times sweeter than sucrose.

Sour substances are all acids, and generally the taste is proportional to the H^+ concentration. Organic acids, however, generally have a stronger sour taste than inorganic acids, probably because they penetrate the sensory cells more easily.

Salt taste is elicited by anions of metal salts, as well as some organic salts.

Bitter substances include a variety of organic compounds such as the alkaloids caffeine, morphine, nicotine, quinine and strychnine; urea, aspirin and the inorganic salts of magnesium, calcium and ammonium.

The application of pure solutions to the surface of the tongue demonstrates that it is most sensitive to sweet and salt at its tip, to sour at its edge and to bitter at its back (Figure 8.33). It should be noted, however, that this distribution is not exclusive since the tongue is, for example, also quite sensitive to bitter substances on its tip and edges. There are no discernible structural differences between the taste buds in different parts of the tongue. Individual sensory cells may be sensitive to one, two, three or even all four primary tastes.

Individual sensory cells discharge at particular frequencies determined by the type and concentration of specific substances. A particular taste sensation is achieved by a specific frequency pattern produced by the discharge of several receptor cells. This mechanism can also explain how the four 'primary' tastes can lead to an appreciation of an almost infinite variety of tastes that are potentially available.

Overall, the tongue is generally most sensitive to bitter substances and least sensitive to salt and sweet substances.

Different tastes appear to stimulate the sensory cells by different mechanisms. In all cases, the molecules dissolve in the saliva and interact with the surface membranes of the gustatory hairs. Salty substances open Na^+ channels, Na^+ enters the cell, thereby depolarizing it and generating a **receptor potential**. The H^+ in sour substances closes K^+ channels and cause depolarization. Sweet and bitter substances combine with specific membrane receptors which then influence ion channels. The generation of action potentials in the sensory nerve fibres is then probably stimulated by neurotransmitter released by the sensory cells. Taste receptors are of the rapidly adapting type.

Gustatory pathways

Taste buds on the anterior two-thirds of the tongue connect with fibres of cranial nerve VII (facial); those on the posterior one-third of the tongue are associated with fibres of cranial nerve IX (glossopharyngeal) (Figure 8.33). Loss of function of the facial nerve, therefore, results in impaired taste of sweet, sour and salty foods, whereas loss of function of the glossopharyngeal nerve diminishes bitter tastes. Pharyngeal taste buds send impulses to the brain in cranial nerve X (vagus).

Fibres from all three nerves enter the medulla oblongata and combine to form the **tractus solitarius**, most of which terminate in the **nucleus tractus solitarius** (Figure 8.35).

Second-order neurones then cross over and pass up through the brain stem to the **ventral posterior nucleus of the hypothalamus**, from which fibres travel to the **primary gustatory area** in the parietal lobe

Adaptation of receptors (page 215), in Ch. 7, Sensory Processing.

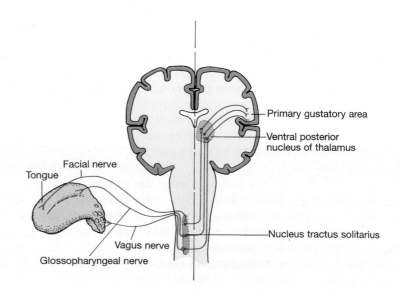

Figure 8.35 Gustatory pathways. Sensory neurones from taste buds on the anterior and posterior parts of the tongue and the pharynx are carried by the facial, glossopharyngeal and vagus nerves to the nucleus tractus solitarius in the brain stem. From here the pathway crosses over and ascends to the ventral posterior nucleus in the thalamus. Projection fibres connect the thalamus with the primary gustatory area of the cerebral cortex.

Primary gustatory area

Ventral posterior nucleus of thalamus

Facial nerve

Tongue

Nucleus tractus solitarius

Vagus nerve

Glossopharyngeal nerve

of the cerebral cortex (see Figure 5.10). Taste is perceived in this area (also called the parietal operculum), which lies at the posterior end of the lateral sulcus close to the area where other sensations from the tongue are perceived.

The nuclei tractus solitarius are the relay points for parasympathetic pathways to the salivary glands and the stomach. These pathways stimulate reflex salivation, gastric secretion and gagging and vomiting. Other ascending pathways synapse in the hypothalamus which effects a higher level of autonomic control.

See also **Salivation** (page 544), **Control of the secretion of gastric juice** (page 553), and **Vomiting** (page 558), in Ch. 15, Digestion and Absorption of Food.

Other sensations influencing taste

The presence of food in the mouth stimulates several different sensory receptors simultaneously: these convey a range of information about the nature of the food, which collectively can be interpreted as its taste.

The olfactory cells in the nose are stimulated by the chemicals in the food much more strongly than the taste buds. Temperature is conveyed by the thermal receptors, texture by mechanoreceptors, and spicy food such as hot curry stimulates nociceptors and causes pain.

SMELL (OLFACTION)

The sense of smell is much less important to humans than to animals. The parts of the brain concerned with smell in animals, the rhinencephalon, are dominant structures, whereas in humans, much of the rhinencephalon has become part of the limbic system and the olfactory areas of the cerebral cortex are relatively small structures (see Figure 5.10).

The senses of taste and smell are closely associated. Much of the enjoyment obtained from food, for example, is derived as much from its odour as from its taste. When olfactory sensation is impaired, for example during a head cold, food 'tastes' very bland.

Like taste, smell also has a protective function; for example, food that is 'going bad' has a repellent odour.

The olfactory receptors are located in the olfactory mucosa, which lines the roof of each nasal cavity. The olfactory receptors are stimulated by airborne chemicals. Action potentials are transmitted to the olfactory areas of the brain.

Olfactory mucosa

The olfactory mucosa occupies an area of about 2.5 cm² on the roof of the nasal cavity, extending down a short distance on to the surface of each superior nasal concha. It does not lie in the air stream that enters the nose during normal respiration, although the sudden, sharp inspirations that accompany 'sniffing' carry molecules up to the sensory cells (Figure 8.36).

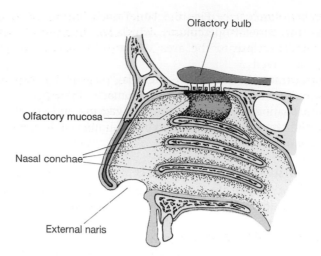

Figure 8.36 The location of the olfactory mucosa in the roof of the nasal cavity.

The olfactory epithelium is somewhat thicker than the respiratory epithelium which lines the nasal cavities and it is composed of three types of cell. These are the olfactory receptor cells, supporting or sustentacular cells and basal cells (Figure 8.37).

The **olfactory receptor cells** are bipolar sensory neurones with a cell body lying basally within the epithelium and a process that terminates in a small knob or olfactory vesicle, from which up to 20 long cilia (**olfactory hairs**) project above the epithelium (Figure 8.37). The cilia do not move and usually lie flat in the layer of mucus. Basally, each cell gives rise to a slender unmyelinated axon; this joins with other axons to form

Figure 8.37 Ultrastructure of the olfactory mucosa. The olfactory receptor cells are bipolar neurones, which are stimulated by odorants that dissolve in the mucus covering the epithelium. Bowman's glands secrete mucus. The basal cells divide and replenish the receptor cells and the supporting cells.

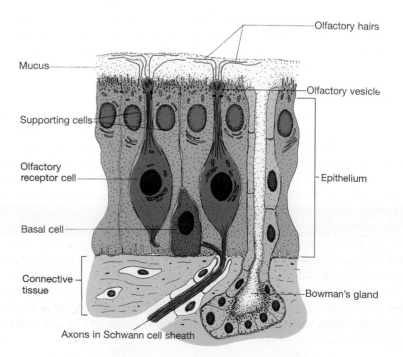

small bundles, which penetrate the bone. Each bundle of axons (not each axon) then receives a Schwann cell sheath. Bundles of axons pass through holes in the ethmoid bone and enter the olfactory bulb, where they synapse.

The **supporting** (**sustentacular**) **cells**, which lie between the receptor cells, are irregular columnar cells with nuclei lying close to their apical surfaces, which have numerous microvilli.

The **basal cells** divide and replenish both the supporting and the receptor cells every 60 days on average. The olfactory epithelium is unique in the human body because its nerve cells are routinely replaced.

The olfactory epithelium also contains the openings of the Bowman's glands, which lie in the connective tissue beneath. Bowman's glands secrete mucus on to the surface of the olfactory epithelium.

Stimulation of olfactory receptors

It is not clear exactly how olfactory receptors react with airborne odorous substances (**odorants**) and generate action potentials, although the first stage is that the chemicals dissolve in the mucus and bind to receptor proteins on the surface membranes of the cilia. There is a protein in the mucus that combines with hydrophobic odorants and presents them to the ciliary receptors.

The receptor cells emit a basal frequency of action potentials. The binding of odorants opens ion channels (usually Na^+) which causes depolarization and an increased firing rate. A few odorants cause hyperpolarization and a reduced firing rate.

A number of primary odours have been suggested, analogous to the primary tastes. One classification recognizes seven odours: camphoraceous, floral, musky, peppermint, ethereal, pungent and putrid. Other research work has indicated a much longer list of primary odours.

Individual receptor cells respond more strongly to one odour than to another. It is presumed that the discrimination of up to 4000 substances of which humans are capable depends upon the pattern of impulses generated by the olfactory epithelium as a whole.

Olfactory pathways

There are around 100 million receptor cells in each olfactory epithelium all of which give rise to axons that travel in about 20 bundles of the **olfactory nerve** (**cranial nerve I**). The nerve bundles pass through the cribriform plate in the ethmoid bone at the base of the skull to the **olfactory bulbs**. Within the bulbs, these axons synapse with the dendrites of second-order neurones (mitral and tufted cells), in structures known as **olfactory glomeruli** (Figure 8.38).

There is evidence that different odorants stimulate different glomeruli, indicating that sensory processing starts in the olfactory bulbs before reaching the cerebral cortex. This situation is analogous to retinal processing of visual information.

The olfactory bulbs also contain granule cells that release the neurotransmitter GABA, which inhibits the mitral cells. The granule cells also have neural connections with higher parts of the brain. This affords a possible mechanism whereby adaptation to odours is so rapid.

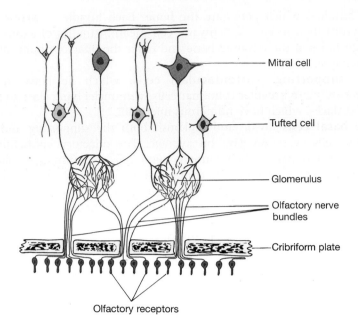

Mitral cell

Tufted cell

Glomerulus

Olfactory nerve bundles

Cribriform plate

Olfactory receptors

Figure 8.38 The principal neural connections within the olfactory bulb.

See also **Olfactory areas** (page 150) and **Limbic system** (page 155), in Ch. 5, The Brain.

From the olfactory bulb, mitral cell fibres pass into the olfactory tracts and from there to various sites on the medial aspect of the temporal lobe, principally the **primary olfactory cortex** and the **amygdala**.

The two olfactory bulbs have cross connections through the anterior commissure.

Pathways to the olfactory cortex mediate the conscious analysis of smells, whereas those to the amygdala feed into the limbic system and hypothalamus and are responsible for responses to the smell of food such as licking the lips and salivating, as well as learning whether particular smells are pleasant or unpleasant.

Loss of smell (anosmia)

Impaired function anywhere from the olfactory mucosa to the olfactory cortex can cause anosmia. Replenishment of olfactory receptor cells requires zinc, and consequently zinc deficiency can cause anosmia, as can inflammation of the nasal cavity. Head injuries can damage the olfactory nerves or the pathways to the olfactory cortices. Irritation of the olfactory pathways can cause uncinate fits, which involve olfactory hallucinations.

Autonomic and somatic motor activity

9

Autonomic motor function

The term 'autonomic' means 'functioning automatically or involuntarily'. The autonomic nervous system (ANS) regulates those functions not directly under voluntary control, such as blood flow, movements and secretions of the gut, sweating and release of glucose from the liver.

The ANS can be defined more precisely as the motor or efferent system that connects the CNS with smooth muscle, cardiac muscle and some glands. This definition effectively excludes somatic motor pathways to skeletal muscle, even though skeletal muscles do act in an involuntary fashion in reflexes such as the knee-jerk, withdrawing the hand from a painful stimulus and quiet respiration.

Structural organization of the autonomic nervous system

The ANS consists of two-neurone pathways, so that there is a synapse between the CNS and effector (see Figure 4.3). Synapses are located within ganglia outside the brain or spinal cord. The ratio of preganglionic (B fibres) to postganglionic neurones (C fibres) is not, however, 1:1 because there are more postganglionic than preganglionic neurones. Autonomic pathways, therefore, are divergent. Preganglionic neurones are myelinated whereas postganglionic ones are unmyelinated.

The hypothalamus is the major area of the brain that regulates autonomic activity. This has neural connections with specialized 'centres' in the brain stem that coordinate activities such as blood circulation, swallowing and vomiting. Higher centres of the brain, particularly the limbic lobe of the cerebral cortex, can also stimulate autonomic activity by neural connections with the hypothalamus.

Although the ANS is usually defined as a motor system, many of its activities are reflex and are therefore initiated by impulses in sensory neurones, which are then relayed in the spinal cord or in the regulatory centres in the brain.

The ANS is subdivided into two divisions, the parasympathetic and the sympathetic, which have clear anatomical and functional differences.

See also **Peripheral nerve fibres** (page 103), in Ch. 3, Tissues.

The hypothalamus is part of the Limbic system; see page 155 in Ch. 5, The Brain.

PARASYMPATHETIC NERVOUS SYSTEM

The parasympathetic nervous system has a craniosacral outflow from the CNS. Figure 9.1 shows the distribution of the principal parasympathetic pathways in **cranial nerves III (oculomotor)**, **VII (facial)**, **IX (glossopharyngeal)** and **X (vagus)**.

The only points of emergence from the spinal cord are in the **pelvic splanchnic nerves** arising from **segments S2**, **S3** and **S4**. The cell bodies of the preganglionic neurones are found in the lateral columns of the grey matter in this part of the spinal cord.

Parasympathetic ganglia are generally located near to, or lie within, the innervated organs. This means that the postganglionic fibres are relatively short compared with the preganglionic fibres.

In the cranial region of the system there are four ganglia: the **ciliary, pterygopalatine, submandibular** and **otic**. These are the synapse

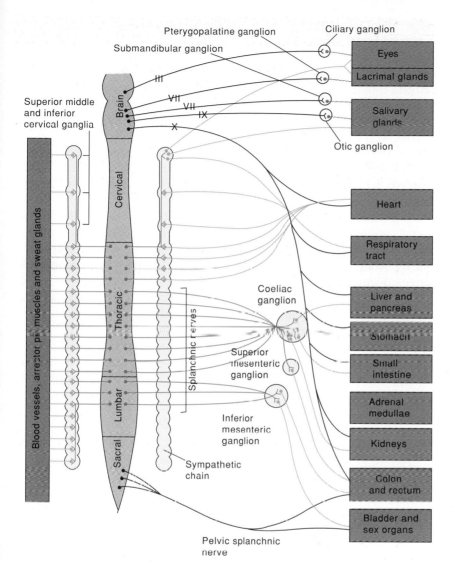

Figure 9.1 Plan of the autonomic nervous system. The system is bilaterally symmetrical, but the innervation of some parts of the body is shown only on the left-hand side, that of others only on the right-hand side.
Sympathetic pathways: green
Parasympathetic pathways: purple
Postganglionic neurones: paler colours.
In many cases parasympathetic ganglia are within the innervated organs.

points in pathways to the eyes, the lacrimal glands, the salivary glands and the oral and nasal mucosae.

The vagus nerves have a particularly extensive distribution, including the heart, respiratory tract, liver, pancreas, kidneys and the gastro-intestinal tract as far as the proximal colon. The ganglia are located within the organs themselves. e.g. the intramural plexuses in the gastrointestinal tract.

The distal colon, rectum, bladder and sex organs are supplied by the pelvic splanchnic nerves. The ganglia either lie within the organs them-selves, or there are very small ones found where the parasympathetic fibres meet branches of the sympathetic pelvic plexuses.

SYMPATHETIC NERVOUS SYSTEM

Figure 9.1 shows that the sympathetic pathways emerge from the **thoracic** and **upper lumbar segments** (L1 and L2 and sometimes L3) of the spinal cord. The system therefore has a thoracolumbar outflow.

Sympathetic ganglia are located relatively near to the spinal cord, either in two interconnected **sympathetic chains** or **trunks** (paravertebral ganglia) on either side of the vertebral column, or in **collateral ganglia** (prevertebral ganglia) next to the abdominal aorta. The principal collateral ganglia are named the coeliac (2), superior mesenteric and inferior mesenteric because they are located near to the origins of the arteries with the same names.

As sympathetic ganglia lie close to the CNS, the preganglionic fibres are relatively short compared with the postganglionic fibres. This contrasts with the relative proportions of the two types of parasympathetic neurones.

The preganglionic sympathetic neurones have their cell bodies in the lateral columns of the grey matter in the thoracolumbar region of the spinal cord. The axons leave in the anterior roots of the spinal nerves and then enter the sympathetic chains in the **white rami communicantes** (Figure 9.2).

The latter are so named because they contain myelinated axons. Thereafter the preganglionic sympathetic fibres may:

1. pass up or down the chain before synapsing;
2. synapse immediately in a ganglion of the sympathetic chain;
3. not synapse in the chain at all, but pass through it into a splanchnic nerve to a collateral ganglion. This is the pathway to the gastrointestinal tract.

Figure 9.2 Sympathetic pathways from the spinal cord. Preganglionic fibres leave the cord in the ventral root of the spinal nerve and may then either pass up or down the chain before synapsing, synapse immediately within a ganglion of the sympathetic chain (in this case the postganglionic fibre passes back into the spinal nerve through the grey ramus communicans) or not synapse in the chain at all, but instead pass through it and out into a splanchnic nerve, and synapse in a collateral ganglion.

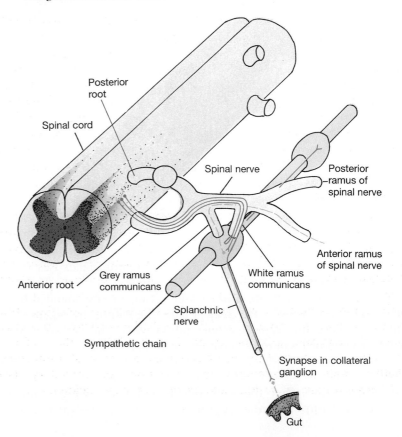

The postganglionic neurones also follow a variety of routes. They may:

4. pass back to the spinal nerve in a **grey ramus communicans** (postganglionic neurones are unmyelinated and so appear grey), and then travel in the posterior or anterior branches of the spinal nerves; this is the route taken to blood vessels, sweat glands and hairs in areas supplied by the spinal nerves;
5. be distributed alongside blood vessels;
6. ascend or descend the sympathetic trunk before leaving, as in (4) or (5).

It may be noted from Figure 9.1 that many organs receive fibres from both sympathetic and parasympathetic divisions; this is termed **dual innervation**.

The distribution of the sympathetic system is more widespread than that of the parasympathetic system, however, so that sweat glands, arrector pili muscles and most blood vessels receive only sympathetic innervation. This is also true of the adrenal medullae, which are supplied by preganglionic sympathetic fibres.

Neurotransmitters in the autonomic nervous system

The neurotransmitter released by the preganglionic fibres in both parasympathetic and sympathetic nervous systems is **acetylcholine**. The transmitter–receptor interaction is excitatory, so that all autonomic ganglia are collections of excitatory synapses.

Small doses of the drug **nicotine** bind with the nicotinic receptors in autonomic ganglia and stimulate postganglionic autonomic activity (see Figure 4.15). In larger doses such as those obtained by heavy smokers, nicotine blocks activity in the postganglionic neurones. The effects of nicotine, therefore, are diverse, in that it can stimulate or inhibit the parasympathetic or sympathetic nervous systems. Other **ganglion-blocking drugs** such as hexamethonium reduce activity in the postganglionic autonomic neurones in the same way as high doses of nicotine.

The neurotransmitters at the neuroeffector junctions differ in the two divisions of the ANS. In the parasympathetic system, the postganglionic fibres release acetylcholine, whereas in the sympathetic system they release noradrenaline. Sweat glands are exceptions, however, since they are supplied by sympathetic postganglionic fibres that secrete acetylcholine. As usual at synapses and neuroeffector junctions, the neurotransmitters are rapidly removed by enzymes, in this case **cholinesterase** for acetylcholine, and **monoamine oxidase** and **catechol-O-methyl transferase** catalyse the breakdown of noradrenaline

The sympathetic and parasympathetic systems exert opposing influences upon their target organs, and the fact that the two divisions release different chemicals into the tissue largely explains the different responses. The nature of the tissue receptors, however, also influences whether individual responses are excitatory or inhibitory (see *Acetylcholine receptors in the tissues* and *Adrenergic receptors*, below).

See also **Inactivation of neurotransmitters** (page 132), in Ch. 4, Cellular Mechanisms of Neural Control.

Actions of the autonomic nervous system

Both divisions of the ANS maintain basal levels of activity; this is referred to as **parasympathetic** and **sympathetic tone**. Alteration to the basal state, therefore, involves a change in the balance of activity between the two divisions. For example, at rest the heart is controlled by both divisions of the ANS, although the parasympathetic nervous system is dominant. When someone becomes more active or anxious, sympathetic activity increases and parasympathetic activity decreases. Both of these actions, therefore, result in an increase in heart rate and strength of contraction.

The actions of the sympathetic nervous system are generally more widespread and concerted than those of the parasympathetic system, and this is directly related to differences in their anatomical pathways. The chains of interconnecting ganglia on either side of the spinal cord provide an outflow to all parts of the body, which then respond simultaneously. Furthermore, the ratio of postganglionic to preganglionic neurones is higher in the sympathetic nervous system. Parasympathetic innervation is more restricted. It does not supply the skin, most blood vessels or the adrenal medullae. In contrast to the sympathetic pathways, parasympathetic pathways are generally separate from one another and therefore their actions are more discrete.

Those organs that receive only sympathetic innervation, such as most blood vessels, are controlled by an increase or decrease of sympathetic tone; vasodilation is caused by a decrease in sympathetic tone and vasoconstriction by an increase.

ACTIONS OF THE PARASYMPATHETIC NERVOUS SYSTEM

Overall, the parasympathetic nervous system promotes inactivity and the build up of food reserves by digestion. Someone asleep after a big meal is '**resting and refuelling**' and demonstrates the effects of a dominant parasympathetic nervous system.

The vagus nerves have an extensive distribution and therefore often affect many sites at once, for example, the cephalic phase of the control of gastric secretion stimulates the flow of pancreatic juice and bile, as well as gall bladder contraction.

Many parasympathetic pathways, however, are separate from one another, with the result that activity can be local to one area e.g. lacrimation, pupillary reflexes.

Table 9.1 lists the actions of the parasympathetic nervous system in particular sites. The actions follow the general pattern of rest and refuelling in the digestive glands, the heart, and the gastrointestinal tract. Elimination of urine and faeces by micturition and defaecation are promoted by the parasympathetic nervous system.

The PNS also promotes secretion by glands in the respiratory tract and by the lacrimal glands. Blood vessels generally lack parasympathetic innervation, with the exception of the coronary arterioles (where neural control is minor), the 'blush' area of the face, and the clitoris and penis. Parasympathetic stimulation causes vasodilation in all these areas.

Table 9.1 Effects of sympathetic and parasympathetic activity

Site	Sympathetic	Parasympathetic
Eye		
Iris	Pupil dilation (contraction radial muscle)	Pupil constriction (contraction circular muscle)
Ciliary muscle	Relaxation (suspensory ligaments tighten, lens flattens – far vision)	Contraction (suspensory ligaments relax, lens becomes more convex – near vision)
Lacrimal glands	—	Secretion
Salivary glands		
Secretory cells	Scant, viscous secretion	Copious watery secretion
Arterioles	Vasoconstriction	—
Heart		
SA node	↑Rate of firing	↓Rate of firing
Atria	↑Force of contraction	↓Force of contraction
Ventricles	↑Force of contraction	—
Arterioles		
General	Vasoconstriction	—
Skeletal muscle	Vasoconstriction (α) Vasodilation (β)	
Coronary	Vasoconstriction (α) Vasodilation (β)	Vasodilation
Face	Vasoconstriction	Vasodilation
Veins	Venoconstriction	—
Bronchi		
Smooth muscle	Bronchodilation	Bronchoconstriction
Glands	↓Secretion	↑Secretion
Gastrointestinal tract		
Smooth muscle	↓Peristalsis	↑Peristalsis
Sphincters	Constriction	Relaxation
Glands	↓Secretion	↑Secretion
Pancreas		
Exocrine cells	↓Secretion	↑Secretion
Islets of Langerhans	↓Insulin secretion ↑Glucagon secretion	↑Insulin secretion
Gall bladder	Relaxation	Contraction
Liver	↑Glycogenolysis	—
	—	↑Bile secretion
Adipose tissue	↑Lipolysis	—
Kidneys		
Juxtaglomerular cells	↑Renin secretion	—
Urinary bladder		
Detrusor muscle	Relaxation	Contraction
Trigone and sphincter	Contraction	Relaxation
Skin		
Sweat glands	↑Sweat secretion (cholinergic)	—
Arrector pili muscles	Contraction	—
Uterus		
Pregnant	Contraction	Variable
Non-pregnant	Relaxation	—
Clitoris/vagina	Contraction of vagina	Erection of clitoris (vasodilation)
Penis	Ejaculation	Erection (vasodilation)
Adrenal Medullae	↑Adrenaline and noradrenaline secretion (cholinergic)	—

See also **Receptors** (page 126), in Ch. 4, Cellular Mechanisms of Neural Control.

Acetylcholine receptors in the tissues

Stimulation of parasympathetic pathways leads to the release of acetylcholine at the neuroeffector junctions. The chemical is 'bound' to muscarinic receptors on the effector cells. Once in position, the complex alters the permeability characteristics of the effector cell membrane, rendering it more or less excitable. In most sites the effect is inhibitory, but in the gastrointestinal tract the effect is increased glandular secretion and motility of the wall; in the bladder, the responses result in micturition.

Parasympathomimetic drugs such as pilocarpine can be used to intensify the effects of the PNS by combining with muscarinic receptors in a similar way to acetylcholine. Other drugs (Table 9.2) can bind with muscarinic receptors and 'block' them from acetylcholine, and thereby inhibit parasympathetic responses.

ACTIONS OF THE SYMPATHETIC NERVOUS SYSTEM

The sympathetic nervous system causes physiological changes associated with physical exercise such as stimulating the heart, raising blood pressure and releasing adrenaline. It is also more active when one is frightened or anxious, causing changes such as dilated pupils and the raising of skin hairs giving the appearance of 'gooseflesh' (piloerection).

Walter Cannon suggested in the 1920s that the sympathetic system was stimulated in states of emergency in '**fright**, **fight** or **flight**' and that there was generalized activity in the system, the '**sympathetic discharge**'. The widespread actions of the sympathetic nervous system are dependent upon the anatomical arrangement of the chains of ganglia, whereby all parts of the body are interconnected and consequently act 'in sympathy'.

Table 9.1 summarizes the effects of sympathetic stimulation at various named sites. It can be seen that the responses are generally associated with fear and/or physical exercise, and that the effects of sympathetic activity are generally opposite to those of the parasympathetic system.

Table 9.2 Drug actions on the parasympathetic nervous system	
Action	*Examples*
Cholinergic stimulants	
1. Stimulate acetylcholine	Black-widow-spider venom
2. Stimulate muscarinic receptors	Methacholine Pilocarpine
3. Inhibit cholinesterase	Neostigmine Pyridostigmine
Cholinergic blockers	
Block muscarinic receptors	Atropine Hyoscine

There are a few anomalies, however. With regard to pupil size, the sympathetic system causes dilation, whereas the parasympathetic system causes constriction. The two effects, however, are not brought about by the same set of muscles. Pupillary dilation is caused by contraction of the radial muscles in the iris, whereas pupillary constriction is the result of contraction of the circular muscle in the iris. Both divisions stimulate salivation, albeit with different results. Parasympathetic stimulation causes a copious, watery secretion while sympathetic stimulation brings about the production of small amounts of very viscous saliva. This effect is intensified by vasoconstriction of arterioles supplying the salivary glands, since it restricts the amount of fluid available to them.

The sympathetic system is dominant during physical exercise, and it has a strong effect on the circulatory system. The heart rate and stroke volume are increased, both of which increase cardiac output and thus systolic arterial blood pressure. There is generalized vasoconstriction, but the coronary arterioles and those in active skeletal muscle dilate (mainly due to local chemical changes as well as circulating adrenaline). Sympathetic stimulation also causes venoconstriction and thus increases venous return during exercise. Overall, sympathetic activity increases cardiac output, which enhances blood flow generally, and the blood is directed towards the heart and active skeletal muscle and away from other areas not involved in the exercise. These adjustments result in the active areas receiving oxygen and nutrients in the blood at the increased rate at which they are used. Similarly the carbon dioxide, heat and metabolites are removed by the increased blood flow. The circulatory changes, therefore, maintain the constancy of the environment around the cardiac and skeletal muscle cells.

The sympathetic system has an inhibitory effect on the gastrointestinal tract so that peristalsis is inhibited and the sphincters constrict. Activity is further reduced by vasoconstriction, which reduces the blood supply.

Sexual activity is affected by the sympathetic nervous system. It causes ejaculation in men and vaginal and uterine contractions in women during orgasm.

See also **Cardiovascular responses to physical exercise** (page 425), in Ch. 12, Circulation of Blood and Lymph.

SYMPATHOMIMETIC ACTIONS OF ADRENALINE AND NORADRENALINE

The sympathetic system innervates the adrenal medullae. The preganglionic neurones release acetylcholine which combines with nicotinic receptors on the glandular cells and stimulates the release of adrenaline and noradrenaline (in a ratio of about 4:1). The glands, therefore, are analogous to postganglionic sympathetic neurones. Once noradrenaline and adrenaline are released into the blood they intensify the effects of sympathetic stimulation and prolong its action between five and 10 times. The hormones are said to have a **sympathomimetic effect**, i.e. they mimic the effects of sympathetic neurone stimulation.

The circulating hormones are able to control parts of the body that lack sympathetic innervation.

Adrenergic receptors

There are two main types of adrenergic receptor found in the tissues, alpha (α) and **beta** (β). They may be further subdivided into **alpha₁, alpha₂, beta₁** and **beta₂-adrenoceptors**. More recently, a beta₃-adrenoceptor has been identified on adipocytes. The different receptors are distributed unevenly in different tissues. Furthermore, noradrenaline and adrenaline have different affinities for the receptors. Noradrenaline combines strongly with alpha-adrenoceptors, but only weakly with beta-adrenoceptors, whereas the reverse is the case for adrenaline, which combines strongly with beta-adrenoceptors and less strongly with alpha-adrenoceptors.

Table 9.3 summarizes the major effects of adrenaline and noradrenaline combining with alpha- or beta-adrenoceptors. Beta₁-adrenoceptors are present in cardiac muscle, where their activation increases activity. Beta₂-adrenoceptors are stimulated strongly by adrenaline and very little by noradrenaline. Beta₂-adrenoceptors are generally associated with smooth muscle relaxation, e.g. vasodilation in skeletal muscles and coronary arterioles, intestinal relaxation, and bronchodilation. Beta₂-adrenoceptor stimulation is also associated with metabolic changes such as the breakdown of glycogen to glucose and its release from the liver (glycogenolysis). Both of these metabolic actions and the release of free fatty acids from stored triglycerides in adipose tissue (lipolysis) increase the nutrients available for active muscles. Beta₂-adrenoceptor activation can double the metabolic rate.

The sympathomimetic actions of adrenaline resulting from its action on beta-receptors, therefore, are especially powerful in stimulating the

---

Table 9.3 Actions of adrenergic receptors

Alpha-adrenoceptors	Beta-adrenoceptors
Alpha₁-adrenoceptors	*Beta₁-adrenoceptors*
Intestinal relaxation	Increased heart rate
Pregnant uterus contraction	Increased stroke volume
Pupil dilation	*Beta₂-adrenoceptors*
Vasoconstriction	Ciliary muscle relaxation
Bladder, trigone and sphincter contraction	Vasodilation of coronary and skeletal muscle arterioles
Thick viscous salivation	Bronchodilation
Palms sweating	Intestinal relaxation
Vasoconstriction	Bladder wall relaxation
Intestinal sphincter contraction	Non-pregnant uterus relaxation
Piloerection	Increased glucagon secretion
Ejaculation	Glycogenolysis
Glycogenolysis	Increased metabolic rate
Alpha₂-adrenoceptors	*Beta₃-adrenoceptors*
Platelet aggregation	Lipolysis
Vasoconstriction	

Table 9.4 Drug actions on the sympathetic nervous system

Action	Examples
Adrenergic stimulants	
1. Stimulate noradrenaline release from postganglionic neurone endings	Amphetamine Ephedrine Tyramine
2. Stimulate alpha-receptors	Phenylephrine
3. Stimulate beta-receptors	Adrenaline Isoprenaline
4. Stimulate beta$_1$-receptors	Dobutamine
5. Stimulate beta$_2$-receptors	Salbutamol
6. Inhibit uptake of noradrenaline	Tricyclic antidepressants Cocaine
7. Inhibit MAO	Tranylcypromine Phenelzine
Adrenergic blockers	
1. Inhibits synthesis and storage of noradrenaline in postganglionic neurone endings	Reserpine
2. Inhibits the release of noradrenaline from postganglionic neurone endings	Guanethidine
3. Block alpha-receptors	Phenoxybenzamine Phentolamine
4. Blocks all beta-receptors	Propranolol
5. Blocks beta$_1$-receptors	Sotalol Alprenolol

heart, diverting blood to the heart and skeletal muscles, stimulating metabolism in general and glycogenolysis and lipolysis in particular.

Adrenaline also acts on the central nervous system, causing increased respiration, muscle tremor and increased strength of contraction, and feelings of fear and anxiety.

There are a whole range of drugs that act on the sympathetic nervous system, either altering the secretion or release of noradrenaline or stimulating or blocking the adrenergic tissue receptors. Table 9.4 summarizes the mechanisms of drug action and gives examples of specific drugs in each category.

Excess sympathetic vasoconstriction (Raynaud's phenomenon)

An exaggerated vasoconstrictor response, usually on exposure to cold, can be seen in individuals displaying **Raynaud's phenomenon**. The intense vasoconstriction causes the fingers and toes to become pale, ischaemic and consequently cyanotic and painful. In severe cases the tissue can actually die (**gangrene**). Alleviation of the symptoms can be achieved by cutting the sympathetic supply to the fingers and toes, so that the arterioles dilate.

THE AUTONOMIC NERVOUS SYSTEM AND STRESS

Stress can be described as the physical and psychological responses to a stimulus which is generally, but not always, unpleasant. The stimulus is the **stressor**, the resultant psychophysiological state is the **stress**. Some of the physiological changes involved are the result of changes in the level of activity of the ANS. Stressors such as pain, fear, anticipating or experiencing an unpleasant event are perceived by the cerebral cortex, which then stimulates the hypothalamus (Figure 9.3).

Figure 9.3 Actions of the sympathetic nervous system in stress.

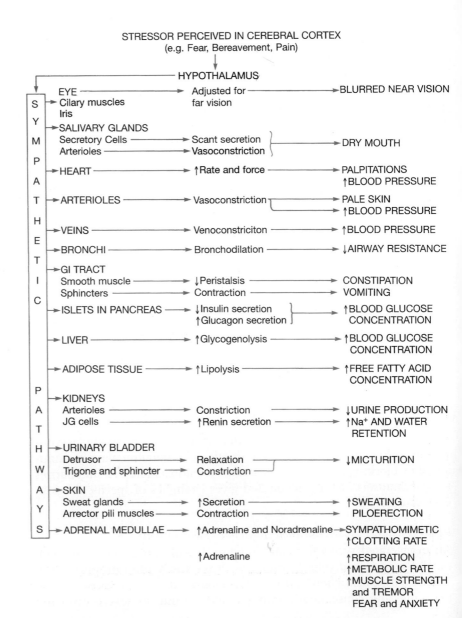

A typical 'alarm' response to a stressor involves mass discharge of the sympathetic nervous system. A cat which is threatened arches its back, its hair stands on end, its pupils dilate, its heart beats harder and faster, and so on. Its appearance can indeed appear frightening, and the physiological responses prepare the animal for flight or fight.

In humans, many of the responses are the same as those seen in other mammals: increased heart rate and force (palpitations), pale sweating skin, gooseflesh, dilated pupils, release of glucose from the liver – all mediated by increased sympathetic activity supported by the release of adrenaline and noradrenaline from the adrenal medullae.

Depending on the nature of the stressors, these responses may either maintain homoeostasis or disturb it. If the stress response involves physical activity such as running away or fighting, then clearly a rise in blood pressure will increase blood flow to active muscles. Similarly, many of the changes will tend to restore homoeostasis. Following a haemorrhage, for example, peripheral vasoconstriction tends to keep central arterial pressure up and maintains blood flow to the vital centres in the brain. However inactivity during stress, such as sitting worrying or grieving, will tend to disrupt homoeostasis by raising blood pressure, blood glucose and fatty acid concentrations, inhibiting digestion etc. Clearly there is the potential here for disturbances to health, and such a situation may therefore lead to stress-related illness. Although 'stress' is a rather vague term and, it can be argued, is present to some degree in everyone all the time, there are a number of conditions in which excessive stress has been implicated as a causative factor. They include hypertension, arteriosclerosis, constipation, diverticulitis, duodenal peptic ulcer and diabetes mellitus.

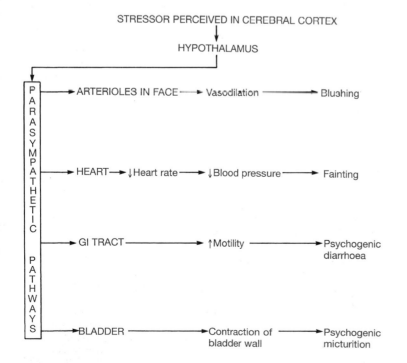

STRESSOR PERCEIVED IN CEREBRAL CORTEX
↓
HYPOTHALAMUS

PARASYMPATHETIC PATHWAYS

→ ARTERIOLES IN FACE —→ Vasodilation ————→ Blushing

→ HEART —→ ↓Heart rate ——→ ↓Blood pressure ———→ Fainting

→ GI TRACT ————————→ ↑Motility ———→ Psychogenic diarrhoea

→ BLADDER ———————→ Contraction of bladder wall ——→ Psychogenic micturition

Figure 9.4 Stress responses mediated by the parasympathetic nervous system.

There are occasions, particularly in fearful or anxious situations when the parasympathetic system becomes dominant (Figure 9.4).

Strong parasympathetic stimulation of the heart (a **vasovagal attack**) reduces cardiac activity and therefore blood pressure. The resultant fall in cerebral blood flow can cause 'fainting' (syncope), a loss of consciousness due to hypoxia. Falling down or putting the head down improves the blood flow to the brain and can restore consciousness. Someone who remains upright after fainting, so that the cerebral blood flow remains low, can experience violent muscular contractions (convulsions) of an epileptic nature.

Other examples of physiological responses to strong PNS stimulation in stress are uncontrolled micturition or defaecation (**psychogenic micturition** or **diarrhoea**). Vasodilation in the arterioles supplying the face results in a red face or **blushing**.

An additional major physiological response to stressors is the release of cortisol from the adrenal cortices.

See also **Cortisol and stress** (page 642), in Ch. 16, Endocrine Physiology.

Somatic motor function

See also **Peripheral nerve fibres** (page 103), in Ch. 3, Tissues.

Somatic motor neurones connect the CNS with skeletal muscle (see Figures 4.2, 4.3). The nerve fibres are type Aα, the most thickly myelinated and fastest-conducting (up to 120 m/s) in the body.

Action potentials are transmitted across the neuromuscular junctions into the skeletal muscle fibres which, following a series of intracellular events (excitation–contraction coupling), then contract.

This chapter analyses the events causing skeletal muscle contraction and the control of voluntary movement by the brain. Reflex movements are covered in other chapters.

Reflex movements involving skeletal muscles are covered in **Spinal reflexes** (page 200), in Ch. 6, The Spinal Cord; **Rotational movements of the eyeballs** (page 233), in Ch. 8, The Special Senses; **Blinking** (page 234), in Ch. 8, The Special Senses; **Attenuation reflex** (page 250), in Ch. 8, The Special Senses; and **Reflex control of ventilation** (page 459), in Ch. 13, Respiration.

Skeletal muscle fibres

Skeletal muscles are composed of specialized fibres which, in the case of the sartorius muscle, may be up to 30 cm long. Their diameter varies from 10–100 µm. They are cylindrical and contain many hundreds of peripheral nuclei.

All skeletal muscle fibres are not identical and they are classified as either **twitch** (fast) or **tonic** (slow) fibres. Action potentials from somatic motor neurones are transmitted across the neuromuscular junction to twitch fibres, propagated along the length of the fibres and cause an 'all-or-nothing' contraction.

See also **Skeletal muscle** (page 98), in Ch. 3, Tissues.

Tonic fibres, on the other hand, do not propagate action potentials and therefore depend upon repeated neural stimulation for contraction. They represent a very small proportion of the total number of muscle fibres in mammals. The following account of skeletal muscle activity relates to twitch fibres only.

The all-or-nothing principle is described in **The action potential** (page 117), in Ch. 4, Cellular Mechanisms of Neural Control.

Twitch fibres are generally classified into three groups: red, intermediate and white. **Red, slow-twitch fibres** contain the red protein myoglobin, which provides an intracellular oxygen store, and have a high density of mitochondria and low stores of glycogen, but relatively large stores of triglyceride. They are therefore suited to oxidative metabolism and sustained muscular contraction. **Intermediate, fast-twitch fibres** also contain large amounts of myoglobin and mitochondria, but have intermediate amounts of glycogen and triglycerides. Such fibres are functionally as well as structurally intermediate, being capable of both oxidative metabolism and anaerobic glycolysis. **White, fast-twitch fibres** are larger than the red ones, have fewer mitochondria but are rich in glycogen and glycolytic enzymes; they have a low fat content. They are therefore specialized for anaerobic glycolysis, which gives a fast, but small, supply of ATP. Since they fatigue rapidly they are most effective in providing brief bursts of muscle activity.

Whole muscles contain a mixture of both fibre types, but postural muscles, which exhibit slow tonic contractions, have a higher proportion of red fibres while muscles that bring about rapid movements of part of the body have a higher proportion of white fibres. Muscles with a high proportion of red or intermediate fibres contain extensive capillary networks, whereas those in muscles containing largely white fibres are sparse.

> Anaerobic glycolysis is explained in **Glucose oxidation** (page 595), in Ch. 15, Digestion and Absorption of Food.

MYOFIBRILS

When viewed with a light microscope, a dark and light banding pattern

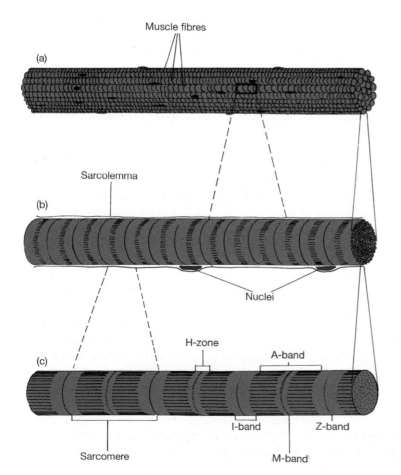

Figure 9.5 Skeletal muscle.
(a) Bundle of muscle fibres.
(b) Individual fibre. **(c)** Myofibril.

Muscle fibres

(a)

Sarcolemma

(b)

Nuclei

(c)

H-zone

A-band

I-band

Z-band

Sarcomere

M-band

(striations) can be seen across a muscle cell (Figure 9.5). This is dependent upon the presence of long cylindrical myofibrils, which run parallel to the long axis of the cell. Each myofibril exhibits the banding pattern and, since the bands are in register across the cell, the whole cell appears striated. There are alternate dark and light bands; the dark ones are known as **A-bands**, because they are anisotropic (strongly rotate the plane of polarized light), while the light ones (**I-bands**) are isotropic (weakly rotate the plane of polarized light). In stained preparations, too, the A-bands appear darker, since they take up stain more strongly than

Figure 9.6 Electron micrograph of skeletal muscle. (Reproduced with permission from Fawcett, D. W. (1993) *Bloom and Fawcett: A Textbook of Histology*, Chapman & Hall, London.)

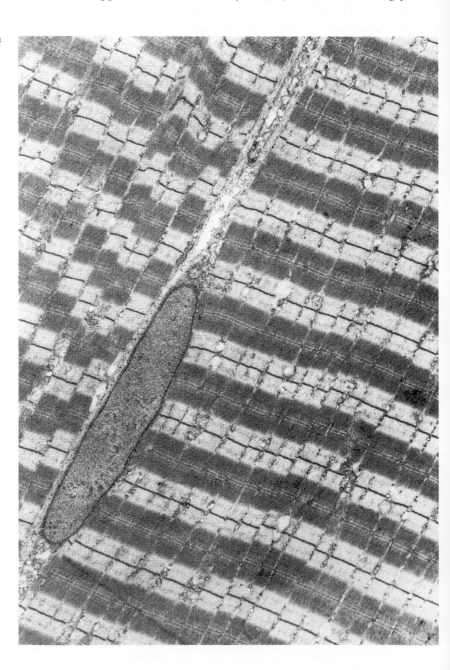

the I-bands. The I-bands are bisected by a dark **Z-line** or disc (*Zwischenscheibe*).

The electron microscope further reveals that the A-bands have a pale central region known as the **H-band** or H-zone, which itself has a dark **M-band** (or M-line) crossing it. The repeating units from Z-line to Z-line are called **sarcomeres**, consisting of one half of each of two I-bands separated by an A-band (Figure 9.6). Each myofibril may be visualized as a column of disc-like sarcomeres.

The cross-striations of the myofibrils result from the very regular arrangement of the **myofilaments** which they contain. There are two types of myofilament, thick (mainly myosin) and thin (mainly actin).

The large number of **mitochondria** present between the myofibrils, and under the sarcolemma, reflects the high rate of production and usage of ATP.

T-TUBULES AND SARCOPLASMIC RETICULUM

The **sarcolemma** (surface membrane) is invaginated into the cell to form structures called **T-tubules**, which run transversely across the cell and around each myofibril. As these tubules are an extension of the sarcolemma, they contain extracellular fluid. Each sarcomere contains two such tubules which cross the cell at each A–I band junction (Figure 9.7).

The smooth endoplasmic reticulum in skeletal muscle cells is called **sarcoplasmic reticulum** and runs longitudinally around each myofibril. A T-tubule runs between adjacent sections of sarcoplasmic reticulum and on either side of it there are dilated tubules of the sarcoplasmic reticulum, known as **terminal cisternae**. In section a structure known as a **triad** can be seen, consisting of two terminal cisternae with a T-tubule in between (Figure 9.7).

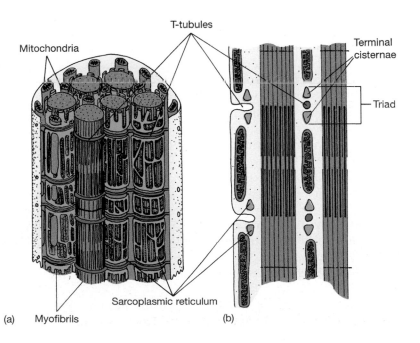

T-tubules

Mitochondria

Terminal cisternae

Triad

Sarcoplasmic reticulum

(a) Myofibrils

(b)

Figure 9.7 **(a)** Arrangement of myofibrils and tubular systems in a muscle fibre. **(b)** Longitudinal section to show the relationships between the banding pattern and the tubular systems.

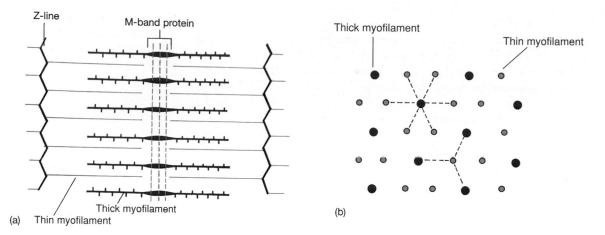

(a)   (b)

Figure 9.8 Arrangement of myofilaments within a sarcomere. **(a)** Longitudinal. Thick myofilaments are held in position centrally by M-band protein. Thin myofilaments are anchored at one end to the Z-line.   **(b)** Transverse section through an A band. Each thick myofilament is surrounded by six thin myofilaments and each thin filament is surrounded by three thick ones.

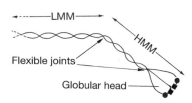

Figure 9.9 A myosin molecule. LMM – light meromyosin, forming the 'tail'; HMM – heavy meromyosin, forming the neck and 'head'. The binding sites for ATP (●) and actin (■) are shown on the head region.

MYOFILAMENTS

If a myofibril is cut through at an A-band and the cut surface is examined, it can be seen that the myofilaments are arranged in a very regular pattern. Each thick filament is surrounded by six thin filaments and each thin filament is surrounded by three thick ones (Figure 9.8).

The principal protein comprising the **thick myofilaments** is myosin. Each myosin molecule has a long tail region composed of light meromyosin (LMM), which consists of two helical polypeptide chains wound around each other, and a neck and head region composed of heavy meromyosin (HMM). The neck region is also helical and the head is double and globular. There are two flexible regions (like hinge joints) at the LMM–HMM junction and between the neck and the head. Each head has a binding site for ATP and a separate site for combining with actin, thus each HMM molecule has two binding sites for ATP and two for actin (Figure 9.9).

The myosin molecules are arranged head to tail, with the tails forming the thick filament and the head and neck parts sticking out from the main axis and forming **cross-bridges**. The orientation of these cross-bridges is very regular. Each filament has cross-bridges sticking out in pairs opposite each other and each pair is orientated 120° with respect to adjacent pairs. Every fourth pair is thus orientated in the same direction. The arrangement means that there are cross-bridge positions all along the thick filaments that correspond with the arrangement of the six thin filaments that surround it (Figures 9.8, 9.10). At the M-band the myosin molecules are orientated tail to tail and anchored in position by the M-band protein.

The **thin myofilaments** consist mainly of the protein **actin**. The globular molecules (**G-actin**) form a polymer of fibrous actin (**F-actin**), which resembles two strings of beads twisted around each other to form a double helix. There are seven G-actin molecules per twist in each chain (Figure 9.11).

There is a second protein, **tropomyosin**, running alongside the groove between the two strands of F-actin. Tropomyosin consists of two

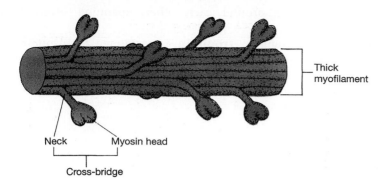

Figure 9.10 Arrangement of myosin molecules to form a thick myofilament. Consecutive molecules are rotated 120°.

Thick myofilament

Neck   Myosin head

Cross-bridge

(a)

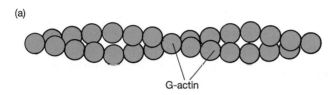

G-actin

(b)

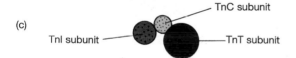

Single alpha helix

Figure 9.11 Components of a thin myofilament. **(a)** Fibrous actin formed from a double helix of individual globular molecules. **(b)** Tropomyosin. **(c)** Troponin complex. TnT (binds to tropomyosin) TnC (binds to Ca^{2+}) TnI (binds to actin and inhibits its binding to myosin). **(d)** Thin filament assembled. **(e)** Cross-section of a filament showing the location of two troponin complexes and two tropomyosin helices on either side of the actin helix.

(c)

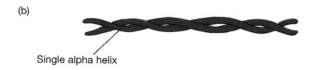

TnC subunit

TnI subunit   TnT subunit

(d)

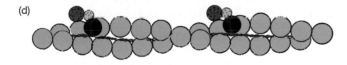

(e)

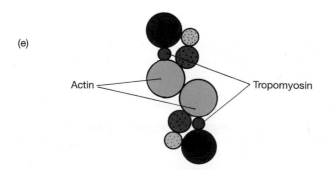

Actin   Tropomyosin

alpha-helices wound around each other, spanning seven G-actin molecules.

A third protein complex, **troponin**, is positioned about one-third of the distance along from the end of each tropomyosin molecule (Figure 9.11). Troponin has three subunits, TnT (binds to tropomyosin); TnC (binds to Ca^{2+}) and TnI (binds to actin and inhibits the interaction between actin and myosin).

Sliding filament theory

The sliding filament theory of muscle contraction dates from around 1950 and is attributed to the scientists Hugh and Andrew Huxley and Jean Hanson. It was observed that, when a muscle contracts and the sarcomeres reduce in length, the I-bands become narrower but the A-bands do not, and that, if a resting muscle is stretched, then the H-zones increase in size. These observations can be explained in terms of a varying degree of overlap between thick and thin filaments. When a muscle contracts, the thin filaments slide in between the thick ones and towards the M-band. Conversely, if the muscle is stretched, the thin filaments slide away from the M-band and increase the length of the H-zone (Figure 9.12). The force of contraction (**tension**) is developed by

Figure 9.12 Changes in the banding pattern with contraction and relaxation of muscle.
(a) When the muscle is contracted the thin myofilaments overlap thick ones – the I band is narrow and there is no H band. **(b)** The muscle is partially contracted and there is some overlap between myofilaments – the I band is wider and the H zone is apparent.
(c) The muscle is relaxed and there is very little overlap between myofilaments – the I band is wide and so is the H zone.

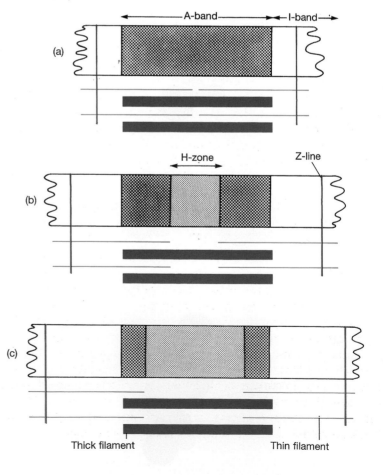

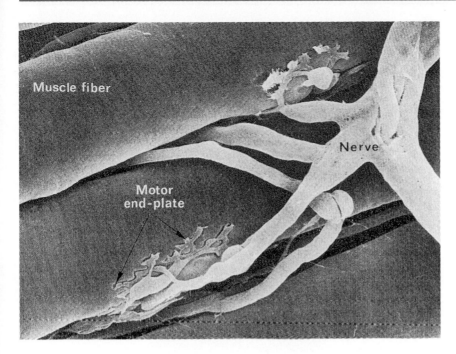

Muscle fiber

Nerve

Motor
end-plate

Figure 9.13 Scanning electron micrograph of a motor neurone (labelled 'nerve') and two end-plates on adjacent muscle fibres. (Reproduced with permission from Fawcett, D. W. (1993) *Bloom and Fawcett: A Textbook of Histology*, Chapman & Hall, London.)

the cross-bridges in the overlap region. The thin filaments are pushed towards the M-band by the repeated movement of the cross-bridges making and breaking contact with them, like oars in a boat with water.

Neuromuscular junction

The somatic motor neurones that innervate skeletal muscle cells terminate in structures called **motor end-plates**. Each axon branches towards its end and each branch supplies a separate muscle fibre (Figure 9.13). When the neurone is stimulated, the impulses pass along each of the branches to the muscle fibres, which then contract in unison.

The term 'motor end-plate' is used to describe either 1) the specialized area of muscle cell lying beneath the terminal branches of each axon branch (it contains several nuclei and numerous mitochondria), or 2) the axon branch together with the underlying structure; in this case the term **sole plate** is used to identify the area of muscle. Each axon terminal is unmyelinated, lies in a trough (**primary synaptic cleft**) formed by an invagination of the sarcolemma, and is covered by Schwann cells (Figure 9.14). The primary synaptic cleft itself has **secondary synaptic clefts**, which increase the surface area.

The axon terminals contain large numbers of vesicles containing the neurotransmitter **acetylcholine**. There are also large numbers of mitochondria present, which provide the ATP required for the release of acetylcholine into the synaptic clefts and the reuptake of choline, which is then recycled. The sarcolemma lining the clefts contains closely packed particles which are believed to be acetylcholine receptors. Molecules of the enzyme **cholinesterase**, which are attached to the sarcolemma, break down the neurotransmitter to choline and acetate.

(a)

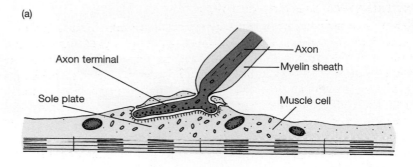

(b)

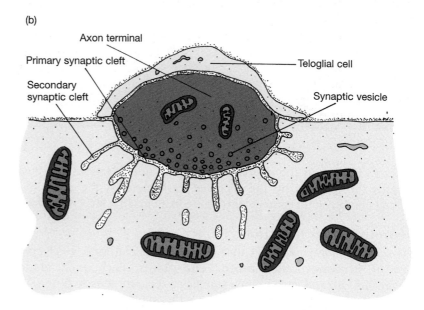

Figure 9.14 Neuromuscular junction. **(a)** Axon terminal and sole-plate. **(b)** Section through the motor end-plate to show synaptic clefts and the relationship between the axon terminal and the surface of the muscle fibre.

Motor units

A motor unit is a group of muscle fibres of the same type that are innervated by a single motor neurone and therefore contract in unison. On average, there are about 100 muscle fibres in a single unit, but the numbers in individual units vary widely. Thus, small, rapidly-acting muscles, which are under fine control (such as those in the larynx, fingers and controlling eye movements), contain motor units of only a few fibres, whereas large, slow-acting muscles, which are only capable of gross movements (e.g. hip muscles), contain motor units of several hundred fibres.

The fibres of one motor unit do not form a discrete structure within a muscle, but are spread throughout, each fibre being surrounded by members of other units. Contraction of a single or small group of units, therefore causes shortening of the whole muscle and not merely a part of it.

Excitation–contraction coupling

Each muscle fibre has its own motor end-plate, usually located centrally on the fibre. An active neurone transmits action potentials along its axon to the terminals. Each action potential causes some of the vesicles in the axon terminals to fuse with the neurone membrane and release a quantity of acetylcholine into the synaptic cleft. The neurotransmitter diffuses across the cleft, combines with receptor sites on the sarcolemma and increases its permeability to ions. This results in Na^+ entering the muscle cell and initiating an action potential in the sarcolemma. The action potentials are transmitted rapidly over the sarcolemma and into the muscle fibres by means of the T-tubules. The presence of action potentials in the T-tubules cause the adjacent terminal cisternae to release Ca^{2+} into the sarcoplasm.

Troponin and tropomyosin are known as regulatory proteins because in resting muscle they prevent the combination of actin with myosin to form actomyosin, i.e. they prevent the cross-bridges of the thick filaments from attaching to the thin filaments surrounding them.

When Ca^{2+} ions are released into the sarcoplasm they bind to the troponin subunit TnC and the inhibitory action of the regulatory proteins is lifted so that actin and myosin combine. It is thought that the inhibitory action of the regulatory proteins is effected by tropomyosin physically covering the myosin-binding sites on the actin molecules, and that the troponin complex holds the tropomyosin in position.

When Ca^{2+} is bound to TnC, the troponin subunits are drawn closer together and slightly away from the myofilament so that tropomyosin rolls further into the groove between the two F-actin strands and exposes the binding site for myosin (Figure 9.15).

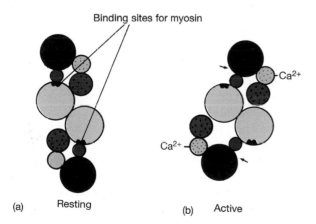

Binding sites for myosin

Ca^{2+}

Ca^{2+}

(a) Resting   (b) Active

Figure 9.15 The relationships between the components of thin myofilaments in resting and active muscle in cross-section.
(a) Resting muscle – tropomyosin covers the myosin-binding sites on the actin molecules. **(b)** Active muscle – Ca^{2+} binds to TnC and the troponin subunits draw away from the filaments, tropomyosin rolls further into the groove thereby exposing the myosin binding site.

The head of the cross-bridge can then make contact with the two nearby actin molecules. Ca^{2+}, therefore, is pivotal in enabling contraction to take place.

The energy for contraction is derived from the breakdown of ATP (actually Mg.ATP) in the myosin heads. The energy released is used to bend the myosin head from its resting 'low-energy' position, through 45° into the 'high-energy' or 'cocked' position, perpendicular to the thin myofilament (Figure 9.16).

Figure 9.16 The contraction cycle. **(a)** Before contraction begins, Mg.ATP binds to the myosin head, which is orientated at an angle of 45°, pointing towards the M-band (low-energy configuration). **(b)** Mg.ATP is immediately broken down to Mg.ADP and phosphate (P) by myosin ATPase in the head. The energy released causes the head to bend some 45° into the 'high-energy' or 'cocked' position, so that it is perpendicular to the thin myofilament. **(c)** When Ca^{2+} binds to troponin, the myosin head binds to the nearby actin myofilament. **(d)** The myosin head tilts towards the tail of the cross-bridge and pushes the thin myofilament towards the M-band. Once the head is tilted, ADP and P dissociate from it. **(a)** Another molecule of ATP can now combine with the myosin head causing it to dissociate from the thin myofilament.

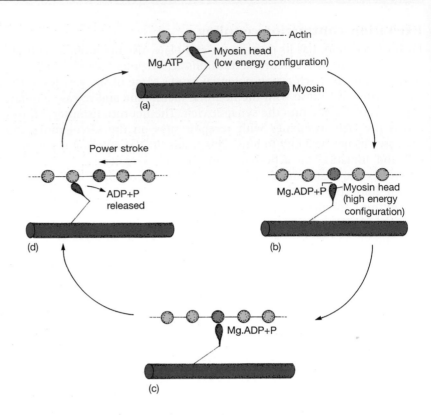

When Ca^{2+} binds to troponin, the myosin head binds to the nearby actin myofilament and then tilts towards the tail of the cross-bridge, pushing the thin myofilament towards the M-band. The power stroke which moves the thin myofilament towards the M-band, therefore, consists of the head of the cross-bridge changing from the 'high-energy' perpendicular position to the 'low-energy' tilted position.

The precision of neural control is dependent upon its being of short duration, so that a single nerve impulse does not result in an inappropriately long muscle contraction. Two mechanisms serve to keep the response to each impulse short. Cholinesterase rapidly destroys acetylcholine in the synaptic cleft and Ca^{2+} ions are 'pumped' back into the sarcoplasmic reticulum. Muscle contraction, therefore, only takes place as long as action potentials continue to arrive at the motor end-plate and maintain a raised intracellular Ca^{2+} concentration.

Sources of energy for muscle contraction

There are three energy-producing systems that power muscle contraction; the one used depends upon the duration of the contraction. The three systems are the phosphagen system, the glycogen–lactic acid system and the aerobic system (Figure 9.17).

The **phosphagen system** uses creatine phosphate as an energy source. Creatine phosphate is an energy-transferring compound like ATP, containing even more energy and present in large amounts in muscle. Creatine phosphate in the muscle cells is broken down to form creatine and PO_4^{3-}, the energy liberated in the reaction being transferred to ATP and subsequently used to drive the contractile apparatus. This process takes less than 10 s and is used for short bursts of activity, such as a 100 m sprint.

The **glycogen–lactic acid system** employs the breakdown of stored glycogen to glucose (glycogenolysis) Without using oxygen (anaerobic) glucose is converted to lactic acid, with the production of a small amount of ATP. This process provides energy for up to about 1.5 min.

The **aerobic system** requires the presence of oxygen, (aerobic conditions) for glucose oxidation to CO_2 and H_2O with the liberation of 38 molecules of ATP per molecule of glucose. This process can proceed as long as glucose and oxygen are available, and is employed by muscles that are contracting continuously or exercising over long periods.

> ATP synthesis is explained in **Glucose oxidation** (page 595), in Ch. 15, Digestion and Absorption of Food.

Strength of muscle contraction (tension)

The strength of muscle contraction may be varied in two ways, by the **recruitment** of additional motor units and by summation of the contractions of individual motor units.

The greater the number of motor units that are stimulated simultaneously then the greater the tension will be. A weak stimulus excites the motor units with the smallest number of muscle fibres first. As the stimulus gains in strength, other larger units are recruited until all the motor units in the muscle are contracting simultaneously. This happens because the smallest motor units are stimulated by the smallest motor neurones, which are also the most excitable. Increasing stimulation of muscle therefore enables smooth contractions to be developed as motor units are recruited sequentially.

When an action potential causes a motor unit to twitch the duration of the action potential (0.4 ms) is much shorter than the duration of the twitch (25–75 ms). It is therefore possible for a second action potential to arrive at the myoneural junction before the contraction caused by the previous action potential is over. In this case the contraction initiated by

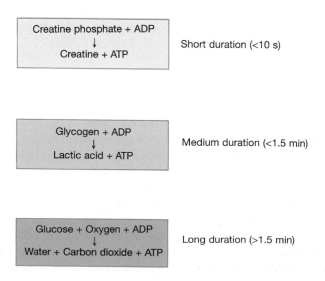

Creatine phosphate + ADP
↓
Creatine + ATP   Short duration (<10 s)

Glycogen + ADP
↓
Lactic acid + ATP   Medium duration (<1.5 min)

Glucose + Oxygen + ADP
↓
Water + Carbon dioxide + ATP   Long duration (>1.5 min)

Figure 9.17 Sources of energy for muscular contraction.

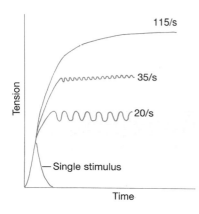

Figure 9.18 Summation of tension generated by muscle contractions, showing the effect of a single stimulus and then increasing the frequency of stimuli. The very high frequency of 50/s induces sustained contraction known as tetanus. (Modified from Astrand, P. and Rodahl, K. (1986) *Textbook of Work Physiology*, McGraw-Hill, New York.

the second action potential is added to that initiated by the first and therefore the tension developed is higher. This effect is called **summation** (Figure 9.18). If the frequency of stimulation is increased to about 50/s then the muscle tension does not fall between successive stimuli, so that a sustained contraction known as **tetanus** is achieved.

Isotonic and isometric contractions

Isotonic contraction produces external work (e.g. lifting a weight or pedalling a bicycle). The load (weight or resistance of the bicycle wheels) produces a constant tension in the muscle, which shortens.

Isometric contraction, on the other hand, does not involve shortening of muscle fibres, and the muscle tension rises during the contraction. This type of contraction occurs if the external work is either too great, (e.g. trying to push open a stiff window), or offers resistance (e.g. pressing the hands together). Muscle contractions that hold joints stationary or maintain an upright posture are isometric.

Rigor mortis

Several hours after death, muscles contract as a result of the loss of the ATP molecules that separate the cross-bridges between actin and myosin in relaxed muscle. Approximately one day later, enzymes released by lysosomes in the muscle cells start to break down the contractile molecules and the muscle relaxes again.

Muscle atrophy and hypertrophy

The nerve supply to muscle is essential for its maintenance because muscle activity helps maintain its integrity; denervated muscle atrophies. Lower motor neurone damage leads to atrophy of the muscle cells; the consequences of temporary denervation can be minimized by electrical stimulation and physiotherapy. Muscles which are unused for a period of time, such as when a limb is encased in plaster, atrophy rapidly.

On the other hand, repeated use of particular muscles (e.g. in weight training) causes them to increase in size. This is due to hypertrophy of the existing cells and not to an increase in number. Protein is laid down within the fibres and there is replication of myofibrils and associated enzymes. Muscles can also increase in length. In this case, sarcomeres are added to each end of the muscle.

Androgens (**anabolic steroids**) stimulate muscle hypertrophy, a property manifested in athletes and body builders.

Effects of training upon skeletal muscle

The **mechanical efficiency of muscle contraction** equals work output/ work + heat output. Training improves the capacity of slow and fast fibres to perform more efficiently. Intense exercise, which employs largely anaerobic metabolism, increases the mass and strength of fast fibres; aerobic exercise, on the other hand, causes enlargement of slow fibres.

Maximal, slow isometric contractions performed only five times a day, three times a week are usually sufficient to induce a rapid increase in muscle strength, though without improvements in aerobic capacity and endurance. This increase in strength is thought to be due initially to a more efficient activation of motor units. Enlargement of muscle fibre diameter, with the production of more myofibrils, follows more slowly. This type of strength training does not improve capillary circulation, which explains the muscles' poor endurance. Weight lifters and others with greatly enlarged muscles often cannot perform endurance exercise for even quite short periods without lactic acid build up.

Aerobic exercise increases the number of mitochondria (and therefore of respiratory enzymes) present in the muscle cells which enables them to resist fatigue. The vascularity of muscle tissue also increases, which enables more oxygen and food molecules to be carried to the cells and carbon dioxide and other metabolic wastes to be carried away.

Muscular dystrophies

There are a number of quite rare muscle diseases which result in progressive muscular weakness. In the most common, **Duchenne-type muscular dystrophy**, there may be atrophy of some muscle tissues but hypertrophy of others, due to fat accumulation; in both cases the ability to contract effectively is reduced. Muscular weakness usually affects the pelvic muscles early on so that walking becomes increasingly difficult. Involvement of the respiratory muscles usually leads to death.

Impaired neuromuscular transmission (myasthenia gravis)

Myasthenia gravis is one of the commoner muscular diseases and results from the inactivation of acetylcholine receptors on the motor end-plates by autoantibodies. It is characterized by muscle weakness that is exacerbated by repeated contraction. Muscles with the smallest motor units are involved first, with the ocular muscles being most often affected. Drooping of the eyelid and double-vision are therefore common symptoms. The disease may progress to involve the facial muscles and neck muscles so that chewing and swallowing become difficult. Subsequently the limb muscles may be affected, so that even the slightest activity results in extreme fatigue. If the respiratory muscles also become affected then death may ensue.

Neural control of voluntary movement

An apparently simple movement, such as picking up a ball, includes movements of the wrist, the lower and upper arms and the shoulder, as well as postural adjustments. Most movements involve relaxation as well as contraction of a number of muscle groups.

Somatic motor neurones, controlled by the CNS, initiate muscle contraction in the skeletal muscle fibres within muscles. There are three levels of control of motor activity within the CNS:

1. areas that have neural connections with the spinal cord;
   a. the motor areas of the cerebral cortex;
   b. some brain stem nuclei;
2. the basal ganglia and cerebellum, which regulate and coordinate movements effected by the cortical areas and brain stem nuclei;
3. the spinal cord, which generates walking movements (Figure 9.19).

See also **Reciprocal inhibition** (page 199), in Ch. 6, The Spinal Cord.

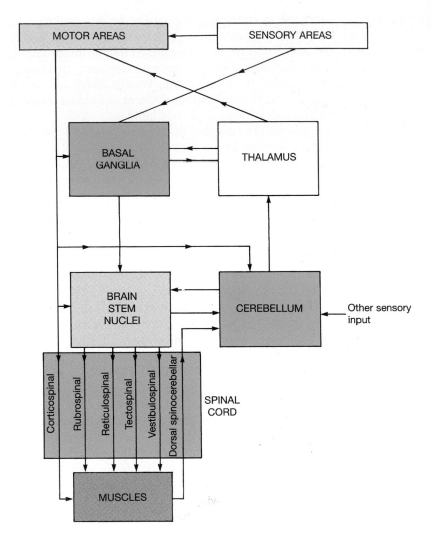

Figure 9.19 Schematic diagram of the major brain areas involved in the control of voluntary movement. Motor areas of the cerebral cortex and brain stem nuclei [pink] send projection fibres into the spinal cord and connect with somatic motor neurones to the muscles. The basal ganglia and cerebellum [blue] regulate and coordinate movements effected by the cortical areas and brain-stem nuclei. The spinal cord [green] contains neural circuits that generate walking movements, which are regulated by the projection areas.

See Ch. 5, The Brain, for further information on parts of the brain.

Level 1a

The cortical areas concerned with the conscious control of motor activity are the primary motor cortex, the premotor area and the supplemental motor area.

Planning an action appears to be initiated in the **supplemental motor area**. It has been shown that the blood flow increases in this part of the brain prior to a movement being carried out, whereas blood flow in the primary motor cortex only increases when the movement is actually taking place.

Sensory inputs are of major importance in the planning stage, since it is usually necessary to direct an action to a particular point. When throwing a ball, for example, the brain needs to know the ball's target as well as the position of the parts of the body involved in the action. Sensory information is obtained from a variety of sensory areas: the visual cortex, the primary somatic sensory, vestibular and auditory areas. The **posterior parietal cortex** receives all this information, which is then relayed to the **premotor cortex**, which calculates the relationships between the various parts of the body and also their positions relative to their surroundings. The premotor cortex passes signals into the **primary motor cortex**, which then initiates activity in appropriate muscle groups, principally via the corticospinal and rubrospinal tracts.

The **corticospinal tract** (Figure 9.20) begins as upper motor neurones in several parts of the cerebral cortex: the primary motor cortex, the premotor and supplemental motor areas as well as the somatic sensory areas.

Fibres from the sensory cortical areas terminate in sensory nuclei in the brain stem and spinal cord. As many as 80% of corticospinal fibres are thought to originate in the primary motor cortex, descend through the internal capsule to the medulla oblongata, where about 80% cross over, forming the medullary pyramids, before entering the lateral white matter of the spinal cord.

See also **Descending (motor) pathways** (page 196), in Ch. 6, The Spinal Cord.

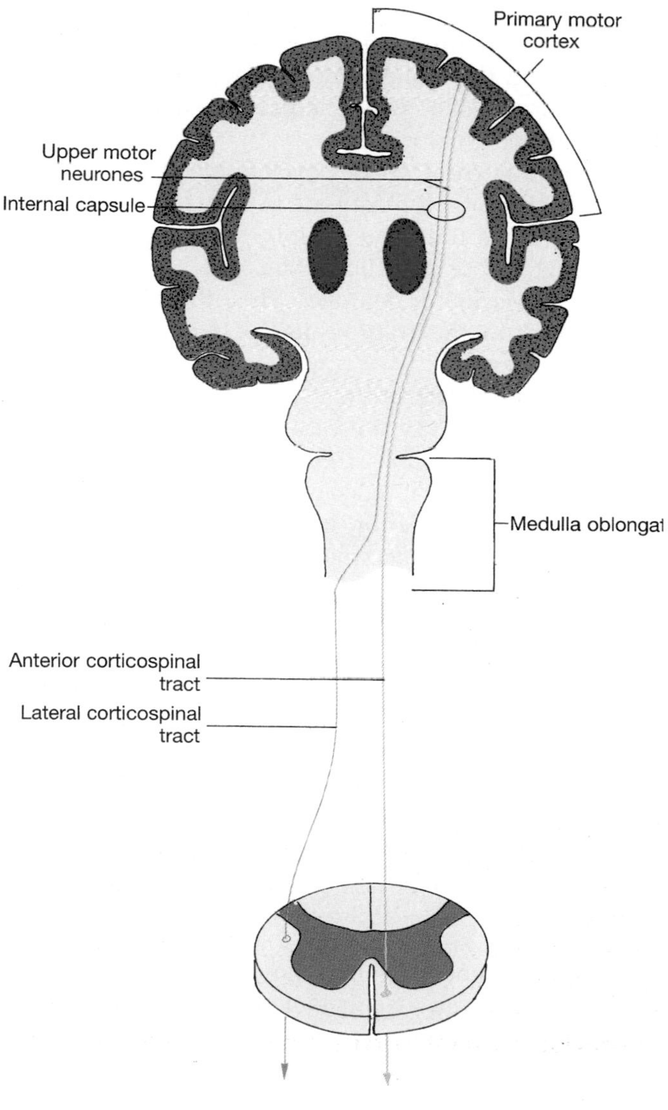

Figure 9.20   The corticospinal tracts arise in the cerebral cortex (mostly the primary motor cortex) as upper motor neurones and pass down through the internal capsule. About 80% of upper motor neurones cross over in the medulla oblongata (5% do not) and descend in the lateral corticospinal tracts; 15% of the fibres descend uncrossed in the anterior corticospinal tract. (See also Figure 6.10.)

Collateral fibres from the upper motor neurones synapse with nerve cell bodies in the basal ganglia, brain stem nuclei and cerebellum. Each vertical column of cell bodies in the motor cortex functions as a unit that stimulates either a single muscle or a group of synergistic muscles.

Most upper motor neurones synapse with interneurones in the intermediate grey matter of the contralateral side of the spinal cord, which then relay with lower motor neurones in the anterior horns. The lower motor neurones are then distributed to the muscles in the spinal nerves.

The neural pathway between the motor cortex and the muscles of the hands and feet, however, does not include interneurones. The upper motor neurones synapse directly with the lower motor neurones in the lateral region of the anterior horns. The hands, which are capable of fine movements and have a high degree of representation on the motor cortex, are therefore controlled directly by the motor cortex.

See also **Spinal nerves** (page 188), in Ch. 6, The Spinal Cord.

Level 1b

The brain stem nuclei that have neural links with muscles are the **red nuclei**, the **reticular nuclei** and the **vestibular nuclei**, all of which are concerned with the maintenance of the body in a vertical position; and the superior colliculi, which initiate movements of the eyes and upper body towards visual stimuli.

The **rubrospinal tract** crosses over in the medulla oblongata and runs parallel to the corticospinal tract in the lateral white matter of the spinal cord; its fibres terminate mainly on interneurones in the grey matter, although those that innervate the hands and feet synapse directly on the lower motor neurones. The rubrospinal tract parallels the corticospinal tract in the transmission of motor signals to individual muscles, mostly flexors.

The **reticulospinal tracts** from the brain stem are concerned with the regulation of antigravity muscles, i.e. muscles of the spinal column and the extensors of the limbs. The reticular nuclei in the pons varolii are the origins of the medial reticulospinal tracts, which terminate in the medial region of the anterior horns and stimulate the antigravity muscles. The reticular nuclei, which lie in the medulla oblongata, give rise to the lateral reticulospinal tract and inhibit the antigravity muscles.

See also **Reticular formation** (page 164), in Ch. 5, The Brain, and **Muscle tone** (page 204), in Ch. 6, The Spinal Cord.

The vestibular nuclei give rise to the **vestibulospinal tracts**, which convey signals to antigravity muscles on the same side, thereby maintaining equilibrium in response to signals from the vestibular apparatus. As the head is tilted, the tone of antigravity muscles increases.

The **tectospinal tract** arises in the superior colliculus of the tectum of the midbrain. It crosses over and terminates in the medial part of the anterior horns in the spinal cord at cervical and upper thoracic levels. The tract mediates movement of the eyes, head and trunk towards visual stimuli.

Level 2

The regulation and coordination of movements is achieved by the cerebellum and basal ganglia. Neither of these have efferent connections with the spinal cord; rather they moderate the activity of the motor areas of the cerebral cortex and brain stem.

The **cerebellum** contributes to the planning of the sequence of muscle contractions bringing about a movement, as well as monitoring and making corrective adjustments as the movement takes place. Extensive sensory input is relayed to the cerebellum, principally via the **dorsal spinocerebellar tracts**, which appraise it of the length and tension of muscles, the positions and rates of movement of parts of the body and the forces acting on the surfaces of the body (from mechanoreceptors in the skin). The sensory information about actual body movements is compared with information about intended body movements from the motor and premotor cortices via the corticopontocerebellar fibres from the opposite side, and from olivocerebellar, vestibulocerebellar and reticulocerebellar tracts from the brain stem.

The parts of the body are represented somatotopically in the cerebellar cortex, and in turn they are connected to the same somatotopic areas of the motor cortex (via ventral intermediate thalamic nuclei, see Figure 5.14), the red nucleus and the reticular formation. The actions that these areas control can thereby be modified. The cerebellum also connects with the other regulatory areas, the basal ganglia, via the thalamus.

The **basal ganglia** receive afferents from all parts of the cerebral cortex and in turn influence motor activity in the premotor cortex via the thalamus. The basal ganglia assist the cortex in carrying out subconscious patterns of movement which have been learned. The ganglia receive input from the motor cortex and sensory information from the posterior parietal cortex. In an activity that involves sequential contraction and relaxation of a number of muscles, like writing, individual muscles are not directed consciously. Instead the motor cortex 'instructs' the basal ganglia to 'write'; the basal ganglia then send sequences of impulses back to the cortex, via the thalamus, which instructs the groups of muscles which are directly involved in the action to form the letters. The basal ganglia are also able to modify movements so that, in this case, letters can be varied in size.

Level 3

The spinal cord contains neural circuits that cause **walking movements**, and these are regulated by the vestibular, red and reticular nuclei in the brain stem, as well as the motor cortex.

See also **Standing and walking** (page 206), in Ch. 6, The Spinal Cord.

Impulses from the projection areas can modify spinal activity in a number of ways. They may:

- promote the normal patterns of activity in the cord, e.g. the brain directs the body to walk, which requires reciprocal activity in the flexors and extensors of each leg, as well as the maintenance of balance;
- change the intensity or duration of some part of the neural activity, e.g. a limp is incorporated into a walking pattern;
- inhibit existing cord patterns and replace them with new ones, e.g. a walk is replaced by a hop.

For more about postural reflexes, see **Vestibular pathways** (page 264), in Ch. 8, The Special Senses.

Changing the pattern of movement from walking to hopping, or indeed any other form of locomotion, is accompanied by modification of the postural reflexes so that the body remains upright.

Summary

To summarize: the decision to move all or part of the body is initiated in the supplemental motor area, but is implemented by the motor cortex and the brain stem nuclei. These areas are regulated by the basal ganglia and the cerebellum. The posterior parietal cortex directs attention towards sensory stimuli. The movement may employ existing pathways within the spinal cord or new ones may be initiated.

UPPER MOTOR NEURONE LESIONS

Damage to an upper motor neurone caused, for example, by haemorrhage, a thrombus or an embolus in the internal capsule of the brain, results in paralysis with increased muscle tone (**spastic paralysis**) due to the unopposed stimulation of intact lower motor neurones by subcorticospinal neurones. Deep tendon reflexes are also exaggerated and the plantar reflex becomes extensor, so that when the sole of the foot is stroked there is dorsiflexion of the big toe and the other toes fan out (**Babinski reflex**).

LOWER MOTOR NEURONE LESIONS

Lower motor neurones (somatic motor neurones) emerge from the spinal cord and innervate peripheral muscles. If the lower motor neurone is damaged by being crushed or cut, for example, then there is no output to the muscles so that all stimulation is absent, resulting in complete lack of muscle tone (**flaccid paralysis**). Tendon reflexes are absent and the plantar reflex is either absent or flexor.

A '**broken neck**', in which adjacent cervical vertebrae are pushed out of line, results in both upper and lower motor neurone incapacity. Muscles whose nerves leave the cord below the point of damage become rigidly paralysed, whereas those whose nerves originate within the damaged area have a flaccid paralysis.

See also **Subcorticospinal (extrapyramidal) tracts** (page 197), in Ch. 6, The Spinal Cord.

See also **Plantar reflex and the Babinski sign** (page 207), in Ch. 6, The Spinal Cord.

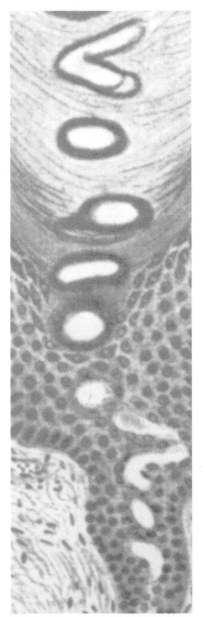

The skin and the regulation of body temperature

The skin

The skin, or integument, forms the external surface of the body and extends inwards as the lining of the external auditory meatus and the vestibule of the nasal cavity. The skin is the largest single organ of the body, comprising 5–6% of total body weight.

The frictional properties of the skin surface enable the feet to grip the ground and the fingers to hold and manipulate even quite small objects. The position of the skin, on the surface of the body, enables sunlight to convert 7-dehydrocholesterol to vitamin D3.

The presence of a variety of sensory receptors in or just under the skin conveys information, particularly relating to the external environment.

The structure of skin gives protection to the underlying tissues from damage due to mechanical, chemical, thermal, photic or osmotic causes, and forms a barrier to invasion by microorganisms. A limited amount of absorption, particularly of lipids, can occur through the skin, and a small quantity of water constantly diffuses out.

Alterations in the quantity of blood flowing through the skin affects its temperature and consequently the amount of heat lost from the body. The skin, therefore, has an important role to play in the regulation of body temperature.

The skin comprises two principal layers: the superficial epidermis and the deeper dermis or corium (Figure 10.1). Beneath the skin lies the hypodermis or superficial fascia, which is formed from loose areolar connective tissue in some parts, and adipose tissue in others.

The epidermis

Cells in the deepest layers of the epidermis are constantly dividing and thereby pushing the more superficial cells outwards. The surface cells are constantly being rubbed off (forming the major component of house dust) and replaced by the cells beneath. The epidermis contains the

> For more about vitamin D see **Regulation of blood calcium and phosphate concentrations** (page 630), in Ch. 16, Endocrine Physiology.

Figure 10.1 Longitudinal section of the skin, showing the keratinized and germinative zones of the epidermis and the papillary and reticular layers of the dermis.

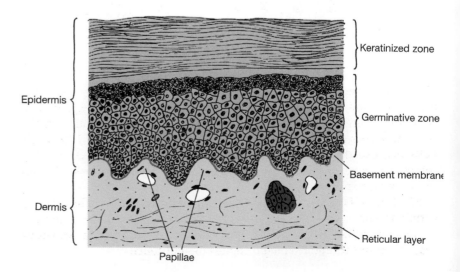

protein **keratin**, which imparts many properties to the skin: toughness, flexibility and resistance to bacterial penetration and water loss.

The majority of cells in the epidermis are involved in the production of keratin and are therefore known as **keratinocytes**. These cells are organized into two zones: the deeper germinative zone and the superficial keratinized zone. Within each zone there are two or three layers of cells.

Macrophages, known in the skin as **Langerhans cells**, are also present in the epidermis. Their long processes extend between the keratinocytes. The presence of macrophages offers immunological protection very near to the surface of the body.

> The role of macrophages in immunity is discussed in Ch. 11, Blood, Lymphoid Tissue and Immunity.

THE GERMINATIVE ZONE

The germinative zone consists of a layer of cuboidal or columnar cells on the basement membrane, the **stratum germinativum** (or stratum basale); and a layer of variable thickness above, the **stratum spinosum** (Figure 10.2).

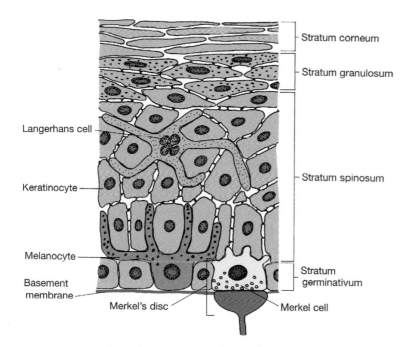

Figure 10.2 Arrangement of keratinocytes, melanocytes, Langerhans cells and Merkel cells in the epidermis of the skin.

The germinative zone is so named because it is in this layer that the cells divide and replenish those sloughed off from the surface. Cell division occurs principally in the stratum germinativum, but also in the stratum spinosum. The cells in this layer have been named **'prickle' cells** because they appear to have spines all over their surfaces. The spines are actually filament-filled cytoplasmic extensions and desmosomes, which anchor the cells together.

Merkel cells are scattered among the keratinocytes of the stratum germinativum. Each cell is hemispherical and lies next to a sensory nerve ending in the dermis. The two structures make up a **Merkel's disc**, a sensory receptor which responds to light touch.

THE KERATINIZED ZONE

The deepest layer of the zone of keratinization is called the **stratum granulosum** because the flattened cells synthesize granules of the protein **keratohyalin**. As the cells move nearer to the surface their lysosomes rupture and destroy the cells' organelles. In the epidermis of the palms of the hands and the soles of the feet a clear layer, the **stratum lucidum**, may be seen. This consists of a thin transparent layer of cells, which lack organelles but contain a mass of keratohyalin filaments. The superficial layer of cells, the **stratum corneum**, consists of dead, anucleate cells known as **squames**, which are full of the protein keratin.

The thickness of the epidermis is generally 0.07–0.12 mm, but reaches a thickness of 1.4 mm on the soles of the feet. The transit time from a cell starting in the deepest layer to being rubbed off the surface is between 15 and 30 days.

The dermis

Below the epidermis lies the dermis; this layer may be up to 3 mm thick on the soles of the feet. The dermis is attached to the subcutaneous tissue, the hypodermis.

The dermis consists of two layers, the upper **papillary layer**, containing papillae which interdigitate with the folds of the epidermis, and the lower **reticular layer**. The papillary layer consists of loose connective tissue containing fibroblasts, mast cells and macrophages. The reticular layer is thicker and consists of irregular dense connective tissue. Both layers contain elastic fibres, and collagen fibres that help to anchor the dermis to the epidermis.

The collagen fibres thicken with age and collagen synthesis decreases. Elastic fibres increase in number and in thickness, and cross-linking of collagen fibres causes skin to lose its elasticity and become wrinkled.

The dermis contains a rich blood supply as well as numerous nerve fibres and sensory endings. In addition, hair follicles and sweat and sebaceous glands are abundant (Figure 10.3).

Skin colour

Skin pigmentation is mainly due to the presence of **melanin**, a polymer of the amino acid tyrosine, which is synthesized by **melanocytes**, cells found in the germinative layer of the epidermis (Figure 10.2). The pigment is formed close to the nucleus and then migrates along the many branches of the cell in membrane-bound vesicles and is secreted at their endings. The melanin is then taken up by keratinocytes and is deposited in a layer in the parts of the cells closest to the skin surface. This affords protection against the effects of sunlight.

The skin-darkening effect of exposure to the ultraviolet waves in sunlight is caused initially by a darkening of the melanin already present, a relatively short-lived effect. This is followed by an increase in the rate of melanin synthesis, and lastly by an increased number of melanocytes.

Melanin protects against damage by ultraviolet light, which can cause sunburn and skin cancer. Freckles and pigmented moles contain accumulations of melanin. Darker-skinned races have similar numbers of

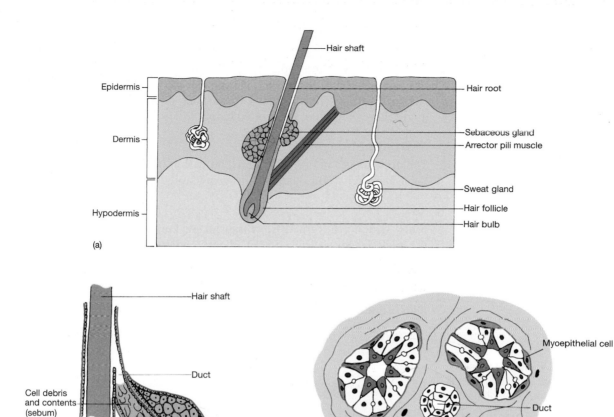

Figure 10.3 **(a)** Skin appendages: hair, arrector pili muscle, sebaceous gland and sweat glands. **(b)** A sebaceous gland secreting sebum into a hair follicle. **(c)** Section through a sweat gland showing the dark (glycoprotein-secreting) and light (serous-fluid-secreting) cells in the coiled body surrounded by contractile myoepithelial cells. The primary secretion of sweat is secreted by the clear cells into the intercellular canaliculi.

See also **Cyanosis** (page 470), in Ch. 13, Respiration.

melanocytes as those who have paler skin, but there is more melanin within each cell. Complete absence of melanin (**albinism**) occurs as a recessive Mendelian character. The number of melanocytes decreases with age, so that by the age of 70 years the cell population has typically halved, rendering the elderly more susceptible to damage from ultra-violet light.

The amount of **carotene**, a yellow/orange pigment, in the stratum corneum and adipose cells of the dermis and superficial fascia affects skin colour. Carotene is present in carrots and so people who eat a lot of these vegetables can have an orange tinge to the skin.

The relative amounts of reduced haemoglobin (dark red) and oxyhaemoglobin (bright red) in the superficial venous plexuses also affect skin colour. In **cyanosis**, there is less oxyhaemoglobin and conse-quently the skin in the nail beds and the mucous membranes appears bluish in colour.

See also **Jaundice** (page 569), in Ch. 15, Digestion and Absorption of Food.

See also **Clotting** (page 328), in Ch. 11, Blood, Lymphoid Tissue and Immunity.

In jaundice, a condition in which plasma bilirubin concentration is elevated, the pigment is deposited in the skin, which then takes on a yellow or orange hue.

Bruises, which are typically 'black and blue', but can also appear red or yellow, result from the leakage of blood into the tissue spaces (**haematoma**). The changing appearance of a bruise results from the gradual breakdown of the clotted blood.

Skin appendages

The appendages of the skin, which lie within or project from it, comprise nails, hair, sebaceous glands and sweat glands.

NAILS

Nails, which are formed from translucent keratinized squames, support the digital pads at the ends of fingers and toes. Each nail comprises a **free border**, a **body** which overlies skin, and a **root** which is inserted into a groove of skin (Figure 10.4).

Except for the free border, the edges of the nail are overlapped by folds of skin (**nail folds**). The **cuticle** (eponychium) is formed from

Figure 10.4 Structure of a nail. **(a)** Surface view. **(b)** Longitudinal section through the distal phalanx.

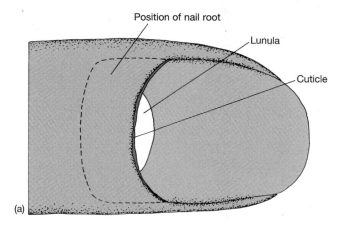

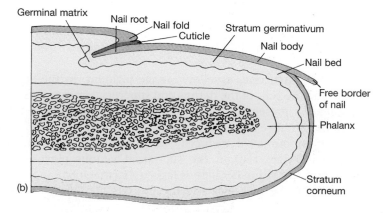

stratum corneum which extends from the nail fold covering the root of the nail and partially covers the white, crescent-shaped **lunula**.

The **nail bed** which lies underneath the body of the nail comprises the germinative zone overlying the vascular dermis. This gives nails their usual pink colour; they can look blue in hypoxia, however, because of the relative lack of bright red oxyhaemoglobin.

Under the root and the lunula, the thickened germinative zone is called the **germinal matrix**. It is here that epidermal cells are produced that eventually become the nail.

Nails grow at about 0.5 mm per week, quicker in summer and faster in fingers than toes. Growth can be disturbed in illness, giving rise to transverse ridges or white flecks.

HAIRS

Hairs are flexible, threadlike structures, composed principally of keratin. They are found in the skin covering most parts of the body except for the lips, nipples and parts of the external genitalia, the dorsal surface of the distal phalanges and the undersurfaces of the feet and hands. Skin without hairs is known as **glabrous skin**. In the eyelids, the hairs do not project beyond the surface of the skin.

Each hair comprises a root, which lies in the skin, and a shaft which projects from the skin (Figure 10.3). Hair shafts have three layers: the inner medulla, the cortex and the cuticle (Figure 10.5). The **medulla**

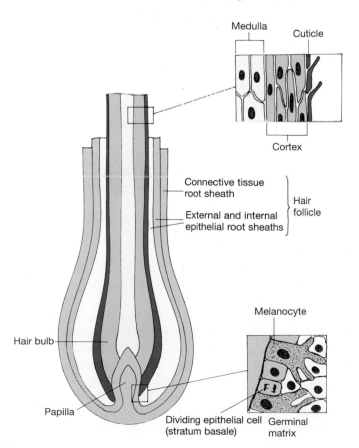

Figure 10.5 Structure of a hair in longitudinal section. The hair root, which lies in the skin, is expanded at its deepest point into a hair bulb. The hair follicle, comprising the connective tissue and epithelial root sheaths, surrounds the hair root. Growth of the hair occurs from the germinal matrix covering the dermal papilla The shaft of the hair, which protrudes from the skin, consists of an outer cuticle, cortex and inner medulla.

contains polyhedral cells with air between and sometimes within them. Fine body hair lacks the medullary layer. The **cortex** consists of several layers of elongated cells which are joined to form flattened fibres containing pigment granules in dark hair or air in white hair. The outer **cuticle** is a single layer of overlapping flat cells, which contain a lot of keratin. Where the cuticle wears away at the tips of the hairs, the fibres of the cortex are exposed and are called 'split ends'.

The **hair follicle** is an invagination of the epidermis and superficial part of the dermis, although some follicles extend into the subcutaneous tissue. Follicles have a funnel-shaped opening at the skin surface, and run obliquely (straight hair) or in a curve (curly hair) through the skin, with a dilated end, the **hair bulb**.

One or more sebaceous glands open into each follicle near the skin surface.

The dermis of the skin projects into the follicle as a **papilla** which contains blood vessels and nerve endings. These are stimulated if the hair is bent. The outer coat of the follicle is fibrous, continuous with the dermis, and contains blood vessels and nerve fibres. The inner coat next to the hair root has two layers, the external and internal root sheaths.

During the fifth and sixth months of foetal life, the skin is covered by fine primary hairs (**lanugo coat**), which are mostly shed by birth and replaced by secondary (**vellus**) hairs. Secondary hairs are replaced by **terminal hairs** in the eyebrows, beard, pubic hair, scalp, axillary hair, and male chest hair. Beard and pubic hairs are thicker than the rest.

Scalp hair varies in shape, such that straight hair is round in cross-section, wavy hair oval and curly hair flat.

Hair growth occurs in the bulb of the follicle. Cells covering the papilla form the **germinal matrix** and the dividing cells push those next to them outwards. As in the epidermis, the cells become keratinized as they move towards the surface. The keratin produced in hairs is harder than that in the epidermis, and as a result the hair cells do not desquamate.

Hairs grow about 1.5 mm per week (fine) and 2.2 mm per week (coarse). Each hair lasts from between 4 months (eyelashes, axillary hair) to 4 years (scalp). They fall out and are replaced, after a break, with new growth from the germinal matrix.

After 40 years of age, new hair growth is slower than the shedding of old hair and so the hair becomes thinner. The terminal hairs are replaced by vellus hairs.

Male baldness (**alopecia**) is an inherited condition caused by a change in testosterone receptors in the hair follicles that inhibits follicular growth. Eunuchs are never bald.

Arrector pili muscles originate in the superficial layer of the dermis and insert into the outer coat of hair follicles, below the sebaceous duct (Figure 10.3). The muscle is found on the side towards which the hair slopes, so that when the muscle fibres contract, the hair is elevated. The skin over their origin is depressed and around the hair it is elevated, giving the appearance of '**goose flesh**' characteristic of cold or emotional states. Piloerection is stimulated by the sympathetic nervous system (see also *Mechanisms counteracting a fall in body temperature*, below).

SEBACEOUS GLANDS

Sebaceous glands are associated with hairs in the skin all over the body, being particularly abundant on the scalp and face. Like hairs, therefore, they are absent from the palms and soles.

Each gland has a single large duct and several alveoli comprising a basement membrane and epithelial cells (Figure 10.3). The outer cells are small and polyhedral; the inner cells are larger and contain fat. In the centre of the gland the cells disintegrate and their fatty contents and cell debris constitute the secretion, **sebum**. Sebaceous ducts usually open into hair follicles but some open directly on to the skin surface. Sebum lubricates hair and skin, partially waterproofs skin and has some bactericidal action.

An accumulation of sebum in a duct initially forms a **whitehead** and, as the sebum dries and becomes oxidized, it becomes a **blackhead**. If sebaceous glands become infected, usually by the bacterium *Staphylococcus*, the inflammatory response forms **pimples** or 'spots'. An outbreak of such infected glands (**acne**) often occurs during puberty, when testosterone production rises and stimulates sebum secretion. After puberty, sebum is secreted continuously.

SWEAT GLANDS

Sweat (sudorific) glands are subdivided into two types known as eccrine (or merocrine) and apocrine glands. The terminology refers to secretion without a loss of cytoplasm from the cell (eccrine) or with a loss of cytoplasm (apocrine). This distinction is no longer thought to apply to the glands, neither of them being apocrine glands, but the names persist.

Eccrine sweat glands are distributed widely in the skin all over the body, being particularly plentiful on the palms and the soles.

Each gland is a single tube, the deep part of which is coiled into an oval or spherical ball lying in the deeper layers of the dermis or hypodermis.

The duct of the gland is convoluted in the deeper layers of the dermis, becoming straighter as it approaches the surface (Figure 10.3).

Sweat glands are two-layered: the outer thin layer is areolar tissue, continuous with the superficial stratum of the dermis. The inner layer consists of epithelial cells. The coiled body has cuboidal or polyhedral cells, classified as **dark** (glycoprotein-secreting) and **clear** (serous fluid-secreting) cells, which contain glycogen. **Myoepithelial cells** are found around the epithelial cells. As these can contract, it is likely that they contribute to the process of expelling sweat from the gland.

Sympathetic cholinergic neurones innervate the coiled part of the glands and stimulate sweating; this generally happens if body temperature rises. The glands can also be stimulated by adrenaline and noradrenaline circulating in the blood, which accounts for the '**cold sweat**' that can accompany emotional states.

Sweat is produced in two stages; the clear cells in the coiled portion of the sweat gland secrete fluid into the intercellular canaliculi (Figure 10.3). This primary fluid has a similar ionic composition to plasma, and it is modified as it passes through the duct portion, principally by the absorption of Na^+ and Cl^-.

Glands (page 77), in Ch. 3, Tissues.

Apocrine sweat glands are found in the axillae, eyelids, areolae and nipples, around the anus and on the external genitalia. The ducts of the glands usually open into the distal ends of hair follicles. These glands, which are larger than eccrine sweat glands, are not involved in temperature regulation. They produce a viscous, milky secretion by exocytosis, not by membrane-bound vesicles as the name 'apocrine' suggests. Components in apocrine sweat, together with their bacterial degradation products, give rise to '**body odour**'. Some of these chemicals are thought to act as **pheromones**, i.e. chemical signals that are sexually attractive. Apocrine sweat glands are innervated by both sympathetic and parasympathetic nerve fibres. They are stimulated during stress.

The **ceruminous glands** found in the skin lining the external auditory meatus are modified apocrine sweat glands. Their waxy secretion, **cerumen**, probably repels insects and prevents the entry of airborne particles into the ear.

Skin circulation

Small arteries take the blood into a sheet-like plexus, the **rete cutaneum**, situated at the junction of the dermis and hypodermis beneath (Figure 10.6).

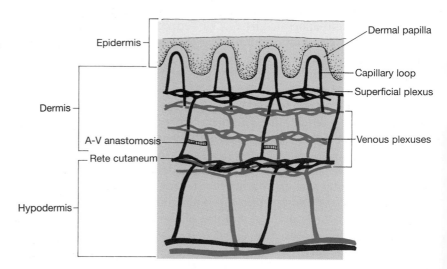

Figure 10.6 Distribution of blood vessels in the skin. The epidermis does not contain blood vessels. The dermis, however, contains small arteries, arising from deeper larger vessels, which supply an arterial plexus (the rete cutaneum) that in turn supplies the superficial plexus. The veins in the dermis are arranged in two superficial plexuses which drain into a deep venous plexus. Arteriovenous anastomoses are present in the lower dermis. When these contract, blood drains from the venous plexuses and the skin cools.

From here vessels pass towards the surface of the dermis, giving off branches to hair follicles, sebaceous glands and sweat glands. Close to the junction of the dermis and epidermis, they form a superficial plexus, from which capillary loops pass towards the surface in dermal papillae. These capillaries supply the epidermis, which does not contain blood vessels.

Venous plexuses are found at various levels in the dermis; they drain into a deep venous plexus at the junction of the dermis and superficial fascia and from there into large veins in the hypodermis.

Arteriovenous anastomoses are present in the lower dermis. In some parts of the body (hands, feet, lips, nose, ears) they are highly muscular. These direct connections between the arteries and veins allow relatively large volumes of blood to flow into the venous plexus in the deep layers of the skin. The anastomoses contain smooth muscle fibres, which are regulated by sympathetic vasoconstrictor pathways originating in the temperature-regulating centre in the hypothalamus. When the anastomoses are dilated, blood fills the deep venous plexus, warming the skin and increasing heat loss to the environment. When constricted, the anastomoses allow little or no blood into the deep venous plexus and body heat is conserved. In this situation, however, the extremities become extremely cold.

The superficial arterioles are also regulated by the sympathetic nervous system, increased activity causing vasoconstriction, decreased activity causing vasodilation.

When heat or cold is applied locally to the skin, thermoreceptors respond by sending impulses to the spinal cord, initiating a spinal reflex resulting in vasodilation or vasoconstriction, respectively.

Overall, skin blood flow may be as low as 1 mL/100 g/min in cold conditions, rising to 150 mL/100 g/min if body temperature rises.

Although the nervous system is the main regulator of skin circulation, local factors such as heat and cold and the accumulation of metabolites also affect skin blood flow.

Local factors affecting arteriolar radius are illustrated in Figure 12.26 in Ch. 12, Circulation of Blood and Lymph.

In extreme cold, vasodilation occurs, which is probably a combination of inactivation of the sympathetic nerve endings combined with the action of local metabolites that have accumulated during the period of vasoconstriction. The increased blood flow warms the tissues and prevents damage.

Nerve supply of the skin

The dermis abounds with a variety of sensory receptors conveying sensations of light touch, strong pressure, hair-pulling, heat, cold and pain.

Skin sensory receptors and sensory pathways from them are covered in Ch. 7, Sensory Processing.

With the exception of the first cervical spinal nerves, each pair of spinal nerves innervates an area of skin known as a dermatome. The dermatomes are not completely discrete areas, they overlap with those innervated by adjacent spinal nerves.

Nerve fibres enter the skin from the hypodermis and supply the sensory receptors, blood vessels, sweat glands, hair follicles and arrector pili muscles. There are plexuses around the hairs and in the dermal papillae.

See also **Spinal nerves** (page 188), in Ch. 6, The Spinal Cord.

Motor innervation of the skin is primarily from the sympathetic nervous system. Vasoconstrictor, noradrenergic fibres innervate skin arterioles and arteriovenous anastomoses. When stimulated, these fibres therefore reduce the amount of blood in the skin and cool it. Vasodilation is generally caused by a reduction in sympathetic tone to the arterioles.

Eccrine sweat glands are innervated by sympathetic sudomotor cholinergic neurones, which stimulate sweating.

Arrector pili muscles are innervated by sympathetic noradrenergic neurones causing piloerection.

Regeneration and healing of skin

Damage to the skin leads to the destruction of blood vessels and leakage of blood into the damaged area. Constriction of blood vessels and clotting of the blood then seals off the cut and prevents further blood loss.

The cells of the epidermis undergo mitotic proliferation and generally the wound is covered over with a thin layer of cells within 24 hours. At this stage the wound site is very weak and inflamed.

Within about 2 days there are active **fibroblasts** within the wound and new capillary buds enter from nearby vessels (Figure 10.7).

This tissue, which replaces the blood clot, is known as **granulation tissue** because of the granular appearance of the capillary buds growing

See also **Haemostasis** (page 326) and **Inflammation** (page 356), in Ch. 11, Blood, Lymphoid Tissue and Immunity.

Figure 10.7   Repair of a skin wound.   **(a)** A blood clot seals the wound. Phagocytes invade the tissue.   **(b)** Granulation tissue forms from capillary buds growing into newly synthesized connective tissue.   **(c)** Capillaries reduce in number, new collagen fibres form scar tissue and strengthen the area.

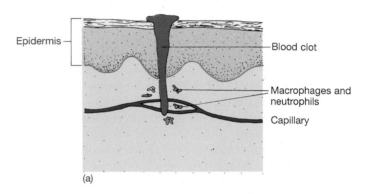

(a)

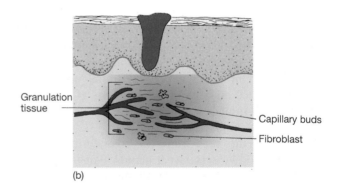

(b)

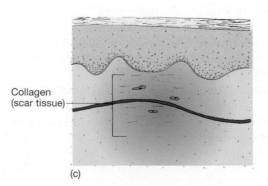

(c)

into it. At first, the fibroblasts lie perpendicular to the wound track but later they come to lie across it. As fibroblastic growth increases, the proportion of intercellular **collagen** also increases forming a **scar** the capillaries reduce in number and the wound becomes pale. The collagen fibres shorten and the scar reduces in size.

The regulation of body temperature

The internal temperature of the body, the 'core' temperature, does not normally vary by more than 0.6°C. Body temperature is usually measured with a thermometer under the tongue, and oral temperature is normally found to lie between 36.7 and 37°C. Measurements of rectal temperature are generally some 0.6°C higher, suggesting that it is nearer to the core temperature.

Although core temperature is regulated within about 0.6°C, variations are routinely observed. There is a generally a peak between 1700 and 1900 h each day and a trough at night and in the early morning. There is a rise in temperature of 0.3–0.5°C at ovulation, which is then maintained until one or two days before menstruation. During pregnancy, body temperature shows a slight increase in the first 4 months, followed by a fall of 0.5–1°C thereafter. Heavy exercise, extremes of atmospheric temperature or fever may cause body temperature to rise or fall outside the normal range. Infants and young children generally have a higher mean body temperature than adults.

Skin temperature is not maintained within such a narrow band as core temperature, and it rises and falls according to ambient temperature. This effect results in a corresponding rise or fall in the rate of heat loss from the skin, an important means of regulating body temperature.

Heat is produced continuously by the body as a consequence of metabolic activity. As a result, temperature regulation is usually an operation that stimulates mechanisms that result in heat loss.

Physical mechanisms of heat loss

Most heat is lost from the body surface. About 60% is lost by radiation of infra-red waves. A much smaller percentage is lost by **conduction**, either to surfaces in contact with the body (such as a chair, the floor or a bed), or to the layer of air next to the skin. As molecules in the air become warm it becomes lighter, and **convection** currents are set up that carry the heat away. All these mechanisms rely on the ambient temperature being lower than skin temperature. As ambient temperature rises, therefore, these mechanisms alone may be insufficient to maintain a steady core temperature.

There is a continuous 'insensible' loss of water through the incompletely waterproof layers of the skin. **Evaporation** of water from the skin surface takes heat away from the body (2.4 kJ per gram of water). 'Sensible' loss of water by sweating also results in heat loss by evaporation. The amount of water in the atmosphere affects the rate of evaporation, so that in humid conditions, the evaporative loss is reduced, and

> Units of temperature are explained in **Temperature** (page 12) and units of energy in **Energy** (page 29), in Ch. 1, Molecules, Ions and Units.

> Infra-red radiation is explained in **Electromagnetic radiation** (page 30), in Ch. 1, Molecules, Ions and Units.

one can feel uncomfortably hot. Sweating is under physiological control and is therefore an important mechanism by which heat loss can be regulated, particularly in conditions of high ambient temperature or if body temperature rises due to infection.

Hypothalamic control of body temperature

The core temperature of the body is controlled by a **temperature-regulating 'centre'** in the hypothalamus. A bilateral area in the posterior hypothalamus receives information concerning the temperature of various parts of the body and sends out impulses to the structures that are able to modify heat loss or gain, as appropriate (Figure 10.8).

The major thermosensitive receptors (the **central receptors**) are found in the preoptic and anterior hypothalamic nuclei of the hypothalamus. The receptors are mostly heat-sensitive, but about one-third are cold-sensitive.

Peripheral thermoreceptors are found in the skin and some deeper structures, e.g. the spinal cord and great veins. In contrast to the central receptors, these receptors respond mainly to a fall in temperature.

See also **Hypothalamus** (page 153), in Ch. 5, The Brain.

Figure 10.8 Responses to a fall in body temperature.

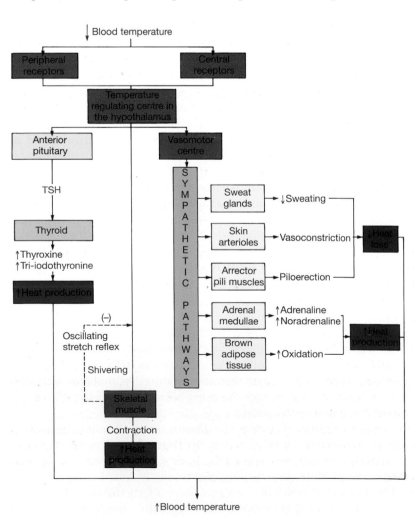

The hypothalamic temperature-regulating centre acts like a thermostat that initiates heat-losing activities should the body temperature start to rise, and initiates heat-gaining and reduces heat-losing activities should it start to fall.

Mechanisms counteracting a rise in body temperature

A rise in body temperature stimulates physiological mechanisms that lead to an increase in heat loss: vasodilation and sweating.

VASODILATION

If the temperature of the blood flowing into the hypothalamus starts to rise, the hypothalamus increases the frequency of impulses that have an inhibitory influence on the vasomotor centre. As a result, the frequency of impulses along the sympathetic vasoconstrictor fibres to the arterioles in the skin is reduced and so vasodilation occurs.

The extra blood passing through the skin warms it, thereby increasing the temperature gradient between the body and its surroundings, and heat is subsequently lost by radiation, conduction and convection.

See also **Blood flow and its control** (page 403), in Ch. 12, Circulation of Blood and Lymph.

SWEATING STIMULATED BY THE HYPOTHALAMUS

The hypothalamus stimulates sweating via sympathetic neurones to sweat glands on all parts of the skin surface. The postganglionic sympathetic neurones to sweat glands are known as sudomotor neurones, and they are unusual in being cholinergic. The stimulated sweat glands then secrete fluid on to the skin surface. It is the evaporation of this fluid that carries heat away. It is estimated that as much as 1.5 L of fluid can be lost per hour through sweating. This represents 3600 J of heat.

Acclimatization of sweating

One of the processes by which individuals become 'acclimatized' to a hot climate is a substantial increase in the volume of sweat produced (from a maximum rate of about 0.7 L/h normally to 2 L/h after acclimatization). Furthermore, the amount of sodium chloride lost in the sweat reduces, an effect mediated by the increased secretion of **aldosterone**. This is stimulated by a fall in plasma volume due to the loss of fluid by excessive sweating. Aldosterone has a similar action on the ducts of sweat glands as it has on kidney tubules i.e. it promotes Na^+ reabsorption and K^+ secretion.

See also **The adrenal cortices** (page 637), in Ch. 16, Endocrine Physiology, and **Role of aldosterone in the regulation of sodium and potassium balance and blood volume** (page 505), in Ch. 14, Renal Control of Body Fluid Volume and Composition.

REFLEX SWEATING INDUCED BY A LOCAL RISE IN SKIN TEMPERATURE

Should one particular part of the body become hot, for example by putting a hand in hot water, local vasodilation and sweating occur, mediated by nerve pathways through the spinal cord. Sensory fibres from thermoreceptors transmit impulses to the cord; vasodilation is caused by reduced activity in the sympathetic noradrenergic fibres to skin arterioles; sweating is caused by increased activity in the sympathetic cholinergic fibres to sweat glands.

Heat stroke

If the limits of the heat-lowering mechanisms are exceeded, for example in very humid and hot conditions, then heat stroke can occur. Body temperatures above 41°C can directly damage tissues and cause local haemorrhages. The principal effects of a high body temperature are dizziness, abdominal distress and delirium. Excess loss of body fluid from sweating can result in hypovolaemic shock.

Mechanisms counteracting a fall in body temperature

A fall in body temperature can be counteracted in two ways: by reduced heat loss and by increased heat production.

REDUCED HEAT LOSS

If the blood flowing into the hypothalamus is relatively cool, the vaso-motor centre becomes more active so that there is an increase in sympathetic vasoconstrictor activity in the skin (Figure 10.8). The resultant reduction of blood flow cools the skin and thereby reduces the rate of heat lost by radiation, conduction and convection.

Constriction of the arteriovenous anastomoses in the skin of the extremities prevents blood flow into the plexuses, which then become relatively empty and the skin cools (see also *Skin circulation*, above). The rate of heat loss from areas with arteriovenous anastomoses is therefore reduced considerably, although the cost of this is ischaemia, which can be painful and in more extreme conditions can lead to frostbite, in which the skin actually freezes.

As body temperature falls, so sweating is inhibited.

A characteristic sign of cooling the body is that the skin hairs stand on end (**piloerection**). The arrector pili muscles are stimulated by sympathetic fibres and pull on the hairs. The resultant puckering of the skin around each hair gives the characteristic 'goose flesh' appearance. In humans, the value of this effect is limited to it being a sign that someone is cold, whereas in animals with a thick coat of hair the amount of air trapped in it is increased, and this enhances the insulating properties of the fur coat.

INCREASED HEAT PRODUCTION

In addition to the mechanisms that reduce heat loss if body temperature falls, several mechanisms increase the rate of heat production by the body. When the hypothalamus is cooled, the usual inhibitory influence from the anterior hypothalamic-preoptic area upon the hypothalamic 'shivering centre' in the posterior hypothalamus is reduced. In addition, impulses from peripheral cold receptors stimulate the centre. The shivering centre stimulates activity in the motor pathways to the skeletal muscles, which then contract and cause the characteristic 'tense' muscles seen in individuals who feel cold. Following this initial phase, more powerful contractions occur that shake the body (**shivering**). The precise mechanism which governs shivering is not understood, but it is likely that the stretch reflex is involved (being inhibited when the muscles contract and stimulated when they relax). Because the process

See also **Ischaemic pain** (page 215), in Ch. 7, Sensory Processing.

of muscle contraction produces heat, shivering can increase heat production up to five-fold when the body is cooled.

The hormones **thyroxine** and **tri-iodothyronine** are released when the body is cooled and increase metabolic rate and therefore heat production. The effect, however, is slow in onset and therefore of doubtful value in the process of temperature regulation.

The general increase in sympathetic activity that occurs in cool conditions also results in the release of **adrenaline**, which increases metabolic rate, particularly in children.

Another source of heat when the body is cooling down is mediated by the sympathetic stimulation of **brown fat**. The rate of oxidation in these cells is increased, with a corresponding increase in heat production. This source of heat is particularly important in neonates, who have a higher proportion of brown fat than in later life.

> **Metabolic actions of T_3 and T_4** (page 625), in Ch. 16, Endocrine Physiology.

Hypothermia

If the body is exposed to extreme or prolonged cold and the core temperature drops below about 29°C, then the regulatory mechanisms are unlikely to be able to restore the normal core temperature. As body temperature falls, metabolic rate is reduced which means that the body cells produce very little heat; respiratory and cardiovascular activities reduce. At around 33°C, muscle rigidity replaces shivering and amnesia and mental confusion occur. By 30°C, tendon reflexes are lost, unconsciousness is likely and respiratory and heart rates become irregular.

Hypothermia can also be caused by hypothyroidism, alcohol intoxication, heavy sedation or circulatory failure.

Fever (pyrexia)

The hypothalamic thermostat can be reset by chemicals called **pyrogens**. These substances are secreted by bacteria and leucocytes when the body is infected. In this case, the thermostat is reset at a higher level than normal and, since the body temperature will, at that time, be lower than this new level, the heat-gain mechanisms come into play. Vasoconstriction, inhibition of sweating and shivering occur, all of which raise the body temperature to the new level. If at the higher temperature the pyrogens are destroyed, the thermostat is reset to its usual lower value and heat-loss mechanisms become apparent. Vasodilation and profuse sweating cause cooling of the body back to the level of the reset thermostat.

Thus in a fever, a period of feeling cold (chills) with a pale, dry skin and shivering is followed by a point at which the fever breaks (crisis) and the person becomes warm and flushed and sweats profusely.

of muscle contraction (shivering) that may can increase heat production up to five-fold when the body is cooled.

The hormones thyroxine and tri-iodothyronine increase basal metabolic rate and enhance heat production. The effect, however, is slow in onset and therefore should take a day or two to operate here completely.

The appeal to our initial problem is clearly that of heat stimulus also results in the release of adrenaline which increases metabolic rate, particularly in children.

Blood, lymphoid tissue and immunity

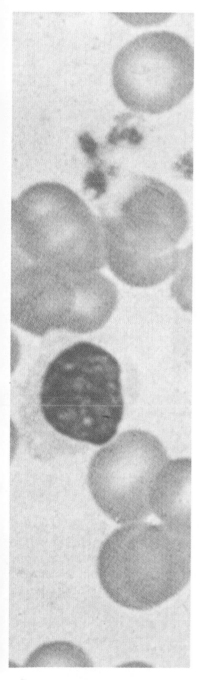

BLOOD

Blood is an opaque liquid, with a viscosity three to four times that of water. It comprises cells and cell fragments (**formed elements**) suspended in fluid (**plasma**). When blood is centrifuged, it separates into a layer of plasma above a thin layer of white cells (**leucocytes**) and cell fragments (**platelets** or **thrombocytes**) and a large lower layer of red cells (**erythrocytes**) (Figure 11.1).

Figure 11.1 The components of blood separated by centrifugation.

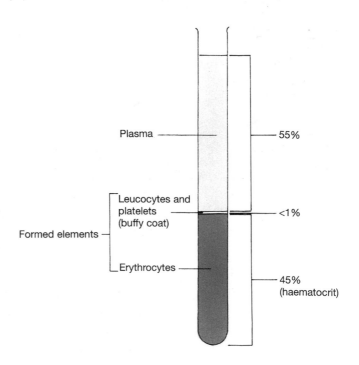

Plasma —— 55%

Leucocytes and platelets (buffy coat) —— <1%

Formed elements —

Erythrocytes —— 45% (haematocrit)

Blood is slightly alkaline, the pH of arterial blood being around 7.4 whereas that of venous blood is about 7.37. The colour of blood is due to the presence of the pigment haemoglobin and varies with the amount of oxygen or H^+ combined with it: oxyhaemoglobin (HbO_2) is bright red, whereas reduced haemoglobin (HHb) is dark red. Blood volume is approximately 70 mL/kg body weight (5 L in a 70 kg adult: 3 L of plasma and 2 L of formed elements).

Blood transports respiratory gases, nutrients, waste products, hormones and heat from one part of the body to another. The white cells and antibodies in the blood defend the body against injurious agents such as microorganisms and toxins. Blood loss from a damaged blood vessel is reduced by the ability of blood to clot and seal the wound. The continuous exchange of water and solutes between plasma and interstitial fluid maintains the internal environment of cells within very narrow limits.

See also **Composition and exchange of constituents between compartments** (page 32), in Ch. 2, Cells and the Internal Environment.

Plasma

Plasma is a straw-coloured, watery fluid, rich in protein. It contains ions, nutrients (principally amino acids, glucose, lipoproteins and vitamins), products of protein breakdown (urea and creatinine) and nucleic acid breakdown (uric acid), as well as enzymes and hormones. Oxygen and carbon dioxide are also carried in the plasma. Plasma is also the medium by which heat is transferred to the surface of the body, from where it is lost by a combination of radiation, conduction, convection and evaporation.

Table 11.1 shows the concentration of the major constituents of blood plasma. Protein is the single largest organic component and Na^+ and Cl^- are the most abundant ions. Table 11.2 summarizes the actions of the major electrolytes in plasma and the effects on the body of alterations in their concentrations.

Transport of respiratory gases by the blood (page 451), in Ch. 13, Respiration.

Physical mechanisms of heat loss (page 317), in Ch. 10, The Skin and the Regulation of Body Temperature.

Table 11.1 Typical concentrations of solutes in plasma (excluding vitamins and hormones)

Ions	(mmol/L)	Respiratory gases	(mmol/L)
Na^+	142	O_2	0.1
K^+	4	CO_2	1
Ca^{2+}	2.5	**Plasma proteins**	(g/dL)
Mg^{2+}	1	Total	7.3
Cl^-	100	Albumin	4.5
HCO_3^-	27	Globulins	2.5
$HPO_4^{2-}/H_2PO_4^-$	1	Fibrinogen	0.3
SO_4^{2-}	1	**Waste products**	(mmol/L)
Nutrients	(mmol/L)	Creatinine	0.09
Glucose	5.6	Urea	5.7
Lipids	7.5	Uric acid	0.3
Amino acids	2	Bilirubin	0.003–0.018

Plasma proteins

Plasma proteins are classified as albumin and globulins (alpha, beta – including fibrinogen – and gamma).

Proteins are large molecules and therefore do not generally cross capillary walls in large numbers to enter the tissue spaces. They therefore exert an osmotic pressure across the capillary wall, which promotes the passage of water into the blood. Although albumin represents about 60% by weight of the total plasma protein content, its contribution to the osmotic pressure exerted by the plasma proteins is nearer 80%. This is because albumin molecules are smaller than the other plasma

See also **Proteins** (page 22), in Ch. 1, Molecules, Ions and Units.

See also **Formation and re-absorption of interstitial fluid** (page 409), in Ch. 12, Circulation of Blood and Lymph.

Table 11.2 Functions and effects of deficiency and excess of plasma electrolytes

Ion	Functions	Deficiency	Excess
Na^+	Maintenance of ECF volume and OP	Decreased BP	Increased BP Cellular dehydration Confusion, coma
	Neuromuscular activity	Muscular weakness	
K^+	Neuromuscular activity	Cardiac arrhythmias	Bradycardia Cardiac arrest/arrhythmias
		Muscular weakness	Muscular weakness, paralysis
	exchanges with H^+ in cells Competes for excretion with H^+	Alkalosis	
Ca^{2+}	Clotting	Poor clotting	
	Reduces cell membrane permeability to Na^+	Increased nerve and muscle activity	Nausea, vomiting Loss of muscle tone Confusion, coma
Mg^{2+}	Neuromuscular activity	Twitching, tremors cardiac arrhythmias	Depressed neuromuscular activity
	Essential for many enzymes to function		
Cl^-	Maintenance of ECF volume and OP	Decreased BP	Increased BP Cellular dehydration Confusion, coma
	Exchanges with HCO_3^- formed in red cells	Alkalosis (HCO_3^- retention)	Acidosis (HCO_3^- loss)
HCO_3^-	Acid-base balance CO_2 carriage	Acidosis	Alkalosis

See **Osmotic pressure** (page 14) and **Buffers** (page 15), in Ch. 1, Molecules, Ions and Units.

proteins, so that there are a greater number per gram, exerting a correspondingly higher osmotic pressure.

Plasma proteins contribute to the buffering capacity of the blood by taking up H^+.

Some protein molecules are involved in blood clotting: others (primarily the gamma-globulins) are antibodies (see *Acquired (specific) immunity*, below). The alpha- and beta-globulins act as carriers for many substances, including minerals and hormones.

Haemostasis

If a blood vessel becomes damaged, a series of mechanisms is stimulated that reduce or stop the blood loss. The term **haemostasis** is used to describe these mechanisms, which comprise three main events:

- vasoconstriction;
- formation of a temporary platelet plug;
- clotting.

Haemostasis is most effective in the microcirculation; because of its high pressure, it is particularly difficult to stop the flow of blood from damaged arteries into the tissues. Loss of blood from veins, on the other hand, can be reduced by the pressure of the accumulated blood in the tissues. Blood in the tissues is called a **haematoma**.

Vasoconstriction

If a blood vessel is damaged there is an immediate local constriction, which reduces blood flow and therefore blood loss. There are several mechanisms that contribute to this vasoconstriction, including the direct effect of trauma causing muscle spasm, a neural reflex initiated by nociceptors, and the release of various chemicals from the damaged tissue and from platelets (Figure 11.2). Thromboxane A_2, a derivative of arachidonic acid is a powerful vasoconstrictor released from platelets.

Vasoconstriction can restrict blood loss from a wound for some 20–30 minutes, during which time firstly the platelet plug and then the clot has time to form.

Platelet plug

Platelets (thrombocytes) are small disc-shaped elements, 2–4 μm in diameter, numbering 150 000–400 000/mm³ (see Figure 11.10). They are formed in the bone marrow as anucleate fragments of large cells called megakaryocytes, (see *White blood cells (leucocytes)*, below).

Damage to the endothelium exposes the underlying collagen, to which blood platelets respond by swelling, becoming irregular in shape and sticking to the blood vessel wall. The adherence of the platelets to

Figure 11.2 Formation of a platelet plug initiated by exposure to collagen in the blood vessel wall, enhanced by von Willebrand factor (vWF) released from platelets and endothelium. Platelet aggregation is accelerated by platelet ADP and thromboxane A_2 and inhibited by endothelial factors nitric oxide (NO) and prostaglandin I_2. (PGI$_2$) Platelet serotonin and thromboxane A_2 enhance the vasoconstriction phase of haemostasis.

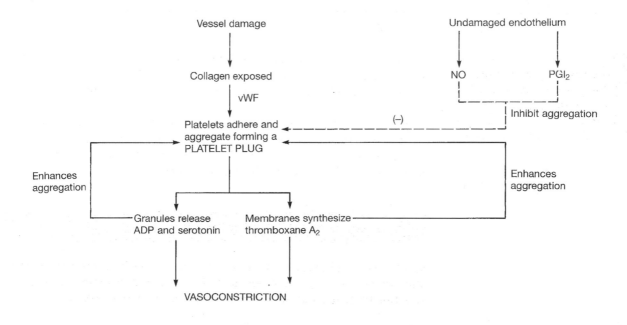

collagen is facilitated by **von Willebrand factor**, which is secreted by both endothelial cells and platelets (Figure 11.2).

The phospholipids in the surface membrane of platelets contain **platelet factor**, which is involved at several points in the clotting process. Platelets contain secretory vesicles (granules), inside which are several chemicals, including ADP and **serotonin**, which play a pivotal role in haemostasis. **Thromboxane A₂** is synthesized from phospholipids in the surface membrane of the platelets. It stimulates the release of serotonin and ADP from the platelets and increases platelet aggregation. Serotonin is a vasoconstrictor, while ADP (along with thromboxane A₂) attracts other platelets, leading to the formation of a platelet plug within 1 minute. This plug temporarily prevents blood loss.

Aspirin inhibits thromboxane A₂ and regular low dosage is thought to reduce the incidence of myocardial infarctions and cerebrovascular accidents caused by thrombi.

There is a positive feedback cycle between platelets sticking to the endothelial wall and further platelets being attracted to the area. The cycle is limited by the inhibitory action on platelet aggregation of the prostaglandin called prostacyclin, or **prostaglandin I₂** (**PGI₂**), and **nitric oxide**. Both these chemicals are released from endothelium adjacent to the wound.

Platelet plugs can effectively block holes in small blood vessels, without the formation of a clot. In larger wounds, however, the platelet plug is replaced by a clot.

> For other actions of nitric oxide see **Vasoactive substances released by vascular endothelium** (page 408), in Ch. 12, Circulation of Blood and Lymph.

Clotting

A blood clot consists of strands of the insoluble protein **fibrin**, which is formed from the soluble beta-globulin **fibrinogen**. Fibrinogen is converted to fibrin monomer which is then itself polymerized to form a loose gel of fibrin threads. Fibrin is then enzymatically converted to a dense network which forms the basis of the clot (Figure 11.3).

Clots usually form within 3–6 minutes of the blood vessel being damaged and retract after about 20 minutes, which produces a firmer seal.

The characteristic ability of plasma to clot on standing is dependent upon the presence of fibrinogen, calcium ions and a group of proteins known as the **coagulation** or **clotting factors**.

The mechanism by which fibrinogen is converted to fibrin involves a 'cascade' of reactions, which require a number of plasma factors (Table 11.3). The conversion of fibrinogen to fibrin is catalysed by **thrombin**,

Figure 11.3 The final stage of clot formation.

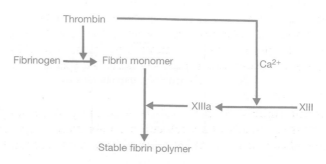

Table 11.3 Blood clotting factors (numbered according to the sequence of their discovery rather than their involvement in the clotting pathways)

Factor	Name (Alternative name)
I	Fibrinogen
II	Prothrombin
III	Tissue factor (thromboplastin)
IV	Ca^{2+}
V	Proaccelarin (labile factor or platelet accelerator)
VI	Discovered to be the same as Factor V
VII	Proconvertin (serum prothrombin conversion accelerator)
VIII	Antihaemophilic factor
IX	Christmas factor (plasma thromboplastin component)
X	Stuart-Prower factor (Stuart factor)
XI	Plasma thromboplastin antecedent
XII	Hageman factor
XIII	Fibrin stabilizing factor
PF	Platelet factor

which in turn is produced from **prothrombin** (Factor II) in the presence of several substances, collectively called **prothrombin activator**, and consisting of Ca^{2+}, Factor V, activated Factor X and platelet factor (PF) or tissue factor (Factor III) (Figure 11.4).

Two different pathways, the intrinsic and the extrinsic, can lead to the activation of factor X and then to the formation of prothrombin activator (Figure 11.4). Once thrombin is present, the clot forms within 10–15 s. Thrombin catalyses the activation of Factor V, so accelerating the whole process by positive feedback.

INTRINSIC PATHWAY

The term 'intrinsic' is used to describe that part of the clotting pathway which uses only factors present within the plasma. If the lining of a large blood vessel is damaged and the collagen in its wall is exposed to the blood, then Factor XII is activated and the platelets release PF. The activation of Factor XII is followed by a series of reactions culminating in the conversion of prothrombin to thrombin by prothrombin activator. Clotting brought about by this pathway takes 1–6 min.

EXTRINSIC PATHWAY

The extrinsic pathway (Figure 11.4) is initiated by blood mingling with damaged tissue, usually in a small cut or an abrasion. A lipoprotein and phospholipid complex (Factor III) released from the tissue (and therefore

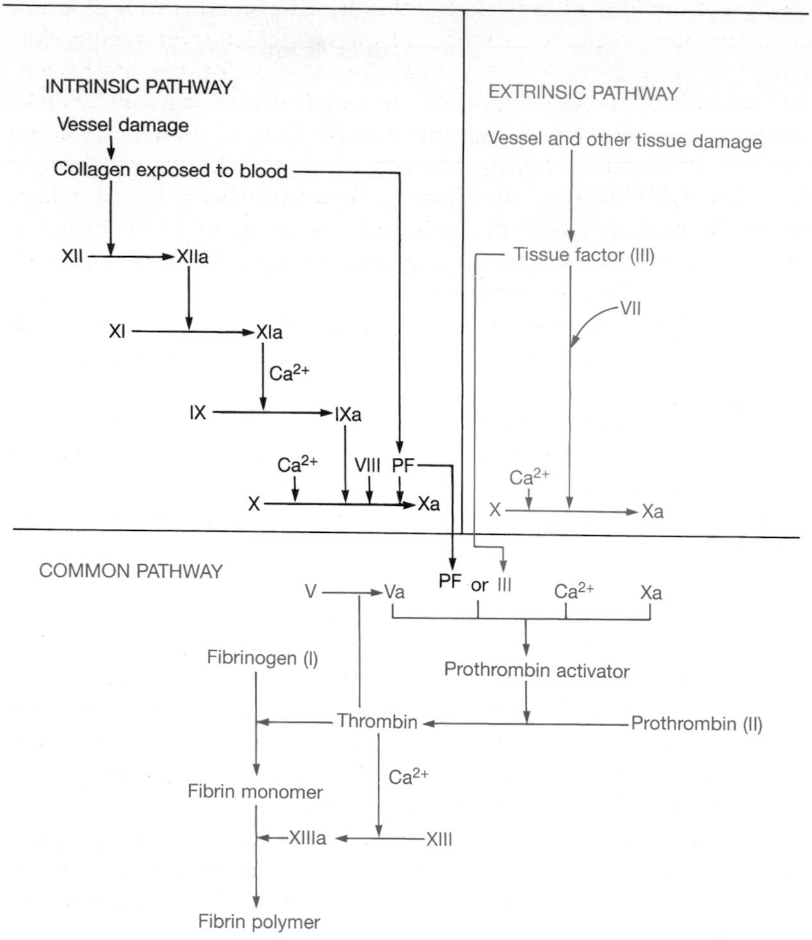

Figure 11.4 Clotting pathways. The intrinsic pathway is initiated by the exposure of blood to collagen in a damaged blood vessel wall and the release of platelet factor (PF). It involves a cascade of chemical reactions terminating in the activation of Factor X. The extrinsic pathway is initiated by the mixing of blood with damaged tissue, which releases Factor III and together with Factor VII and Ca^{2+} activates Factor X. The final common pathway starts with the formation of prothrombin activator and finishes with the formation of insoluble fibrin threads.

extrinsic to the plasma) joins with Factor VII, which, in the presence of Ca^{2+}, brings about the activation of Factor X. The conversion of prothrombin to thrombin is then common to both the extrinsic and the intrinsic pathways. The extrinsic pathway, however, is very much quicker than the intrinsic one, taking as little as 15 s.

CLOT RETRACTION

Soon after a clot has formed, it begins to reduce in size and serum is expressed from it. Serum is plasma with little or no clotting factors in it. Clot retraction is brought about by platelets. As long as they are present in the clot, they continue to release Factor XIII, which tightens the fibrin threads. Platelets also contain the contractile proteins actin, myosin and thrombosthenin, and these enable the platelets to pull on the fibrin threads and thereby further tighten the clot.

ANTICLOTTING MECHANISMS

The formation of a clot is important in the prevention of blood loss from the body but the formation of clots within healthy blood vessels is potentially dangerous. There are a number of ways in which spontaneous clotting within vessels is prevented and any clots that do form are destroyed.

The smooth endothelial lining of the blood vessels, together with its glycocalyx layer, repel platelets and clotting factors, thereby avoiding activating the intrinsic clotting pathway. The endothelial cells have a protein on their surface membrane, **thrombomodulin**, to which thrombin binds. This action not only reduces the quantity of thrombin present in the blood, but also activates a plasma protein, **protein C**, which inactivates Factors V and VIII.

Thrombin levels are also reduced in other ways: by binding to the fibrin threads of a clot, or to a plasma globulin, **antithrombin III (ATIII)**.

Heparin is an anti-clotting agent secreted by basophils and mast cells (and added to blood samples). It combines with ATIII, forming a complex which inhibits the actions of thrombin, IXa, Xa, XIa and XIIa.

Activated clotting factors are removed from the circulation by Kupffer cells in the liver.

FIBRINOLYSIS

Plasmin (fibrinolysin) is a proteolytic enzyme that brings about the breakdown of fibrin and fibrinogen. The enzyme plays a very important role in the circulation, as well as in the tissues, in removing clots. Small clots are formed frequently within small blood vessels and if they were not removed occlusion of the vessel would result.

Plasmin is formed from an inactive precursor in plasma called plasminogen, by the action of tissue plasminogen activator released from the blood vessel wall (Figure 11.5). Plasmin also digests other clotting factors II, V, VIII and XII.

Mechanisms which break down the clot, therefore, begin as soon as the clot is formed since plasminogen is trapped within it. The complete breakdown of a clot can, however, take several days.

Plasmin is inhibited by another plasma protein, **antiplasmin**, which binds to it.

Plasmin activity, therefore, is controlled by tissue plasminogen activator, which stimulates it and causes the slow breakdown of blood clots, and antiplasmin, which inhibits it.

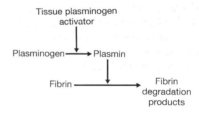

Figure 11.5 Formation and action of plasmin. The concentration of fibrin degradation products can be used as a clinical test for thrombosis.

EFFECTS OF PLATELET DEFICIENCY (THROMBOCYTOPENIA)

Thrombocytopenia is a condition in which there is excess bleeding, particularly from small blood vessels. The cause is a platelet count that is lower than about one-third of the normal value. This leads to a reduction in the formation of platelet plugs, which manifests itself as many purple blotches resulting from small haemorrhages under the skin. A second consequence of a lack of platelets is that clot retraction is impaired. The condition is treated by blood transfusion or by removal of the spleen (splenectomy), which normally removes platelets from the blood.

See also **The malabsorption syndrome** (page 587), in Ch. 15, Digestion and Absorption of Food.

DEFICIENCIES OF BLOOD CLOTTING FACTORS

Most of the clotting factors are synthesized by the liver. It follows, therefore, that impaired liver function can result in defective clotting and therefore excessive bleeding.

Vitamin K deficiency, which in turn may be due to malabsorption of fat from the gut, results in reduced synthesis of clotting Factors II, VII, IX and X.

Haemophilia is a condition in which there is excess bleeding caused by the deficiency of a specific clotting factor. Some 85% of cases of haemophilia are classic haemophilia or haemophilia A, caused by **Factor VIII deficiency**. The remaining 15% (haemophilia B) are caused by **Factor IX deficiency**. The cause of either type of haemophilia is a recessive trait carried on the X chromosome. This means that a female child born with haemophilia has the haemophilia gene on both X chromosomes. If only one chromosome has the affected gene, she would be a carrier and have no haemophiliac symptoms. Male children, however, who only have a single X chromosome, will have haemophilia if that chromosome has the affected gene. Haemophilia, therefore, is much more common in men than in women.

Untreated haemophilia can cause severe and prolonged bleeding as a result of even quite minor trauma. Until recently, treatment consisted of replacement by injections of purified Factor VIII extracted from human blood, or by plasma transfusion. Unfortunately, some recipients have contracted viral conditions, including hepatitis and HIV, from contaminated blood. Factor VIII can now be produced from bacteria by genetic engineering techniques and this is reducing the incidence of cross-infection.

THROMBI AND EMBOLI

A **thrombus** is a blood clot formed within the cardiovascular system by two principal causes: altered endothelium or very slow blood flow. Once the thrombus has formed, blood flowing over it can break pieces off and carry them in the circulation as **emboli**.

See also **Ischaemic heart disease** (page 390), in Ch. 12, Circulation of Blood and Lymph.

Thrombus formation due to altered endothelium occurs in arteriosclerosis, trauma or infection.

Slow blood flow can cause thrombus formation because of the local accumulation of clotting factors. These would otherwise be removed by faster flowing blood and be broken down in the liver.

Prolonged bed rest can precipitate clot formation, if the blood flow, particularly in the legs, is very slow. The lack of leg movements reduces the action of the skeletal muscle pump, which normally promotes venous return. Some clots that develop in the leg veins can extend their whole length and beyond into the common iliac vein and inferior vena cava. If an embolus breaks free from this huge clot, it is likely to flow through the right side of the heart and out into one or both pulmonary arteries. The severity of the resultant **pulmonary embolism** depends upon where the embolus lodges in the pulmonary circulation. The nearer to the arterial inflow the more likely the condition is to be fatal.

Red blood cells (erythrocytes)

A total of 99% of all the formed elements in blood are erythrocytes. They constitute about 45% of whole blood (about 42% in women and 47% in men) (Figure 11.1). The fraction of blood consisting of red blood cells (RBCs) is known as the **haematocrit**, a major determinant of blood viscosity. The red pigment in erythrocytes is the iron-containing protein **haemoglobin**, which contributes to the carriage of both oxygen and carbon dioxide. Haemoglobin is also a blood buffer.

See also **Buffers** (page 15), in Ch. 1, Molecules, Ions and Units.

Red blood cells (RBCs) are biconcave discs, without nuclei, measuring about 1 μm thick in the centre, 2 μm at the edges, and about 7.5 μm in diameter (Figure 11.6).

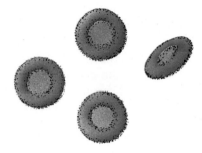

Figure 11.6   Erythrocytes.

This shape results in a high surface-area-to-volume ratio, which facilitates diffusion of oxygen and carbon dioxide across the membrane. RBCs contain a fibrous protein (**spectrin**) attached to the inner surface of the cell membrane. Spectrin makes the cells flexible and able to change shape, particularly when squeezing through the small capillaries. Erythrocytes contain few organelles and, since there are no mitochondria, ATP production is anaerobic.

See also **Glycolysis** (page 595), in Ch. 15, Digestion and Absorption of Food.

The RBC count is around 5 million per cubic millimetre of blood – 4.8 million/mm^3 in women (4.8 × 10^{12}/L), 5.4 million/mm^3 (5.4 × 10^{12}/L) in men.

Haemoglobin A

The concentration of haemoglobin in blood is about 15 g/dL (14 g/dL in women and 16 g/dL in men).

Haemoglobin consists of one subunit of **globin** and four subunits of the red pigment **haem** (Figure 11.7).

Globin is made up of four amino acid chains and the haem comprises iron and protoporphyrin. The most common form of haemoglobin, (haemoglobin A) contains two alpha and two beta amino acid chains. It is estimated that there are around 250 million molecules of haemoglobin inside each RBC.

About 98% of the oxygen and 6% of the carbon dioxide in blood is transported by the RBCs, attached to haemoglobin.

See also **Transport of respiratory gases by the blood** (page 451), in Ch. 13, Respiration.

When oxygen combines with haemoglobin in the lungs, it becomes loosely attached to the iron, which is in the ferrous form, forming

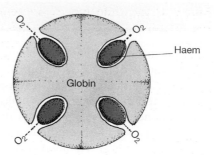

Figure 11.7 Structure of the haemoglobin molecule. Globin comprises four amino acid chains, each forming a 'pocket' containing one molecule of haem. Each haem can combine with one molecule of dissolved oxygen.

See also **Gas exchange** (page 449), in Ch. 13, Respiration.

See also **Cyanosis** (page 470), in Ch. 13, Respiration.

See also **Effects of smoking on respiratory functions** (page 471), in Ch. 13, Respiration.

The inheritance of haemoglobin S is explained in **Alterations in chromosome number or structure** (page 65), in Ch. 2, Cells and the Internal Environment.

See also **Foetal haemoglobin** (page 454), in Ch. 13, Respiration.

oxyhaemoglobin (HbO_2). In the tissues, oxygen is easily released from the iron and then diffuses out of the RBCs into the plasma and from there to the cells.

Carbon dioxide combines with amino groups in the globin part of the molecule, forming carbaminohaemoglobin ($HbCO_2$). In the lungs, some of the carbon dioxide is released from carbaminohaemoglobin, dissolves in the plasma and then diffuses into the alveoli before being exhaled.

The buffering action of haemoglobin depends upon its ability to act as an H^+ acceptor, forming reduced haemoglobin (HHb). Excess HHb (cyanosis) changes the colour of circulating blood to a darker red, which can appear blue through the skin.

The gas carbon monoxide (CO), which is present in vehicle exhaust fumes and cigarette smoke, combines with haemoglobin to form the cherry red compound **carboxyhaemoglobin** (HbCO).

OTHER FORMS OF HAEMOGLOBIN IN SICKLE CELL ANAEMIA AND THALASSAEMIA

In the condition called **sickle cell anaemia**, one glutamic acid molecule in each of the two beta chains of HbA is replaced by valine, forming **haemoglobin S** (HbS).

At low oxygen partial pressures, HbS forms long, sharp crystals that make the red blood cells sickle-shaped and can rupture them. The sickle shape hinders the passage of erythrocytes through capillaries, leading to blockage, clotting and ischaemic pain. The fragility of the red blood cells results in a low red cell count.

A sickle cell 'crisis' involves a form of positive feedback in which tissue hypoxia causes sickling of the RBCs and consequent blockage of blood vessels, which further increases the hypoxia.

The **thalassaemias**, like sickle cell anaemia, are also conditions in which the structure of the globin part of the haemoglobin is altered, leading to fragile erythrocytes that rupture easily and therefore result in anaemia.

Production of red blood cells (erythropoiesis)

In the foetus, RBCs are initially produced by the yolk sac; later the liver becomes the predominant site of production, and the spleen also contributes. By the end of gestation, the site of red cell production has changed to the bone marrow.

During childhood, most bones contain erythropoietic tissue, but the number of sites reduces as the child grows. By adulthood, RBCs are produced only in the marrow of skull bones, vertebrae, ribs, sternum, pelvis and the proximal ends of the femur and humerus. This reduction in erythropoietic activity parallels the reduction in demand for RBCs. During childhood and adolescence, blood volume and erythropoiesis increase, whereas in adulthood, blood volume, and therefore the rate of erythropoiesis necessary to replace lost RBCs, remains relatively constant.

All blood cells originate from stem cells in the bone marrow. which are capable of becoming any type of blood cell. These 'uncommitted' stem cells (or **pluripotent haemopoietic stem cells**) are able to divide and produce daughter cells, some of which will differentiate to become stem cells 'committed' to a particular cell line. The undifferentiated daughter cells maintain a pool of uncommitted stem cells in the bone marrow.

The committed stem cell that results in the production of erythrocytes is called a **colony-forming unit-erythrocyte** (CFU-E). It is about 18 μm in diameter with a large nucleus and cytoplasm that stains dark blue with basic dyes (Figure 11.8).

Each CFU-E divides and one daughter cell differentiates into a proerythroblast which is smaller than its precursor and its nucleus occupies a smaller proportion of the total cell volume. These trends towards smaller cells and nuclei continue with successive cell types in the series (**early, intermediate** and **late erythroblast**). Haemoglobin synthesis begins in the early erythroblast and is complete by the late erythroblast stage, in which the cytoplasm stains red.

When erythroblasts divide, both daughter cells differentiate into the next cell type, so that a greater number of cells is produced by each division.

The late erythroblast loses its nucleus and thereby becomes a biconcave cell called a **reticulocyte**. These cells are so named because they contain remnants of endoplasmic reticulum and clumps of ribosomes (the site of haemoglobin synthesis).

The reticulocytes enter the blood by squeezing between the endothelial cells of the sinusoids in the bone marrow (diapedesis). The cells lose their endoplasmic reticulum and mature into **erythrocytes** in one or two days. If the rate of erythropoiesis rises, so does the reticulocyte count in the blood. From proerythroblast to erythrocyte takes 3–5 days, and so therefore, does replenishment of RBCs lost by blood donation, or the enhancement of the haematocrit induced by high altitude.

HORMONAL CONTROL OF ERYTHROPOIESIS

For the RBC count to remain constant, the rate of production of new cells must equal the rate of destruction of old cells. The rate of production is indirectly controlled by tissue hypoxia caused by a fall in either the oxygen content of the blood or its rate of delivery to the tissues.

The oxygen content of the blood falls if the RBC count falls, for example following a haemorrhage or due to anaemia, at very high altitudes or if oxygenation of blood in the lungs is reduced, for example in lung disease.

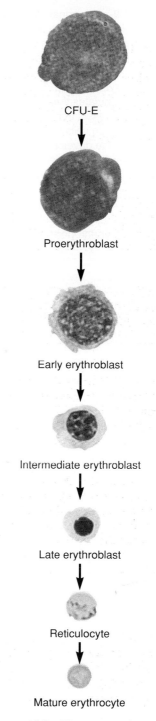

CFU-E

Proerythroblast

Early erythroblast

Intermediate erythroblast

Late erythroblast

Reticulocyte

Mature erythrocyte

Figure 11.8 The stages of erythrocyte production in bone marrow from a colony-forming unit erythrocyte (CFU-E) to a mature erythrocyte . (Reproduced by courtesy of D. M. Quincey.)

Figure 11.9 Hormonal control of erythropoiesis. Tissue hypoxia, which can be caused by either hypoxaemia or reduced blood flow, stimulates the release of the hormone erythropoietin. The hormone stimulates the production of proerythroblasts from the committed stem cells (CFU-E), and accelerates the development of erythrocytes from its precursors. The resulting rise in erythrocyte count raises the oxygen content of the blood, which exerts a negative feedback effect on the rate of secretion of erythropoietin.

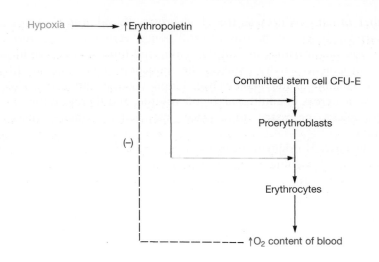

See also **Causes of respiratory hypofunction** (page 464), in Ch. 13, Respiration.

The rate of delivery of oxygen to the tissues falls, for example, in heart failure.

Hypoxia acts as a stimulus for the increased production of a circulating hormone, **erythropoietic factor** (**erythropoietin**). The probable sequence of events is shown in Figure 11.9.

The stimulus increases the rate of release of erythropoietin from the kidneys. Erythropoietin is probably synthesized in the mesangial cells at the pole of the glomerulus (see Figure 14.6). The kidney is thought to be responsible for some 80–90% of erythropoietin production, with the liver making up most of the rest. Adrenaline and noradrenaline and some prostaglandins also stimulate erythropoietin production.

Erythropoietin stimulates the conversion of the committed stem cells, CFU-E, to proerythroblasts, as well as their more rapid passage through the erythroblast stages to form erythrocytes. After the few days necessary for this to occur, the RBC count increases, hypoxia is reduced and, by negative feedback, so does the rate of production of erythropoietin.

HIGH ERYTHROCYTE COUNT (POLYCYTHAEMIA)

If the rate of RBC production exceeds the rate of destruction, then the RBC count increases. This condition is called erythrocytosis or polycythaemia. The cause is only rarely due to a primary increase in erythropoietin synthesis (e.g. due to a renal tumour) or increased bone marrow activity (e.g. due to bone marrow cancer). Polycythaemia more commonly occurs in response to hypoxia caused, for example, by high altitude, haemorrhage or reduced cardiac or respiratory function.

EFFECTS OF NUTRITIONAL DEFICIENCIES ON ERYTHROPOIESIS (ANAEMIAS)

Both **vitamin B₁₂** and **folic acid** are required for the synthesis of DNA, and if insufficient is present, then inadequate numbers of RBCs are produced, resulting in anaemia. The cells produced in these conditions are abnormally large (megaloblasts instead of erythroblasts); the mature cells, macrocytes, are fragile and oval instead of biconcave discs, and their survival time is reduced. This type of anaemia is called **mega-loblastic anaemia**.

Lack of vitamin B_{12} may be due to poor absorption in the small intestine or, more rarely, to an inadequate dietary supply. Absorption of vitamin B_{12} requires **intrinsic factor**, which is produced by the gastric glands and combines with the vitamin when it is in the stomach. The complex is resistant to digestion and travels through the duodenum and jejunum to the ileum, where it is absorbed. In the absence of intrinsic factor, therefore, vitamin B_{12} is liable to be digested and not absorbed, giving rise to a condition called **pernicious anaemia**. The liver stores relatively large amounts of vitamin B_{12}, so a deficiency may not be manifested for some months.

Folic acid deficiency due to an inadequate intake can occur because the vitamin is easily destroyed by cooking. Folic acid deficiency is common in pregnant women and older people.

Deficiency of both vitamin B_{12} and folic acid can result from malabsorption in the small intestine, in, for example, sprue.

Iron is required for the synthesis of haemoglobin, because, although the iron released from worn-out red cells is largely recycled, there is a small loss in the faeces, urine, sweat and sloughed off skin cells (about 1 mg/day). Menstrual losses in women average a further 1 mg/day.

Iron is absorbed in the ferrous form, attached to a protein, in the duodenum and jejunum. Although there may be a large amount of iron in the diet, only a few milligrams are absorbed daily. The rate of iron absorption appears to be controlled by the intestinal epithelium itself and depends upon the total iron balance in the body. For example, if there is an excess of iron in the body, then any additional iron remains in the mucosal cells and is lost when the cells are shed.

Following absorption from the small intestine, iron combines with the plasma protein **transferrin**, a beta-globulin, which binds to receptors on the cell membrane of erythroblasts. The iron–transferrin complex is taken into the cells by endocytosis. Iron is stored in the liver mainly as **ferritin**, which is formed by the combination of iron with the protein **apoferritin**. Any excess iron is deposited in the hepatocytes as insoluble haemosiderin.

Iron-deficiency or **hypochromic anaemia** can result from an inadequate dietary intake of iron, malabsorption in the small intestine or lack of transferrin in the blood. There is a reduced RBC count, and the cells contain very little haemoglobin.

Destruction of erythrocytes

The average lifespan of a RBC is 120 days. The lack of a nucleus means that replacement of essential proteins, such as enzymes, cannot occur. Old, fragile erythrocytes tend to rupture in 'tight spots' of the circulation, particularly the spleen. The phagocytic macrophages engulf these ageing cells and the haemoglobin is broken down into haem and globin. The iron from the haem and the amino acids from the globin are used again in the marrow, whereas the protoporphyrin part of the haem is broken down to **bilirubin**. This is taken up by the liver cells and is eventually excreted in the bile.

Dietary sources of vitamins and minerals are given in Table 15.2, in Ch. 15, Digestion and Absorption of Food.

Iron absorption is described in **Absorption of ions, water and vitamins** (page 585), in Ch. 15, Digestion and Absorption of Food.

See also **Bilirubin** (page 569), in Ch. 15, Digestion and Absorption of Food.

Blood groups

Red blood cell membranes contain glycoproteins or glycolipids with antigenic properties, i.e. they can induce the production of antibodies. Although there are some 30 different varieties of red blood cell antigen, only two, the **ABO** and **Rh** (**Rhesus**) systems, are particularly hazardous if incompatible blood is transfused.

ABO BLOOD GROUPS

> See also **Inheritance** (page 54), in Ch. 2, Cells and the Internal Environment.

Individuals are classified as type A, B, O or AB blood group, which is determined by three alleles: A, B (both dominant) and O (recessive).

Antibodies are not formed against the individual's own red blood cell antigens, rather to the A or B antigens that he or she lacks, so that blood group A individuals produce anti-B antibodies in the plasma and blood group B individuals produce anti-A antibodies. Blood group O individuals have both anti-A and anti-B antibodies, whereas blood group AB individuals have neither (Table 11.4).

Antibody production starts around 2–3 months after birth, probably in response to A and B antigens found in bacteria populating the respiratory and alimentary tracts.

A, B and O blood groups were discovered by Karl Landsteiner in 1901, AB a year later. Subsequently group A has been subdivided into group A_1 (80%) and A_2 (20%).

Blood group A_1 individuals have both A and A_1 antigens, whereas A_2 individuals have only A antigen. The anti-A antibodies found in blood group O and B individuals actually consist of anti-A and anti-A_1 components.

If erythrocytes are mixed with serum containing the antibody to them the cells clump together (**agglutinate**) as a result of the antigen–antibody reaction. Blood groups may be tested in this way, by mixing the cells with two sera, one containing anti-A, the other anti-B antibodies. If the cells agglutinate only with the anti-A serum, then the blood must be group A. If the cells also agglutinate with anti-B serum, then the blood is group AB. If the cells only agglutinate with anti-B serum, then the blood must be group B. If neither antiserum causes agglutination, then the blood is group O. The agglutination reaction between blood group antigens and their antibodies gives rise to the alternative names **agglutinogens** and **agglutinins**, respectively.

Table 11.4 ABO blood groups – these percentage distribution figures are typical of caucasian populations; black and Asian populations have a lower percentage of group A individuals and a higher percentage of AB and B groups than white populations

Phenotype	Genotype	A and B antigens on cells	Antibodies in serum	% distribution (caucasian)
A	AA or OA	A	anti-B	41
B	BB or OB	B	anti-A	9
AB	AB	AB	—	3
O	OO	—	anti-A and anti-B	47

Table 11.5 Transfusion reactions

Recipient	Incompatible donors (donor cells agglutinate)	Compatible donors
O	A, B, AB	O
A	B, AB	O, A
B	A, AB	O, B
AB	—	O, A, B, AB

Blood transfusion

If incompatible blood is transfused, then the donor's cells are agglutinated by the recipient's antibodies. Antibodies from the donor's blood are so diluted that they are unlikely to cause agglutination of the recipient's cells.

Table 11.5 shows which transfusions cause agglutination and which do not.

Theoretically, blood group O (whose cells lack both A and B antigens) can be transfused into a recipient with any blood group and is consequently called the universal donor, whereas blood group AB (which lacks both anti-A and anti-B antibodies) does not cause agglutination in any of the other types and is therefore called the universal recipient.

The consequences of agglutination can be very severe. Agglutinated cells block small vessels in the circulation and are then destroyed by phagocytes, which liberate haemoglobin into the blood. This in turn leads to a rise in plasma bilirubin concentration and **jaundice**.

The haemoglobin released from the agglutinated cells passes through the glomerular membrane into the kidney nephrons, where it can precipitate and occlude the tubules. The resultant **acute renal failure** can be fatal.

Agglutination also reduces the number of circulating erythrocytes and therefore causes anaemia and hypoxia.

In practice, whenever it is possible prior to a transfusion, the compatibility of the donor and recipient's bloods is tested. The donor's cells are mixed with the recipient's serum and if no agglutination occurs then the two bloods are compatible.

In the absence of compatible blood, an emergency expansion of blood volume can be achieved without whole blood, or even plasma, by using solutions of molecules that will retain fluid in the blood. Such **plasma expanders** include protein (albumin) and polysaccharide (Dextran).

Alternatively, infusions of isotonic solutions of electrolytes with the same composition as plasma can be given, e.g. Ringer's solution.

Rh BLOOD GROUPS

A great number of antigens are included in the Rhesus system of blood groups. The system was first studied in Rhesus monkeys and consequently named after them. The principal antigens of the system (Rhesus

See also **Jaundice** (page 569), in Ch. 15, Digestion and Absorption of Food.

See also **Renal failure** (page 516), in Ch. 14, Renal Control of Body Fluid Volume and Composition.

See also **Hypoxia** (page 469), in Ch. 13, Respiration.

Table 11.6 Sets of genotypes in the Rh blood group system. Each individual contains two sets, one from each parent. An Rh⁻ individual has the genotype cde/cde, whereas an RH⁺ individual has at least one C, D or E gene in one of the two sets

Rh-positive sets	Rh-negative set
Cde	cde
cDe	
CdE	
CDe	
cDE	
CdE	
CDE	

factors) are identified as C, D, and E, the most potent being D. Individuals are classified as either 'Rh-positive' or 'Rh-negative', commonly meaning RhD positive or negative, but for transfusion purposes a donor is Rh-positive if s/he has any of the antigens, C, D or E. Some 85% of caucasians are RhD-positive and 15% are RhD-negative.

Rhesus factors, like the ABO system, are inherited. They differ, however, in that they are inherited by genes on three separate loci as opposed to one locus as in the ABO system. The alleles are C and c, D and d and E and e. The genes given capital letters are dominant over those with small letters. Each individual inherits one allele from each parent at each locus (Table 11.6). A Rhesus-negative person always has the genotype cde/cde, whereas a Rhesus-positive person has one or more dominant genes among the six.

In contrast to the ABO system, Rhesus antibodies are not automatically produced against the antigens that an individual lacks, but only when exposure to 'foreign' cells occurs. Should, therefore, Rh⁺ blood be transfused into a Rh⁻ recipient, antibodies would not be formed immediately and cause agglutination. Rather, the process resembles vaccination, whereby the immune system becomes sensitized and produces antibodies in response to subsequent exposure to antibodies.

Haemolytic disease of the newborn (erythroblastosis foetalis)

If an RhD⁻ mother carries an RhD⁺ foetus, then the mother's 'exposure' to the D antigen may well not occur until parturition. At this time some foetal red cells cross the placenta and induce the production of anti-D antibodies by the mother. In a subsequent pregnancy with an RhD⁺ foetus, the mother's anti-D antibodies cross through the placenta to the baby and cause agglutination and haemolysis of the baby's RhD⁺ red blood cells. The excess breakdown of the haemoglobin results in jaundice. The bilirubin can pass through the foetal blood–brain barrier and is deposited in the brain (**kernicterus**), where it causes neurological damage. Erythropoiesis is stimulated by the hypoxia and an increased number of erythroblasts are found in the circulation subsequently. Rh antigens other than D can also occasionally cause haemolytic disease of the newborn.

There are two ways in which this disease can be prevented: by administering a serum containing anti-Rh antibodies or by transfusing the baby's blood.

If the mother is given anti-Rh antibodies before or shortly after birth, these remove any Rh⁺ cells and thereby remove the antigenic stimulus for the mother to produce a lot of anti-Rh antibodies.

The baby's blood can be transfused before birth with a compatible type, to replace any erythrocytes that have already been destroyed by antibodies. After birth, the baby can be given one or two exchange transfusions, whereby its blood is replaced with Rh⁻ blood, so avoiding any antigen–antibody reactions. After some 6 weeks, the baby's own Rh⁺ erythrocytes will have replaced the transfused ones, and any of the mother's antibodies will have disappeared.

White blood cells (leucocytes)

Leucocytes defend the body against microorganisms and remove old or defective cells. The blood is simply a means of conveying these cells to their sites of action in the tissues. The total leucocyte count is usually between 4000 and 11 000 per cubic millimetre ($4–11 \times 10^9$/L). The number of leucocytes in blood reflects their level of activity in the tissues, although it only represents a small percentage of the total number of leucocytes in the body. Leucocyte numbers rise during bacterial or viral infections or allergic reactions. A high leucocyte count is known as **leucocytosis**.

Several types of white cell escape from the blood into the tissues by squeezing between the endothelial cells in the capillaries. This process is known as **diapedesis** and is facilitated during inflammation. Once in the tissues, these leucocytes move by amoeboid motion, i.e. by means of cytoplasmic flow within limb-like processes (pseudopodia). The cells move towards chemicals in areas that have been damaged or invaded by microorganisms (positive chemotaxis).

Classification of leucocytes

The five types of leucocyte can be classified in various ways. Three of them, neutrophils, eosinophils and basophils, are named according to the staining characteristics of their granules. They are known collectively as **granulocytes**.

The cells which lack granules (**agranulocytes**), comprise lymphocytes and monocytes.

Alternatively, leucocytes can be classified according to function as:
- cells mainly involved in non-specific immunity: phagocytic cells (monocytes, neutrophils and eosinophils) and mediator cells (basophils);
- cells mainly involved in specific immunity: lymphocytes.

Table 11.7 shows the typical cell counts and percentage distribution of leucocytes in blood. During acute inflammation the neutrophil count can increase to 25 000/mm^3.

The cells are illustrated in Figure 11.10.

Table 11.7 Count and percentage distribution of leucocytes in blood		
Cell type	Number/mm³	% of total leucocytes
Neutrophils	3000–7000	50–70
Lymphocytes	1500–3000	20–40
Monocytes	100–700	2–8
Eosinophils	100–400	1–4
Basophils	20–50	0.5

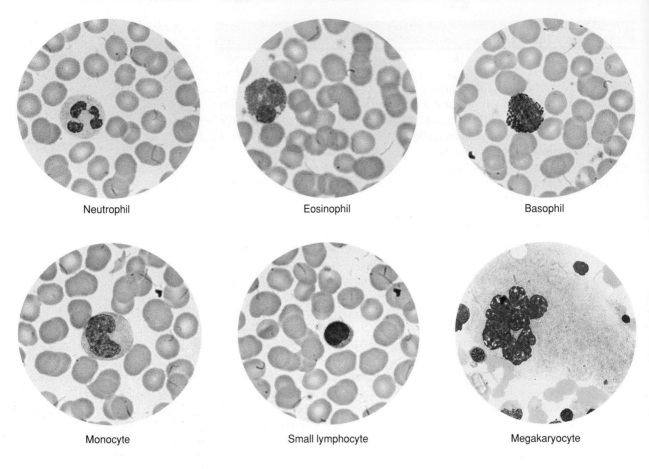

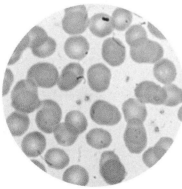

Platelets

Figure 11.10 White cells and platelets in blood. Megakaryocyte in bone marrow. (Reproduced by courtesy of D. M. Quincey.)

Neutrophils

Neutrophils (neutral-loving) have granules, some of which take up the red, acid dye eosin, others the blue, basic dye methylene blue. The combined effect of the two dyes produces a lilac colour. The granules are actually **lysosomes** containing hydrolytic enzymes and peroxidases. Other, non-staining granules contain proteins called **defensins** or **phagocytins**. When the vesicles containing defensins combine with the phagosomes containing microorganisms, the defensins become spear-shaped peptides and pierce the microorganism.

Neutrophils are about 10–12 μm in diameter in dried blood smears, but only 7 μm in circulating blood. They are polymorphonuclear, with up to six lobes in the nucleus, more lobes developing with age. They are the biggest group of leucocytes.

A particular characteristic of neutrophils is that they respond quickly and migrate from the blood to sites of inflammation. They are phagocytic in the tissues, particularly with respect to **bacteria** and some **fungi**. Arachidonic acid in the cell membrane is the precursor of a group of compounds called **leukotrienes** which:

- promote adhesion of neutrophils to the endothelium prior to migrating from the blood;

- chemically attract other neutrophils, eosinophils and monocytes;
- increase the permeability of postcapillary venules;
- cause bronchoconstriction in asthma.

Eosinophils

Eosinophils contain large granules (**lysosomes**) that stain red with eosin. They are about 12 μm in diameter in blood smears and about 9 μm when circulating. The nucleus typically has two lobes.

The cell count of eosinophils is relatively low compared with neutrophils (Table 11.7). Eosinophils have a specific role in combating **parasitic worms**. If a worm invades the respiratory or intestinal mucosa, it is too large to be phagocytosed and eosinophils surround it, releasing lysosomal enzymes, which then digest it from the outside.

The eosinophil count rises in **allergic reactions**, when they phagocytose antigen–antibody complexes and inactivate some inflammatory chemicals.

Basophils

Basophils are relatively scarce in blood (Table 11.7). Their large granules stain blue-black with methylene blue and generally obscure the nucleus, which can appear lobular in section, but is actually U- or J-shaped. Basophils are structurally similar to the mast cells found in connective tissues, although they are not thought to be the same cells and they develop separately in the bone marrow. The granules contain the chemicals **histamine** and **heparin**. Histamine causes vasodilation and increased capillary permeability during inflammation. Heparin is an anticlotting agent.

Basophils are slightly smaller than neutrophils and eosinophils, with a diameter of about 10 μm in blood smears.

> Mast cells are described in **Areolar (loose) connective tissue** (page 80), in Ch. 3, Tissues.

Lymphocytes

The principal circulating lymphocytes are 4–7 μm in diameter, and are designated small lymphocytes. Other circulating forms (medium lymphocytes) are 7–11 μm in diameter. The main structural feature of lymphocytes is their large, spherical nucleus, with a surrounding rim of cytoplasm that stains light blue.

The two major categories of small lymphocyte are **B lymphocytes** and **T lymphocytes**. B lymphocytes are responsible for the production of antibodies, which mediate the humoral immune response. There are several subpopulations of T lymphocytes: some regulate the activity of B lymphocytes by means of chemicals called **lymphokines**, others are toxic to foreign cells, giving rise to a cell-mediated immune response. B and T lymphocyte function is covered in *Acquired (specific) immunity*, below.

Natural killer (NK) cells are a type of large lymphocyte that circulates in blood and lymph. They attack cancer cells and virus-infected cells (see *Cells involved in innate immunity*, below).

Monocytes

Monocytes are the largest of the blood cells, measuring up to 17 μm in dried blood smears, 9–12 μm in circulation. The nucleus is kidney-shaped and the cytoplasm stains grey-blue. These cells migrate into the tissues, enlarge, and become **macrophages** (literally, 'big eaters') over a period of about 8 hours. They are slower but more powerful than neutrophils in their response to inflamed tissue, and are therefore particularly important in combating chronic infections such as tuberculosis. In addition to their phagocytic role, macrophages stimulate lymphocytes to mount specific immune responses (see Figures 11.21, 11.26).

Cytokines

Cytokines are proteins or polypeptides secreted by leucocytes, which regulate immune responses. Lymphokines are secreted by lymphocytes, monokines by monocytes and macrophages. Some chemicals are secreted by more than one leucocyte, and therefore the generic name cytokine has been adopted.

Some cytokines act locally, others circulate and act in tissues remote from their site of production.

Principal cytokines are:

- **interleukins**, secreted by T lymphocytes and macrophages, which stimulate T and B lymphocytes;
- **colony-stimulating factors**, secreted by macrophages and T lymphocytes, which stimulate leucopoiesis;
- **interferons**, secreted by lymphocytes, which are antiviral;

Figure 11.11 Major cell types involved in the development of leucocytes and platelets. Cell types in the [beige] area are confined to the bone marrow, whereas those in the [pink] area circulate.

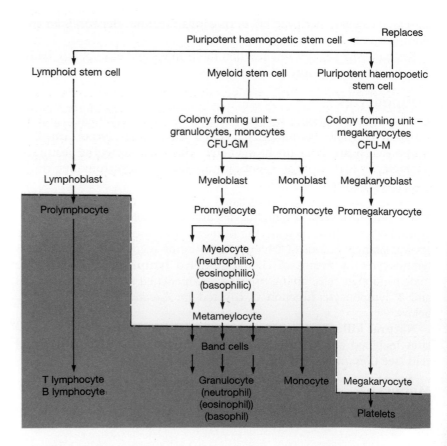

- **tumour necrosis factor**, secreted by macrophages and lymphocytes, which kills foreign cells;
- **chemotactic factors**, secreted by a variety of cells, which attract cells to or repel them from sites of inflammation.

Production of white blood cells (leucopoiesis)

All white blood cells originate from the same uncommitted stem cells in the bone marrow as red blood cells. Megakaryocytes, which produce platelets, also originate from the same stem cells.

Figure 11.11 summarizes the stages through which the leucocytes pass before maturation.

The uncommitted stem cell (pluripotent haemopoietic stem cell) divides and differentiates into two types of stem cell: **lymphoid** and **myeloid**. Some daughter cells of the uncommitted stem cell do not differentiate and thereby maintain the pool of uncommitted stem cells.

The **lymphoid stem cells** divide and differentiate into **lymphoblasts** and then into **prolymphocytes**. Some prolymphocytes leave the bone marrow and are processed in the thymus gland to become mature, immunocompetent T lymphocytes (Figure 11.12).

It is less clear where maturation into B lymphocytes occurs, except in birds, where it occurs in an organ called the bursa of Fabricius (hence the name B lymphocyte). In humans, who lack such an organ, B-lymphocyte maturation probably occurs principally in the bone marrow itself (the **bursa equivalent**). Each immunocompetent T or B cell has several thousand surface receptors to which one specific antigen can bind. The T and B lymphocytes then populate peripheral lymphoid tissue and, when stimulated by antigen-binding, can transform into lymphoblasts (immunoblasts), which gives rise to large numbers of small and medium lymphocytes.

The **myeloid stem cells** are the precursors of platelets and all leucocytes except lymphocytes. The first cell division and differentiation gives rise to two **colony-forming units**: one for granulocytes and monocytes (CFU-GM) and one for megakaryocytes (CFU-M). Thereafter, division and differentiation produces **myeloblasts**, **monoblasts** and **megakaryoblasts**, followed by **promyelocytes**, **promonocytes** and **promegakaryocytes**.

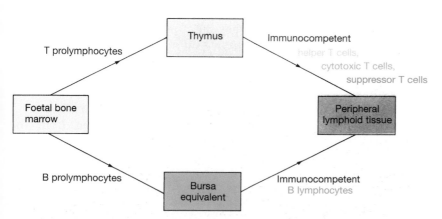

Figure 11.12 Origin of T and B lymphocytes.

Granulocytes develop along three separate lines after the promyelocyte stage, firstly into neutrophilic, eosinophilic and basophilic **myelocytes**, when their distinctive granules appear. Cell division stops at this stage, and the cells mature into **metamyelocytes** and then **band cells**, during which process the nuclei curve and then become lobed. The mature granulocytes are stored in the bone marrow forming a pool which is rapidly mobilized into the blood by infection, tissue damage and other immune responses.

Promonocytes divide and develop into **monocytes**, a small pool of which remain in the bone marrow. Monocytes enter the circulation before populating the tissues as macrophages.

The cytoplasm of **megakaryocytes** becomes subdivided by membranes prior to the formation of cellular fragments, the platelets, which are released into the blood.

CONTROL OF LEUCOPOIESIS

Leucopoiesis is controlled by several polypeptide cytokines, called **colony-stimulating factors** (CSFs). The principal sources of these are macrophages and T lymphocytes. One cytokine, multi-CSF (interleukin-3), enhances the production (and activity of the mature cells) of neutrophils, monocytes and megakaryocytes; granulocyte-monocyte-CSF stimulates the production of both neutrophils and monocytes; whereas monocyte-CSF and granulocyte-CSF only stimulate the production of a single cell type.

The synthesis and secretion of CSFs are stimulated by a variety of chemicals activated during the immune responses mediated by leucocytes. Since many leucocytes die in the tissues as a result of combating infection, the stimulation of leucopoiesis ensures replacement stocks in the bone marrow.

Life span of leucocytes

The bone marrow and lymphoid tissue contain a large pool of leucocytes, which spend a relatively short time in the blood when they are 'mobilized' prior to combating infection or tissue damage. Some estimates suggest that there are 10 times more granulocytes in the marrow than there are in the circulation.

Granulocytes typically spend a few hours in the circulation and a few days in the tissues, where they die. During infection, their time in the blood and the tissues may be much shorter than this.

Monocytes may also spend less than 1 day and no more than 3 days in the blood, but once in the tissues they enlarge and transform into **macrophages**. Their phagocytic activity and survival time in the tissues is greater than granulocytes; they can last for months or years.

Lymphocytes are added continuously to the blood from the lymphatic circulation. They usually spend only a few hours in the blood before entering the tissues (including lymphoid tissue), from where they are drained in the lymph. The life-span of lymphocytes may be days or years.

Decreased leucocyte count (leucopenia)

Gamma-rays, benzene or drugs, including thiouracil, chloramphenicol or barbiturates, can damage the bone marrow, with the result that its production of leucocytes (and sometimes erythrocytes) ceases.

In view of the major role that the leucocytes play in the defence mechanisms of the body, a cessation of their production leads to death within a few days if treatment is not given. In the short term, the areas of the body in contact with the external environment will be unable to combat invasion by microorganisms. These areas include the respiratory and alimentary tracts, eyes, urethra and vagina. They may become ulcerated within 2 days, with subsequent spread of bacteria into the underlying tissues.

Increased numbers of abnormal leucocytes (leukaemia)

There are various types of leukaemia, conditions in which there is uncontrolled growth of cancerous cells in the myeloid or the lymphoid series. The abnormal leucocytes do not function effectively, with the result that infections are common.

Myelogenous leukaemia begins in the bone marrow, but spreads to other areas which then also produce bizarre, usually undifferentiated leucocytes. The production of red blood cells and platelets is usually reduced, causing anaemia and a tendency to excessive bleeding. The bone marrow can enlarge and erode and weaken the bone, causing pain.

Lymphogenous leukaemias begin in lymphoid tissue and, like the myelogenous leukaemias, then spread to other areas where they destroy the tissue and use excessive amounts of nutrients. This leads to weakness and depletion of tissue.

LYMPHOID TISSUE

Individual lymphocytes circulate in the blood and lymph and populate connective and epithelial tissues. Lymphoid tissue, on the other hand, contains lymphocytes that are packed tightly together, often supported by a network of reticular fibres. Such tissue is found in lymph nodes, nodules in the intestine (see Figure 15.46), the spleen, the thymus and the tonsils. The term **peripheral lymphoid tissue** refers to all such tissue except that in the thymus and bone marrow.

Lymph nodes

Lymph nodes are found along the path of the lymphatic vessels and are particularly abundant in the groin, axilla and neck, as well as along the large blood vessels in the thorax and abdomen (Figure 11.13).

They act as filters, removing cellular debris and microorganisms from the lymph. Antigens within macrophages stimulate immune responses, including the formation of more lymphocytes.

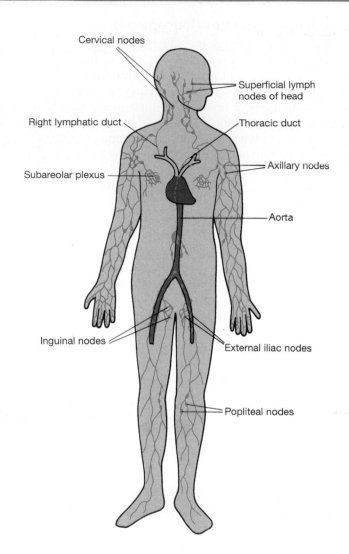

Figure 11.13 Distribution of the major groups of lymph nodes.

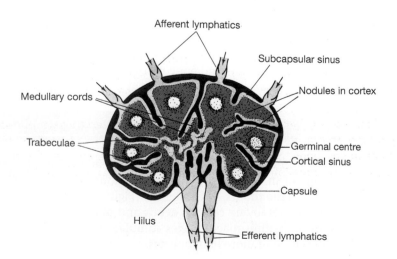

Figure 11.14 Section through a lymph node.

Lymph nodes are small, bean-shaped structures of variable size, (0.1–2.5 cm long), with a small indentation (**hilus**) on the concave surface. Each node consists of a collagenous capsule which is continuous with partitions (**trabeculae**) lying within the node (Figure 11.14).

A fine network of reticular fibres supports large numbers of lymphocytes, plasma cells and macrophages, which fill much of the node. Lymph nodes are divided into a superficial cortex and inner medulla.

Lymph enters the node through several **afferent lymphatic vessels** on the convex surface and flows into the subcapsular sinus, through the cortical sinuses which lie peripheral to the follicles, and also percolates between the lymphocytes. The lymph drains from the medulla into the **efferent lymphatic vessels**.

Small arteries and veins pass through the hilus into the lymph node. There are extensive capillary networks in the cortex of the node.

The outer cortex contains spherical nodules of tightly packed lymphocytes. Some nodules have a paler-staining **germinal centre**, the site of production of new B lymphocytes and the plasma cells they give rise to. The plasma cells produce antibodies, which then leave the lymph node in the lymph. T lymphocytes populate the remaining lymphoid tissue, which extends to the central region as medullary cords. Macrophages are particularly abundant in the reticular tissue in the medulla, as well as in the germinal centres.

Lymphocytes (mainly T) are carried to the node in arterial blood and enter the substance of the node in postcapillary venules and via the afferent lymphatic vessels. They leave the lymph node in the efferent lymphatics and are returned to the blood by way of the thoracic and right lymphatic ducts (Figure 11.13).

Reactive lymph nodes (swollen glands)

Should an area of the body become infected, some antigenic material (free or within phagocytes) will be delivered to lymph nodes nearby via the lymph draining the area. The antigens stimulate the inflammatory response and the nodes become painful.

Some antigens stimulate the production of B lymphocytes and plasma cells (see *Humoral immunity*, below). Antibody-producing, large lymphocytes emerge in the efferent lymph after about 5 days. These cells populate successive lymph nodes in the lymphatic pathway, where they differentiate into plasma cells, the main antibody-producing cells.

Other antigens stimulate cell-mediated responses (see *Cell-mediated immunity*, below), in which case the T lymphocytes, particularly in the deep cortex of the lymph nodes, proliferate.

Swollen, painful lymph nodes are therefore found in the path of the lymphatic drainage of the area and can be a guide to the location of infection in the body. Swollen but pain-free lymph nodes can be the result of cancer spreading via the lymphatic circulation and infiltrating the nodes.

See also **Structure and distribution of lymphatic vessels** (page 401) and **Formation and flow of lymph** (page 415), in Ch. 12, Circulation of Blood and Lymph.

Tonsils

There are openings on the surface of the tonsils, located near the entrance to the pharynx (see Figure 13.2) through which microorganisms can gain entrance to the lymphoid tissue within. The subsequent inflammation and proliferation of lymphocytes can cause very painful swollen tonsils, but also provides a means of stimulating the production of memory cells (see *Acquired (specific) immunity*, below), thereby strengthening the body's resistance to future infective agents.

Spleen

The spleen is the largest lymphatic organ in the body, weighing about 150 g, measuring about 12 cm long, 7 cm broad and 4 cm deep. It is roughly oval in outline, with a domed upper and flattened lower surface. It is located in the left side of the abdominal cavity, occupying the space between the fundus of the stomach and the diaphragm (Figure 11.15). It has a soft consistency and is very vascular.

Figure 11.15 Locations of the spleen and thymus.

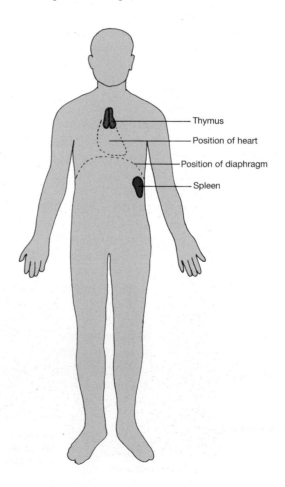

Thymus

Position of heart

Position of diaphragm

Spleen

The principal functions of the spleen are:
- production of blood cells;
- destruction of erythrocytes and platelets;
- removal of bacteria from the blood.

Although all these functions are vitally important, they are also carried out by other organs. The spleen is relatively easily ruptured if subjected to a blow, and it is then usually surgically removed. Following the period of recovery after splenectomy, there may be an increased susceptibility to infection, especially in children, but no other particular deleterious effects.

The human spleen, unlike its counterpart in many animals, has little ability to store blood. Generally the blood vessels can increase in diameter to accommodate an increased volume of blood and muscular constriction will result in its expulsion. However, since the capsule contains little muscle, large-scale storage and expulsion is not possible.

The spleen is covered by a fibroelastic capsule, which is itself largely covered by peritoneum. Projecting into the spleen from the capsule are **trabeculae**, which provide a supporting framework for internal structures.

The splenic artery splits into five or more branches just before entering the inferior surface of the spleen. These smaller vessels further divide and travel within the trabeculae as **trabecular arteries** (Figure

Figure 11.16   Fine structure of the spleen showing the islands of lymphoid tissue (white pulp) in the red pulp comprising venous sinusoids, pulp veins and splenic cords containing blood cells.

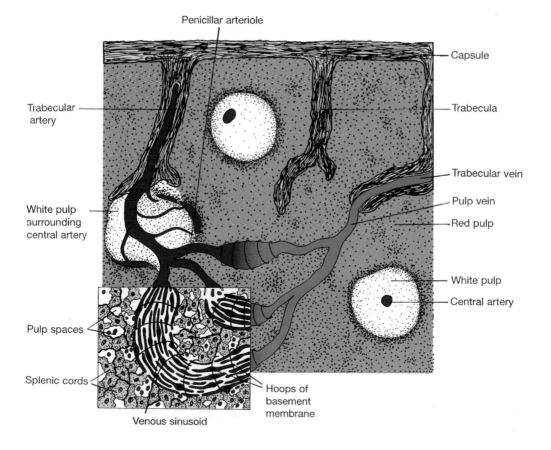

11.16). Within the spleen, the trabecular arteries lead into arteries, which become invested with lymphoid tissue like the nodules in lymph nodes, known as **white pulp**. In section the artery appears to be buried in the middle of a mass of lymphoid tissue and is referred to as the **central artery**.

The tissue between the islands of white pulp is known as **red pulp** because of the large number of red blood cells in the spaces between venous sinusoids. The spaces are occupied by **splenic** or pulp **cords**, which comprise reticular fibres and reticular cells together with blood cells.

The central artery in the white pulp branches into several thin penicillar arterioles which supply capillaries and venous sinusoids in the red pulp. The sinusoids are lined by mildly phagocytic, fusiform endothelial cells surrounded by basement membrane, arranged in bands; the whole structure resembles an elongated barrel. The clefts between the endothelial cells allow blood cells to leave or re-enter the circulation.

The venous sinusoids drain into pulp veins, which converge on to trabecular veins and then on to branches of the splenic vein.

Whether blood flows from the penicillar arteries into capillaries and out into the splenic cords before flowing back into the venous sinusoids (open circulation hypothesis), or directly from capillaries to venous sinusoids (closed circulation hypothesis) is not known.

In the foetus, blood cells are produced within the spleen, but this ceases at birth. In children and adults the spleen is one of several sites of lymphocyte production.

T lymphocytes in the white pulp, following appropriate antigenic stimulation, proliferate and migrate into the spaces in the red pulp before passing into the blood in the sinusoids.

B lymphocytes are found in the germinal centres of the white pulp and, in the presence of particular antigens, transform into antibody-producing plasma cells.

> See also **Bilirubin** (page 569), in Ch. 15, Digestion and Absorption of Food.

The macrophages in the cords of the red pulp and the marginal zones of the white pulp engulf fragments of old, abnormal or broken erythrocytes. Haemoglobin is broken down and the resultant bilirubin is taken up by the cells of the liver before being discharged in the bile. The iron and amino acids are recycled during the synthesis of new erythrocytes.

In addition to their role in the removal of erythrocytes, macrophages also remove aged platelets and are very active in removing bacteria from the blood that passes through the red pulp.

Thymus

In proportion to total body weight, the thymus is largest at birth. Its actual weight steadily increases to a maximum of about 40 g at puberty and then it gradually shrinks and may weigh as little as 10 g in old age. Clearly then, the main activities of the thymus occur early in life, during which time it processes immature lymphocytes into T lymphocytes (Figure 11.12), which then populate lymphoid tissue elsewhere.

The thymus is located in the upper thorax, anterior to the great vessels where they emerge from the heart (Figure 11.15). It consists of two unequal pyramidal lobes, their precise shape being determined by the surrounding organs.

Each lobe is covered by a delicate fibrous capsule from which project short septa that penetrate the substance of the organ and divide it into lobules, each of which has a dark-staining cortex and a much lighter medulla. The medullae of adjacent lobules are linked by cords of medullary tissue.

Histologically, the organ is made up of an irregular framework of epithelial cells supporting lymphocytes and other cells (Figure 11.17).

This contrasts with the framework of reticular fibres found in other lymphoid tissues. In the cortex, the cells are tightly packed together and consist principally of large lymphoblasts, which are continuously producing new lymphocytes. About 90% of the lymphocytes die within the organ, only lasting about 3–5 days; the remaining 10% enter the circulation. Macrophages in the cortex remove the dead cells.

The medulla contains fewer, less closely packed lymphoblasts and young lymphocytes. In addition, scattered throughout the medulla are the mysterious **Hassall's corpuscles** composed of concentric layers of

Figure 11.17 Fine structure of the thymus, showing the lobules containing a dark-staining cortex and paler medulla. T-lymphocytes are produced in the cortex. The medulla contains Hassall's corpuscles, which are concentric layers of epithelial cells. Their function is unknown.

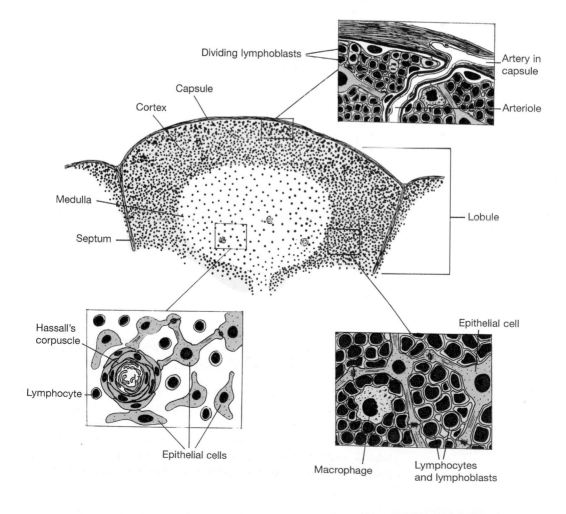

Dividing lymphoblasts

Capsule

Cortex

Artery in capsule

Arteriole

Medulla

Septum

Lobule

Hassall's corpuscle

Lymphocyte

Epithelial cells

Epithelial cell

Macrophage

Lymphocytes and lymphoblasts

epithelial cells. The innermost cells usually become anucleate and resemble the surface cells of the epidermis.

The **blood supply** of the thymus is derived from branches of the internal thoracic arteries. Arteries lie within the septa, giving rise to arterioles that enter the lobules. Like lymph nodes, the thymus contains postcapillary venules, which lie mainly in the corticomedullary border, from where they drain into interlobular veins in the septa and from there to a single thymic vein which drains into the left brachiocephalic vein.

The epithelial cells in the thymus produce a number of peptides or 'thymic hormones', the functions of which are poorly understood. They are **thymopoietin, thymic humoral factor** and **thymosin**. Their actions are probably confined to promoting the differentiation and proliferation of T lymphocytes in the thymus, so that the term 'hormone', though commonly used, is rather misleading.

Maturation of T lymphocytes in the thymus

The thymus produces immunologically competent T lymphocytes, which then populate peripheral lymphoid tissue. The prolymphocytes released from the bone marrow are attracted chemotactically to the thymic cortex as a result of the secretion of **thymotaxin** by subcapsular epithelial cells. The maturation of the cells is controlled by cytokines secreted by macrophages and epithelial cells within the thymus (see *Cytokines*, above).

The immature T cells divide and differentiate into different subpopulations of T lymphocytes: **helper T cells, cytotoxic T cells** and **suppressor T cells**, with different surface proteins: 1) major histocompatibility (MHC) proteins and 2) receptors. During this process, the maturing T lymphocytes migrate into the medulla, towards the centre of the gland.

All cell membranes (except red blood cells) of an individual have the same proteins, unique to each person, known as **major histocompatibility (MHC) proteins**, class I. During thymic processing, cytotoxic and suppressor T cells acquire class I MHC proteins on their surface and helper T cells acquire class II MHC proteins.

Each T cell also acquires surface receptors that can bind to a fragment of a foreign antigen (**epitope**) complexed with MHC protein. Only T cells with receptors that recognize and react to self-MHC complexed with foreign epitopes survive. Those reacting to self-epitopes die in large numbers in the thymus. By this means, T cells are selected that combine with foreign antigens presented by the body's own cells.

Immunocompetent T lymphocytes pass out of the postcapillary venules in the thymus and are deposited in peripheral lymphoid tissue, principally the spleen, lymph nodes and tonsils, where they give rise to colonies of mature cells. T-cell activation and specific immunological roles in sites outside the thymus are described in *Cell-mediated immunity*, below.

Absence of the thymus from the neonate leads to a failure of normal development of the spleen and lymph nodes, a great reduction in the number of circulating T lymphocytes and severe immunodeficiency.

IMMUNITY

The term 'immunity' refers to the mechanisms by which the body is able to resist or defend itself against the potential damage caused by toxins and microorganisms. It is usual to subdivide these mechanisms into 1) **innate (non-specific) immunity** and 2) **acquired (specific) immunity**. Innate immune mechanisms are rapid responses to any foreign substance, whereas acquired immune responses vary according to the nature of the specific 'foreign' substance involved.

Innate (non-specific) immunity

Surface barriers

The skin and those internal surfaces that have a direct link with the exterior form barriers which prevent the entry of foreign organisms and chemicals.

The protein keratin present in the epidermis of the skin offers a physical barrier to microorganisms and chemicals. The mucous membranes lining the respiratory, alimentary, urinary and reproductive tracts also offer a physical barrier and the mucus that covers them traps potential invaders. In addition, the respiratory tract lining is ciliated so that the mucus is moved out of the body, a process reinforced by coughing and sneezing.

A number of body fluids have antimicrobial properties by virtue of their acidity, including sweat, sebum and gastric juice. The enzyme lysozyme (which breaks down bacterial walls) is found in lacrimal fluid, nasal secretions and saliva.

The presence of microbial flora on the skin and internal linings of the body inhibits the growth of more harmful microorganisms.

Cells involved in innate immunity

Should foreign substances or toxins gain entry through breaks in the surface barriers, some leucocytes are able to mount a rapid defensive attack on them. These cells are: 1) phagocytes and 2) natural killer (NK) cells.

The principal **phagocytic cells** are the neutrophils and macrophages. The foreign material is taken into the cell, forming a small vacuole or phagosome, which then fuses with a lysosome (see Figure 2.14). The lysosomal enzymes digest and destroy the foreign material. Neutrophils also produce defensins which spear the prey (see *Neutrophils*, above) and secrete oxidizing chemicals into the surrounding interstitial fluid. Such chemicals also kill the neutrophils themselves. Macrophages, on the other hand, are not killed following phagocytosis. The process of **opsonization**, in which the foreign material is coated with opsonins such as antibodies and a component of complement, facilitates the process of phagocytosis (Figure 11.18).

NK cells attack **cancer cells** and **virus-infected cells**. Their action

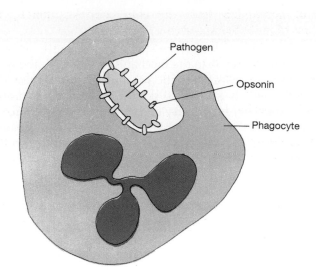

Figure 11.18 Opsonins enhance phagocytosis by coating the pathogen and facilitating its uptake by the phagocyte. Major opsonins are antibodies and a component of complement.

contrasts with that of the T lymphocytes, which require an initial exposure to specific antigens prior to mounting an effective response on subsequent exposures.

Inflammation

Inflammation comprises the responses to tissue injury described by Aulus Celsus in the 1st century as:

- rubor (redness);
- calor (heat);
- tumor (swelling);
- dolor (pain).

See also **Oedema** (page 411), in Ch. 12, Circulation of Blood and Lymph.

The redness and heat are caused by local vasodilation, which increases blood flow to the area. The swelling (oedema) is caused by a rise in capillary hydrostatic pressure due to the vasodilation, together with an increase in capillary permeability, which causes an increased filtration of protein-rich fluid from the blood into the interstitial fluid.

The pain is caused by stimulation of nociceptors by:

- the pressure of fluid;
- chemical stimulation by bacterial toxins and chemicals leaking from damaged cells
- chemicals released during the inflammatory response, such as histamine and bradykinin, potentiated by prostaglandins.

For pain stimuli see **Nociceptors** (page 214), in Ch. 7, Sensory Processing.

The extra fluid in the tissues can dilute harmful chemicals as well as bringing with it nutrients and oxygen and proteins. Some of the proteins are involved in the immune responses, others cause clotting (the deposition of fibrin threads), which isolates the area and consequently reduces the spread of infection from it.

LEUCOCYTE MIGRATION

Injured cells release leucocytosis-inducing factors, which stimulate the release of neutrophils from the bone marrow, thereby raising the neutrophil count in blood within a few hours.

The increased blood flow delivers phagocytes to the damaged area at an increased rate. The increased filtration of fluid out of the blood slows the blood flow and neutrophils begin to stick to the sides of the capillaries (margination or pavementing) within 1 minute of tissue damage. Margination is aided by several inflammatory chemicals. The increased capillary permeability facilitates neutrophil migration from the blood, which they do by squeezing between the endothelial cells (diapedesis). The phagocytes move by positive chemotaxis towards chemicals such as the breakdown products of damaged tissue, kinins and components of complement.

The macrophages already present in the tissues multiply and become mobile and they are joined by additional cells that migrate from the blood (as monocytes) an hour or so after the neutrophils. The transformation of monocytes into the powerfully phagocytic macrophages in the tissues takes 8–12 h.

The neutrophils, then, are the first phagocytes to be mobilized and they engulf infectious or damaged tissue. In many cases they are short-lived in the tissues. If vast numbers of them are involved they contribute to the formation of **pus** (dead neutrophils, pathogens, broken down tissue). The more powerful macrophages arrive later; they are capable of phagocytosing the neutrophils as well as the microorganisms, particularly those that can live within cells.

Eosinophils are also phagocytic and they are mobilized particularly in parasitic infections, as well as in allergic reactions.

HISTAMINE

Histamine is found in the basophils of the blood and the mast cells in the tissue, as well as in platelets. The mast cells are probably the major source of histamine, which is released by mechanical disruption of the cells (along with tissue damage generally) as well as by chemicals released from neutrophils and by complement (Figure 11.19).

Histamine is a vasodilator and thereby increases blood flow. It also loosens the junctions between the endothelial cells of capillaries, thereby facilitating the exudation of protein and cells from the blood into the surrounding tissue. Histamine released into interstitial fluid causes itching.

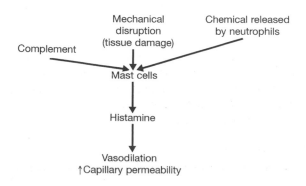

Figure 11.19 Actions and release of histamine in inflammation.

KININS

The kinins (e.g. bradykinin) are polypeptides that are normally present in an inactive form as the plasma protein **kininogen**. They are split off from kininogen under the action of the activated enzyme **kallikrein**, which is present in plasma and in interstitial fluid. Kallikrein, in turn, is activated by chemicals released during the inflammatory process. When capillary permeability is increased, the plasma kininogen leaks out and becomes activated in the tissues. Both kallikrein and bradykinin are rapidly inactivated by enzymes, and therefore do not persist very long in the tissues.

The kinins cause chemotaxis and pain as well as enhancing vasodilation and increasing capillary permeability.

COMPLEMENT

The complement system consists of plasma proteins named C1–C9, factors B, D and P and several regulatory proteins. C1–C9 are normally present in an inactive form and activation may be initiated by an antigen–antibody complex (classical pathway) or by an alternative pathway, where the initiation process involves only non-specific immune mechanisms (Figure 11.20).

The alternative pathway is initiated by plasma proteins (factors B, D and P) interacting with polysaccharides in the wall of some (not all)

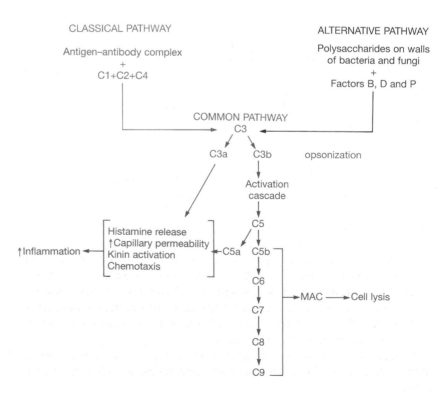

Figure 11.20 Activation and actions of complement. **Classical pathway** (specific immunity): complement is activated by the interaction between an antigen-antibody complex and complement proteins C1, C2 and C4 (complement fixation). **Alternative pathway** (non-specific immunity): complement is activated by the interaction between plasma proteins (Factors B, D and P) with polysaccharides on the cell wall of some bacteria and fungi. **Common pathway:** C3 is cleaved into C3a and C3b. C3b binds to the target cell membrane and activates the remaining complement proteins as well as enhancing phagocytosis (opsonization). C5–C9 form the membrane attack complex, (MAC) causing lysis of the target cell. C3a and other complement proteins enhance histamine release, increase capillary permeability, activate kinins and promote chemotaxis.

bacteria and fungi. This interaction activates C3 by splitting it into C3a and C3b. C3b binds to the target cell membrane and the remaining complement proteins are activated in sequence, like the activation of clotting factors.

Collectively the complement proteins amplify inflammation, phagocytosis and cell lysis. C3b enhances phagocytosis by binding to the target cell and to the phagocyte (opsonization), thereby bringing the two together (Figure 11.18). C5b–C9 form the **membrane attack complex**, a hole in the target cell's membrane through which its contents leak out, causing lysis of the target cell. C3a and C5a enhance histamine release, increase capillary permeability, activate kinins and promote chemotaxis.

INTERFERONS

Viral invasion of the body causes the production of a protein, interferon, particularly by lymphocytes. This cytokine can migrate and bind to the cell membrane of other host cells, where it stimulates the synthesis of antiviral proteins. There are several different forms of interferon, including gamma-interferon (γ-interferon), produced by lymphocytes, which also activates macrophages and mobilizes natural killer cells. Interferon has been used clinically to treat hepatitis C (sexually transmitted) and Kaposi's sarcoma, a cancer contracted by some AIDS patients.

PROSTAGLANDINS

Prostaglandins are derivatives of arachidonic acid, a fatty acid found in the phospholipids of cell membranes. They amplify the inflammatory response, principally by sensitizing the blood vessels of the microcirculation to the effects of other mediators of inflammation such as histamine and the kinins. They also increase pain by potentiating the actions of histamine, kinins and serotonin.

Non-steroidal anti-inflammatory drugs (**NSAIDs**), including aspirin, exert their effects by inhibiting the synthesis of prostaglandins.

> Prostaglandins are also discussed with regard to: hyperalgesia (page 223) in Ch. 7 Sensory Processing; vasodilation (page 408) in Ch. 12 Circulation of Blood and Lymph; semen (page 666) and parturition (page 675) in Ch. 17 Sex and Reproduction.

TRIPLE RESPONSE

If the skin is stroked firmly with a sharp instrument, a type of inflammatory response known as the triple response is elicited. The response comprises a thin red line, a red flare (1–2 cm wide) and a weal.

The red line appears within 3–15 s and is due to vasodilation caused by direct mechanical stimulation of the arterioles.

The red flare appears between 15 and 30 s and is caused by the axon reflex. Stroking the skin stimulates sensory nerve endings (dendrites) that generate action potentials. The impulses, in addition to being propagated towards the CNS, are also propagated at the branch points back into the skin. The dendrites release a histamine-like substance, which causes vasodilation of arterioles in the area.

The weal develops in 3–5 minutes along the red line. It is a line of oedema caused by increased capillary permeability following tissue trauma.

Acquired (specific) immunity

Specific immune responses can be regarded as the body's third line of defence against potentially harmful substances or organisms; the first being the surface barriers and the second the non-specific responses of inflammation and phagocytosis. As the name 'acquired immunity' suggests, specific immune responses do not offer immediate protection, rather, a first exposure initiates mechanisms by which the body acquires protection to subsequent exposures.

In specific defence mechanisms, the body reacts to 'foreign' antigens (usually proteins) in one of two ways: 1) **humoral immunity**, which is mediated by circulating antibodies; and 2) **cell-mediated immunity**, which is mediated by circulating cells.

Figure 11.21 Humoral immunity: **primary response**. Free bacteria bind to antibodies on the surface of B lymphocytes in lymphoid tissue (or a macrophage may 'present' the bacterium to the B lymphocyte), which transform into a dividing cell, the immunoblast. The daughter cells differentiate into plasma cells and memory B cells, which can 'recognize' the antigen on subsequent exposure. The plasma cells synthesize antibodies, which then circulate to the infected site and bind to antigen. The antigen–antibody complex can directly neutralize free antigen, but the major actions are enhancing the actions of other immune responses: phagocytosis, natural killer cell activity and complement. B lymphocyte transformation is also stimulated by several interleukins secreted by activated helper T cells. These are activated by interleukin I secreted by macrophages, which present the antigen to the helper T cells.

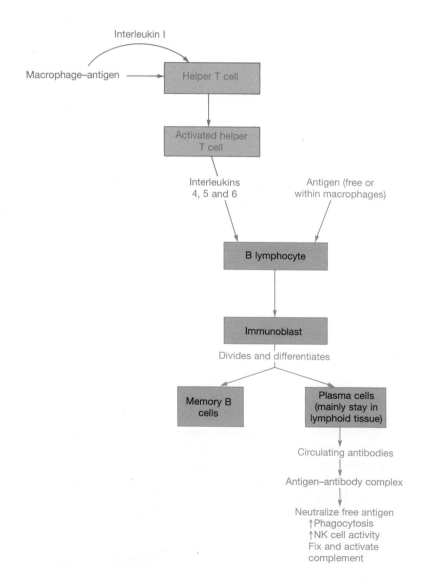

Humoral immunity

Humoral immunity involves the production of circulating antibodies by plasma cells, which are themselves derived from B lymphocytes. It is the method by which bacteria, viruses and toxins in extracellular fluids are counteracted.

Following their phagocytosis in the tissues, bacteria are carried by macrophages in the lymph to the lymph nodes; some bacteria are also carried free in the lymph. Free bacteria bind to antibodies on the surface of B cells, or alternatively the macrophage may 'present' the bacterium to the B cell which then transforms into an **immunoblast**, a dividing cell. The daughter cells differentiate into **plasma cells** and **memory B cells**. (Figure 11.21).

Memory B cells can last for weeks, months or years and they 'recognize' the antigen on subsequent exposure. The plasma cells synthesize **antibodies** for about 4–5 days and then they die. The antibodies circulate to the infected site.

Only a few of the B cells in the lymph node are capable of responding to a given antigen. They are a clone of cells, genetically programmed to synthesize a particular antibody and no other.

B cell activation is enhanced by a type of T lymphocyte called helper T cells. In the lymphoid tissue, the macrophage processes and then 'presents' a fragment of the antigen (epitope) on the bacterial surface to a helper T cell. The macrophage also secretes interleukin 1, a cytokine which activates the helper T cell. The helper T cell then enlarges, secretes another cytokine, interleukin 2, and divides, producing a clone of activated helper T cells. These secrete several interleukins, including interleukin 2, 4, 5 and 6. Interleukins 4, 5 and 6 stimulate the B cells to divide and differentiate into immunoblasts, then plasma cells and memory B cells.

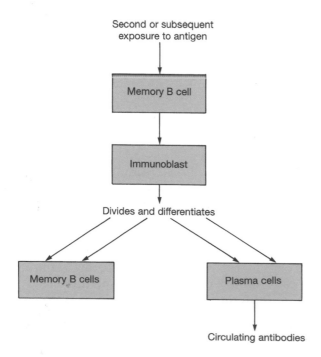

Figure 11.22 Humoral immunity: **secondary response**. On a subsequent exposure to the same antigen, the memory B cells transform into immunoblasts which repeatedly divide and differentiate into plasma cells and memory B cells. This results in the production of a greater number of antibodies by more plasma cells in a shorter time than in the first exposure.

On a subsequent exposure to the same antigen, the memory cells transform into immunoblasts, which repeatedly divide and differentiate into plasma cells and memory B cells (Figure 11.22). This results in the production of a greater number of antibodies by more plasma cells in a shorter time than in the first exposure. This principle is exploited in **vaccination**, where the body is exposed to the antigen in the vaccine in a dead or attenuated form. Should the microorganism invade the body at a later date, memory cells will respond to combat the infection more effectively. The first exposure results in the smaller, slower primary response, taking about a week before the first antibodies appear (Figure 11.23). Antibodies continue to be produced for several months. Subsequent exposures result in the larger secondary response, taking only 2 days for high levels of antibodies to appear in the blood.

Figure 11.23 Primary and secondary (humoral) immune responses. The first exposure to antigen results in a rise in the concentration of antibodies in the blood after about a week (latent period). Antibodies continue to be produced for several months. Subsequent exposures result in the larger secondary response, taking only about two days for high levels of antibodies to appear in the blood. Antibodies are produced for a longer period in secondary responses than primary ones.

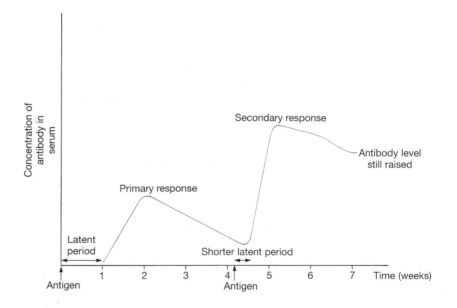

ANTIBODIES

Antibodies are proteins which are capable of combining with a specific antigen. They constitute the gamma-globulin fraction of plasma proteins. They have two longer heavy chains and two shorter lighter chains, joined together by disulphide links (Figure 11.24).

Part of the antibody molecule has a different amino acid sequence from any other antibody (variable portion) and it is this region which combines with a specific antigen in a 'lock and key' type of mechanism. As each antibody has two variable regions, each antibody can combine with two antigens. Each Y-shaped molecule is called an **antibody monomer**. Some antibodies are linked together by a structure known as a J chain, in pairs (**dimer**) or groups of five (**pentamer**).

Antibodies or **immunoglobulins (Ig)** are subdivided into five classes according to their molecular weights: IgG, IgA, IgM, IgD and IgE.

IgG are the most abundant antibodies in the plasma. They are

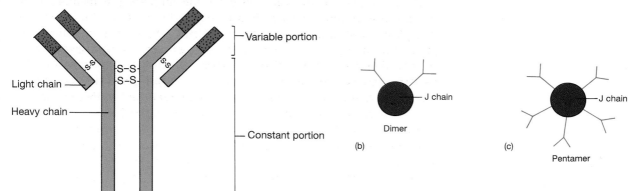

Figure 11.24 Antibody structure. **(a)** Each antibody (immunoglobulin) has four polypeptide chains: two longer heavy chains and two shorter lighter chains, joined together by disulphide (–S–S–) links. The variable portion of each chain combines with a specific antigen. Each antibody can combine with two antigens. Each of these Y-shaped structures is known as an antibody monomer. **(b)** The monomers of IgA antibodies are linked together in pairs by a J chain to form a dimer. **(c)** IgM antibodies circulate as pentamers – five monomers linked by a J chain.

monomers and the only antibodies that are capable of diffusing across the placenta and conferring immunity on the neonate for the first few months of life. IgG antibodies are present in colostrum and are subsequently absorbed from the baby's intestine. IgG can also diffuse into interstitial fluid. These antibodies are mainly concerned with combating bacterial infection, during which they fix and activate complement and enhance phagocytosis of microorganisms by acting as opsonins.

IgA antibodies are present as dimers in many secretions, including tears, nasal fluid, saliva and colostrum and breast milk. They are also present in lymphoid tissue lining the respiratory, alimentary and urinary tracts – areas particularly vulnerable to invasion by microorganisms. The antibodies may act by preventing adherence of microorganisms to mucosal cells, thereby preventing penetration.

IgM antibodies, together with IgG, account for the major defence against bacteria and viruses in extracellular fluids. The IgM molecule circulates in blood as a large pentamer and is therefore confined within the blood. IgM antibodies cause agglutination (anti-A and anti-B blood group antibodies are included in this group) and complement fixation. IgM antibodies are the first to be produced. Some surface receptors of B lymphocytes are essentially 'fixed' IgM monomer antibodies.

The **IgD** group of antibodies is only present in small amounts in the blood. IgD monomers are found on B lymphocytes as surface receptors and stimulate lymphocyte activity.

IgE antibodies, like IgD antibodies are monomers, but are found in very small amounts in the blood. They are secreted by plasma cells in the skin and the respiratory and gastrointestinal tracts. They bind to mast cells and basophils and stimulate the secretion of histamine. In some allergic reactions, such as asthma and hay fever, this effect can be very pronounced. IgE antibodies stimulate eosinophils to combat parasitic infections.

Antibodies can combine with bacterial toxins, thereby directly neutralizing them prior to their phagocytosis. They can also combine with some viral surface molecules and prevent them from binding to and subsequently entering the host cells.

Antibodies bind to antigens on the surface of microorganisms and then act by physically linking the microorganism with several other substances that can kill it: macrophages, NK cells or complement.

IgG or IgM antibody, when bound to antigen, activates the classical complement pathway (Figure 11.20). C1 binds to the constant portion of the antibody and is thereby 'fixed' to the target cell. The activated complement molecules enhance phagocytosis and inflammation, and the membrane attack complex kills the foreign cells.

Cell-mediated immunity

Cell-mediated immunity involves T lymphocytes with antibody-like receptor molecules on their surfaces combating primarily the body's own cells that have become infected with viruses, fungi or bacteria, and also transplanted tissue. Cancer cells, which probably arise daily by the alteration of the genes of normal cells, are also attacked by T lymphocytes.

T cells, like B cells, are activated by the binding of antigen to their surfaces in peripheral lymphoid tissue. However, in the case of T cells, the epitope must be complexed with the **major histocompatibility (MHC) proteins** on cell membranes. All an individual's cell membranes (except those of red blood cells) have the same unique proteins, known as major histocompatibility (MHC) proteins. Most cells have MHC class I proteins, but on the surface of macrophages, B lymphocytes, helper T cells and a few other cells MHC class II proteins are found.

For antigen binding, helper T cells require the epitope to be complexed with MHC class II protein, whereas cytotoxic T and suppressor T cells require MHC class I proteins complexed with epitope. This requirement is known as **MHC restriction** and is acquired during T-cell maturation in the thymus.

The antigen-binding of the immunocompetent **cytotoxic T cell** results in its transformation into an **immunoblast** followed by cell division and differentiation into **activated cytotoxic T cells** as well as **memory cytotoxic T cells** (Figure 11.25). The activated cytotoxic cells circulate in the blood and lymph and bind to the antigen–MHC I protein complex displayed on the surface of infected or foreign cells.

The cytotoxic T cell, once bound to the target cell surface, secretes a protein, **perforin**, which inserts into the target cell membrane and causes the formation of pores in it. Solutes and water enter the target cell, causing it to lyse. This action is analogous to that of complement. Cytotoxic T cells also secrete several cytotoxic chemicals into the target cells.

The memory T cells that are also produced as a result of antigenic stimulation cause a much greater and faster response to a second exposure to the antigen.

The avoidance of rejection of donor organs transplanted into a recipient is achieved firstly by matching the blood groups and the MHC proteins as closely as possible (75% or more). In addition to this, recipients are given immunosuppressive therapy with drugs and X rays.

The antigen-binding of the immunocompetent **helper T cell** results

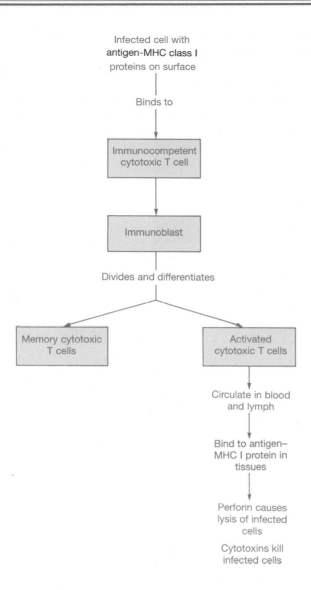

Infected cell with
antigen-MHC class I
proteins on surface

Binds to

Immunocompetent
cytotoxic T cell

Immunoblast

Divides and differentiates

Memory cytotoxic
T cells

Activated
cytotoxic T cells

Circulate in blood
and lymph

Bind to antigen–
MHC I protein in
tissues

Perforin causes
lysis of infected
cells

Cytotoxins kill
infected cells

Figure 11.25 Cell-mediated immunity. Activation of cytotoxic T cells. The antigen is presented complexed to MHC class I protein on the surface of an infected cell. Antigen–antibody binding stimulates the cell to transform into an immunoblast, which divides and differentiates, giving rise to clones of memory cells and activated cytotoxic T cells. These cells can bind to infected cells having the same antigen–MHC I protein on their surfaces. Bound cytotoxic T cells secrete a protein, perforin, which causes lysis of the target cell, and cytotoxins.

in transformation into an immunoblast followed by cell division and differentiation into **activated helper T cells** as well as **memory helper T cells** (Figure 11.26). The activated helper T cells can then bind to the same antigen–MHC II protein complex displayed on the surface of B cells, and secrete interleukin 2 and other cytokines, which stimulates other helper T cells, cytotoxic T cells and B cells.

The mechanism of activation of **suppressor T cells** is not clear, but is probably a combination of free antigen binding and antigen presentation complexed to MHC proteins.

Suppressor T cells are complementary in their actions to helper T cells. They release cytokines that suppress T and B cells, and are responsible for inhibiting the immune responses after antigen has been inactivated or destroyed.

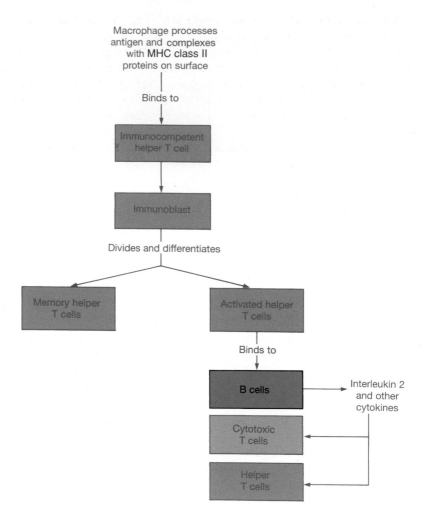

Figure 11.26 Cell-mediated immunity. Activation of helper T cells. The antigen is presented complexed to MHC class II protein on the surface of a macrophage. Antigen–antibody binding stimulates the cell to transform into a dividing cell, the immunoblast giving rise to clones of memory cells and activated helper T cells. These cells bind to the same antigen–MHC II protein on the surface of B cells and secrete the cytokine interleukin 2 which stimulates other helper T cells, cytotoxic T cells and B cells.

Immunodeficiency

Immunodeficiency may be congenital or acquired.

Two congenital conditions are congenital thymic aplasia, in which the thymus fails to develop, and severe combined immunodeficiency disease, in which there is a deficit of both B and T lymphocytes. Children with these conditions have little or no protection against disease combated by either humoral or cell-mediated immunity.

Acquired immunodeficiency conditions include Hodgkin's disease (cancer of the lymph nodes) and acquired immune deficiency syndrome (AIDS).

Acquired immune deficiency syndrome (AIDS)

AIDS is thought to have first arisen in the late 1970s in the heterosexual population of Africa. The symptoms have two forms: 1) **AIDS related complex** (**ARC**); and 2) **full-blown AIDS**.

ARC symptoms include severe weight loss, fever, lethargy and swollen lymph nodes, symptoms typical of infections in general.

Full-blown AIDS shows the symptoms of ARC, together with opportunistic infections such as **Pneumocystis pneumonia**, caused by a fungus, and **Kaposi's sarcoma**, a cancer-like condition that affects blood vessels and causes purple lesions of the skin. AIDS ends in death due to cancer or infection between a few months and 8 years after it starts.

AIDS is caused by the **human immunodeficiency virus** (**HIV**), commonly transmitted (from blood or semen) via:

- blood transfusions;
- blood-contaminated needles;
- sexual contact, particularly when the mucosa is torn and bleeds;
- across the placenta to the baby during delivery or via breast milk.

There is no evidence that AIDS is transmitted through intact skin, food, saliva, sweat, tears, faeces, urine or vomit.

HIV is a retrovirus which has RNA rather than DNA as its primary genetic material. It attacks helper T cells. Once the virus is inside a host cell, a viral enzyme transcribes the viral RNA into DNA, which is then integrated into the host cell's chromosomes. The drug **zidovudine** (formerly called azidothymidine, AZT) blocks the action of this enzyme. Replication of the virus inside the cell causes the cell's death. The destruction of helper T cells results in a deficit of antibodies, together with cytotoxic T cells that do not respond to viral antigen.

From infection by HIV to the development of AIDS commonly takes about 10 years. During the first 5 years the virus multiplies, the person stays asymptomatic and helper T cell count stays normal (1000 cells/mm^3 blood). After that the count drops to about half and symptoms of ARC begin.

Autoimmunity

If the immune system loses its ability to distinguish self from non-self, autoantibodies appear in the blood and T cells are processed that are capable of attacking host tissues. This can occur after the destruction of some of the body's tissues, releasing antigens, some of which combine with other proteins (e.g. bacterial or viral) to form new 'foreign' antigens.

There are various reasons why autoimmunity occurs:

- The structure of a host antigen is changed.
- Antigens normally hidden from immune scrutiny are released into the circulation.
- Antibodies mounted against a foreign antigen may also react with a host antigen.
- There may be failure of negative clonal selection in the thymus of T lymphocytes recognizing self.
- There may be a deficiency of suppressor cells.

There are several sites in the body where potential antigens are isolated from immune surveillance, e.g. sperm cells, lens and cornea of the eye, and thyroid follicles. Should these tissues become damaged and/or inflamed, and the antigens are released into the blood, then they are recognized as non-self by the immune cells.

Table 11.8 gives some examples of sites subjected to an autoimmune attack and the names of the diseases associated with them.

Table 11.8 Examples of autoimmune diseases and the sites of tissue damage

Disease	Site of autoantigen/tissue damage
Autoimmune thrombocytopenia	Platelets
Glomerulonephritis	Basement membrane of glomerulus
Juvenile diabetes	Islets of Langerhans
Lupus erythematosus	Many different body tissues
Multiple sclerosis	Myelin sheaths of neurones
Myasthenia gravis	Acetylcholine receptors in skeletal muscle
Rheumatic fever	Joints, heart
Rheumatoid arthritis	Joints

Allergy (hypersensitivity)

In allergic or hypersensitive immune responses, the environmental antigen is relatively harmless but the immune response is inappropriately large and results in inflammation and damage to the tissues. Antigens that cause allergy are called **allergens**. The responses are either antibody-mediated (types I, II and III) or cell-mediated (type IV).

Type I hypersensitivity

Type I hypersensitivity responses occur immediately and typically subside within half an hour, although a late-phase reaction may follow which lasts many hours or days, during which large numbers of leucocytes, attracted by chemotaxis, migrate to the area, prolong the inflammation and can damage the tissue.

Large quantities of **IgE** antibodies (also called sensitizing antibodies or **reagins**) are produced against the allergens in genetically susceptible individuals. The allergen binds with a specific IgE reagin, which also attaches to **basophils** and **mast cells**, causing them to secrete histamine and **heparin** and synthesize various chemicals including **slow-reacting substance of anaphylaxis** (a mixture of leukotrienes), eosinophil and neutrophil **chemotactic substances** and a **protease**. These chemicals cause vasodilation, chemotaxis of neutrophils and eosinophils, tissue damage by the protease, increased capillary permeability and oedema by histamine and contraction of smooth muscle cells by the slow-reacting substance of anaphylaxis.

Such responses are known as **anaphylactic reactions** and may be local or systemic. If an allergen such as a bee sting circulates it causes widespread release of chemicals from mast cells and basophils. The widespread vasodilation and fluid loss from circulation may cause **anaphylactic shock**. Noradrenaline can be used to reverse these effects by its vasoconstrictor action.

Local anaphylactic reactions include urticaria, hay fever and asthma. In urticaria (nettlerash) the allergen invades the skin causing a red flare and swelling and itching. In some individuals, urticaria is caused by non-allergic stimuli such as cold or pressure on the skin. In hay fever, where the allergen–reagin reaction occurs in the nose, resulting in vasodilation, swelling and increased secretions in the nasal cavity linings. In asthma, where the allergen–reagin reaction occurs in the bronchioles of the lungs, the slow-reacting substance of anaphylaxis being the major cause of bronchospasm.

Type II hypersensitivity

The antigen in type II hypersensitivity is bound to the surface of a body cell. **IgG** and **IgM** antibodies are produced and bind to the antigen, resulting in tissue damage, stimulating phagocytosis and complement fixation. The response usually occurs within 1–3 h. Drug reactions, haemolytic disease of the newborn and autoimmune conditions fall into this category.

Type III hypersensitivity

Type III hypersensitivity is similar to type II hypersensitivity except that the antigen circulates freely and the antigen–antibody complex causes inflammation wherever it lodges. Farmer's lung, nephritis and autoimmune conditions can result.

Type IV hypersensitivity

Type IV hypersensitivity takes 1–3 days to develop (delayed hypersensitivity). The response involves increased secretion of cytokines by helper T cells. The cytokines act as inflammatory mediators and activate macrophages. The first exposure causes sensitization, so that subsequent exposures cause an even bigger response.

Such responses are seen as skin eruptions in response to certain chemicals (allergic contact dermatitis), the Mantoux test for tuberculosis, and rejection of transplants.

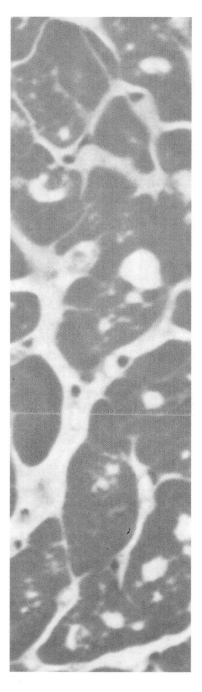

Circulation of blood and lymph

12

Every cell in the body requires a constant supply of life-sustaining food materials and oxygen. In addition, waste products, including carbon dioxide, are removed continuously. The circulation of blood and lymph provides a means by which both of these functions are fulfilled.

The heart pumps blood from its two sides into two different subsections of the circulation (Figure 12.1). The **systemic circulation** carries oxygenated blood from the left side of the heart to the rest of the body and the **pulmonary circulation** carries blood from the right side of the heart through the lungs, where it is oxygenated.

Figure 12.1 Plan of the circulation. The right atrium of the heart receives venous blood ([blue]) from the upper and lower body and the right ventricle pumps blood into the pulmonary circulation to the lungs, where it gains oxygen and loses carbon dioxide. The left atrium receives oxygenated blood ([red]) from the lungs and the left ventricle pumps it into the systemic circulation to the rest of the body.

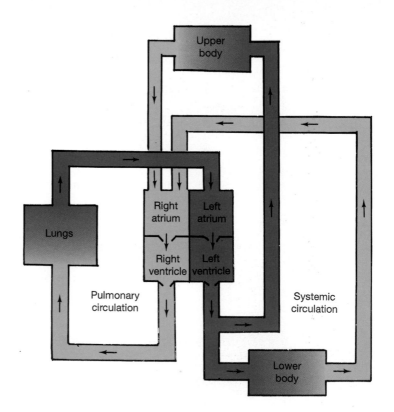

A continuous, though varied, rate of blood flow to the tissues is maintained by the pumping action of the heart which pushes blood into the arteries. Blood flows from the tissues towards the heart, in the veins.

In the tissues, some 20 L per day of fluid is filtered out of the smallest blood vessels, the capillaries, into the interstitial fluid (Figure 12.2). About 90% of this volume is reabsorbed directly back into the blood and the remaining 10% drains into the lymphatics, which return it to the venous system (Figure 12.3).

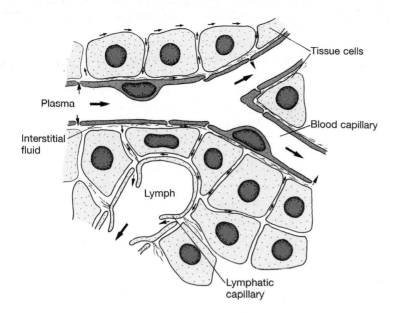

Figure 12.2 The circulation of fluids in the tissues. Fluid is filtering into the interstitial spaces on the lefthand side of the diagram (representing the arterial end of the capillary bed) and returning to the blood on the right (representing the venous end). About 10% of the fluid flows into the lymphatic capillaries.

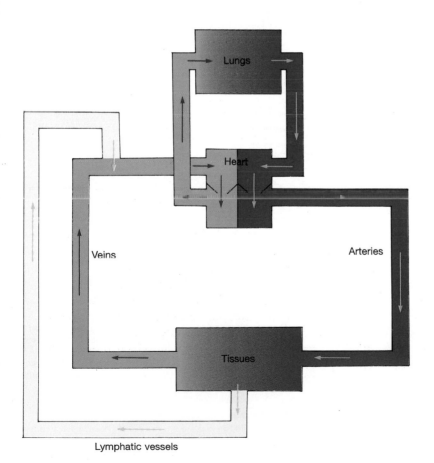

Figure 12.3 The relationship between the cardiovascular and lymphatic circulations. Blood is pumped from the heart to the tissues in arteries and returns to the heart in veins. About 2 litres of fluid per day flows from the tissues into the lymphatic vessels and then back to the venous circulation.

Structure of the heart

The heart is a small, muscular organ, conical in shape and with four chambers, two **atria** and two **ventricles**. In adults it weighs 300–400 g, generally being rather heavier in men than in women; there is a tendency for the heart to increase in weight with age in both sexes. When contracted it is about the same size as an adult's clenched fist. The heart is located in the thoracic cavity immediately above the diaphragm and between the lungs, in the inferior portion of the central section of the thoracic cavity, known as the **mediastinum**. One-third of the heart lies to the right of the sternum and two-thirds to the left. Its base is uppermost and is attached to the major blood vessels. The apex of the heart is directed downwards and to the left so that the wall of the right ventricle lies on the diaphragm.

The pericardium

The heart is enclosed by a conical, fibroserous sac, which also contains the roots of the great vessels. This sac is known as the pericardium and consists of an outer, fibrous layer, which is continuous with the external coat of the great vessels, and an inner, double, serous layer. Each serous membrane comprises a single layer of simple squamous epithelium (mesothelium) supported by a thin layer of fibroelastic connective tissue.

The fibrous pericardium is anchored to adjacent structures at various points. Inferiorly, it is anchored to the diaphragm and anteriorly to the sternum. This limits the extent to which the heart can move within the chest cavity. Lining the fibrous layer is the parietal layer of the serous

Figure 12.4 Longitudinal section through the human heart. The atria have been displaced slightly so that all four chambers can be seen in the same plane.

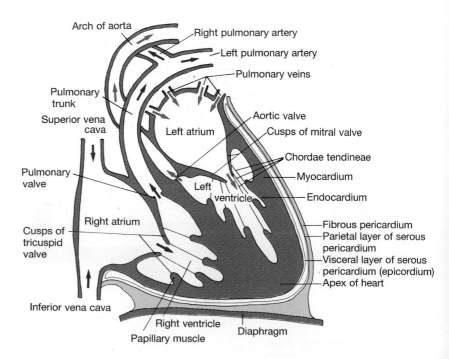

pericardium, which is continuous with the visceral layer covering the heart (epicardium) (Figure 12.4).

As the heart beats, it changes in size and moves within the pericardium. The two serous layers are able to slide over one another, lubricated by a small amount of fluid.

Atria

The two atria lie at the top of the heart and are separated by an oblique interatrial septum. The right atrium lies in front of the left.

The **right atrium** receives blood from the superior and inferior venae cavae; only the inferior vena cava exhibits a (poorly developed) valvular opening. It is a thin-walled cavity which, on contraction, generates only a slight increase in the pressure of the blood. The **coronary sinus**, the vessel which carries blood from the heart's own circulation (see *Coronary circulation*, below), drains into the right atrium between the opening of the inferior vena cava and the tricuspid valve. The lower part of the opening of the coronary sinus is covered by a semicircular valve. The **left atrium** is smaller than the right, but has a thicker wall. It receives blood from the lungs via the pulmonary veins.

Ventricles

The **right ventricle** extends from the right atrium but does not reach the apex of the heart. The wall is much thinner than that of the left and, because its chamber wraps around the left ventricle, its cavity is crescent-shaped (Figure 12.5).

The **right atrioventricular orifice** is a large, oval opening between the right atrium and ventricle. It is surrounded by a fibrous ring to which

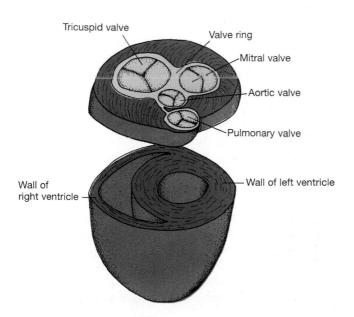

Tricuspid valve
Valve ring
Mitral valve
Aortic valve
Pulmonary valve
Wall of right ventricle
Wall of left ventricle

Figure 12.5 Cross-sections through the heart to show the valves above and the ventricles below.

the three cusps (also known as flaps or leaflets) of the **tricuspid valve** are attached. The cusps have smooth atrial but roughened lower (ventricular) surfaces. The margins and lower surfaces are attached to the ventricular wall by a number of delicate cords, the **chordae tendineae**. These are anchored to two irregular columns of muscle, the **papillary muscles**, which project from the ventricle wall. When the ventricles contract, the papillary muscles contract just before the rest of the wall and pull on the chordae tendineae. This prevents eversion of the atrioventricular valves when blood pressure rises within the ventricle, and prohibits backflow of blood into the atria.

The **pulmonary valve**, which guards the entrance of the pulmonary trunk, has three semi-lunar cusps. These are sac-like and close by being filled with blood when arterial pressure is above that in the ventricle. A high pressure in the ventricle opens the valve by flattening the cusps against the arterial wall, thereby allowing blood to flow out of the heart.

The **left ventricle** is longer than the right and extends to the apex of the heart. Its walls are approximately three times thicker than those of the right ventricle and its cavity is circular or oval in transverse section. The thicker wall is able to contract more strongly than that of the right ventricle and therefore generate a far higher pressure.

The **left atrioventricular** or **mitral orifice** is guarded by the **mitral valve** that is similar to the tricuspid valve but has only two, unequally-sized cusps. They are anchored to papillary muscles by chordae tendineae and prevent regurgitation of blood back into the left atrium during ventricular contraction.

The **aortic valve** is similar in structure to, but rather more robust than the pulmonary valve.

Structure of the heart wall

The heart is covered by the serous layer of the pericardium. This is firmly attached to the muscular wall of the heart and is termed **epicardium**. The contractile part of the wall, to which the epicardium is attached, is known as the **myocardium** and forms the bulk of the heart wall. It is lined by **endocardium**, which is composed of a layer of elastic tissue lined by a single layer of endothelium.

The cardiac muscle cells of the myocardium are branched and striated and are interconnected, forming a network through which action potentials can pass easily. The cells of the atria are separated from those of the ventricles by the fibrous tissue sheet that contains the heart valves. There are therefore two separate networks, or functional syncytia, which are connected only through the atrioventricular bundle (see *Conduction system and innervation of the heart wall*, below). Within each syncytium the cells are arranged in complex double-layered spirals.

In cardiac muscle cells the **T-tubules** cross the cell at the level of the Z lines and longitudinal tubules of the **sarcoplasmic reticulum** run parallel to the contractile myofibrils (Figure 12.6). These tubules have small dilations (**saccules**), which lie close to a T-tubule.

See also **Cardiac muscle** (page 99), in Ch. 3, Tissues.

T-tubules and the arrangement of the sarcoplasmic reticulum in skeletal muscle cells are described in **Skeletal muscle** (page 98), in Ch. 3, Tissues.

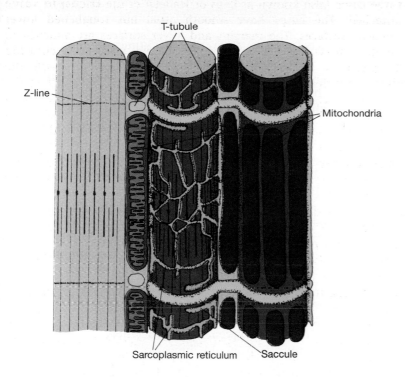

Figure 12.6 Fine structure of cardiac muscle showing the T-tubules and sarcoplasmic reticulum.

Conduction system and innervation of the heart wall

The conducting system of the heart consists of specialized muscle cells in the sinoatrial (SA) node, the atrioventricular (AV) node, the AV bundle and its right and left branches, together with the branching network of Purkinje fibres beneath the endocardium (see Figure 12.10).

The **SA node**, or **pacemaker**, is a narrow structure located immediately beneath and medial to the opening of the superior vena cava in the wall of the right atrium. It measures 10–20 mm by 3 mm and is about 1 mm thick.

The **AV node** is somewhat smaller and lies in the interatrial septum, just above the tricuspid valve. From the node, a slender bundle of fibres, the **AV bundle**, or bundle of His, passes through the fibrous sheet separating the atria from the ventricles into the interventricular septum. The AV bundle then divides into right and left branches (bundles of Purkinje fibres), which travel just beneath the endocardium down to the apex of the heart before supplying the papillary muscles and then the myocardium. **Purkinje fibres** are large diameter cardiac muscle cells, which transmit action potentials faster than ordinary cardiac muscle.

The heart receives parasympathetic fibres from the Xth cranial (vagus) nerve from the medulla oblongata of the brain. The sympathetic supply arises in the upper thoracic region of the spinal cord and fibres pass to the heart via the cervical sympathetic ganglia. Both sympathetic and parasympathetic fibres innervate the atria but the ventricle receives sympathetic fibres only.

The cardiac cycle

The heart contracts (or beats) an average of 75 times a minute when the body is at rest. With each beat each side of the heart pumps out 60–70 mL of blood (when sitting, it is higher when lying down), leaving about 40–50 mL behind.

The term **cardiac cycle** refers to the series of electrical and mechanical events that take place in the heart during one complete heart beat. Both atria and both ventricles contract (**systole**) and relax (**diastole**) during the cycle and pump blood into the systemic and pulmonary divisions of the cardiovascular system. Figure 12.7 illustrates the sequence and duration of the events in the cardiac cycle.

In each cycle deoxygenated blood enters the right atrium from the organs above and below the heart, via the superior and inferior venae cavae respectively. Blood flows passively at first and is then pumped through the AV valve into the right ventricle when the atrium contracts. The ventricle itself then contracts, closing the AV valve and causing a rise in pressure that forces open the pulmonary valve and carries blood into the pulmonary trunk and then to the lungs via the left and right pulmonary arteries.

At the same time as deoxygenated blood enters the right atrium, oxygenated blood returns from the lungs to the left atrium via the pulmonary veins and then into the thick-walled left ventricle through the AV valve. Ventricular contraction causes a large rise in pressure, which closes the AV valve and then opens the aortic valve, enabling blood to enter the aorta and pass around the body.

The events taking place in the two sides of the heart are essentially identical, the only difference being in the magnitude of the pressures generated in the two ventricles. On the left side **maximum ventricular pressure** is around 120 mmHg, whereas on the right it is only about 25 mmHg.

Figure 12.8 shows the events taking place in the left side of the heart during the cardiac cycle.

Atrial pressure

Pressure within the atrium rises (a) as blood enters passively from the pulmonary veins; the AV valve is shut. A slight dip in the pressure curve is caused by the closure of the aortic valve.

Towards the end of atrial filling, the ventricle starts to relax so that its pressure falls. When atrial pressure exceeds that in the ventricle the AV valve is pushed open (1). Some 70–80% of the blood in the atrium then flows passively into the ventricle. As blood leaves the atrium the intra-atrial pressure drops, although during this phase of the cardiac cycle it is still higher than that in the ventricle (b). Atrial systole causes a rise in the pressure of the blood remaining within the atrium and forces most of it into the ventricle (c).

Ventricular systole follows atrial systole, and immediately ventricular pressure rises above that in the atrium. This causes the AV valve to close (2). It is this closure which brings about the brief increase in atrial pres-

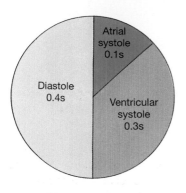

Figure 12.7 A typical resting cardiac cycle (0.8 s) comprising diastole (relaxation) (0.4 s), followed by atrial systole (contraction) (0.1 s) and then ventricular systole (contraction) (0.3 s).

Units of pressure are explained in **Pressure** (page 12), in Ch. 1, Molecules, Ions and Units.

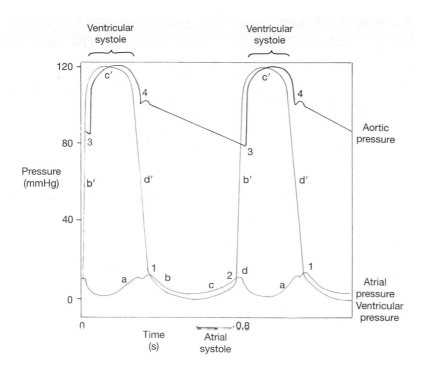

Figure 12.8 Pressure changes during the cardiac cycle: left side only. (Note that more than one cycle is shown – two ventricular systoles are included.) a–d = atrial pressure curve; a'–d' = ventricular pressure curve; 1 = AV valve opens; 2 = AV valve closes; 3 – Aortic valve opens; 4 = Aortic valve closes.

sure (d). Atrial diastole causes a sharp drop in atrial pressure and this is then followed by a steady rise as blood again enters from the pulmonary vein (a). A small peak in atrial pressure corresponds with the opening of the aortic valve.

Ventricular and aortic pressures

The rise in pressure that accompanies ventricular systole closes the AV valve (2). The chamber is full of blood, but this blood is not able to enter the aorta because the high pressure in that artery prevents the aortic valve from opening. Thus ventricular systole does not immediately pump blood out of the heart, but causes the intraventricular pressure to rise very rapidly (b'). Contraction of the ventricular muscle without accompanying shortening is described as **isometric contraction**.

Once ventricular pressure rises above that in the aorta, the aortic valve opens (3) and blood flows out of the heart (c').

Some 70% of the stroke volume is ejected rapidly during the first one-third of systole, whereas the remaining 30% is ejected more slowly. During the last two-thirds of systole, ventricular pressure falls slightly below aortic pressure. At a heart rate of 75 beats/min, systole lasts for a total of 0.3 s.

At the beginning of ventricular diastole, intraventricular pressure falls further below that in the aorta and the aortic valve closes (4). Ventricular pressure continues to fall rapidly (d') and once it has dropped below that in the atrium the AV valve opens (1). Although the ventricle is now receiving blood from the atrium, its pressure falls because it is enlarging as it relaxes (b). The ventricular pressure then starts to rise during atrial systole (c) when blood is pumped into the fully relaxed chamber. At a heart rate of 75 beats/min, diastole lasts for 0.5 s.

The muscular activity of the heart causes it to move within the chest cavity. In diastole the heart is soft, but in systole the ventricles harden, causing an increase in the anteroposterior and a decrease in the transverse diameters. The apex of the heart scarcely moves since it is anchored to the central tendon of the diaphragm. The base of the heart, however, moves downwards and forwards during ventricular systole.

Volume changes

When the body is at rest, each ventricle fills during diastole to a volume of 100–120 mL (**end-diastolic volume**). During systole 60–70 mL is ejected, leaving 40–50 mL behind (**end-systolic volume**).

Heart sounds

The actions of the heart in the cardiac cycle give rise to a sequence of sounds, which can be heard with the aid of a stethoscope. The first sound ('lub') is recorded when the cusps of the AV valve come together as ventricular pressure builds up. The second heart sound ('dup') is due to closure of the aortic and pulmonary valves.

Initiation and conduction of the cardiac impulse

All cardiac muscle cells are **myogenic**, that is they are able to generate action potentials and accompanying rhythmic contractions. The resting potential of cardiac muscle cells is about −90 mV and the action potential about +20 mV. Atrial cells remain depolarized for 0.2 s, ventricular cells for 0.3 s, much longer that skeletal muscle fibres, so that the potential plateaus (Figure 12.9).

Like skeletal muscle fibres, cardiac muscle cell membranes contain Na^+ and K^+ channels, as well as Ca^{2+} channels, which remain open for much longer. When the cell is stimulated, the Na^+ channels open first, followed by the Ca^{2+} channels, through which both Ca^{2+} and Na^+ enter down their concentration gradients. However, K^+ channels are closed, so that rapid

Figure 12.9 The action potential in a ventricular muscle cell.

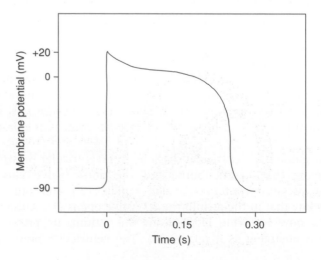

repolarization is not possible and the cell remains depolarized. Once the Ca^{2+} channels close, the K^+ channels open and repolarization does then occur. Ventricular cells have a long absolute refractory period (0.3 s), which corresponds to the length of time the Ca^{2+} channels are open; additionally there is a relative refractory period of about 0.05 s. Atrial cells have correspondingly shorter refractory periods (0.15 and 0.03 s). The long refractory period of cardiac muscle lasts about as long as its contraction and therefore prevents summation of contractions and tetanus.

Different parts of the heart have different natural rhythms, and if these rhythms were not coordinated, the heart would not function as an effective pump. The cells of the sinoatrial (SA) node have the highest rate of activity of any in the heart, generating about 100 impulses per minute. The SA node acts, therefore, as a 'pacemaker', since these impulses effectively swamp any that are generated at other sites in the heart.

The cells of the SA node have a resting potential of only -55 to -60 mV, largely because they are especially leaky to Na^+. When the cells are excited only slow Ca^{2+} channels can open (the Na^+ channels are closed by the inactivation gates at membrane potentials below -60 mV), so that the action potential is slow to develop. The cells are self-exciting because the inward leakage of Na^+ causes a rising potential which, when it reaches a threshold of -40 mV, causes the Ca^{2+} channels to open and initiate an action potential. Inactivation of these channels after 0.1–0.15 s and increased opening of the K^+ channels causes a rapid loss of K^+ and hyperpolarization. Na^+ then begins to leak in again and the potential drifts up and initiates another action potential.

From the SA node impulses are transmitted through the atrial syncytium and as each cell receives an impulse it starts to contract. Conduction is rapid, so that both atria contract virtually simultaneously. The impulse is received by the AV node 0.04 s after leaving the SA node (Figure 12.10).

From the AV node the impulse is conducted through the fibrous sheet that separates the atria from the ventricles and into the interventricular septum by means of the AV bundle. This is the only connection between the cells of the atria and those of the ventricles. Conduction of the

Summation and tetanus are explained in **Strength of muscle contraction** (page 297), in Ch. 9, Autonomic and Somatic Motor Activity.

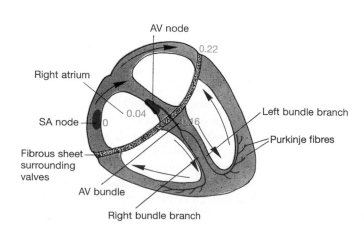

Figure 12.10 Spread of excitation through the heart. Figures indicate elapsed time in seconds.

impulse from the AV node to the end of the bundle takes about 0.12 s, some three times longer than it takes for the impulse to travel from the SA node to the AV node. This delay ensures that the atria finish contracting before the impulse is transmitted through to the ventricles. The cells of the AV node and atrioventricular bundle are narrower than typical cardiac muscle cells and slow to excite because their resting potentials are lower; they also have fewer intercalated discs, so that resistance to the flow of ions is greater.

The AV bundle divides into two main branches and each gives off smaller branches, which distribute the impulse throughout the myocardium. These Purkinje fibres have a much larger diameter than cardiac muscle cells and transmit impulses at a velocity of 2.5 m/s, which is five times faster. All parts of the ventricular myocardium are thereby stimulated to contract virtually simultaneously so that effective ejection of blood occurs during systole.

Conduction of an impulse from the SA node throughout the myocardium takes about 0.22 s.

Contraction of cardiac muscle cells

Action potentials enter each cell by means of the T-tubules. These potentials stimulate the sarcoplasmic reticulum to release Ca^{2+} into the sarcoplasm, which initiates the contractile process (as in skeletal muscle).

However, the amount of Ca^{2+} released from the sarcoplasmic reticulum alone would not be large enough to sustain maximal contraction; additional quantities are released extracellular fluid stored in the T-tubules (which have a total volume 25 times that in skeletal muscle).

CARDIAC ARRHYTHMIAS

The rhythm of the heart can be irregular and caused by:

- a different part of the heart beginning to act as a pacemaker, either the AV node (generating **nodal rhythm**), or another part of the myocardium (**ectopic focus**);
- a block in the transmission of impulses between atria and ventricles (**heart block**);
- impulses passing back and forth over the same part of the myocardium, causing uncoordinated, ineffective contractions (**fibrillation**).

Should an area of the heart become hyperexcitable and generate action potentials at a rate faster than the SA node, **extrasystoles** occur, heartbeats additional to those caused by the SA node. An area other than the SA node acting as pacemaker is known as an ectopic focus. Should the AV node act as a pacemaker, since its natural rhythm is slower than that of the SA node the heart rate is also reduced.

As the AV bundle is the only path by which action potentials can be transmitted from the atria to the ventricles, any impairment in AV-node or AV-bundle function delays transmission. Impairment may be caused by reduced blood flow (ischaemia), inflammation or compression by scar tissue and results in varying degrees of 'heart block'. An artificial pacemaker can be used to compensate for heart block.

EFFECTS OF ALTERED CONCENTRATIONS OF EXTRACELLULAR Na^+, K^+ AND Ca^{2+} ON HEART ACTIVITY

Since the heart beat is dependent upon the generation of action potentials, it is predictable that alterations of the ionic concentrations of the internal environment of the cardiac muscle cells will alter cardiac activity.

A rise in Na^+ concentration blocks the transport of Ca^{2+} into cardiac muscle cells, thereby reducing their contraction and heart rate. A fall in Na^+, on the other hand, causes tachycardia.

A rise in K^+ concentration reduces (makes less negative) the resting membrane potential of cardiac muscle cells and also reduces the size of the action potential, which can result in a weakened contraction and slowed heart. Heart block and cardiac arrest can result. A fall in K^+ concentration weakens the heart and causes arrhythmias.

Low Ca^{2+} in extracellular fluid reduces the amount of Ca^{2+} in the T-tubules and therefore depresses the heart rate, whereas high Ca^{2+} stimulates cardiac contraction, resulting in spastic contraction.

Electrocardiogram

Depolarization and repolarization of the cardiac muscle cells sets up electrical currents in the body fluids which can be detected by attaching electrodes to the surface of the skin on opposite sides of the heart. Such a recording is known as an electrocardiogram (**ECG**).

Conventionally three sets of electrodes are used which are attached as follows: lead I (electrodes on right and left arms), lead II (electrodes on right arm and left leg), and lead III (electrodes on left arm and left leg). The leads are attached to a measuring device (electrocardiograph) and the ECG recorded. Slightly different records are obtained depending upon the lead which is chosen. Figure 12.11 illustrates a typical lead I ECG.

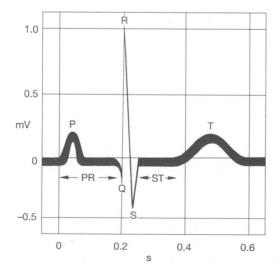

Figure 12.11 Typical lead 1 electrocardiogram.

The asymmetrical orientation of the heart means that it takes different amounts of time for the electrical currents passing through the heart to reach the two wrists. Therefore, for a brief moment in time, a charge difference can be recorded between them.

Depolarization of the atria is indicated by a small **P wave**, which is followed by a short interval during which time the atria are in a state of contraction. The wave and the short interval are together referred to as the **P–R interval**, which lasts 0.1–0.2 s. Atrial repolarization then occurs but is masked by the **QRS complex**, which signals the start of ventricular contraction.

Repolarization of the ventricular fibres begins 0.15 s after initial depolarization but may not be completed for 0.3 s; as a result, the accompanying **T wave** is usually more prolonged and flatter than the QRS complex.

Notice that the trace is flat during some of the P–R interval and the whole of the S–T interval, even though the atria in the first case and the ventricles in the second are in a state of contraction. A wave is only observed at the beginning of depolarization or repolarization.

A wave of excitation passes from the SA node, which lies close to the base of the heart, towards the tip of the ventricles, the apex. The electrodes attached to the surface of the body record this wave as it radiates out from the heart through the body fluids. In a lead I record, because the right arm is nearest to the base of the heart it receives the wave first and becomes negative with respect to the left arm electrode, which is positive. The two electrodes are connected to the recording device so that an upward deflection is given when the right arm electrode is negative; thus a positive R wave is observed on the ECG.

It is evident from the above that it is the direction the wave of excitation takes that determines the direction of deflection on the ECG.

The negative Q wave is generated when the wave of excitation passes across the interventricular septum from left to right. This is because the left-hand side of the septum depolarizes slightly ahead of the right. The negative S wave results from the wave travelling through the outer ventricular wall back towards the base. The ventricular repolarization wave moves towards the apex and gives rise to a positive T wave.

Clinical measurement of the ECG can be a more complicated procedure than that covered here. In addition to the three limb locations, as many as six on the chest may be used for the attachment of electrodes and, as a result, many different ECG 'pictures' may be obtained. Such pictures may be employed in the analysis of heart function; for example, a prolonged P–R interval indicates heart block.

Cardiac output

The volume of blood pumped out by each ventricle during 1 minute is known as the cardiac output. It is dependent upon the volume of blood ejected from the heart at each beat (**stroke volume**) and the number of beats during one minute (**heart rate**).

Thus: cardiac output = stroke volume × heart rate

e.g. cardiac output = 65 mL/beat × 75 beats/min
= 4875 mL/min ≈ 5 L/min

These figures represent average values obtained from men aged between 30 and 60 years of age, measured at rest and in the sitting position. Equivalent average values for stroke volume and cardiac output in women are slightly lower than those in men.

An increase in cardiac output can be brought about by an increase in heart rate or an increase in stroke volume, or both. For example, a young athlete undergoing maximal exercise can attain a heart rate of 200 beats/min and a stroke volume of 150 mL/beat, resulting in a cardiac output of 30 L/min.

Heart rate

The spontaneous rhythm of the heart is modified by the autonomic nervous system even under resting conditions. The sinoatrial node is innervated by both sympathetic and parasympathetic fibres, which exert a continuous, though varied, influence upon heart rate.

Stimulation of the parasympathetic fibres reduces the heart rate (**bradycardia**) and prolonged stimulation may cause the heart to stop beating completely. Blocking impulse transmission in the fibres with drugs or by surgery will, on the other hand, lead to an increase in the resting heart rate.

Stimulation of sympathetic nerves induces an increase in heart rate (**tachycardia**), whereas a reduction in their activity will result in a slowing of the heart. Since the resting heart rate is about 75 beats/min and the SA node alone elicits a rate of about 100 beats/min, it is evident that, at rest, the parasympathetic system is dominant.

The autonomic pathways to the heart originate in a diffuse network of nerve fibres situated in the medulla oblongata. Some of these fibres initiate parasympathetic activity and this region is therefore known as the **cardioinhibitory centre**. Another area, the **vasomotor centre**, is responsible for initiating vasoconstriction and an increase in heart rate through the sympathetic system.

Several hormones alter heart rate. Adrenaline increases heart rate by combining with beta$_1$-adrenoceptors on the cells of the SA node, causing an increase in Na$^+$ permeability. Thyroxine directly increases the excitability of heart muscle and enhances the action of adrenaline. Cortisol also exerts a stimulatory influence on cardiac muscle cells, probably by enhancing the action of adrenaline. A rise in body temperature increases the metabolic rate of the cells of the SA node and, therefore, increases heart rate.

Stroke volume

At rest each ventricle ejects 60–70 mL of blood (stroke volume), leaving about the same volume behind (end-systolic volume).

There are two ways by which stroke volume can be increased beyond the resting value. One is by increasing the rate of filling of the heart which thereby increases the volume of blood available for pumping

Sympathomimetic actions of adrenaline are described on page 281, in Ch. 9, Autonomic and Somatic Motor Activity. Thyroxine and cortisol functions are covered in **Tri-iodothyronine (T3) and thyroxine (T4)** (page 624) and **Cortisol and corticosterone (glucocorticoids)** (page 639), in Ch. 16, Endocrine Physiology.

(end-diastolic volume). The second is by the ventricles contracting more strongly and consequently expelling more blood during each cardiac cycle and leaving less behind (end-systolic volume).

INCREASED END-DIASTOLIC VOLUME

A rise in the rate of filling of the heart (venous return) results in a greater volume of blood in the ventricles at the end of diastole, i.e. there is an increase in end-diastolic volume. This causes the cardiac muscle cells in the myocardium to be stretched which enables them to contract with increased force. The increased force of contraction allows the heart to eject a greater volume of blood, i.e. stroke volume increases. Factors increasing venous return are covered in *Venous circulation*, below.

In addition, if heart rate increases there is less time available during each beat for cardiac filling and emptying. The rapid relaxation of the heart in diastole produces a drop in pressure, which helps to suck blood into the ventricles, with a consequent increase in end-diastolic volume. This effect is only observed with heart rates of up to about 120–130 beats/min, however, and above these rates there is insufficient time for effective refilling and emptying so that stroke volume begins to fall.

It is clear that these cardiac adjustments are mediated through volume increases. The heart contracts more strongly when cardiac volumes are raised and the muscle cells in the wall are stretched. The relationship between the degree of stretch of the muscle wall and the amount of work they produce is summarized by the Frank–Starling law of the heart: 'the force of contraction is proportional to the length of the muscle cells'. This means that, within physiological limits, the heart adjusts its output of blood, keeping pace with inflow and thereby avoiding excessive amounts of blood being either retained in the venous system or shunted into the arterial system.

DECREASED END-SYSTOLIC VOLUME

Changes in stroke volume may also be brought about under the influence of the sympathetic nervous system, which innervates the cardiac muscle cells in the ventricles. Noradrenaline from sympathetic nerve endings has little effect alone, whereas circulating adrenaline from the adrenal medullae increase the contractility of cardiac muscle cells. Thus, for a given initial cell length, adrenaline increases the strength of contraction and the final cell length is reduced. The increased strength of contractions leads to more complete ejection of blood and less blood is left in the heart at the end of each beat. The end-systolic volume, then, is reduced and stroke volume is raised.

Cardiac reflexes

Changes in arterial blood pressure and/or blood gas composition initiate a number of autonomic reflexes which have the effect of altering cardiac output and consequently maintain homoeostasis.

The components of the cardiac reflexes are arterial sensory receptors, the cardiovascular centre in the medulla oblongata and a number of effectors that include the heart itself, the walls of blood vessels and the adrenal medullae.

CARDIOVASCULAR CENTRE

The cardiovascular centre consists of two functional components, the **vasomotor centre** and the **cardioinhibitory centre**. The vasomotor centre is further subdivided into a **depressor** and a **pressor** area. The vasomotor centre is connected to the heart by sympathetic motor pathways, whereas the cardioinhibitory centre has parasympathetic connections with the heart.

BARORECEPTOR REFLEX

Baroreceptors are spray-type nerve endings found in the walls of many of the major arteries of the thorax and neck, as well as in the heart itself. The receptors actually respond to stretch of the blood vessel (or heart) walls, which is itself caused by an increase in blood pressure.

The major baroreceptors are found in the wall of the aortic arch and in the carotid sinuses (the dilated proximal section of each internal carotid artery) (Figure 12.12).

Nerves from the baroreceptors (**vagi** from the aortic receptors and **Hering's nerve**, which leads to the **glossopharyngeal nerves**, in the case of the carotid sinuses) exhibit tonic activity. Thus, at rest there is a low frequency of impulses passing to the medulla. If arterial blood pressure falls, there is a reduction in the level of stimulation of the baroreceptors and the frequency of impulses in the nerves falls. This reduces

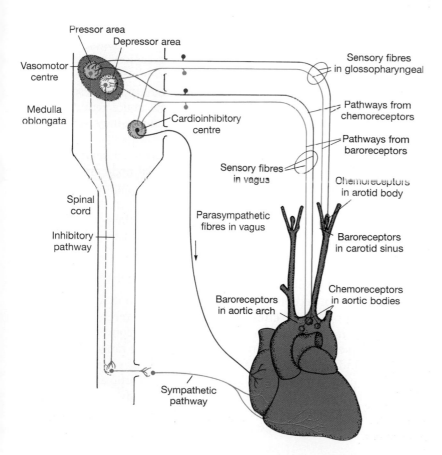

Figure 12.12 Cardiac baroreceptor and chemoreceptor reflex pathways. Baroreceptors in the aortic arch and carotid sinuses send impulses via sensory neurones to the cardioinhibitory centre and the depressor area of the vasomotor centre located in the medulla oblongata in the brain stem. Chemoreceptors in the aortic and carotid bodies send impulses via sensory neurones to the pressor area of the vasomotor centre. The pressor area has neural connections with the sympathetic nerves to the heart; the depressor area inhibits sympathetic pathways in the spinal cord; the cardioinhibitory centre is linked to the heart by parasympathetic fibres in the vagus nerves.

stimulation of both the depressor area of the vasomotor centre and the cardioinhibitory centre.

The depressor area is connected by inhibitory neurones to preganglionic sympathetic fibres in the spinal cord; when stimulated they reduce the actions of the pressor area. When the depressor area is inhibited, therefore, the number of impulses from the pressor area travelling in the sympathetic nerves to the heart rises. Inhibition of the cardioinhibitory centre decreases vagal discharge to the heart. The combined effects of the two centres, therefore, is an increase in heart rate and stroke volume, thereby increasing cardiac output and raising blood pressure.

The baroreceptor reflex is therefore an important means by which transient falls in blood pressure can be countered.

A rise in blood pressure stimulates the baroreceptor reflex, which, in this case, results in a reduction in cardiac output and a fall in blood pressure. The reflex thereby limits the extent by which blood pressure can rise.

In the long term, the responsiveness of the reflex to the level of blood pressure may change. For example, in a person with high blood pressure (**hypertension**) the initial increased baroreceptor response diminishes with time, so that the hypertension continues.

The baroreceptor reflex also involves responses in blood vessels and the adrenal medullae. These are discussed in *Control of arterial blood pressure*, below.

The walls of the atria contain stretch receptors (baroreceptors) that are particularly important in the detection of changes in blood volume. An increase in blood volume stimulates the atrial receptors, leading to reflex dilation of the afferent arterioles of the glomeruli of the kidneys. At the same time, the hypothalamus reduces ADH output. There is consequently an increase in glomerular filtration rate and a reduction in the amount of water reabsorbed by the tubules of the kidney, resulting in a fall in blood volume.

Stretching the right atrium also leads to an increased heart rate. This is the result of both a direct action on the sinoatrial node and, to a lesser extent, the **atrial (Bainbridge) reflex**, in which impulses travel from the atrial baroreceptors to the cardiovascular centre in the medulla and then back to the heart via sympathetic (in which there is an increased frequency of impulses) and parasympathetic fibres (a reduced frequency of impulses).

CHEMORECEPTOR REFLEXES

A second group of receptors, which usually plays only a minor part in cardiac regulation, is the **chemoreceptors**. These receptors respond to lowered oxygen, raised carbon dioxide or raised H^+ concentration caused by, for example, a very low arterial pressure in the range 40–80 mmHg. They are found in the **aortic** and **carotid bodies**, spherical structures some 1–2 mm in diameter that project from the aortic arch and carotid bifurcation on small stalks (Figure 12.12). Each body has a small artery that supplies it with blood and, though they are very small, their blood supply is relatively enormous, about 2000 mL/100 g tissue. They monitor

See also **Regulation of nephron function** (page 501), in Ch. 14, Renal Control of Body Fluid Volume and Composition.

Table 12.1 Approximate distribution of the cardiac output in an adult 65 kg male (at rest)

	Weight		Blood flow		% cardiac output
	kg	%	mL/min	mL/100 g/min	
Heart	0.4	0.6	210	52	4
Brain	1.4	2.2	650	46	13
Abdominal organs	4.0	6.2	1210	30	24
Skin	3.6	5.5	430	12	9
Kidneys	0.3	0.5	950	317	19
Skeletal muscle	31.0	47.7	1030	3	21

the rate of delivery of dissolved gases, rather than the absolute amount in the blood. The aortic and carotid chemoreceptors send impulses to the medulla via the vagi and glossopharyngeal nerves respectively to the pressor area of the vasomotor centre. The latter then increases sympathetic discharge to the heart, causing a rise in heart rate. This increases blood flow to the chemoreceptors, reduces the stimulus and maintains homoeostasis.

Distribution of the cardiac output

The distribution of blood to the different tissues and organs of the body is generally a reflection of their different levels of metabolic activity. Thus the kidneys, which have a combined weight of approximately 300 g, receive 19% of the cardiac output, whereas skeletal muscles (31 kg) at rest only receive about 21% (Table 12.1). Descriptions of the regional blood supply to various parts of the body are given in the appropriate chapters, together with accounts of the mechanisms by which these blood flows are regulated.

Coronary circulation

The myocardium of the heart is supplied principally by two coronary arteries, which arise from sinuses situated above the cusps of the aortic valve at the root of the aorta (Figure 12.13).

The arteries distribute branches over the surface of the heart in the epicardium and then enter the myocardium. The **left coronary artery** supplies the wall of the left ventricle with oxygenated blood, whereas the **right coronary artery** supplies the right ventricle and a portion of the left ventricle. Venous blood from the left ventricle drains via the coronary sinus into the right atrium; some blood from the right ventricle also drains into the right atrium through the anterior cardiac veins.

Blood flow through the coronary system represents about 4% of the output from the left ventricle (approximately 70 mL/100 g/min at rest).

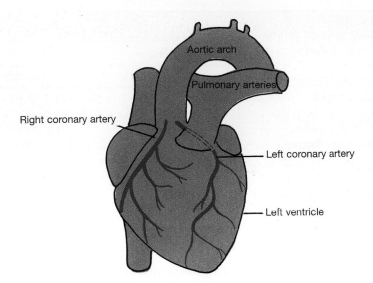

Figure 12.13 Distribution of the coronary arteries over the surface of the heart.

This flow is intermittent, since during systole compression of the coronary vessels by the surrounding muscle inhibits the free passage of blood through the myocardium, especially in the left side.

Although the coronary arterioles are innervated by both divisions of the autonomic nervous system, blood flow through the coronary system is thought to be regulated primarily by local factors, namely the oxygen levels of the blood and the presence of metabolites. When the body is at rest, heart muscle extracts about 65% of the oxygen from the blood in the coronary vessels. This is near to the maximum amount that can possibly be removed. In exercise, when the oxygen requirement of the cardiac muscle is increased, there is an increased blood flow, which provides the extra oxygen. A four- or five-fold increase in blood flow can occur and the stimulus for this increased blood flow is probably reduced oxygen level. The exact mechanism by which low oxygen (hypoxia) promotes vasodilation, thereby increasing blood flow, is not completely understood. It has been suggested that hypoxia promotes the release of vasodilator substances, e.g. adenosine, from the surrounding tissues.

It will be recalled that sympathetic activity causes increased activity of the heart. Although sympathetic stimulation of the coronary blood vessels causes slight vasoconstriction, this effect is masked during exercise by vasodilation caused by local metabolic factors. In addition, circulating adrenaline combines with beta$_2$-adrenoceptors in coronary arterioles and causes vasodilation.

Ischaemic heart disease

Currently, the principal cause of death in Western countries is recorded as ischaemic heart disease (IHD). Ischaemia means 'reduced blood flow', and in this case it is due to arteriosclerosis of the coronary arteries. This involves the deposition of various substances, principally cholesterol, in the inner layers of blood vessel walls. The fatty plaques (**atheromatous plaques**) protrude into the vessel lumen thereby partially occluding it and reducing the blood supply to the cardiac muscle. The plaques can become invaded by connective tissue (fibrosed) and calcium can be deposited, which results in a hardening of the blood vessel wall (sclerosis), with a consequent loss of elasticity.

ANGINA PECTORIS

The term 'angina pectoris' literally means 'pain of the chest' and the condition is a result of insufficient coronary blood flow. Usually, the pain occurs if the person carries out some kind of physical activity. In this situation, the heart muscle uses more oxygen than it does when the body is in the resting state and produces more carbon dioxide and other metabolites. In IHD the reduced blood supply results in hypoxia and possibly tissue damage. The resultant rise in lactic acid, bradykinin and prostaglandins probably stimulate nerve endings and cause pain. The pain can be referred to areas other than the chest, down the left arm and up to the chin.

> The physiology of pain is discussed in Ch. 7 Sensory Processing.

MYOCARDIAL INFARCTION (HEART ATTACK)

An atherosclerotic plaque can cause a clot to form around it, particularly if the plaque has broken through into the lumen of the vessel, thereby exposing a 'foreign' surface to the blood. The clot may completely occlude the vessel and deprive the cardiac muscle distal to it of blood. The severity of the consequences depends upon where the blockage occurs and how effective the alternative (collateral) circulation is in the affected site. If cardiac muscle is deprived of blood to a point where it cannot function and dies (necrosis), then it is said to be infarcted.

Myocardial infarction can cause death in several different ways. Cardiac output can be insufficient to keep the body tissues alive, either because the infarcted area is sufficiently large to impair the heart's pumping ability, or because the area has ruptured. If the heart ruptures, the leaked blood accumulates within the pericardium and presses on the heart (**cardiac tamponade**) thereby preventing the flow of blood through the chambers. Myocardial infarction can lead to irregular, ineffective ventricular contractions known as **ventricular fibrillation**. This is another cause of an inadequate cardiac output.

The damaged heart has a reduced ability to pump blood returning to it from the systemic and pulmonary circulations. This can lead to vascular congestion and pulmonary oedema. The latter can prevent oxygen uptake and result in inadequate oxygenation of the blood.

Heart failure

The constant beating of the heart maintaining a continuous blood supply to the tissues is clearly an essential requirement for life. If the function of the heart is impaired, then it follows that the activity of the body as a whole is threatened.

As the heart effectively consists of two pumps, there are two types of heart failure, right-sided and left-sided. These two conditions may occur either separately or together.

Left-sided heart failure is a condition in which the left ventricle cannot maintain a cardiac output high enough to maintain the metabolic needs of the tissues.

In **right-sided heart failure**, the heart is unable to keep pace with venous return so that there is pooling of blood in the venous system with resultant fluid congestion in the tissues.

Physiological causes of heart failure

The immediate physiological causes of heart failure fall into three principal categories: decreased filling, overwork and impaired cardiac muscle function.

DECREASED FILLING

If either ventricle does not receive sufficient blood during diastole, the stroke volume will clearly be reduced. If the left or right atrioventricular orifice becomes narrowed, the flow of blood between atrium and ventricle on the affected side will be reduced. **Valvular stenosis**, often a result of rheumatic fever, can cause heart failure of this type. Stenosed valves become thickened and stiffened and the orifice is narrowed. Thus mitral stenosis is a cause of left-sided failure, whereas tricuspid stenosis can lead to right-sided failure.

OVERWORK

A second type of heart failure is due to overwork because of an increase in end-diastolic volume (increased **preload**), so that the heart is constantly having to pump out extra blood. **Regurgitation** of blood through a faulty valve can lead to such a situation. If an AV valve cannot close properly during ventricular systole then some of the blood is pumped back into the atrium, rather than out of the heart. The consequence of this is atrial enlargement and an increase in the volume of blood passing from atrium to ventricle. The ventricle thus has to pump out the regurgitated blood as well as the usual stroke volume. Mitral regurgitation can be caused by stenosis, calcification, rupture of the chordae tendineae or dilation of the left ventricle, which weakens the valve. (Left ventricular dilation, in turn, can be caused by hypertension or aortic regurgitation.)

Cardiac failure due to overwork can also be caused by the ventricle having to overcome increased resistance to the ejection of blood (increased **afterload**). It may be caused, for example, by aortic stenosis, hypertension on the left side, pulmonary stenosis or pulmonary artery hypertension on the right side.

IMPAIRED CARDIAC MUSCLE FUNCTION

Heart failure most commonly occurs because the myocardium itself is impaired, as a result, for example, of ischaemic heart disease (see *Heart failure*, above).

Effects of heart failure

CONGESTION AND OEDEMA

Left-sided heart failure

In left-sided heart failure, because the outflow of blood from the left ventricle is impaired, the outflow of blood from the left atrium is reduced in turn (Figure 12.14).

The increased volume of blood and accompanying rise in pressure within the atrium promote enlargement, which leads to hypertrophy of the muscle cells. The rise in atrial pressure also affects pulmonary blood flow, so that the pressure in the pulmonary veins is raised, leading to **pulmonary congestion**. Fluid exudes from the capillaries into the limited amount of interstitial space in the alveolar walls and, more seriously, into the air-containing spaces of the alveoli themselves (**pulmonary oedema**), thereby impeding gas exchange. The accumulation of fluid also makes the lungs less compliant and therefore more difficult to inflate. This makes the work of breathing more difficult and so the person has uncomfortable breathing (**dyspnoea**).

Left-sided heart failure may lead to failure of the right side. The pulmonary arterioles may constrict, thereby raising pulmonary artery pressure. This presents an increased afterload to the right ventricle with resultant hypertrophy.

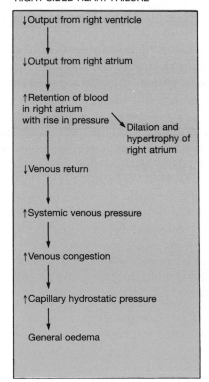

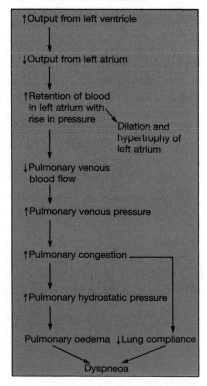

Figure 12.14 Development of congestion and oedema in right-sided and left-sided heart failure.

Right-sided heart failure

In right-sided heart failure, there is again ventricular impairment and resultant atrial enlargement. The heart fails to keep pace with venous return, causing a damming of blood in the systemic veins and a consequent increase in systemic venous pressure. This, in turn, impairs the venous flow from the tissues, so that they become congested and enlarged, leading to generalized oedema.

REDUCED CARDIAC OUTPUT

If the left ventricle fails, a direct consequence is that cardiac output is reduced. If the right ventricle fails, blood flow to the lungs is reduced and therefore blood flow back from the lungs to the left side of the heart is also reduced, so that cardiac output will be affected secondarily.

Reduced cardiac output can result in hypoxia and resultant underfunctioning of tissues generally. The poor blood flow in the tissues causes peripheral cyanosis ('cyan' – blue colour). This condition is due to blood containing a smaller amount of bright red oxyhaemoglobin than usual and a larger amount of reduced haemoglobin, which is a darker red. When such blood flows through vessels which are close to the body surface, e.g. in the lips and nail beds, it appears bluish in colour.

PAIN

Myocardial ischaemia causes pain. If the coronary arteries are narrowed due to arteriosclerosis, then pain in the chest (angina pectoris) results (see *Angina pectoris*, above). Angina can also be caused by hypertrophy of cardiac muscle cells. In this case the blood supply is unchanged, but the demands of the tissue are increased. The pain of a myocardial infarction is more severe than angina and it is not relieved by rest

INCREASED BLOOD VOLUME

In both left-sided and right-sided heart failure, there is accompanying fluid retention by the body. There are several likely mechanisms by which this occurs.

Whether the cause of the problem is primarily on the right or the left side of the heart, cardiac output is reduced. This reduces blood flow to the kidneys and thereby reduces the glomerular filtration rate, leading directly to a reduction in urine output and fluid retention.

The reduced renal blood flow also increases the release of renin from the juxtaglomerular cells, activates angiotensin and increases aldosterone secretion. Sodium ion and water reabsorption are thereby both increased.

A reduction in blood pressure leads to an increase in the secretion of ADH· from the posterior pituitary gland and thereby increases water reabsorption from the collecting ducts in the kidneys.

See also **Regulation of nephron function** (page 501), in Ch. 14, Renal Control of Body Fluid Volume and Composition.

Structure of blood vessels

Blood is pumped from the heart into the major **arteries** of the body. These branch to form increasingly smaller arteries and eventually **arterioles**. The latter are continuous with a close-meshed network of minute vessels, the **capillaries**. Blood then passes into larger **venules**, which join with one another to form **veins**; these unite to form the largest veins, which carry blood back to the heart.

With the exception of capillaries, all blood vessels are composed of three major layers, the tunica intima (inner), tunica media (middle) and tunica adventitia (outer) (Figure 12.15).

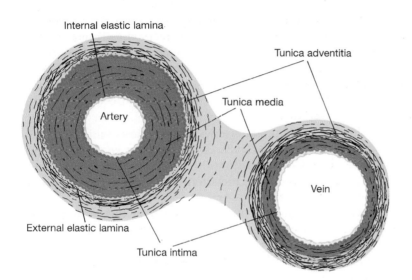

Figure 12.15 Cross-section through a muscular artery and a vein. Both vessels have walls that are made of three layers or tunicae: adventitia, media and intima In arteries, the tunica media contains sheets of elastic fibres, two of which, the internal and external elastic laminae, separate it from the other two layers. The walls of veins are considerably thinner than those of the corresponding artery, and the three layers are difficult to distinguish.

The **tunica intima** is composed of two primary layers. The inner layer consists of endothelium, which provides a smooth lining to the vessel that prevents blood clotting and facilitates blood flow; it also synthesizes several vasoactive substances. The outer layer of the tunica intima is composed of connective tissue containing elastic and collagen fibres.

The **tunica media** is the muscular layer of blood vessels. It is composed of smooth muscle cells and connective tissue fibres wound spirally. Contraction of the smooth muscle cells consequently reduces the diameter of the vessel.

The **tunica adventitia** is a connective tissue layer containing elastic and collagen fibres, continuous with the surrounding structures.

The composition and relative proportions of these three layers in the different blood vessels confer varying degrees of distensibility and contractility.

Elastic arteries (1–2.5 cm in diameter)

These vessels, e.g. the aorta and pulmonary artery, receive blood in bursts from the heart. During systole, when additional blood is added to the arteries, the vessels distend, while during diastole they recoil. This means that the flow of blood through the vessels is continuous despite the pulsatile nature of the heart beat.

The high degree of distensibility of these vessels is afforded by the large proportion of elastic fibres in the tunica media. These fibres are arranged in concentric sheets separated by smooth muscle and collagen fibres. Additional elasticity is conferred on the vessel by internal and external elastic laminae. The **internal elastic lamina** consists of a perforated sheet of elastic tissue forming the subendothelial layer of the tunica intima. The outermost layer of the tunica media constitutes the **external elastic lamina**.

Muscular arteries (0.1–1 cm in diameter)

These vessels, which include the brachial, femoral and radial arteries, distribute the blood under high pressure to the tissues. The walls are therefore strong and less elastic. The tunica media and tunica adventitia are generally thinner than those of elastic arteries and the tunica media contains a higher proportion of muscle cells.

Microcirculation

Blood flows from muscular arteries into arterioles within the tissues and then via metarterioles to capillaries, the smallest vessels of the cardiovascular system. Blood drains from the capillaries into venules and thence to the veins. The arterioles, metarterioles, capillaries and venules constitute the microcirculation.

In **arterioles** (up to 100 μm in diameter) the muscle layer is the predominant feature. Contraction or relaxation of the muscle fibres in the tunica media causes large changes in the diameter of these vessels and consequently they serve to regulate the amount of blood flowing into the capillaries and the pressure of blood behind them in the arterial system.

Branching from the arterioles are **metarterioles**. These vessels contain a discontinuous muscle layer but distally the muscle coat disap-

Figure 12.16 The microcirculation. Oxygenated blood (red) flows from the arteriole into the capillary bed through the arteriovenous anastomosis and, when the precapillary sphincters are open, the capillaries, before draining into the venules. Oxygen is given up to the cells of the tissue (not shown) indicated by the transition from red to blue.

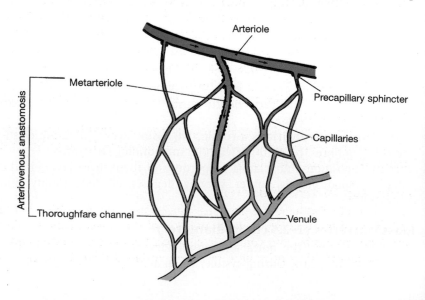

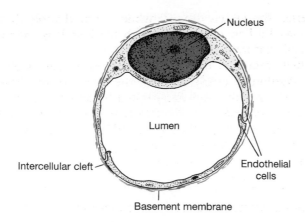

Figure 12.17 Cross section through a capillary. Parts of two endothelial cells are shown.

pears, giving rise to a **thoroughfare channel**, a vessel which is intermediate in structure between a capillary and a venule. The metarteriole and thoroughfare channel together constitute an **arteriovenous anastomosis** between arterioles and venules (Figure 12.16).

Capillaries branch from the metarterioles and, at the junction, one or two muscle cells encircle the capillary to form a contractile precapillary sphincter. Blood flow can therefore proceed either through the arteriovenous anastomosis alone or through the whole capillary bed.

Capillaries (5–7 µm in diameter) are composed of a single layer of endothelium with a little surrounding connective tissue; only one or two endothelial cells form the circumference of the vessel (Figure 12.17). They present, therefore, only a very thin barrier between blood and interstitial fluid. Lipid-soluble materials are able to pass through the cell membranes and the cytoplasm to and from the blood. The paucity of mitochondria is thought to limit cellular activity to passive transport in the main, although the large number of flask-shaped invaginations of the membrane (**caveolae**) suggest that pinocytosis is common. Sometimes, vesicles on opposite sides of a cell fuse to give rise to fused-vesicle channels through which relatively large molecules are able to pass. Some capillaries, such as those in the renal glomeruli, endocrine glands and intestinal villi, are **fenestrated**, i.e. they have pores that are closed by a very thin membrane (this membrane is lacking in the renal glomeruli). Other capillaries lack fenestrations but there are clefts between adjacent cells through which water and solutes can pass. Such clefts are absent from the capillaries of the brain, thus contributing to the 'blood–brain barrier'.

Blood from the capillary beds is drained into the **venules**, the smallest vessels of the venous system (20–30 µm in diameter). These possess very thin walls with indistinct layers.

Veins (up to 3 cm diameter)

The walls of veins have the same three layers as those of arteries, but the thickness of the wall is a lower proportion of the vessel diameter. Veins are more distensible and contain less muscle than arterial vessels and, as a consequence, they offer little resistance to blood flow. Veins can also accommodate relatively large changes in blood volume without a proportional increase in pressure. A 45% rise in the volume of blood within the veins only increases venous pressure by about 20 mmHg.

The larger veins possess pocket-like **valves** on their inner surfaces. These valves aid the unidirectional flow of blood back towards the heart when the vein is compressed by external forces. (see *Venous circulation*, below). If the valves become incompetent, veins become **varicose**, i.e. they have dilated and tortuous sections (**varicosities**). In the anal veins, these are known as **haemorrhoids**.

Distribution of the major arteries

In the systemic circulation, blood leaves the left ventricle in the **ascending aorta**, which passes over and behind the heart as the **aortic arch** and passes down as the **descending aorta**. The aortic arch gives off three major vessels. On the right side, the **brachiocephalic artery** arises and divides to form the **right common carotid** and **right subclavian arteries**. The **left common carotid** and **subclavian arteries** arise independently, directly from the aortic arch (Figure 12.18). Each subclavian artery arches laterally over the upper surface of the first rib, when it becomes known as the **axillary artery**. A little further down, below the armpit, it becomes the **brachial artery**, which divides at the elbow to form the **radial** and **ulnar arteries**, carrying blood to the forearm and hand.

Each common carotid divides into two branches, the **internal** and **external carotid arteries**. The internal branch supplies oxygenated blood to the cerebral hemispheres, communicating with the corresponding vessel on the other side through the circle of Willis.

The external branch carries blood to the more superficial structures of the head, i.e. muscle skin and bone.

Once the descending aorta has passed through the diaphragm it becomes known as the **abdominal aorta**. Just below the diaphragm it gives rise to three unpaired arteries, the **coeliac trunk** and the **superior** and **inferior mesenteric arteries**.

A pair of **renal arteries** come off the aorta at right angles and supply the kidneys with blood. Immediately below are the **testicular** (in the male) or **ovarian** (female) **arteries** to the reproductive organs.

The abdominal aorta divides above the pelvis to form the two **common iliac arteries**. Each of these then branches to form a small **internal iliac artery**, which supplies blood to the pelvis, and a large **external iliac artery**, which is the major trunk to the lower limb. In the region of the thigh this vessel becomes the **femoral artery** and behind the knee the **popliteal artery**, before dividing into **anterior** and **posterior tibial arteries**.

The heart also supplies the pulmonary circulation which carries blood from the right ventricle to the lungs. The **pulmonary trunk** passes upwards from the heart, parallel to the ascending aorta, and then divides into **right** and **left pulmonary arteries**, one to each lung.

See also **Cerebral circulation** (page 171), in Ch. 5, The Brain.

See also **Blood supply of the alimentary canal** (page 533), in Ch. 15, Digestion and Absorption of Food.

See also **Pulmonary circulation** (page 437), in Ch. 13, Respiration.

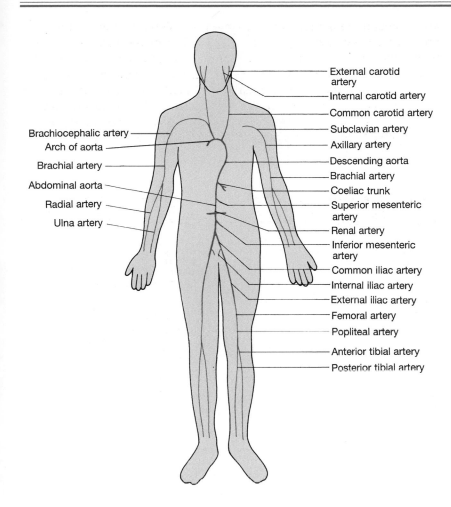

External carotid artery
Internal carotid artery
Common carotid artery
Subclavian artery
Axillary artery
Descending aorta
Brachial artery
Coeliac trunk
Superior mesenteric artery
Renal artery
Inferior mesenteric artery
Common iliac artery
Internal iliac artery
External iliac artery
Femoral artery
Popliteal artery
Anterior tibial artery
Posterior tibial artery

Brachiocephalic artery
Arch of aorta
Brachial artery
Abdominal aorta
Radial artery
Ulna artery

Figure 12.18   Major arteries of the body.

Distribution of the major veins

Blood from the upper regions of the body above the diaphragm drains through the **superior vena cava** into the right atrium, while that from the lower limbs and trunk passes through the **inferior vena cava**.

The **internal jugular vein** is the principal vessel that carries blood from the head and deeper tissues of the neck back towards the heart. The **external jugular vein** drains the superficial tissues of the neck. These two vessels drain into the **brachiocephalic vein**, which then unites with the corresponding vessel on the other side to form the superior vena cava (Figure 12.19). Since the latter is situated to the right of the midline, the left brachiocephalic vein is longer than the right.

In the arm, the main superficial vessels are the **cephalic** and **basilic veins**. The latter unites with the deep-lying **brachial vein** to form the **axillary vein**. This then joins with the cephalic vein to form the **subclavian vein**, which carries blood to the brachiocephalic vein and the heart.

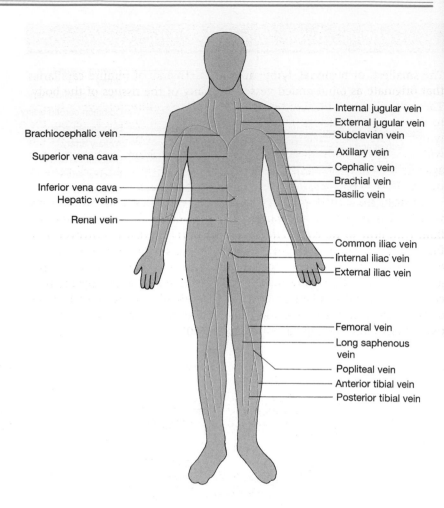

Internal jugular vein
External jugular vein
Subclavian vein
Axillary vein
Cephalic vein
Brachial vein
Basilic vein

Brachiocephalic vein
Superior vena cava
Inferior vena cava
Hepatic veins
Renal vein

Common iliac vein
Internal iliac vein
External iliac vein

Femoral vein
Long saphenous vein
Popliteal vein
Anterior tibial vein
Posterior tibial vein

Figure 12.19 Major veins of the body (broken line = deep veins).

See also **Hepatic circulation** (page 566), in Ch. 15, Digestion and Absorption of Food.

Blood from the foot drains into the **long saphenous vein** and deep-lying **anterior** and **posterior tibial veins**. The last two unite behind the knee to form the **popliteal vein**, which becomes the **femoral vein**. This vessel and the long saphenous unite to form the **external iliac vein**, which, like its counterpart in the arterial system, combines with the **internal iliac**; in this case forming the **common iliac vein**. The left and right common iliacs then unite and give rise to the inferior vena cava.

The major veins draining into the inferior vena cava include those from the kidneys – right and left **renal veins**; and the liver – right and left **hepatic veins**. Blood from most of the abdominal viscera, including the stomach, spleen, pancreas and intestine drains into the **hepatic portal vein** which, along with the hepatic artery, supplies the liver. The liver itself is then drained by the right and left hepatic veins, which carry blood directly to the inferior vena cava.

The lungs are drained by a separate system of blood vessels, the **pulmonary veins**, which carry oxygenated blood into the left atrium. There are two pulmonary veins, one draining each lung.

Structure and distribution of lymphatic vessels

The smallest, or terminal, lymphatics are networks of minute capillaries that originate as blind-ended vessels in many of the tissues of the body. These capillaries drain into larger vessels, which ultimately carry lymph to the cardiovascular system. Small solid masses of lymphoid tissue, the lymph nodes, are distributed throughout in such a manner that lymph will normally pass through one or two before reaching the blood. Other aggregations of lymphoid tissue are found in the walls of the alimentary tract as Peyer's patches, and in the spleen and thymus.

Lymphatic capillaries originate in the tissues and are narrow vessels with extremely thin walls consisting of a single layer of endothelium with little or no connective tissue support. There are, however, fine filaments that serve to anchor the cells to the surrounding tissues. The endothelial cells overlap at their edges and, since they are not firmly joined, molecules are able to pass between them. The arrangement of cells and anchoring filaments creates a series of 'valves', which allow one-way flow of large molecules such as proteins, and debris, from the tissue spaces into the capillaries (Figure 12.20).

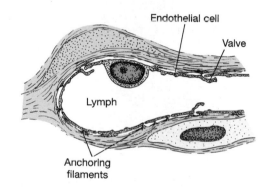

Figure 12.20 Lymphatic capillary. Endothelial cells are anchored by fine filaments, except at areas of overlap. The overlapping free borders of cells gives rise to 'valves' which enable the one-way flow of materials from the tissue spaces into the capillary lumen.

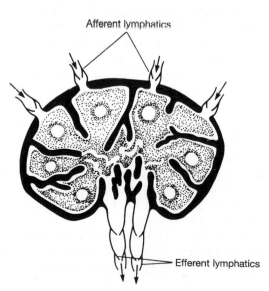

Figure 12.21 Section through a lymph node showing several afferent lymphatic vessels bringing lymph to the node and fewer, larger efferent vessels draining it.

Further details of lymph node structure and function can be found in **Lymph nodes** (page 347), in Ch. 11, Blood, Lymphoid Tissue and Immunity.

Lymphatic capillaries drain into larger **lymphatic vessels**, which have a wall structure similar to that of small veins; there is, for example, a tunica media with a small amount of smooth muscle tissue present in the largest vessels. Valves, similar to those observed in veins, are present in large numbers.

Lymph passes through one or more lymph nodes; there are always **several lymphatic afferent** vessels carrying lymph to the node but fewer **efferent lymphatic vessels** taking it away (Figure 12.21).

Ultimately lymph is carried to the cardiovascular system in the upper thorax. Lymph from the whole body, except the right side of the head and neck, right thorax and the right arm, drains via the **thoracic duct** into the junction of the left subclavian and left internal jugular veins. The upper right hand side of the body drains via the **right lymphatic duct** into the corresponding veins on the right side. Bicuspid valves at the entrances of the thoracic and right lymphatic ducts prevent the regurgitation of blood back into the lymphatic system (Figure 12.22).

Figure 12.22 Distribution of the major lymphatic vessels. Lymphatics in the [green] area drain through the right lymphatic duct into the circulation at the junction of the right subclavian and internal jugular veins, all others drain into the thoracic duct on the left side.

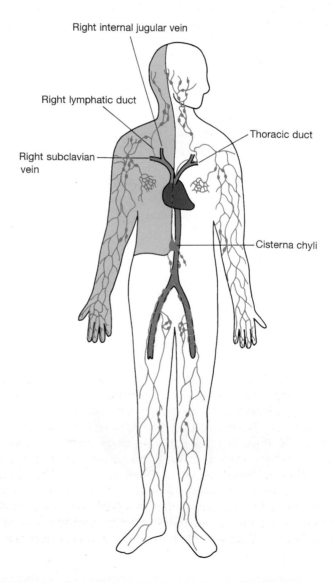

Right internal jugular vein

Right lymphatic duct

Right subclavian vein

Thoracic duct

Cisterna chyli

Virtually all tissues contain extensive networks of lymph capillaries, which lead into increasingly large lymphatic vessels. Unlike arteries and veins, however, lymphatics are not generally named; an exception to this is the **cisterna chyli**, an enlarged lymphatic trunk in the abdomen.

Blood flow and its control

Flow, pressure and resistance

Blood flows from areas of high pressure to areas of low pressure.

Blood flow (Q mL/min) is directly proportional to the difference in the pressure at the start and that at the end of the journey (ΔP).

$$Q \propto \Delta P$$

The other factor which determines the rate of blood flow in a given blood vessel is the frictional resistance (R) offered to the flow of blood by the wall of the vessel. If the resistance is high, it will reduce the rate of blood flow through it. Thus, the rate of blood flow is inversely proportional to the resistance offered to it

$$Q \propto \frac{1}{R}$$

Putting these two equations together:

$$Q = \frac{\Delta P}{R}$$

$$\text{Blood flow} = \frac{\text{pressure difference}}{\text{resistance}}$$

This formula is known as **Poiseuille's law**.

The resistance (R) to blood flow offered by the vessel is determined by three factors; the radius of the vessel (r), the length of the vessel (L) and the viscosity of the blood (η).

$$\text{Resistance} \propto \frac{\text{viscosity} \times \text{length}}{\text{radius}^4}$$

$$R \propto \frac{\eta L}{r^4}$$

Thus a thick fluid (high viscosity) will have a higher resistance than a thin one, a long tube will offer more resistance than a short one and a narrow vessel will offer more resistance than a wide one.

Physiologically, the importance of this formula is that resistance, and therefore blood flow, is markedly affected by small changes in vessel diameter. It can be seen from the formula that resistance is inversely proportional to the fourth power of the vessel radius. Thus doubling the radius will increase blood flow by a factor of 16 (i.e. $2^4 = 2 \times 2 \times 2 \times 2 = 16$). Since the arterioles are structurally adapted for vasoconstriction or vasodilation, it is these vessels that primarily affect the flow of blood to the tissues beyond. They are therefore referred to as **resistance vessels**.

Table 12.2 Mean blood pressures (mmHg) in the systemic circulation; body in horizontal position eliminating regional differences due to gravity

Vessel	Start	End	Pressure drop
Aorta	100	100	negligible
Large arteries	100	96	4
Small arteries	96	85	11
Arterioles	85	30	55
Capillaries	30	10	20
Venules–veins	10	0	10

The pressure of blood in the systemic circulation progressively falls from an average value of about 100 mmHg in the aorta to approximately 0 mmHg in the right atrium. (These are 'gauge' pressures, so that a value of 0 means equal to atmospheric pressure.)

The drop in arterial pressure in each part of the circulation is proportional to the resistance offered to the flow of blood. It can be seen from Table 12.2 that the most dramatic drop in blood pressure occurs as blood flows through the arterioles. They offer about half of the total peripheral resistance of blood vessels.

Arterial and arteriolar circulation

ARTERIAL PULSE

As the heart pumps blood into the arteries during systole, but not during diastole, blood flow through the arterial system is phasic. (The recoil in the elastic arteries that occurs during diastole, however, ensures that blood still flows during this phase.)

The alternating expansion and recoil of elastic arteries sets up a pressure wave (pulse), which travels along the walls of the vessels with the same frequency as the heart beat. Pulse rate, which therefore equals heart rate, can be measured at sites where an artery lies close to the body's surface and can be compressed against a bone. It is most commonly measured in the radial artery at the wrist.

ARTERIAL BLOOD PRESSURE

Blood pressure is a type of **hydrostatic pressure** and is the force exerted by the blood against the blood vessel wall.

Using Poiseuille's law, a definition of mean arterial blood pressure can be obtained:

Pressure = flow × resistance

or

Mean arterial blood pressure (mmHg) =
cardiac output (L/min) × peripheral resistance (PRU).

The peripheral resistance represents the total resistance to blood flow offered by the systemic circulation. It is known as the total peripheral resistance or systemic vascular resistance.

If the pressure difference between two points in a vessel is 1 mmHg, and the flow is 1 mL/s, then resistance is defined as 1 **peripheral resistance unit (PRU)**.

Measurement of blood pressure

'Blood pressure' is conventionally taken as the pressure of blood in the brachial artery, the closest vessel to the heart within which pressure can be measured easily. Two measurements are taken; the first, **systolic pressure**, corresponds to the pressure within the artery when the heart is pumping blood into the aorta, i.e. during systole. The second reading is taken when the heart is relaxed and no blood is being added to the aorta, although blood is still flowing along the brachial artery; this is the **diastolic pressure**.

Blood pressure is conventionally quoted as:

$$\frac{\text{systolic pressure}}{\text{diastolic pressure}} \quad \text{or} \quad \frac{\text{SP}}{\text{DP}}$$

and may be expected to be of the order of 120/80 mmHg in a healthy young adult, at rest. Blood pressures are normally quoted in this way; the equivalent SI measurement is: 16.0/10.6 kPa.

The most accurate measurements of blood pressure are made directly, by inserting the measuring device into a blood vessel or by taking blood from the vessel to the device. Such methods are obviously unsuitable for routine use and so an indirect, or non-invasive, technique is normally used.

The **sphygmomanometer** (developed in 1896 by Riva-Rocci) incorporates a mercury-filled U-tube (manometer) to measure pressure. Although instruments of this type are still used, and will be described here, other more sophisticated automatic and semiautomatic devices with digital or dial read-outs are also now used.

The two limbs of the sphygmomanometer are uneven: one is squat and the other, which bears the pressure scale, is narrow and much longer. The short limb is connected by a tube to a cloth-covered rubber bag or cuff (Figure 12.23).

When measuring blood pressure the cuff is wrapped around the upper arm and the pressure is increased by inflating it, using a rubber bulb. Once the pressure in the cuff is above that in the brachial artery, blood flow to the lower arm will cease. A valve next to the bulb is then opened so that air slowly escapes from the cuff; once the pressure falls just below the systolic pressure in the artery, blood will be able to enter the lower arm during systole, but not during diastole. This may be felt at the wrist (as the arterial pulse) and also heard as a tapping sound when a **stethoscope** is applied over the artery at the inside of the elbow. A manometer reading is taken at the point when the sound first appears/the pulse is first felt; this reading corresponds to systolic pressure.

As the pressure in the cuff continues to fall, blood will be able to pass

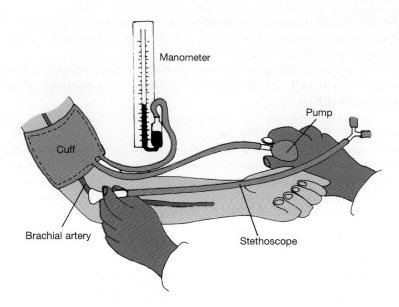

Figure 12.23 Measurement of arterial blood pressure using a sphygmomanometer.

into the lower arm throughout more of the heart's cycle. When the cuff pressure falls just below diastolic pressure the sounds will disappear, or at least change character, becoming muffled (although the pulse will still be felt). At this point the pressure is noted; this reading corresponds to diastolic pressure.

The difference between the two pressures, i.e. SP–DP is referred to as the **pulse pressure** and in this case would be 40 mmHg. The **mean pressure** is the average pressure throughout the cycle, and since systole has a shorter duration than diastole it is a little lower than the arithmetic average of systolic and diastolic pressures. In an individual with an SP of 120 mmHg and a DP of 80 mmHg, the average pressure would be 100 mmHg, while the mean pressure would be about 96 mmHg.

The precise magnitude of blood pressure is dependent upon a large number of factors, not least of which are the conditions under which it is measured. Basal blood pressure can only be reliably measured 10 or 12 hours after a meal, after resting in a warm room for at least 30 minutes. Normally only casual blood pressure is measured.

NEURAL CONTROL OF ARTERIOLE DIAMETER

Arterioles are innervated by noradrenergic sympathetic neurones. There is always some activity in these neurones causing tonic contraction or **vasomotor tone**. Increased activity in the sympathetic fibres causes **vasoconstriction**, whereas decreased activity causes **vasodilation**. In general, neural control of arterioles is concerned with regulating peripheral resistance and hence blood pressure, rather than serving the metabolic needs of the tissues.

Sympathetic discharge to the vessels is controlled by the vasomotor centre in the medulla oblongata (see Figures 12.12 and 12.27). This centre is divided into a depressor and a pressor area. The depressor area is connected by inhibitory neurones (descending in the white matter) to preganglionic sympathetic fibres in the spinal cord. When the centre is active, the inhibitory influence on the preganglionic fibres reduces the rate of impulses travelling to the arterioles, which results in vasodilation. The pressor area is connected by excitatory neurones to the preganglionic sympathetic fibres, so that an increased frequency of impulses in these fibres will increase activity in the peripheral sympathetic neurones and cause vasoconstriction.

In some animals, and possibly in humans, the resistance vessels in skeletal muscles have an additional sympathetic innervation by cholinergic neurones, which cause vasodilation. These neurones are stimulated at the onset of physical exercise, or even before it begins, so that muscle blood flow increases 'in anticipation' of the increased metabolic demands of active skeletal muscle. The control of activity of the sympathetic vasodilator neurones is directly from the hypothalamus and not via the vasomotor centre.

Vascular reflexes

Just as changes in heart rate and stroke volume can be brought about as reflex responses to alterations in blood pressure and blood chemistry (see *Cardiac reflexes,* above) so too are changes in the diameters of arterioles.

A drop in blood pressure not only results in a reflex increase in heart rate but also peripheral vasoconstriction. Thus peripheral resistance is raised, with a consequent rise in pressure.

A decrease in blood oxygen levels and/or a rise in carbon dioxide and hydrogen ion concentration, detected by the chemoreceptors in the carotid and aortic bodies, promotes sympathetic activity, which will induce vasoconstriction. This is in marked contrast to the response to a local rise in carbon dioxide/fall in oxygen levels.

Neural control of arterial blood pressure, below, provides an account of how the cardiac and vascular responses to changes in arterial blood pressure are integrated.

LOCAL CONTROL OF ARTERIOLE DIAMETER

Several local factors that increase or decrease arteriole diameter control the rate of blood flow in specific organs in accordance with their metabolic requirements. An increase in metabolic activity, as for example in skeletal muscle during physical exercise, is accompanied by increased blood flow through the active areas. This phenomenon is known as **active hyperaemia**. There are several possible candidates that have been shown experimentally to mediate this vasodilation directly: they include a fall in oxygen levels, a rise in carbon dioxide, H^+ or K^+ levels, adenosine, adenosine nucleotides and temperature.

A similar effect is observed following the strong vasoconstriction induced by, for example, immersion of the arm in very cold water. During the period of vasoconstriction there is inadequate blood flow to the arm (ischaemia); as a result metabolites produced by the tissues are not removed in the normal way. On removing the arm from the cold water, there follows a period of increased blood flow (**reactive hyperaemia**), producing a warm, red arm. The additional blood flow compensates for the period of deprivation and enables the excess metabolites to be washed away. Once this is achieved the stimuli for arteriolar dilation are removed and blood flow returns to normal.

Histamine, which is released from mast cells during the inflammatory response, is a powerful vasodilator. Bradykinin, formed from a plasma globulin by the action of the enzyme kallikrein, exhibits similar properties. Some prostaglandins (e.g. prostaglandin I$_2$) also have vasodilator properties.

Vasoactive substances released by vascular endothelium

The endothelial lining of blood vessels synthesizes several vasoactive substances. **Endothelium-derived relaxing factor** (**EDRF**) was the name given to an unknown substance or substances one of which has subsequently been identified as **nitric oxide**. Nitric oxide only lasts for a few seconds in the circulation before being chemically degraded; it can, therefore, only act locally.

It is likely that EDRF is secreted continuously by the vascular endothelium of all blood vessels, where it exerts a vasodilating influence. This could be regarded as the equivalent of basal levels of parasympathetic activity, which is largely absent from blood vessels.

EDRF also regulates blood flow into tissues. When the blood flow in the microcirculation increases (by local mechanisms) there is secondary increase in flow in the arteries leading into the tissue. The rise in blood flow increases shear stress caused by the blood dragging against the artery walls, which stimulates the release of EDRF. This causes arterial dilation and further increases blood flow. This mechanism makes changes in the microcirculation much more effective in increasing tissue blood flow.

In several cardiovascular diseases, including arteriosclerosis, the endothelium is impaired, so that EDRF is less effective and microtubular spasm, therefore, more likely.

Another compound released by the vascular endothelium, **endothelin-1**, is a very powerful vasoconstrictor. Its physiological role is currently unknown.

CIRCULATING VASOACTIVE SUBSTANCES

When the sympathetic nervous system is active it stimulates the release of adrenaline and noradrenaline from the adrenal medullae. **Noradrenaline** causes general vasoconstriction, whereas **adrenaline** causes vasoconstriction in most sites but vasodilation in skeletal muscle and coronary arterioles.

Angiotensin II, formed when renin is released from the kidney (when blood volume or pressure falls), causes generalized vasoconstriction.

Antidiuretic hormone (**arginine vasopressin**), released by the anterior pituitary gland, has a pressor (vasoconstrictor) action on arterioles.

Capillary circulation

The structure of capillaries facilitates the exchange of materials between blood and tissues. Blood flow through the tissues is varied according to its metabolic rate.

Blood flow through a tissue can either proceed through the arteriovenous anastomosis alone or through the entire capillary bed. Which route is taken is controlled by the state of contraction of the precapillary sphincters. When these are closed, blood flows through the metarteriole and thoroughfare channel directly from arterioles to venules. As oxygen level falls and metabolites from cells supplied by the capillary bed accumulate, they cause dilation of the precapillary sphincters (in the same way that they cause arteriolar dilation). Once the sphincters are dilated, blood will flow through the capillary bed until the metabolites are washed away, thus removing the stimulus so the sphincters close again. This is an example of **autoregulation**, whereby the perfusion of a tissue is controlled by its own metabolic rate.

In this way blood flow through the microcirculation alternates between the arteriovenous anastomoses alone and the entire capillary bed. This constant change of route is known as **vasomotion**.

The capillaries are passive vessels that simply receive whatever blood is delivered to them, regulated by the arterioles and the precapillary sphincters.

The velocity of blood flow through the capillaries is very slow, allowing sufficient time for the exchange of nutrients and waste products between the blood and the tissues. The movement of substances across the capillary walls is always passive, i.e. by diffusion either through or between the endothelial cells. Because of the passive nature of this exchange, the composition of plasma and interstitial fluid is essentially the same (except for the amount of protein, molecules of which are generally too large to pass out of the blood).

Formation and reabsorption of interstitial fluid

The interstitial fluid that bathes the cells of the body is their immediate source of nutrients and waste disposal route. Interstitial fluid is not, however, static but is continually being produced from the blood by **bulk flow** by filtration through clefts between the endothelial cells. The fluid is subsequently reabsorbed, either directly into the blood vessels or indirectly via the lymphatics. The turnover of fluid is of the order of 20 litres per day (about seven times the total plasma volume).

A mechanism for the formation and reabsorption of interstitial fluid was first suggested by Ernest Starling (1866–1927). Starling hypothesized that there is net **filtration** of fluid out of the blood into the interstitial compartment at the arterial end of capillary beds and a net **reabsorption** of fluid back into the blood at the venous end.

The movement of fluid is caused by a net pressure difference across the capillary wall. There are four individual pressures involved: **capillary hydrostatic pressure, plasma colloid osmotic pressure, interstitial fluid colloid osmotic pressure** and **interstitial fluid hydrostatic pressure** (Figure 12.24).

Figure 12.24 Starling's pressures promoting bulk flow of fluid across capillary walls. IFHP = interstitial fluid hydrostatic pressure (subatmospheric except in oedema); CHP = capillary hydrostatic pressure; IFCOP = interstitial fluid colloid osmotic pressure; PCOP = plasma colloid osmotic pressure.

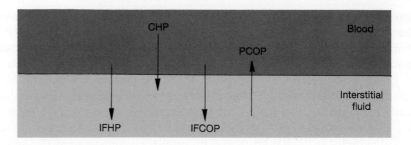

Capillary hydrostatic pressure (CHP)

CHP is simply the pressure of the blood contained within the capillary and represents a force acting outwards across the vessel wall. The value of this pressure depends upon arterial blood pressure, venous blood pressure and the position of the capillary within a capillary bed. A capillary near to the arterial inflow will have a higher pressure than one at a site nearer the venous outflow. This is because the resistance to flow offered by the capillary wall causes the pressure to fall.

Plasma colloid osmotic pressure (PCOP)

PCOP is the osmotic pressure exerted by plasma proteins. The effect of osmotic pressure is to draw solvent towards particles in solution. Thus the particles in plasma tend to draw fluid (strictly water, but solutes will follow by diffusion) into the blood, whereas particles in the interstitial fluid will tend to draw fluid out of the blood into the interstitial compartment.

Since there is considerably more protein in the plasma than in interstitial fluid it is evident that there will be a much greater tendency for water to be attracted into the capillary than for water to be drawn out.

Interstitial fluid colloid osmotic pressure (IFCOP)

IFCOP is the osmotic pressure exerted by protein in interstitial fluid. The amount of protein present in interstitial fluid varies according to the permeability of the capillary wall. Thus in some sites, such as skeletal muscle, there is very little interstitial protein, whereas in the intestine and liver there is a much larger amount present. These regional variations can be attributed to differences in structure of the capillary walls at different sites. Capillaries in skeletal muscle have a thick basement membrane and no fenestrations or pores, while in liver and intestine the basement membrane is much thinner and there are fenestrations. Passage of protein across such a structure is therefore easier.

IFCOP acts to draw fluid from the blood into the interstitial compartment.

Interstitial fluid hydrostatic pressure (IFHP)

IFHP varies according to the volume of fluid present and the distensibility of the compartment. It is now generally held that IFHP is subatmospheric, i.e. a negative pressure, which acts as a force to draw fluid out of the blood.

Three of the four forces (CHP, IFCOP and IFHP) that act across the capillary wall promote filtration, while PCOP is an absorptive force. At the arterial end of capillary beds, the sum of the filtration forces exceeds the absorptive force and therefore there is a net fluid movement out of the blood into the interstitial compartment.

Pressure (mmHg)

CHP	30
IFCOP	8
IFHP	3 (negative)
PCOP	28

Thus the total filtration force across the capillary wall =
$$30 + 8 + 3 = 41 \, \text{mmHg}.$$
This is opposed by the absorptive force $\qquad = 28 \, \text{mmHg}.$
The net filtration pressure is therefore $\quad 41 - 28 \quad = 13 \, \text{mmHg}.$

At the venous end of the capillary beds the capillary hydrostatic has fallen so that the filtration force is significantly reduced. Changes in the other values are small and can be ignored.

Pressure (mmHg)

CHP	10
IFCOP	8
IFHP	3 (negative)
PCOP	28

Thus the total filtration force across the capillary wall =
$$10 + 8 + 3 = 21 \, \text{mmHg}$$

The absorptive force now exceeds the total filtration force, so that the net force becomes absorptive.

The net absorptive force is therefore $28 - 21 = 7 \, \text{mmHg}$

Fluid, therefore, moves from the interstitial compartment back into the blood.

It can be seen that the net pressure forcing fluid out of the blood at the arterial end of a capillary bed is greater than the net pressure causing reabsorption of fluid back into the blood at the venous end (13 mmHg compared with 7 mmHg). The result of this is that more fluid is filtered into the interstitial compartment than is reabsorbed from it into the blood vessels. The excess fluid is reabsorbed into the lymphatic capillaries and returned to the venous system in the neck. The total volume of fluid transported in this way is of the order of 2–4 litres per day.

The pressures across capillary walls in the pulmonary circulation differ from those in the systemic circulation. A comparison of the two is given in Table 13.1.

Oedema

Oedema is the presence of excess fluid in the interstitial compartment. As the fluid accumulates it raises interstitial fluid hydrostatic pressure so that it may become positive. The causes of oedema relate directly to changes in the factors influencing the formation and reabsorption of interstitial fluid. It may be caused, therefore, by an increase in capillary hydrostatic pressure, a drop in plasma colloid osmotic pressure, increased capillary permeability, a rise in interstitial colloid osmotic pressure or obstruction to lymphatic drainage.

PHYSIOLOGICAL CAUSES OF OEDEMA

Raised capillary hydrostatic pressure

The main force promoting filtration of fluid out of the capillary is the hydrostatic pressure of fluid within the vessel. If this is raised then more fluid will be pushed out of the blood into the interstitial compartment. There are two principal ways in which the CHP can be increased, by increased blood flow into the capillary bed or decreased blood flow away from it.

Arteriolar dilation will increase blood flow into capillaries. In the process of inflammation, histamine is released from mast cells and this causes arteriolar dilation. The swelling seen during inflammation is due, in part, to this effect.

High arterial blood pressure (hypertension) does not, as might be expected, result in oedema, because of a form of autoregulation. When arterial blood pressure rises, the supply of blood into the tissues would correspondingly increase if it were not for self-regulating mechanisms that counteract this tendency. One of these, known as the **Bayliss reflex**, results in the contraction of arteries and arterioles after the smooth muscle in their walls is stretched by a rise in the pressure of blood within them.

Any form of **venous obstruction** could result in oedema simply by reducing blood flow away from the capillary and resulting in an excess of blood in the capillaries. The obstruction may be local, such as a **thrombus** (blood clot) or **embolus** (a variety of substances, e.g. air, fat or thrombus, transported to the site in the blood), in which case the resultant oedema would be confined to the area drained by that particular vein. However, a failing heart is another cause of venous obstruction. If the right side of the heart is pumping ineffectively (**right-sided heart failure**), then the venous return from the great veins will be impaired. This will impede the flow of blood from all over the body and cause **generalized oedema**.

Pulmonary oedema can result from **left-sided heart failure**. Blood flow from the lungs in the pulmonary veins is impaired and so therefore is blood flow from the pulmonary capillaries. As the pulmonary bed becomes congested with blood and its hydrostatic pressure rises, excess fluid will eventually be pushed out of the capillaries. As there is very little interstitial space in the lungs, the fluid flows into the alveoli, causing a drowning sensation.

Severe **Na+ and water retention** can occur in kidney disease. Since Na+ concentration is much higher in extracellular than intracellular fluid, the extracellular fluid compartment expands, the osmotic 'pull' of the excess Na+ causing water to be retained. The expansion of blood volume raises venous pressure and thence capillary hydrostatic pressure.

Lowered plasma colloid osmotic pressure

The return of some 90% of the volume of fluid added to the interstitial compartment from the blood vessels is normally brought about by the absorptive pull of plasma proteins. If this plasma colloid osmotic pressure is reduced, then the return of fluid back to the blood will also be reduced and oedema will result.

Plasma protein concentration is dependent upon both its rate of production and its rate of removal. If plasma protein production falls or its rate of removal rises, a fall in concentration will result. A fall in protein synthesis can be caused by a failing liver in conditions such as **hepatitis** or **cirrhosis**. **Malnutritional oedema** results when there is such a low intake of food that plasma proteins are both used as energy sources and replaced at an insufficient rate.

Excessive loss of plasma protein can be caused by kidney disease in which the glomerular membrane becomes more permeable to protein and allows more of it through into the nephrons. Whereas proximal tubules normally reabsorb all of the small amount of protein that filters through the glomerular membrane, an excessive amount results in proteinuria, a lowering of plasma protein concentration and corresponding oedema. The term **nephrotic syndrome** refers to a condition of generalized oedema accompanied by proteinuria and reduced plasma albumin. It is usually caused by **glomerulonephritis**.

Increased capillary permeability

If the capillary wall becomes more permeable, then more fluid will be filtered out into the interstitial compartment and it will contain a greater amount of protein than normal. This is commonly seen in the **inflammatory response**, in which capillaries become more permeable due to the loosening of the junctions between the endothelial cells. Superficial **burns**, in which areas of skin are lost, can be the cause of large losses of protein-rich fluid from inflamed tissue.

Raised interstitial fluid colloid osmotic pressure

The amount of protein in the interstitial compartment affects the osmotic pressure of the fluid and contributes to the filtration pressure that draws fluid into the area. An increase in the amount of protein in the compartment can lead to oedema, as in the inflammatory response. The condition of **myxoedema**, which is caused by a deficiency of thyroid hormones, results in an excess of proteoglycans, mainly hyaluronic acid, in the ground substance of the connective tissue surrounding capillaries. This 'holds' water in the interstitial compartment as a gel. The resultant oedema is different from that resulting from other causes in that it is described as 'non-pitting'. This means that a finger pressed on to the skin will not result in the formation of a pit.

See also **Tri-iodothyronine (T3) and thyroxine (T4)** (page 624), in Ch. 16, Endocrine Physiology.

Blocked lymphatic drainage

Typically, around 10% of the volume of blood transferred from the blood to the interstitium flows into the lymphatics before rejoining the blood in the neck (about 2 litres per day). If, however, the lymphatic drainage is obstructed, then fluid will be unable to flow away and oedema will result. Lymphatic obstruction may be due to inflammatory conditions of the lymphatic vessels themselves, external pressure, such as a tumour, or even surgical excision.

EFFECTS OF OEDEMA

As hydrostatic pressure in the interstitium rises, it reduces net filtration pressure and more fluid flows into the lymphatic vessels (provided that they are not blocked), thereby providing a mechanism that reduces the oedema. This mechanism is limited, however, because if oedema progresses the interstitium is enlarged and the anchoring filaments attached to the lymphatic capillaries come under tension. This causes the endothelial flap valves to remain open and allow fluid back out of the lymphatic capillaries into the interstitial space. In addition, the larger lymphatic vessels are compressed by the raised interstitial fluid hydro-static pressure. Once the latter rises above atmospheric pressure, lymphatic drainage cannot increase sufficiently to drain the excess fluid.

Venous circulation

Veins are known as **capacitance vessels** because they can accommo-date a relatively large increase in blood volume without an equivalent rise in pressure. This is because their thin walls are more distensible than those of arterial vessels.

Increased activity in the sympathetic vasoconstrictor neurones supplying the veins causes **venoconstriction**, which reduces the disten-sibility of the vessel walls and thereby raises venous pressure. The slight reduction in vessel diameter has a negligible effect on resistance to flow, however, and the overall effect of venoconstriction is to increase **venous return**. Venous pressure is low compared with arterial pressure despite the fact that about 60% of the total blood volume is present in the venous system. Pressure in the venules is 10–15 mmHg so that the total pressure drop back to the right atrium is around 10 mmHg, as right atrial pressure is 0–5 mmHg. These values apply when the subject is in the horizontal position.

If the subject stands upright then the pressures in the circulatory system are affected by the weight of blood in the vessels. The pressure in the veins of the feet is approximately 90 mmHg because of the weight of the column of blood between them and right atrium.

Conversely, the neck veins are collapsed by atmospheric pressure (so that the pressure is 0). The non-collapsible sinuses within the skull, on the other hand, contain blood at less than atmospheric pressure, e.g. –10 mmHg in the sagittal sinus. The thoracic veins are not collapsed because intrathoracic pressure is lower than the pressure within these veins.

Venous return from the lower parts of the body to the heart is aided in several ways: the skeletal muscle pump, the presence of valves in the veins, movements of the thorax, and lying flat.

Leg movements compress the veins that run through the muscles and squeeze the blood (**skeletal muscle pumps**). The valves ensure that blood flows towards the heart.

The **valves** are orientated within the veins so that they are flattened

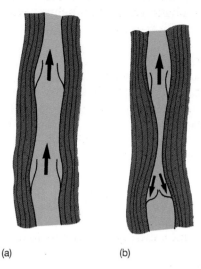

Figure 12.25 The skeletal muscle pump in the legs. **(a)** When the muscle relaxes, the valves are all open and blood flows towards the heart. **(b)** When the muscle contracts blood is squeezed in both directions. The valve nearest to the heart opens and allows blood flow, whereas the valve furthest from the heart closes and prevents backflow of blood.

against the walls of the vessels when blood is moving towards the heart. Backward pressure, on the other hand, causes the sac-like segments of the valves to fill with blood so that back flow is prevented. When the vein is squeezed by muscular contraction, blood therefore moves in one direction only (Figure 12.25).

During **inspiration** the diaphragm descends, raising abdominal pressure. This pressure rise compresses the abdominal veins and propels blood towards the heart. As the intrathoracic pressure falls (as the thoracic volume increases) it aids the flow of blood into the thorax and hence to the heart.

When **lying flat** the gravitational pull on the venous system is greatly reduced so that venous return is improved.

A rough estimate of **central venous pressure** can be made with the subject lying with the head and chest at an angle of 30° to the horizontal. In this position the distended portion of the external jugular veins is clearly visible. The height of the upper limit of distension above the right atrium gives the venous pressure in millimetres of blood.

Alternatively, **peripheral venous pressure** can be measured by inserting a catheter into an arm vein at the level of the right atrium; the catheter is filled with sterile saline connected to a manometer. The mean pressure in the antecubital vein is about 7 mmHg.

Formation and flow of lymph

A major function of lymph is that it drains the tissues of excess fluid and other materials, such as proteins and leucocytes, and returns them to the blood. Approximately 2 litres of lymph is carried to the cardiovascular system every day, about 80% via the thoracic duct. The rate of flow through the system depends upon a number of factors, including its rate of formation, the contractile nature of the lymphatic walls and a number of external forces.

As fluid leaks out of the capillaries of the cardiovascular system, small quantities (some 60–100 g/d) of protein are also carried out. This protein accumulates in the tissue spaces and its presence increases the tonicity of interstitial fluid, which, in turn, leads to the osmotic retention of water. Excess fluid and protein are forced into the blind-ended lymphatic capillaries through the 'valves' in their walls. This is a particularly important mechanism since it provides the only route by which protein can be removed from the interstitial spaces and returned to the blood.

An increase in the pressure of the fluid in the interstitial spaces increases the rate of formation of lymph and results in increased delivery to the cardiovascular system.

The mechanisms that promote the flow of fluid within the lymphatic vessels are similar to those that promote the flow of blood in veins ascending to the heart. That is, the muscle and respiratory pumps tend to draw fluid along the vessels, which, like the veins, have valves ensuring unidirectional flow. Some research has reported that lymph nodes contract periodically, acting as pumps which helps to propel the lymph through the vessels.

In addition, the larger lymph ducts themselves have a smooth muscle component in their walls and this, in conjunction with the valves that are present, helps to propel the lymph towards the cardiovascular system. Increased fluid pressure in a section of a lymphatic between two valves stretches the wall and causes it to contract, forcing lymph into the next segment. Thus lymph is propelled from segment to segment. In the terminal capillaries lymph pressure may be very low, around 3 mmHg, but contraction of the wall of a lymphatic trunk may generate pressures as high as 50 mmHg.

Lymph is similar in composition to blood plasma, apart from the variable amount of protein present. Thus lymph that originates in skeletal muscle only contains about 15% of the amount of protein found in blood plasma, while lymph from the liver contains nearly as much protein as plasma. Lymph originating in the specialized lymphatics (**lacteals**) in the wall of the small intestine contains large amounts of lipid and indeed the lymphatics are the principal route through which dietary fat is taken to the blood. Foreign materials such as bacteria are also found in lymph and are normally removed at the lymph nodes by macrophages.

> The origins and functions of macrophages are considered in **Monocytes** (page 343), in Ch. 11, Blood, Lymphoid Tissue and Immunity.

Integrated cardiovascular function

Determinants of arterial blood pressure

Poiseuille's law relating blood flow to pressure and resistance,

$$Q = \frac{\Delta P}{R},$$

can be applied to the whole systemic circulation (from the aorta to the venae cavae just entering the heart). In this case, the total blood flow is equal to the cardiac output and the pressure drop is equal to mean arterial pressure minus late vena cava pressure,

i.e. $100\,\text{mmHg} - 0\,\text{mmHg} = 100\,\text{mmHg}.$

The resistance part of the equation refers to total peripheral resistance (systemic vascular resistance) which is the combined frictional resistance to blood flow offered by all of the vessels of the systemic circulation.

Thus

$$\text{Cardiac output} = \frac{\text{Mean arterial pressure}}{\text{Total peripheral resistance}}$$

rearranged

Mean arterial pressure = cardiac output × peripheral resistance.

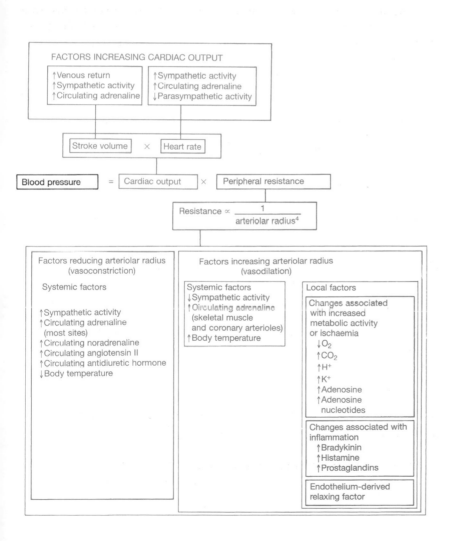

Figure 12.26 Principal determinants of arterial blood pressure.

Therefore, all the factors affecting cardiac output and peripheral resistance will influence arterial pressure. These factors are summarized in Figure 12.26.

Control of arterial blood pressure

Variations in the body's metabolic rate are accompanied by corresponding changes in blood flow, which is itself dependent upon blood pressure. Blood pressure varies considerably depending upon bodily activity so that, for example, during sleep it is low and during vigorous exercise very high. Pressure variations are not, however, as wide as they might be because of the physiological mechanisms which moderate such changes. Arterial pressure is maintained within this restricted range of values by two types of response. There are rapid, short-term effects that moderate changes induced, for example, by standing up quickly after lying down. Such control is mediated by nerve reflexes affecting cardiac output and arteriole diameter. In the long-term, the level of arterial blood pressure is determined by the blood volume, which itself depends on a balance between fluid intake and fluid losses. A 2% increase in blood volume can result in an increase in arterial blood pressure of as much as 50% and, although the rapidly acting control systems will serve to reduce this change, the long-term adjustments will be by increased fluid loss from the kidneys.

NEURAL CONTROL OF ARTERIAL BLOOD PRESSURE

Neural reflex responses to changes in arterial blood pressure, volume and, in some instances, composition are very rapid and therefore promote an equally rapid removal of the stimulus and return to previous levels.

Baroreceptor reflex

The principal action of the baroreceptor reflex is that it brings blood pressure back up when it falls. On standing up after lying down, for example, blood pools in the veins in the lower half of the body. Since more than 60% of the blood is in the veins, this is a very important phenomenon. The consequence of venous pooling is that venous return falls, which leads to an immediate drop in stroke volume and thus cardiac output. The fall in venous return therefore results in a reduction in arterial blood pressure (**postural hypotension**), which initiates the baroreceptor reflex, which in turn raises the pressure again. A similar sequence of events follows a **haemorrhage**.

A fall in arterial blood pressure reduces the frequency of impulses emitted from the baroreceptors. This information is conveyed to the cardiovascular centres, which respond immediately by increasing sympathetic activity and decreasing parasympathetic outflow to the heart, thereby increasing cardiac output and raising blood pressure (Figure 12.27).

Simultaneously there is increased sympathetic discharge to the veins, resulting in venoconstriction, increased venous return and thus increased cardiac output. Sympathetic discharge to the arterioles also

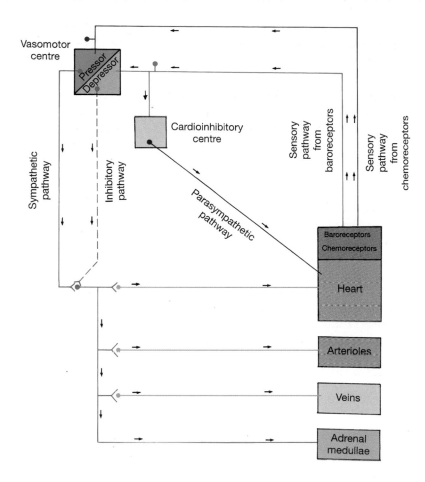

Figure 12.27 Control of arterial blood pressure: baroreceptor and chemoreceptor reflex pathways. Baroreceptors in the aortic arch and carotid sinuses send impulses to the depressor area of the vasomotor centre and cardioinhibitory centre located in the medulla oblongata. Chemoreceptors in the aortic and carotid bodies send impulses to the pressor area of the vasomotor centre, which is linked, via sympathetic pathways, to the heart, arterioles, veins and adrenal medullae. The cardioinhibitory centre is linked to the heart via the parasympathetic nervous system and the depressor area of the vasomotor centre inhibits sympathetic pathways in the spinal cord.

increases, thereby increasing peripheral resistance and raising blood pressure.

Increased sympathetic activity also leads to stimulation of the adrenal medullae, resulting in a rise in blood adrenaline and noradrenaline concentrations for between 1 and 3 minutes. The effect of these hormones is to intensify and prolong the rapid cardiovascular responses induced by neural stimulation. Adrenaline has a more powerful action on the heart than noradrenaline and increases cardiac output. Noradrenaline, on the other hand, promotes vasoconstriction and increases peripheral resistance. Circulating noradrenaline activity alone would actually cause a fall in heart rate. This is a result of a baroreceptor reflex response to the increased blood pressure induced by vasoconstriction.

Pulmonary artery reflex

There are baroreceptors present in the pulmonary arteries that operate over a lower pressure range than those in the systemic arteries. They elicit changes which are essentially the same as those resulting from the baroreceptor reflex, but over the range of pressures prevailing at this site.

This is an additional reflex that supports the baroreceptor reflex.

See also **Pulmonary circulation** (page 437), in Ch. 13, Respiration.

Atrial reflex

There are stretch receptors present in the atria that are variously described as baroreceptors or volume receptors.

Stretch of the atrial walls caused by, for example, increased blood volume, increased venous return or increased systemic arterial blood pressure results in an immediate reflex reduction in sympathetic output, with consequent dilation of peripheral arterioles. As a result there is a fall in peripheral resistance, with an accompanying fall in blood pressure.

Dilation of the renal afferent arterioles increases capillary hydrostatic pressure which raises the glomerular filtration rate so that within minutes there is increased fluid loss in the urine.

Chemoreceptor reflex

If the rate of oxygen supply to, or carbon dioxide or hydrogen ion removal from, the chemoreceptors falls to relatively low levels, then reflex increase in blood pressure is mediated via the medullary cardio-vascular centres in the same way as the baroreceptor reflex, i.e. there is an increased heart activity and generalized peripheral vasoconstriction (Figure 12.27). This chemoreceptor reflex acts as an emergency control system when blood pressure drops below about 80 mmHg.

It may be noted that a local fall in oxygen level (or rise in carbon dioxide or hydrogen ion concentration) causes vasodilation in that area, thereby improving blood flow to that region. The chemoreceptor reflex, on the other hand, causes vasoconstriction, which raises systemic blood pressure and improves blood flow as a whole. So, although the local and reflex responses to a fall in oxygen appear contradictory, they both result in improved blood flow, which will tend to reverse the stimulus and maintain homoeostasis.

CONTROL OF BLOOD VOLUME

The maintenance of blood volume depends upon a balance between fluid input (drinking) and fluid output (in urine, faeces, sweat, expired gas, etc.). Physiologically, output of fluid is controlled by the rate of urine production. Urine volume is regulated principally by two hormonal control systems: antidiuretic hormone and the renin–angiotensin–aldosterone system.

Role of antidiuretic hormone in blood volume regulation

A rise in arterial blood pressure or blood volume stretches the atrial walls and stimulates the atrial receptors so that higher-frequency impulses are conveyed to the hypothalamus, which results in a reduction in anti-diuretic hormone (ADH) secretion rate from the posterior pituitary gland. This leads to a reduction in the reabsorption of water by the kidneys, thereby increasing urinary fluid loss. Thus the reduced blood ADH concentration results in increased fluid loss from the body and reduces blood volume and blood pressure. Conversely, should there be a fall in blood volume and/or pressure, more ADH is released which results in a compensatory increase in fluid retention.

For more details of the actions of ADH and aldosterone see **Regulation of nephron function** (page 501), in Ch. 14, Renal Control of Body Fluid Volume and Composition.

Role of the renin–angiotensin–aldosterone system in blood volume regulation

A fall in renal blood flow (accompanying a fall in arterial blood pressure) results in the release of renin from the juxtaglomerular cells of the afferent arterioles in the kidneys. Renin persists in the circulation for about 1 hour and initiates the sequence of changes that lead to the formation of angiotensin II from angiotensinogen, its precursor in plasma. Angiotensin II stimulates the release of aldosterone from the adrenal cortex and this increases sodium and water reabsorption in the kidneys, which raises blood volume and therefore blood pressure. Angiotensin II has also been shown to possess salt-retaining properties like those of aldosterone and is, in addition, a powerful vasoconstrictor.

The maximal response takes about 20 minutes and is therefore slower to act than the nervous reflexes and action of adrenaline and noradrenaline.

Hypotension and shock

If blood pressure is low (hypotension) then it follows that the blood flow to tissues is reduced. If blood flow is reduced sufficiently to deprive the tissues of an adequate supply of oxygen, then that person can be said to be in a state of shock.

PHYSIOLOGICAL CAUSES OF SHOCK

Shock can be classified according to its physiological causes into three primary groups: hypovolaemic shock (loss of blood volume and therefore cardiac output); vascular shock (loss of vasomotor tone and therefore a reduction in peripheral resistance); and cardiogenic shock (low cardiac output due to a failing heart).

Hypovolaemic shock

Hypovolaemic shock can be caused by haemorrhage, or loss of plasma from severe burns. Excessive **vomiting** or **diarrhoea** can also deplete extracellular fluid volume sufficiently to cause this type of shock.

Vascular shock

Vascular shock is caused by **peripheral vasodilation**, which enlarges the capacity of the cardiovascular system so that the pressure within it falls.

Anaphylactic shock is a type of vascular shock caused by an allergic reaction and is due to a massive inflammatory response initiated by the antibody–antigen reaction. The widespread peripheral vasodilation lowers the blood pressure and the increased capillary permeability causes a loss of blood volume as fluid leaks into the interstitium.

Toxic shock is induced by chemicals, such as endotoxins released by bacteria or drugs like barbiturates and tranquillizers.

Neurogenic shock is due to a massive reduction in sympathetic stimulation of the arterioles. This may occur at various points in the pathway – in the brain (fainting), spinal cord (spinal cord injury), or in the peripheral ganglia (overdose of some antihypertensive drugs).

Cardiogenic shock

Cardiogenic shock occurs when the heart fails, as in myocardial infarction, or if the oxygenation of the blood by the lungs is impaired by, for example, a pulmonary embolus.

EFFECTS OF SHOCK

Someone in a state of shock is likely to exhibit most, if not all, of the following manifestations:
- low blood pressure and rapid pulse;
- pale, cold, sweating skin which has a bluish cast (cyanosis);
- thirst;
- nausea and vomiting;
- increased respiration (hyperventilation);
- restlessness and apprehension, leading to confusion and unconsciousness.

The physiological responses to hypotension help to explain this picture (Figure 12.28).

Figure 12.28 Physiological responses to low blood pressure/shock.

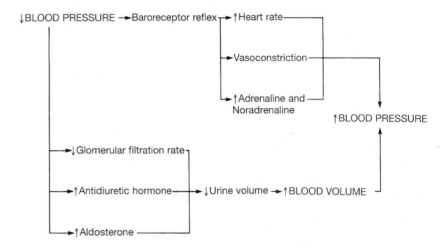

The short term response to a fall in blood pressure is the baroreceptor reflex. This causes an increase in heart rate (rapid pulse) and peripheral vasoconstriction which results in cold, pale skin (pink skin becomes white and brown skin becomes grey).

The release of adrenaline and noradrenaline from the adrenal medullae reinforces the cardiovascular effects of the reflex. Adrenaline has a powerful effect on the heart (beta$_1$-adrenoceptor effect) and causes general vasoconstriction (alpha-adrenoceptor effect). Other effects of the two hormones include sweating and vomiting. In addition, adrenaline increases metabolic rate and, by its action on the central nervous system, stimulates feelings of fear and anxiety, increased ventilation and muscle tremor.

The CNS ischaemic response is initiated when the blood pressure falls below about 50 mmHg and reinforces the effects of the baroreceptor reflex.

The CNS ischaemic response is described on page 173, in Ch. 5, The Brain.

Low blood pressure reduces glomerular filtration and therefore urine production by the kidneys. The low pressure also stimulates the release of antidiuretic hormone from the posterior pituitary gland and this contributes further to the oliguria. Aldosterone secretion by the adrenal cortices is increased and this too leads to a reduction in urine volume.

Reduced cerebral blood flow causes mental disturbances and unconsciousness.

The cardiovascular and renal responses to low blood pressure may, if the shock is not too severe, bring about recovery, particularly if medical treatment related to the cause of the shock is given.

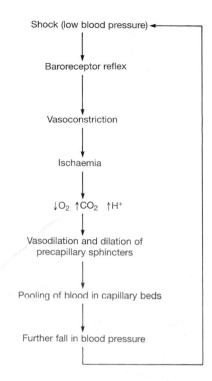

Figure 12.29 Development of refractory shock.

REFRACTORY SHOCK

Severe untreated shock can become irreversible (refractory shock) (Figure 12.29).

Sustained vasoconstriction accompanying the baroreceptor reflex makes the tissues ischaemic so that their local environment becomes low in oxygen (hypoxic), high in carbon dioxide (hypercapnic) and high in other products of metabolism such as hydrogen ions. These changes cause arteriolar vasodilation, as well as dilation of the precapillary sphincters and a consequent pooling of blood in the capillary beds. Blood pressure will thereby be further lowered, which exacerbates the shock; this is an example of positive feedback in the body. In addition, the hypoxia reduces the efficiency of the heart so that cardiac output reduces, further progressing the shock. If the shock persists, the poor perfusion of the vasomotor centre results in its failure, so that the sympathetic responses wane.

The chemical changes resulting from tissue ischaemia also result in: disseminated intravascular coagulation; bacteraemia resulting from increased entry of bacteria into the intestine; a failure of the Na^+–K^+ pump leading to a loss of K^+ from the cells; and a gain of Na^+ and water by the cells.

Hypertension

People with sustained raised blood pressure (hypertension) have an increased risk of experiencing heart attacks (myocardial infarction) and strokes (cerebrovascular accidents) as well as heart failure, liver failure and pain in the legs on exercise (claudication).

Arteriosclerosis is a degenerative disease affecting arteries and arterioles in which the tunica intima is thickened by the deposition of various substances, principally cholesterol. There is a general tendency for this condition to increase with age and hypertension appears to accelerate its development.

ESSENTIAL HYPERTENSION

In the overwhelming majority of cases, the cause of hypertension is unknown and it is designated **essential hypertension**. The condition has a number of characteristics: baroreceptors are reset to a higher level and muscle in the walls of blood vessels becomes more responsive to sympathetic stimulation. In addition, the general level of activity in the sympathetic nervous system may be higher than normal.

SECONDARY HYPERTENSION

Physiologically, high blood pressure can be caused by any factor that increases cardiac output or peripheral resistance. The cause of the hypertension is understood in only a small percentage of cases; this is known as **secondary hypertension**. The most common causes are fluid retention (which raises cardiac output) and vasoconstriction (which raises peripheral resistance).

Some forms of **renal disease** (e.g. glomerulonephritis) can cause hypertension by reducing glomerular filtration rate; or by stimulating the renin–angiotensin system (e.g. renal artery stenosis, renin-secreting tumour or many diseases which cause obstruction to the blood supply, such as inflammation, cyst formation or urinary tract blockage).

Disturbances of some **endocrine glands** can also cause hypertension. Excess secretion by the adrenal cortex, such as is found in Cushing's syndrome and Conn's syndrome, will cause fluid retention and thereby raise blood pressure. Phaeochromocytoma is a tumour of the adrenal medulla which secretes large quantities of catecholamines (adrenaline and noradrenaline). These hormones raise blood pressure by stimulating the heart (beta-adrenoceptor action) and by vasoconstriction (alpha-adrenoceptor action). Hypothyroidism can cause hypertension secondary to the vasoconstriction associated with a fall in body temperature.

PREGNANCY-ASSOCIATED HYPERTENSION

Hypertension can occur in the second half of pregnancy. It resembles essential hypertension in that it covers a variety of conditions and is of unknown origin. The blood pressure is raised due to vasoconstriction. One form of pregnancy hypertension is called **pre-eclampsia** because, if untreated, it may proceed to eclampsia (Greek, *eklampein* – 'to shine forth'), a condition in which convulsions occur. Pre-eclampsia is also associated with proteinuria, caused by alterations to the glomerular membrane which are similar to those seen in glomerulonephritis. The loss of protein leads to oedema.

EFFECTS OF HYPERTENSION

If the pressure of blood in the aorta is raised, the heart has to work harder to pump the blood into the vessel. A compensatory consequence is that the myocardium hypertrophies, i.e. the cardiac fibres increase in size and are therefore able to generate a greater force of contraction. Hypertrophy of the left ventricle is a common consequence of hypertension. This condition predisposes to heart failure (see *Heart failure*, above).

The pathological changes to arterial and arteriolar walls that occur in hypertension have two possible consequences. One of these is that the altered structure predisposes to clot formation, so that the blood vessel may become blocked (occluded) and the tissue beyond the blockage therefore dies (necroses). An **infarction** is necrosis of tissue due to an occluded blood vessel. In the heart this is known as a **myocardial infarction**, whereas in the brain it is a **cerebral infarction**, a type of stroke. A second possibility is that the blood vessel bursts and causes a haemorrhage. In the brain this is another type of stroke.

If the arterial supply to organs is permanently reduced, they become

See also **Tri-iodothyronine (T3) and thyroxine (T4)** (page 624), in Ch. 16, Endocrine Physiology.

Stroke is also discussed in **Cerebrovascular accident (stroke)** (page 174), in Ch. 5, The Brain.

ischaemic and consequently underfunction. **Claudication** (Latin, *claudicatio* – 'limping' or 'lameness') is the consequence of ischaemia to leg muscles on walking. The poor blood flow allows metabolites to accumulate and cause pain. Ischaemia in coronary blood vessels can cause angina and lead to myocardial infarction. Arteriolosclerosis is most common in renal vessels and is therefore a cause of renal failure.

> Renal failure is discussed on page 516, in Ch. 14, Renal Control of Body Fluid Volume and Composition.

Cardiovascular responses to physical exercise

During physical exercise, skeletal muscles increase their metabolic rate and blood flow to them is increased. This is achieved in two principal ways: by an increase in arterial blood pressure, which increases blood flow generally, and by a redistribution of blood from less active regions to skeletal muscle (Figure 12.30).

The **rise in systolic blood pressure** is mediated primarily by an increased cardiac output. The motor cortex stimulates the cardiovascular centres in the medulla (via the hypothalamus), increasing sympathetic activity to the heart and also, more importantly, to the adrenal glands, even in anticipation of exercise. Adrenaline increases the rate and force of contraction of the heart and the resultant increase in cardiac output raises arterial blood pressure.

Increased activity in the vasomotor centre also stimulates constriction in the veins. **Venous return is increased** by this venoconstriction and

> Respiratory changes during exercise are discussed in **Control of ventilation in exercise** (page 462), in Ch. 13, Respiration.

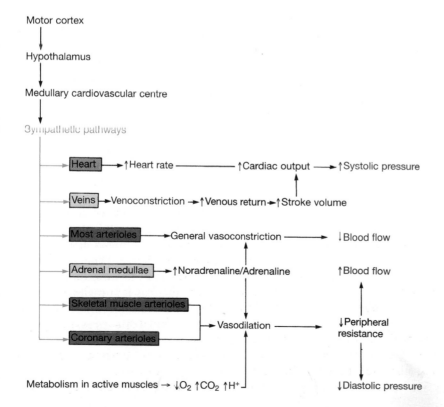

Figure 12.30 Cardiovascular changes during exercise.

Table 12.3 Approximate distribution of blood flow in an adult, at rest and during strenuous exercise

Organ	Rest (mL/min)	% cardiac output	Strenuous exercise (mL/min)	% cardiac output	% charge in blood flow
Brain	650	13	650	4	0
Heart	210	4	650	4	+210
Muscle	1030	21	10780	71	+945
Skin	430	9	1640	11	+280
Kidney	950	19	520	4	−45
Abdominal organs	1210	24	520	4	−57
Other	520	10	340	2	−35
Total	**5000**		**15100**		**+200**

additionally by both the pumping action of the working muscles and the increased respiratory effort associated with physical exercise. An increased venous return will raise cardiac output by the Starling mechanism.

The **redistribution of blood** is initiated by the release of adrenaline, which causes vasodilation in skeletal muscles and in the coronary circulation by acting on beta$_2$-adrenoceptors while the sympathetic nervous system and noradrenaline cause generalized vasoconstriction by their action upon alpha-adrenoceptors.

Arteriolar constriction reduces blood flow to areas such as the gastrointestinal tract and kidneys, thereby increasing the volume of blood available to flow into the active skeletal muscles (Table 12.3). The coronary and cerebral circulations are little affected as they have relatively poor vasoconstrictor innervation.

Once exercise is under way, **vasodilation in skeletal muscle** is maintained by local factors (e.g. the accumulation of metabolites and a fall in oxygen levels). Such local factors also cause relaxation of the precapillary sphincters, so that perfusion of active muscle is greatly increased. The rise in blood pressure also contributes to the increased blood flow.

If the vasodilation in skeletal muscle blood vessels is greater than the vasoconstriction in other areas then the **total peripheral resistance falls**. This means that there will be less increase in mean arterial blood pressure than might be expected because blood is flowing away more easily from the point of measurement. Diastolic pressure, in particular, will reflect any change in peripheral resistance, as it is measured when no blood is being added to the artery. During strenuous exercise, therefore, while systolic pressure always rises, **diastolic pressure often falls**.

Endurance training reduces heart rate and increases stroke volume.

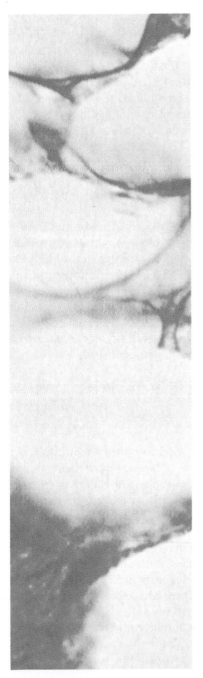

Respiration

13

The process of respiration concerns the means by which oxygen enters the body and carbon dioxide is eliminated. Respiration can be subdivided into five principal areas:
- pulmonary ventilation;
- gas exchange in the lungs;
- transport of oxygen and carbon dioxide in the blood;
- gas exchange in the tissues;
- control of ventilation.

Pulmonary ventilation consists of alternating periods of inspiration and expiration in which inhaled air is added to existing air in the lungs, followed by the exhalation of an equivalent volume of gas containing less oxygen and more carbon dioxide than fresh air.

Inspired air flows through the respiratory tract deep into the lungs, where oxygen is added to the blood and carbon dioxide is removed from it in the air sacs (alveoli) at the end of the conducting passages. Because the two respiratory gases move in opposite directions, the process is known as gas exchange.

Oxygen is carried in arterial blood to the tissues, which take up a variable amount according to their rate of energy expenditure. The carbon dioxide produced by oxidation is returned in the venous blood back to the lungs.

Oxygen is used by all cells in the body in the oxidation of foods, principally glucose and lipids; carbon dioxide is a waste product of this reaction. Biochemically, oxidation is coupled to the synthesis of the chemical adenosine triphosphate (ATP). Each cell has a small store of this compound, which is a source of energy for a variety of its activities.

Arterial oxygen and carbon dioxide concentrations remain remarkably constant despite considerable variation in the body's overall metabolic rate. There are several control mechanisms that match ventilation with the rate of usage of oxygen and production of carbon dioxide.

> Oxidation is covered in **Oxidation/reduction reactions** (page 28) in Ch. 1, Molecules, Ions and Units, and in **Metabolic fate of absorbed foods** (page 594), in Ch. 15, Digestion and Absorption of Food. ATP is described in **Nucleotides** (page 26), in Ch. 1, Molecules, Ions and Units.

The thorax

Most of the structures associated with respiration are found within the cavity of the thorax (Figure 13.1) which is bounded by the vertebral column behind, the twelve pairs of ribs laterally, the sternum in front and the diaphragm below. The upper border is sealed by the tissues of the neck which surround the trachea.

The ribs are attached to the thoracic vertebrae behind and, through the costal cartilages, the first seven pairs are attached to the sternum at the front. The costal cartilages of the eighth, ninth and tenth ribs pass up and fuse with those at the seventh . The eleventh and twelfth ribs do not extend around the front of the chest and are, therefore, not attached to the sternum. They are described as 'floating' ribs.

The rib cage protects the heart, lungs and major thoracic blood vessels. It provides attachment for the muscles of the abdomen, neck and back, as well as the intercostal muscles, which contribute to the process of ventilation. The red bone marrow of the ribs and sternum is one of the major sites of blood cell formation in adults.

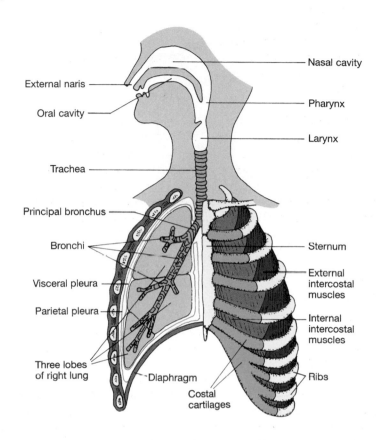

Figure 13.1 The principal organs of respiration. The right-hand side of the chest wall has been removed. The left-hand side illustrates the arrangement of the ribs and musculature.

The conducting airways (anatomical dead space)

The anatomical dead space refers to those parts of the respiratory tract in which gas exchange does **not** occur. It is divided into the upper and lower respiratory tracts. The principal function of the anatomical dead space, apart from acting as a means of conveying the air to and from the areas involved in gas exchange, is one of moistening and cleaning the inhaled air.

Upper respiratory tract

The upper respiratory tract comprises the nasal cavity (or oral cavity if breathing through the mouth) and the pharynx.

NASAL CAVITY

Air enters the respiratory tract via the external nose, whose inferior surface is pierced by two elliptical nostrils (**external nares**). Inside each opening is a **vestibule** lined by skin, with sebaceous and sweat glands; coarse hairs act as filters and help to prevent the entry of foreign bodies. Each lateral wall of the nasal cavity has three bony elevations (superior,

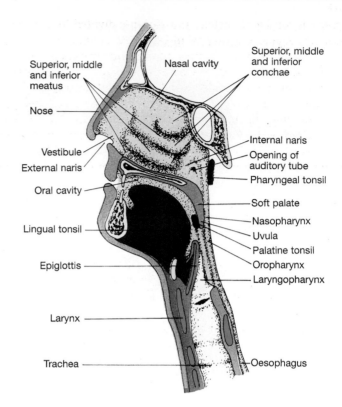

Figure 13.2 Median section through the head and neck showing the upper respiratory tract (nasal cavity and pharynx) and the larynx and upper trachea.

See also **Smell (olfaction)** (page 269), in Ch. 8, The Special Senses.

middle and inferior **nasal conchae**) which separate nasal passages or **meatuses** (Figure 13.2). As the air stream passes over the conchae it is disturbed so that turbulence develops; this allows small dust particles to precipitate out (**turbulent precipitation**). The nasal cavity is divided into two halves by the **nasal septum**, most of which consists of cartilage.

Apart from the vestibules, all other areas of the nasal cavity are lined by **mucous membrane**. In the respiratory region (i.e. most of the cavity) the membrane is covered by pseudostratified ciliated columnar epithelium with many goblet cells. Mucous glands and serous glands are present in the underlying connective tissue, and they secrete around 1 litre of fluid daily. The antibacterial enzyme **lysozyme** is secreted in the watery fluid produced by the serous glands. The goblet cells and mucous glands produce mucus, which lines the nasal cavity and traps dust from the air; this film is moved down and backwards towards the nasopharynx by the action of cilia.

Inspired air is warmed by venous plexuses that lie beneath the epithelium of the inferior nasal conchae.

In the uppermost part of the nasal cavity lies the **olfactory mucosa,** which contains nerve cells sensitive to the presence of inhaled chemicals. This olfactory region is the beginning of the nerve pathway conveying the sense of smell.

PHARYNX

The pharynx is a tube of skeletal muscle. It is divided into three regions the nasopharynx, the oropharynx and the laryngopharynx.

Air passes from the nasal cavities into the **nasopharynx** through two small apertures, the **internal nares** or **choanae**. The nasopharynx lies above the level of the soft palate and is closed off during swallowing, so that it acts solely as a passageway for air. It is lined with ciliated pseudostratified epithelium which moves mucus downwards. The **pharyngeal tonsils**, which consist of lymphatic tissue, are located on the posterior wall; their location enables them to combat inhaled infective agents, although when they become swollen, they become painful and obstruct the passage of air through the nasopharynx.

The auditory tube from each middle ear opens on each lateral wall of the nasopharynx (Figure 13.2).

The oral cavity connects with the **oropharynx** through an archway (the fauces). The **palatine tonsils** are embedded in the lateral walls of the fauces and **lingual tonsils** cover the base of the tongue. The oropharynx acts as a common pathway for air and food and is lined with stratified squamous epithelium, a suitable tissue for an area that is subjected to considerable wear and tear.

The **laryngopharynx**, which lies behind the epiglottis, connects the oropharynx with the oesophagus, which lies posterior to the larynx (Figure 13.2). Like the oropharynx, the laryngopharynx acts as a common pathway for food and air and is also lined with stratified squamous epithelium.

> See also **Tonsils** (page 350), in Ch. 11, Blood, Lymphoid Tissue and Immunity.

Lower respiratory tract

The lower respiratory tract comprises the larynx, bronchi and bronchioles (except those termed 'respiratory bronchioles', which contain alveoli).

LARYNX

The larynx is situated in the upper, frontal region of the neck, between the root of the tongue and the top of the trachea, suspended from the hyoid bone by muscles, ligaments and membranes. It is made up of three pairs of cartilages, the **arytenoids, corniculates** and **cuneiforms** and three single cartilages, the **cricoid, epiglottis** and **thyroid**. The thyroid cartilage is the largest structure of the larynx and is visible externally as the 'Adam's apple'; it wraps around the inner structures in a protective fashion (Figure 13.3).

The cartilages are connected together by **intrinsic muscles** of the larynx. Each muscle is named according to the structures in which it has its origin and insertion. The principal muscles used during sound production (phonation) are the transverse arytenoid (interarytenoid) and the lateral and posterior cricoarytenoids (Figure 13.4).

Internally, the larynx is lined by mucous membrane continuous with that of both pharynx and trachea. The **vocal folds** (vocal cords) run from front to back of the larynx, dividing its cavity. They are covered with stratified squamous epithelium, beneath which lies a layer of

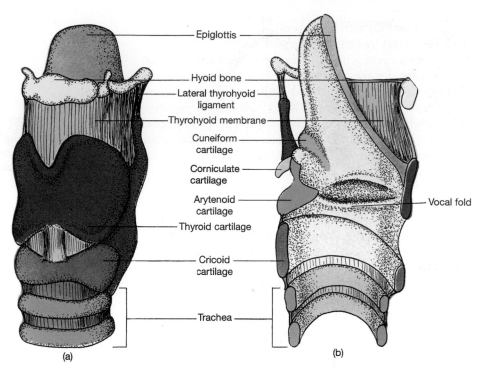

Figure 13.3 The larynx.
(a) Frontal view. **(b)** Lateral internal view.

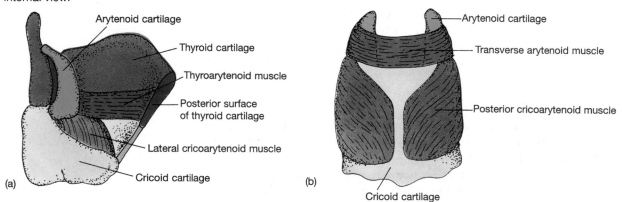

Figure 13.4 Principal laryngeal muscles used during phonation.

connective tissue, the lamina propria, and beneath this, the body of each vocal cord is formed by the **thyroarytenoid muscle**.

In quiet breathing the gap between the vocal cords (the **glottis**) is V-shaped (Figure 13.5), becoming rounded in inspiration. When air is forcibly driven from the lungs the vocal folds vibrate, producing sound in the column of air above. More details of the process of voice production is given in *Vocalization*, below.

The **epiglottis**, a leaf-shaped cartilage attached to the inside of the thyroid cartilage, may be reflected back to close off the air passages during swallowing. Closure of the glottis, however, is a far more effective means of preventing the inhalation of food.

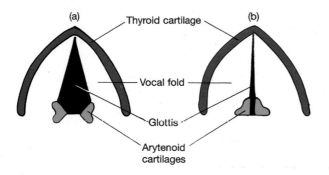

Figure 13.5 The vocal folds **(a)** abducted without speech; **(b)** adducted during speech.

Vocalization

In sound production, or vocalization, air is breathed out in a controlled way, using the expiratory muscles. As air is exhaled, it passes through the vocal tract, which comprises the larynx, pharynx, oral and nasal cavities. The sounds resonate in the air-filled sinuses of the skull.

Vocalization can be divided into two stages: phonation and articulation.

Sounds are generated during **phonation** by vibration of the vocal folds. These sounds are then modified and shaped by the soft palate, tongue and lips in the process of **articulation**.

At the start of phonation, the vocal folds are brought together (adducted) by contraction of the transverse arytenoid muscle and lateral cricoarytenoid muscles (Figure 13.4). This has the effect of reducing the glottis to a linear chink (Figure 13.5).

During expiration, subglottal pressure causes the folds to be forced apart so that air passes between them. This rapid blast of air then creates a drop in pressure which draws the folds together again (**Bernoulli effect**). The folds thus vibrate laterally and open and close the glottis up to 500 times a second.

At the end of phonation, the posterior cricoarytenoid muscle abducts the vocal folds.

The pitch of a sound depends upon the frequency of vibration of the vocal folds. This in turn is determined by their tension, their length (they may increase their length by up to 50%) and their mass per unit length. These factors themselves depend upon the degree of contraction of various intrinsic muscles of the larynx. The folds are stretched and sharpened to produce high pitched sounds and relaxed and thickened to produce sounds that are low in pitch.

The vocal folds give rise to sounds typically varying in frequency from about 60 to about 500 cycles per second (Hz), although some speech sounds reach frequencies of several thousand hertz, and the range depends to some extent upon age and sex. A central vocal frequency of about 100 Hz is typical in men, 200 Hz in women and 250 Hz in children.

The sounds produced in the larynx are shaped by the soft palate, tongue and lips to produce speech, and resonance is added by the oral and nasal cavities, the pharynx and nasal sinuses.

The quality of the sounds is determined by a number of factors, including the position of the vocal folds, the tension in the vocal tract as

See also **Sound** (page 246), in Ch. 8, The Special Senses.

a whole and posture. The nature of the breath support is also of major importance. Loud sounds require increased air pressure below the glottis (usually achieved by keeping the vocal folds closed longer so that subglottal pressure builds up).

TRACHEOBRONCHIAL TREE

The **trachea** continues down from the lower part of the larynx for approximately 10–12 cm, where it divides to give rise to two bronchi. The major part of the wall is formed by 16–20 horseshoe-shaped hoops of hyaline cartilage. Some adjacent hoops are joined by oblique branches; annular ligaments also span the intervals between them. These hoops function to maintain the patency of the airway. The posterior wall of each hoop is absent, being replaced by a thick layer of transverse smooth muscle bundles (**trachealis muscle**). Contraction of this muscle brings about slight narrowing of the airway. The trachea is lined by pseudostratified columnar ciliated epithelium containing goblet cells; in addition, numerous mucous glands are present in the lamina propria. Inhaled dust particles are trapped in the mucus layer and are moved by the cilia to the pharynx at a rate of about 1 cm/min. The mucus is then swallowed or expectorated, thereby eliminating the particles from the body.

The trachea divides at the level of the fifth thoracic vertebra (T5) into two **principal** or **primary bronchi**. The right principal bronchus is wider, shorter and more vertically aligned than the left, which predisposes the right lung to the entry of foreign bodies and the development of infections.

Once the principal bronchi enter the lung substance at the **hilus**, an indentation on the medial surface, their cartilaginous hoops are replaced by cartilaginous plates, which fulfil the same supportive function. The left principal bronchus divides into two smaller bronchi, whereas the right principal bronchus gives rise to three smaller bronchi, one to each lobe. These give rise to **secondary bronchi**, from which several orders

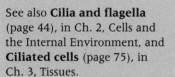

See also **Cilia and flagella** (page 44), in Ch. 2, Cells and the Internal Environment, and **Ciliated cells** (page 75), in Ch. 3, Tissues.

Figure 13.6 Resin cast of the tracheobronchial tree in the lungs.

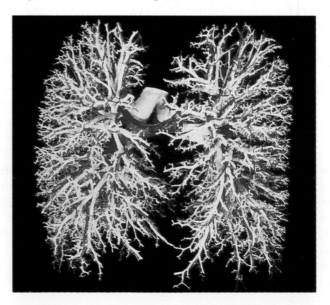

of bronchi and **bronchioles** (with a diameter of 1.0 mm or less) originate. Bronchioles have neither cartilage nor mucous glands in their walls.

The smallest or **terminal bronchioles** (0.5 mm in diameter) form the final branches of the conducting portion of the lung. Figure 13.6 shows the extensive branching of the conducting airways.

The respiratory parts of the lungs

The terminal bronchioles divide to form primary **respiratory bronchioles**, so named because they usually possess outpockets (alveoli) on their walls where gas exchange can occur; they may further subdivide and give rise to secondary respiratory bronchioles. A respiratory bronchiole divides to give rise to a variable number (two to 11) of **alveolar ducts**, each of which, in turn, gives rise to (usually) three **alveolar sacs**. Each sac has numerous terminal alveoli (Figure 13.7).

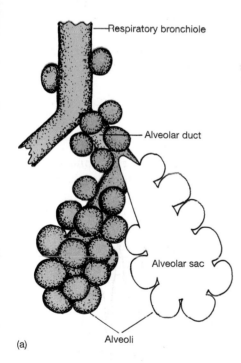

(a)

Figure 13.7 Respiratory portion of the lung. **(a)** The respiratory bronchiole divides to give rise to alveolar ducts and alveolar sacs. **(b)** Fine structure of an alveolus.

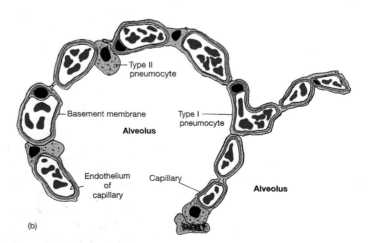

(b)

The **alveolar wall** forms the major part of the respiratory surface of the lung. It is very thin and contains two types of cell (**pneumocytes**), which sit on a fine basement membrane (Figure 13.5). **Type I pneumocytes** are very flat, simple squamous epithelium, and are mainly responsible for gas exchange, while **type II pneumocytes** are cuboidal, and they synthesize and secrete surfactant (see *Intrapleural pressure*, below).

Fine **elastic fibres** surround the alveoli, supporting them. The elastic tissue of the lungs, together with the high surface tension forces within the alveoli, cause the lungs to recoil during expiration (see *Pulmonary ventilation*, below).

Wandering polymorphonuclear cells and lymphocytes may also be observed and, in addition, free cells may be seen in the alveolar spaces; these are phagocytic **dust cells**, which help to remove foreign particles that enter in the inspired air.

The respiratory bronchiole and its associated structures forms the functional unit of the lung called the **primary** or **pulmonary lobule** (5–15 mm diameter). These are aggregated together to form 10 **bronchopulmonary segments**, quite distinct units surrounded by connective tissue continuous with the visceral pleura; each is supplied by a separate **segmental bronchus.**

Small groups (two to five) of bronchopulmonary units then associate to form a **lobe**. The right lung has three lobes, the left has two; each lobe is served by one of the large divisions of a principal bronchus.

Blood supply of the lungs and conducting airways

The lungs as a whole have a double circulation. The **pulmonary circulation** is derived from the pulmonary trunk, which is attached to the right side of the heart and drains via the pulmonary veins into the left atrium. Overall, the pulmonary circulation enables the blood's oxygen to be replenished and carbon dioxide to be eliminated. The alveoli are nourished by the pulmonary circulation.

The **bronchial circulation** nourishes the tissues of the respiratory tract and it is part of the systemic circulation, originating from a number of arteries in the upper thorax.

The lung tissues and the pleural spaces are both drained by the lymphatic system. Both drain independently into nodes at the hilus of the lung.

Bronchial circulation

The bronchial circulation supplies and drains all lung tissue except the alveolar cells, which are nourished by the pulmonary circulation. The volume of the bronchial circulation is very small (less than 1% of the cardiac output); bronchial pressure, however, is much higher than that in the pulmonary circulation.

The bronchial circulation is supplied by the **intercostal, subclavian** and **internal mammary arteries**.

Approximately two-thirds of the bronchial blood flows to the alveoli, where capillaries anastomose with those of the pulmonary system. Mixed bronchial and pulmonary blood then passes into the pulmonary veins and thence to the left atrium. The addition of venous blood from the bronchial circulation to oxygenated blood in the pulmonary veins is know as **venous admixture**. The remaining blood supplies the walls of the extrapulmonary bronchial tree and the visceral pleurae. Blood from these structures passes via the azygous vein to the right atrium.

Although the pulmonary and bronchial circulations normally supply different structures, if either blood supply is impaired for some reason the other can take over. Should a part of the lung become ischaemic due to a blockage in a branch of the pulmonary artery, the bronchial circulation expands and causes an increased flow of blood, which may eventually (after weeks or possibly months) be capable of some gas exchange.

Pulmonary circulation

The **pulmonary trunk** extends for about 4 cm above the right ventricle before dividing into the **right** and **left pulmonary arteries**. These short vessels branch and supply all parts of the lungs. Oxygenated blood drains into two pulmonary veins which connect the hilus of each lung with the left atrium (see Figure 12.4).

All pulmonary vessels have larger diameters than their counterparts in the systemic circulation, and their walls are thinner and more distensible. Thus the compliance of the pulmonary circulation is as great as that of the systemic tree so that it can accommodate the entire output of the right ventricle (which is equal to the output of the left ventricle).

The **pressure** in the pulmonary artery is usually about 25/8 mmHg, with a mean pressure around 16 mmHg. The low hydrostatic pressure in the pulmonary capillaries (about 7 mmHg) prevents the filtration of fluid into the alveolar spaces of the lungs.

The blood vessels of the lungs are perfused unevenly. When the body is vertical, there is a greater volume of blood flowing through the base of the lung than through its apex.

Blood flow through the two lungs is approximately 5 L/min in a resting adult. At any instant, less than 1 litre of blood is contained within the vessels and only 100 mL of this is within the capillary beds involved in gas exchange. Even at rest there is less than 1 second for gas exchange to take place in the alveoli.

Arteriolar dilation can be brought about passively, due to the extreme distensibility of the vessels, or as a reflex response to increased baroreceptor activity. In heavy exercise, blood flow through the lungs can rise to 30 L/min with little increase in pulmonary blood pressure.

Local factors, particularly a fall in oxygen level, cause vasoconstriction. This is unusual as the response in other tissues is vasodilation, which increases blood flow and restores the oxygen level. The pulmonary vasoconstrictor response means that poorly ventilated areas of the lung receive a correspondingly low blood flow, a mechanism which optimizes gas exchange (see *Uneven rates of ventilation and perfusion, below*).

The endothelial lining of the small pulmonary blood vessels contains a converting enzyme which catalyses the conversion of angiotensin I to angiotensin II.

Role of aldosterone in the regulation of sodium and potassium balance and blood volume (page 505), in Ch. 14, Renal Control of Body Fluid Volume and Composition.

Table 13.1 Comparison between average pulmonary and systemic pressures (mmHg) promoting movement of interstitial fluid across capillary walls (figures from Guyton, A.C. and Hall, J. (1996) *Textbook of Medical Physiology*, 9th edn, (W. B. Saunders, Philadelphia)

	Pulmonary	*Systemic*
Filtration forces		
CHP	7	17.3
IFCOP	14	8
IFHP	8 (negative)	3 (negative)
Total	29	28.3
Absorptive force		
PCOP	28	28
Net filtration pressure		
29 − 28 = 1		28.3 − 28 = 0.3

FLUID EXCHANGE IN THE LUNGS

The mechanism of fluid movement across the pulmonary capillary walls is governed by the four pressures identified by Starling.

The process is essentially the same in the lungs as in other capillary beds, except that the values for the pressures are different (Table 13.1). The pulmonary capillary hydrostatic pressure and the interstitial fluid hydrostatic pressure are both lower than those found in systemic capillary beds. Pulmonary interstitial fluid colloid osmotic pressure, however, is higher than that in systemic capillary beds, because more protein leaks out of the pulmonary capillaries.

The net result of all these pressures (+ 1 mmHg) promotes filtration of fluid out of the blood into the interstitium. Fluid is pumped out of the interstitium by the lymphatic system, so that the rate of formation of interstitial fluid from the blood is normally balanced by its rate of removal into the lymphatic system.

Pulmonary oedema

Pulmonary oedema is the presence of excess fluid in the interstitium, or in more severe cases in the alveoli, having leaked through ruptured alveolar walls. The principal causes of pulmonary oedema are a rise in capillary hydrostatic pressure caused, for example, by left-sided heart failure; or increased capillary permeability due to infection, e.g. pneumonia or damage due to the inhalation of toxic fumes such as chlorine gas.

Starling's pressures are explained in **Formation and reabsorption of interstitial fluid** (page 409), in Ch. 12, Circulation of Blood and Lymph.

Oedema (page 411), in Ch. 12, Circulation of Blood and Lymph.

Nerve supply of the lungs

The nerve supply to the lung tissue comprises autonomic pathways to the bronchial smooth muscle and glands.

Sympathetic stimulation of the bronchial smooth muscle results in bronchodilation. This action is due to the neurotransmitter noradrenaline combining with beta$_2$-adrenoceptors in the smooth muscle. The hormone adrenaline, which stimulates beta$_2$-adrenoceptors strongly, is a more powerful bronchodilator. Drugs that stimulate beta$_2$-adrenoceptors, such as salbutamol, are used to induce bronchodilation.

Parasympathetic stimulation of bronchial smooth muscle results in mild vasoconstriction. Parasympathetic stimulation of the glands in the conducting airways results in increased secretion.

Sensory fibres from receptors in the bronchial mucous membrane and the alveoli run alongside the motor fibres. The sensory fibres are involved in several reflexes initiated by mechanical and chemical stimuli, such as the Hering–Breuer reflex and coughing (see *Reflex control of ventilation*, below).

Pulmonary ventilation

During the processes of inspiration and expiration, the lungs are entirely passive. The chest wall and the diaphragm move and pull the lungs with them.

As a result of contraction of the inspiratory muscles, the volume of the thorax increases, the lungs are stretched, intrathoracic pressure drops, and air is drawn into the lungs. In resting expiration, the inspiratory muscles relax, the volume of the thorax reduces, the lungs recoil, intrathoracic pressure rises and air is pushed out of the lungs.

It must be emphasized that the muscles of respiration are of the skeletal type and therefore controlled by somatic motor neurones and not autonomic motor neurones. The confusion can arise because respiration is usually an involuntary activity, but it is one over which conscious control can be exerted.

Pleurae

Each of the lungs is enclosed by two serous membranes (pleurae) in the form of a closed invaginated sac. Each outer membrane (the **parietal pleura**) adheres to part of the chest wall and the diaphragm and each inner membrane (the **visceral pleura**) covers the lung (Figure 13.1).

The free surfaces of the pleurae are smooth and moistened by serous fluid so that they slide over one another during respiration. Under normal circumstances the two free surfaces of the pleurae are in contact and no pleural cavity exists, so that the lungs are attached to the chest wall and the diaphragm by the pleurae. Inflation and deflation of the lungs is, therefore, achieved by movements of the chest wall and the diaphragm.

INTRAPLEURAL PRESSURE

The visceral and parietal pleurae are separated only by a thin film of fluid, the volume of which is regulated by a balance between filtration out of blood capillaries (which forms it) and drainage into blood and lymphatic capillaries (which remove it). The pressure within this pleural cavity is generally subatmospheric (and is sometimes referred to as 'negative' when atmospheric pressure is taken to be zero).

The negative intrapleural pressure is due to the tendency of the lungs and chest wall to pull away from each other, i.e. the chest wall has a tendency to spring outwards and the lungs have a tendency to collapse. If the chest wall is punctured and air enters the pleural cavity, causing the pleurae to separate, then the lung collapses and the chest wall expands. It is consequently, very difficult to ventilate that lung. This condition is called a **traumatic pneumothorax**. If the visceral pleura ruptures, another type of pneumothorax (**spontaneous**) occurs.

The recoil tendency of the lungs is partly due to the presence of elastic connective tissue in the lung tissue framework and partly due to surface tension forces within the alveoli. The latter are lined by a thin layer of moisture and, acting rather like soap bubbles, show a tendency to collapse; this tendency is reduced by the presence of an extremely thin film of lipoprotein, called **surfactant**, which reduces the surface tension in the alveoli. As surfactant is produced late in gestation, some premature babies are born without adequate amounts in their lungs, a condition called **respiratory distress syndrome**. Because of the high surface tension, such babies have great difficulty inflating their lungs.

During inspiration the activities of the respiratory muscles have to overcome the tendency of the lungs to collapse but they are assisted by the natural tendency of the chest wall to recoil outwards. Intrapleural pressure falls from around $-0.5\,\text{kPa}$ to $-1.5\,\text{kPa}$ during resting inspiration (Figure 13.8).

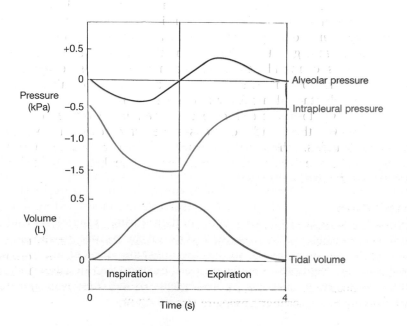

Figure 13.8 Pressure changes in alveoli and pleurae, and volume of air flow during resting inspiration and expiration.

PLEURAL EFFUSION

Usually, there are only a few millilitres of fluid between the two pleural membranes. An excess amount of fluid in the pleural cavity (oedema of the pleural cavity) is called **pleural effusion**. The physiological causes of this condition are the same as those which cause oedema in any site: a rise in capillary hydrostatic pressure, a fall in plasma colloid osmotic pressure, increased capillary permeability, raised interstitial colloid osmotic pressure or blocked lymphatic drainage.

See also **Oedema** (page 411), in Ch. 12, Circulation of Blood and Lymph.

Right-sided heart failure causes pleural effusion by raising capillary hydrostatic pressure. Inflammation of the pleurae (**pleurisy**) increases capillary permeability and interstitial colloid osmotic pressure, both of which result in pleural effusion.

The presence of the excess pleural fluid reduces the adhesion between the lungs and the chest wall and diaphragm, so that breathing becomes more difficult and painful. The pain originates from stimulation of nociceptors in the parietal pleurae, conveyed along the phrenic and intercostal nerves.

Inspiration

The two principal muscles used in inspiration are the diaphragm and the external intercostal muscles.

The **diaphragm** consists of a dome-shaped sheet of striated muscle connected to a central tendon. Stimulation of the muscular component by the two phrenic nerves (which contain fibres from the third, fourth and fifth cervical nerves) causes the diaphragm to flatten. By this means the height of the thoracic cavity can increase by as much as 10 cm.

Irritation of the phrenic nerve results in spasm of the diaphragm (**hiccups**).

The **external intercostal muscles** are stimulated by the intercostal nerves (ventral branches of the first to 11th thoracic nerves). The external intercostal muscles connect the borders of adjacent ribs and their fibres are orientated downwards and forwards (Figure 13.1). Contraction causes the bow-shaped lower ribs to move up and outwards, increasing the anteroposterior and lateral diameters of the thorax.

In quiet breathing, as the volume of the thorax increases, the pressure within it drops to around 0.4 kPa below atmospheric pressure and therefore air flows in from the outside. At the end of inspiration, intrathoracic pressure equals atmospheric pressure (Figure 13.8).

When heavy (forced) breathing occurs, the muscles of the neck may also be active; these include the scalene, sternocleidomastoid and trapezius muscles. Their actions result in greater thoracic volume changes and consequent pressure drop than in quiet breathing, so that a greater volume of air is inspired.

Expiration

Quiet expiration is a passive process caused by the elastic recoil of the lung tissues when the inspiratory muscles relax. The diaphragm moves up and the lower ribs move down and inwards, so reducing the volume of the thorax. This raises the pressure within the alveoli to about 0.4 kPa above atmospheric pressure, and so air is pushed out until alveolar pressure equals atmospheric pressure (Figure 13.8).

In **forced expiration**, contraction of the **abdominal muscles** (external oblique, rectus abdominis, internal oblique and transversus abdominis) increases intra-abdominal pressure and forces the diaphragm up, which actively expels air from the lungs.

The **internal intercostal muscles** also contract during forced expiration. Contraction depresses the ribs and stiffens the intercostal spaces. This action supports the movement of the lower ribs caused by relaxation of the external intercostal muscles. Forced expiration is particularly apparent in strong expiratory efforts such as coughing and singing.

Respiratory measurements

LUNG VOLUMES

The volumes of gas breathed in and out of the lungs under various conditions can be measured using a spirometer. The subject breathes in and out of an air-filled container and a corresponding trace records the volumes breathed (Figure 13.9).

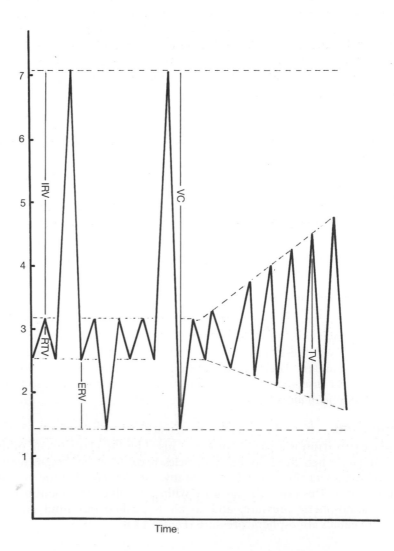

Figure 13.9 Spirometer trace. Inspiration is indicated by an upward trace; expiration by a downward trace. Respiratory volumes: IRV = inspiratory reserve volume; RTV = resting tidal volume; ERV = expiratory reserve volume; VC = vital capacity; TV = tidal volume.

Tidal volume

Tidal volume (TV) is the volume of air that enters or leaves the lungs at each breath. Under resting conditions this becomes the resting tidal volume (RTV).

Inspiratory reserve volume

Inspiratory reserve volume (IRV) is the extra volume of air that can be taken in by maximum respiratory effort over and above a resting inspiration.

Expiratory reserve volume

Expiratory reserve volume (ERV) is the extra volume of air that can be expired by maximum respiratory effort, after the resting tidal volume has been expired.

Residual volume

Residual volume (RV) is the volume of air remaining in the lungs following the deepest possible expiration. As this volume of air cannot be breathed out, it obviously cannot be measured using a spirometer. It can, however, be measured by breathing pure oxygen and collecting the gas displaced from the residual volume. By measuring the quantity of nitrogen so displaced and knowing the composition of alveolar gas, the residual volume can be calculated.

LUNG CAPACITIES

Several types of lung capacity are measured by combining two or more lung volumes.

Inspiratory capacity

Inspiratory capacity (IC) is the maximum volume of air that can be inhaled after a resting expiration; it is the sum of the resting tidal volume and the inspiratory reserve volume.

$$IC = RTV + IRV$$

Functional residual capacity

Functional residual capacity (FRC) is the actual volume of air left in the lungs at the end of a resting expiration; it is the sum of the residual volume and the expiratory reserve volume.

$$FRC = RV + ERV$$

Vital capacity

Vital capacity (VC) is the volume of gas that can be expelled by the deepest possible expiration following the deepest possible inspiration: the sum of the inspiratory reserve volume, the resting tidal volume and the expiratory reserve volume.

$$VC = IRV + RTV + ERV$$

Table 13.2 Mean respiratory values		
	Male (20–30 years) (mL)	*Female (20–30 years) (mL)*
Resting tidal volume	500	400
Inspiratory reserve volume	3100	2000
Expiratory reserve volume	1200	800
Residual volume	1200	1000
Inspiratory capacity	3600	2400
Functional residual capacity	2400	1800
Vital capacity	4800	3200
Total lung capacity	6000	4200
Resting breathing rate (breaths/min)	12	12

Total lung capacity

Total lung capacity (TLC) is the total volume of air that can be held in the respiratory system: the sum of the vital capacity and the residual volume.

$$TLC = VC + RV$$

The examples of lung measurements given in Table 13.2 serve as very rough guides of their sizes.

Lung volumes vary with body size (large people tend to have larger lungs), sex (women generally have smaller lungs than men of the same size) and race (e.g. Chinese people generally have smaller lungs than Caucasian people). The strength of respiratory muscles also affects vital capacity, so that physical training increases its size, whereas conditions that impair respiratory nerve or muscle function reduce it (see Table 13.7).

OTHER MEASUREMENTS OF RESPIRATORY FUNCTION

Minute volume

Minute volume ($\dot{V}$) is the volume of air breathed per minute; it is the tidal volume multiplied by the respiration frequency.

Forced expiratory volume

Forced expiratory volume (FEV) is the volume of gas expelled from the lungs over a timed period (usually 1 second) when the subject makes a maximal expiratory effort starting from a full inspiration.

Airway resistance

The resistance to the flow of air or fluid through a tube is raised by an increase in length or viscosity, and lowered by an increase in the radius of a tube (bronchodilation in this case).

$$R_{aw} = \frac{81\eta}{\pi r^4} \text{ kPa/L/s}$$

Poiseuille's law applies to the flow of air through the respiratory tract as well as to the flow of blood through blood vessels, provided it is smooth (laminar) rather than turbulent.

$$R_{aw} = \frac{P_{res}}{\dot{V}}$$

where P_{res} is the pressure required to overcome resistance to airflow and $\dot{V}$ is the minute volume of air flow. At rest, a typical value in an adult is about 0.2 kPa/L/s.

About half of the total airway resistance occurs in the upper respiratory tract and about 40% in the trachea and bronchi. Any factor that causes narrowing of the bronchi such as histamine, mucus or inflammation, will have a big impact on airway resistance and therefore the ease with which the lungs can be inflated, or more especially deflated. Increased airway resistance causes particular difficulty on exhalation, so that peak expiratory flow rate is reduced and functional residual capacity is increased. This occurs in conditions such as bronchitis, emphysema and asthma, in which the conducting passageways are narrowed.

Peak expiratory flow rate

Peak expiratory flow rate is the maximal flow which can be sustained for a period of 10 ms during a forced expiration starting from total lung capacity. It is usually measured with a peak flow meter.

Lung compliance

Lung compliance (C_L) is a measure of the ease with which lungs can be inflated, and is expressed as a ratio between the change in lung volume and the change in pressure required to produce that volume change. Measurement of compliance involves inflating the lungs in a series of steps and measuring the pressure required to hold the lungs at each step.

$$C_L = \frac{\Delta V}{\Delta P} \text{ L/kPa}$$

Compliance is affected by the elasticity of the lung tissue as well as the surface tension forces in the alveoli.

Reduced lung compliance, leading to an increase in the work of breathing, can be caused by: fluid congestion (e.g. in pulmonary oedema); inflammation (e.g. in pneumonia); the presence of scar tissue (fibrosis); or loss of elastic tissue (e.g. in emphysema). Surfactant deficiency (respiratory distress syndrome) increases the surface tension forces and reduces lung compliance.

Alveolar ventilation

Tidal volume is the total volume of gas inhaled or exhaled per breath. The volumes of air inspired and expired are not usually exactly equal,

Poiseuille's law is applied to the circulation in **Flow, pressure and resistance** (page 403), in Ch. 12, Circulation of Blood and Lymph.

however. This is because the volume of CO_2 added to the lungs from the blood is less than the volume of O_2 taken up by the blood from the alveoli. An adult man at rest consumes about 250 mL O_2 and produces about 200 mL/min. The ratio of the volume of CO_2 produced to the volume of O_2 absorbed is known as the respiratory exchange ratio (R) and is usually less than 1.

Because inspired and expired volumes are different, it is conventional to express ventilation in terms of **expired gas volume**, V_E. Volume per minute is abbreviated with the use of a dot over the V, i.e. $\dot{V}_E$.

The tidal volume can be regarded as consisting of two components, dead space (V_D) and alveolar space (V_A). Only the alveolar gas participates in gas exchange, while pulmonary ventilation is measured by the volume of gas expired per minute ($\dot{V}_E$). Alveolar ventilation equals pulmonary ventilation minus dead space ventilation.

$$V_A = V_E - V_D$$

After a resting expiration, a residual amount of alveolar gas remains in both the alveolar and dead spaces of the lungs (Figure 13.10). This is the **functional residual capacity** and is of the order of 2400 mL in a young adult male. Approximately 150 mL of this volume is dead space. If the

Figure 13.10 Gas mixing.
(a) At the end of expiration, residual alveolar gas is distributed throughout the lungs and dead space. **(b)** On inspiration, dead space gas is displaced by fresh air, a proportion of which also enters the lungs. **(c)** Fresh air mixes with the alveolar gas already in the lungs, but remains unchanged in the dead space. **(d)** On expiration, fresh air is expelled from the dead space, followed by alveolar gas. Thus expired gas is a mixture of alveolar gas and fresh air. The residual alveolar gas will now have the same composition as that in **(a)**.

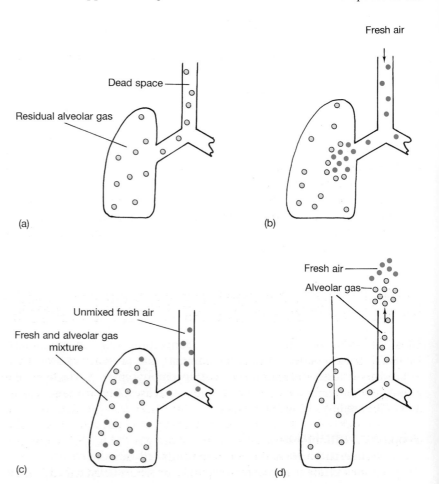

next inspiration were to admit 450 mL of fresh air, then 150 mL of stale air would be displaced into the alveolar region from the dead space, followed by 300 mL of fresh air, leaving the remaining 150 mL of inspired air in the dead space. Thus the percentage of air inspired which actually reaches the alveoli is

$$\frac{300}{450} \times 100 = 66\%$$

This example represents a typical resting value. However, if the inspired volume is increased by physical effort (thereby using some of the inspiratory reserve volume), the percentage of fresh air reaching the alveoli will be greater.

If the inspired volume was 1500 mL, and the dead space volume remained at 150 mL, then the percentage of it reaching the alveoli would be:

$$\frac{1500 - 150}{1500} \times 100 = 90\%$$

The amount of alveolar gas refreshed per breath in the resting example would be:

$$\frac{300}{2400} = \frac{1}{8} = 12.5\%$$

With moderate exercise the amount of alveolar gas refreshed per breath would be:

$$\frac{1350}{2400} \times 100 = 56\%$$

Thus, because of the anatomical dead space and the residual volume of gas remaining in the lungs, alveolar gas is only partially refreshed by each breath of inspired air. The rate of turnover of alveolar gas increases if the tidal volume is increased.

Should the anatomical dead space be increased, for example by breathing through a snorkel, or through tubing attached to an artificial ventilator, then clearly the tidal volume must be increased if alveolar ventilation is to be effective.

Composition of respiratory gas mixtures

Inspired air

In addition to oxygen, inspired or atmospheric air contains N_2, CO_2, water vapour and traces of other gases. In respiratory physiology, the trace gases are usually designated as N_2 because they are regarded as inert. The amount of water vapour present varies with the temperature of the air and is therefore variable in amount. It is usual to express the composition of atmospheric air in terms of dry gas. Table 13.3 shows the percentage composition of the constituent gases in air.

As air travels down the respiratory tract, moisture is added to it from

Table 13.3 Composition of respiratory gas mixtures (vol%)

	Nitrogen (N₂)	Oxygen (O₂)	Carbon dioxide (CO₂)	Water (H₂O)
Atmospheric air (dry)	79.01	20.95	0.04	0.00
Inspired air (saturated)	74.09	19.67	0.04	6.20
Alveolar gas	74.90	13.60	5.30	6.20
Expired gas	74.50	15.70	3.60	6.20

the mucous membrane and it becomes saturated with water vapour, which changes its composition. A comparison of the values in the first two rows of Table 13.3 shows the difference in composition between dry air and saturated air.

Alveolar gas

The gas in the respiratory portion of the lung receives CO_2 from venous blood in the lungs and gives up O_2 to the blood. Its composition will therefore differ from inspired air in that it contains more CO_2 and less O_2. Comparison of the composition of inspired air (saturated) and alveolar gas is made in Table 13.4.

Expired gas

The first portion of gas to be expired is that part which occupied the anatomical dead space; it will therefore have the same composition as atmospheric air because no gas exchange has taken place since the last inspiration.

As expiration proceeds, gas from the alveolar portion of the lung will be expelled, and this, of course, has a different composition from atmospheric air. If the expired gas is collected, its percentage composition is found to lie between that of inspired air and alveolar gas because it is a mixture of the two (Table 13.3 and Figure 13.10).

Table 13.4 Percentage composition and partial pressures of gases in inspired air (saturated)

Gas	% composition	kPa
Nitrogen (N₂)	74.09	75.1
Oxygen (O₂)	19.67	19.9
Carbon dioxide (CO₂)	0.04	0.0
Water (H₂O)	6.20	6.3
Total	100.00	101.3

Gas exchange

The term 'gas exchange' is used to describe the movement of O_2 from the alveoli to the pulmonary blood and the simultaneous movement of CO_2 in the opposite direction. In the tissues, the gases exchange between intracellular fluid and plasma via interstitial fluid. Gas exchange takes place by diffusion of molecules of dissolved gas.

Gases diffuse down a concentration gradient, referred to as a partial pressure gradient.

The following sections describe the nature of partial pressures of gases in a mixture (as in the lungs) and in solution (as in body fluids).

Partial pressures of gases in a mixture

Dalton's law states that if several gases exist together in an enclosure, the total pressure that the mixture exerts is the sum of the partial pressures that each component gas would exert if it were alone in that enclosure.

$$P_T = P_1 + P_2 + P_3 + \text{etc.}$$

where P_T is the total pressure of the gas mixture and P_1, P_2 and P_3 are the partial pressures of the constituent gases 1, 2, and 3.

The partial pressure of a gas is proportional to its percentage composition in the mixture and is therefore determined by multiplying this value by the total pressure of the mixture. Standard atmospheric pressure is 101.3 kPa.

The partial pressure of N_2 with a percentage composition of 74.09 is therefore:

$$P_{N_2} = \frac{74.09 \times 101.3}{100} = 75.1 \text{ kPa}$$

The percentage composition and the partial pressure of the gases in inspired air are given in Table 13.4.

Partial pressures of gases in solution

Gas exchange involves the diffusion of gases between the gas in the alveoli and that in solution in the blood. The partial pressure of a gas dissolved in a liquid is the same as that of the gas above the liquid's surface.

Gases dissolve until the number of molecules escaping from the surface of the liquid equals the number of molecules dissolving in the liquid. The partial pressure of a dissolved gas (**gas tension**) may therefore be regarded as the pressure of molecules of gas attempting to escape from solution.

The volume of gas dissolving in a solution depends both on the partial pressure of the gas above the surface of the liquid (the higher the partial pressure of the gas the greater the force driving molecules into solution), and the solubility of the gas in the particular solvent. A highly soluble gas will have less tendency to escape from solution than a less soluble one and therefore much more will dissolve before the partial pressure of the gas in solution equals the partial pressure of the gas above it.

Diffusion is explained on page 13, in Ch. 1, Molecules, Ions and Units.

Units of pressure are explained in **Pressure** (page 12), in Ch. 1, Molecules, Ions and Units.

These factors are summarized by **Henry's law**, which states that, for a given temperature, the volume of gas (V) going into solution is equal to the partial pressure (P) of the gas above it multiplied by the solubility of the gas in the solvent (S).

$$V = P \times S$$

This can be rearranged to give an expression for partial pressure:

$$P = \frac{V}{S}$$

Thus the partial pressure of a gas in solution is proportional to the volume dissolved and inversely proportional to its solubility. For a particular gas, therefore, the greater the amount of gas dissolved in the plasma, the greater the partial pressure it exerts. This can be seen in Table 13.5. Arterial blood is O_2-rich and has a P_{O_2} of 12.6 kPa, whereas mixed venous blood which is O_2-poor has a P_{O_2} of 5.3 kPa.

Partial pressures of oxygen and carbon dioxide

Arterial blood has a lower P_{O_2} than alveolar gas because a small amount of venous blood (≈ 1–2% of the cardiac output) is added to blood which has equilibrated with alveolar gas in the pulmonary capillaries. This **venous admixture** consists of blood draining poorly ventilated alveoli as well as tissues supplied by the bronchial circulation (see Bronchial circulation, above).

Gas exchange takes place by diffusion down **partial pressure gradients** (Figure 13.11). In the lungs, O_2 diffuses from the alveoli into venous blood down a gradient of 13.3 – 5.3 = 8 kPa. CO_2 diffuses out in the opposite direction from venous blood, which has a partial pressure of 6.1 kPa, into alveolar gas, which has a partial pressure of 5.3 kPa. The gradient for CO_2 is thus 0.8 kPa. As CO_2 diffuses about 20 times faster than O_2, this small gradient is sufficient to move some 200 ml of CO_2 per minute out of the blood.

In the tissues, the gas exchange takes place between the cells and interstitial fluid. As the cells may be some distance from the capillaries, there is usually a lower partial pressure of O_2 in intracellular fluid (typically 3.1 kPa) than in plasma (5.3 kPa) (See Table 13.5).

Table 13.5 Partial pressures of oxygen and carbon dioxide (kPA); the values for intracellular P_{O_2} and P_{CO_2} vary according to the rate of blood flow to the tissue and its metabolic rate

Gas	P_{O_2}	P_{CO_2}
Alveolar gas	13.3	5.3
Arterial blood	12.6	5.3
Mixed venous	5.3	6.1
Intracellular fluid	3.1	6.0

LUNGS

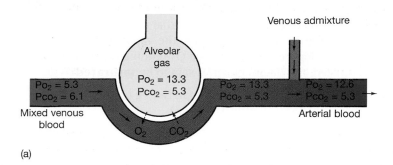

(a)

TISSUES

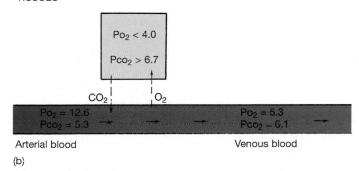

(b)

Figure 13.11 Gas exchange by diffusion down partial pressure gradients (kPa) **(a)** in the lungs and **(b)** in the tissues.

The Po$_2$ in intracellular and interstitial fluid varies according to the match between blood flow and metabolic rate of the cells. If blood flow increases, then interstitial and intracellular Po$_2$ will rise to a maximum of about 5.3 kPa; and if tissue metabolism increases, intracellular Po$_2$ will fall, but generally not below about 2.6 kPa.

The diffusion of CO$_2$ in the tissues takes place down a much smaller gradient than O$_2$, largely because of the relatively high solubility of the gas, which keeps the partial pressure low. The difference in Po$_2$ between intracellular fluid and arterial blood is only about 0.7 kPa; whereas the Po$_2$ gradient is around 9.5 kPa (Table 13.5).

Although Po$_2$ in intracellular and interstitial fluid is affected by changes in blood flow and metabolic rate, the changes are smaller compared with O$_2$. For example, a six fold increase in blood flow only decreases interstitial fluid Po$_2$ from 6.0 to 5.5 kPa.

Transport of respiratory gases by the blood

Oxygen

A total of 98% of the blood's O$_2$ content is combined chemically with the respiratory pigment haemoglobin in the erythrocytes, the remaining 2% being carried in solution.

Haemoglobin A is described on page 333, in Ch. 11, Blood, Lymphoid Tissue and Immunity

Each 100 mL of arterial blood contains only 0.3% mL of O_2 in solution, while in mixed venous blood there is about 0.1 mL O_2 per 100 mL blood. The O_2 carried in solution by the blood is important, however, because it is this alone that exerts the partial pressure or tension.

Each molecule of haemoglobin has the capacity to bind four molecules of O_2 (see Figure 11.7). If all the O_2-binding capacity of the haemoglobin is utilized, the haemoglobin is said to be **saturated**.

100 mL of blood contains approximately 15 g of haemoglobin
1 g of haemoglobin can bind 1.34 mL O_2
therefore the carrying capacity of haemoglobin in 100 mL blood is
$15 \times 1.34 = 20$ mL/100 mL (20 vol%).

Normally, arterial blood contains about 19.5 vol% of O_2 and the haemoglobin is therefore 97% saturated. Mixed venous blood contains about 14.5 vol% of O_2 (72% saturation).

Haemoglobin acts as a store of O_2, combining rapidly with O_2 in the pulmonary capillaries and releasing O_2 in the tissue capillary beds for consumption by the cells. The amount of O_2 carried by haemoglobin depends on the P_{O_2} in solution in the plasma.

OXYHAEMOGLOBIN DISSOCIATION CURVE

A graph plotting the percentage saturation of haemoglobin against P_{O_2} (Figure 13.12) shows that the relationship between the two is not linear but sigmoid.

The construction of the graph can be envisaged by starting with blood containing no O_2 at point zero, and then adding O_2 to the blood in stages and measuring the P_{O_2} of dissolved gas and the percentage saturation at each stage. As O_2 dissolves in the plasma, the P_{O_2} rises. At very low P_{O_2} values, it is difficult for O_2 to combine with haemoglobin, and so the curve is relatively shallow. Between P_{O_2} of about 2–5 kPa, the curve straightens and rises steeply as the addition of more O_2 to the blood raises the P_{O_2}, with a proportional increase in percentage saturation. At higher levels of P_{O_2}, it becomes more difficult to bind O_2 on to haemoglobin, and so the curve forms a plateau.

Moving down the dissociation curve: the upper, flat part covers the range of partial pressures found in oxygenated blood leaving the lungs (P_{O_2} 12.5–14.5 kPa). Arterial P_{O_2} in turn depends on alveolar P_{O_2} and the shape of the curve means that a decrease in alveolar P_{O_2} will not result in much reduction of the percentage saturation of haemoglobin and therefore very little reduction in the amount of O_2 carried by arterial blood. This means that people can tolerate a drop in inspired P_{O_2} caused, for example, by altitude. Since total atmospheric pressure falls progressively above sea level, then P_{O_2} correspondingly falls too. Because of the shape of the oxyhaemoglobin dissociation curve, it is only when climbing extremely high mountains, or flying, that inspired P_{O_2} falls to a level sufficient to cause hypoxia.

The steep part of the dissociation curve covers the range of partial pressures found in reduced or venous blood. At this point on the curve it can be seen that large amounts of O_2 can be dissociated from oxyhaemoglobin with only a small change in blood P_{O_2}. This means that in the

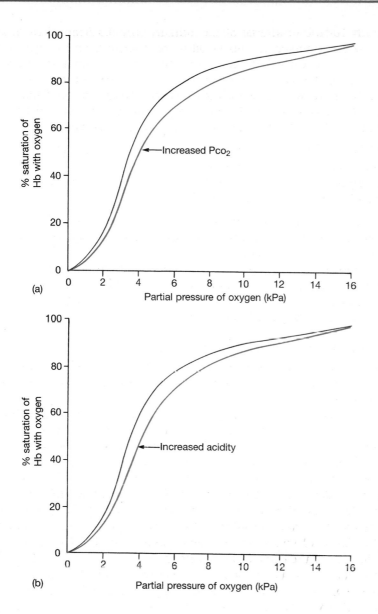

Figure 13.12 Oxyhaemoglobin dissociation curves and the Bohr effect caused by **(a)** raised P_{CO_2} and **(b)** increased acidity.

capillary beds, when O_2 is extracted, the blood P_{O_2} remains high enough to provide a driving force for further O_2 diffusion from the blood to the cells even though the percentage saturation of haemoglobin has dropped.

If the blood becomes more acid and/or has a higher P_{O_2}, the oxyhaemoglobin dissociation curve shifts to the right (the Bohr effect, named after Niels Bohr (1885–1962), Figure 13.12). A rise in blood temperature also shifts the curve to the right. Therefore, for a given P_{O_2}, warmer, more acid blood and blood with a raised P_{O_2} level contains less oxyhaemoglobin. All of these effects accompany an increase in metabolic activity. In exercising muscle cells, for example, when heat, lactic acid and CO_2 are produced, O_2 dissociates from haemoglobin into the plasma and thence to the active cells. The Bohr effect then, means that more O_2 is delivered to cells which have a high metabolic rate.

Foetal haemoglobin

Foetal haemoglobin has a slightly different structure from adult haemoglobin, with the result that it has a higher affinity for O_2. This aids the provision of O_2 to the foetus from blood in the placenta. The increased binding of O_2 to foetal haemoglobin does, however, mean that it is more difficult to unload the O_2 in the tissues.

Myoglobin

Red muscle cells have an additional store of O_2 when it is combined with the pigment myoglobin. The dissociation curve for myoglobin is steeper than and to the left of that for haemoglobin. It can therefore store and release O_2 at relatively low P_{O_2} values, and thereby provide an extra source of O_2 to the cells when the intracellular P_{O_2} has fallen to very low levels, for example in very severe exercise.

See also **Placenta** (page 671), in Ch. 17, Sex and Reproduction.

Carbon dioxide

Mixed venous blood contains a total of about 52 vol% of CO_2. About $4\,mL\,CO_2/100\,mL$ blood is given off at the lungs, leaving an average of 48 vol% of CO_2 in arterial blood.

CO_2 is carried in the blood in three forms: in simple solution; in combination with protein as a carbamino compound ($-NHCOO^-$); and as bicarbonate (HCO_3^-). The percentage distribution is given in Table 13.6.

SIMPLE SOLUTION

CO_2 is more soluble than O_2 in water (2.4 vol% of CO_2 is dissolved in

Table 13.6 Distribution of carbon dioxide between plasma and erythrocytes in venous and arterial blood (% of total carbon dioxide carried)

	Arterial blood	Mixed venous blood
Plasma		
Dissolved	3.2	3.4
Bicarbonate	63.2	61.7
Total	66.4	65.1
Erythrocytes		
Dissolved	2.2	2.3
Bicarbonate	26.4	25.4
Carbamino	5.0	7.2
Total	33.6	34.9
Plasma and erythrocytes		
Dissolved	5.4	5.7
Bicarbonate	89.6	87.1
Carbamino	5.0	7.2

arterial blood compared with 0.3 vol% of O_2). Dissolved CO_2, however, only accounts for 5–6% of the total CO_2 carried. The importance of this small amount of CO_2 in solution is that it exerts a partial pressure which, in turn, determines the amount of diffusion of the gas between fluid compartments. Approximately one molecule in 1000 combines with water in plasma to form carbonic acid. In the erythrocytes, however, the enzyme carbonic anhydrase catalyses the conversion of CO_2 and water to carbonic acid.

$$CO_2 + H_2O \rightleftharpoons H_2CO_3$$

BICARBONATE (HYDROGEN CARBONATE)

Approximately 90% of the total CO_2 carried in blood is in the form of bicarbonate ions. These are produced within the erythrocytes from carbonic acid (formed from CO_2 and water under the influence of carbonic anhydrase).

$$CO_2 + H_2O \overset{\text{carbonic anhydrase}}{\rightleftharpoons} H_2CO_3 \rightleftharpoons HCO_3^- + H^+$$

The H^+ ions produced in this reaction are buffered by oxyhaemoglobin.

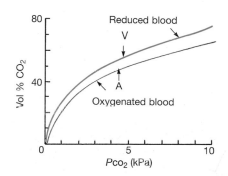

Figure 13.13 The carbon dioxide–blood dissociation curves of oxygenated and reduced blood. The positions of typical venous and arterial blood values are shown as V and A, respectively. The shifting of the curve to the right caused by a raised P_{CO_2} is known as the Haldane effect.

The removal of H^+ by haemoglobin promotes increased dissociation of carbonic acid. The consequent increase in concentration of bicarbonate ions creates a concentration gradient between the erythrocytes and the plasma and therefore bicarbonate ions diffuse out. The movement of bicarbonate ions out of the cell transfers negative charge out, but this is balanced by an equivalent number of chloride ions diffusing into the erythrocyte down a favourable electrochemical gradient (the **chloride shift**).

CARBAMINO COMPOUNDS

The combination of CO_2 with an amino group to form a carbamino compound occurs to a very small extent with plasma protein (less than 1% of total CO_2 carried). A larger proportion of CO_2 is carried in combination with amino groups on haemoglobin (Table 13.6).

The CO_2 combines with different chemical sites on haemoglobin from O_2; however, the two gases do not readily coexist on the same molecule so that the addition of CO_2 to blood favours dissociation of oxyhaemoglobin, an appropriate effect for gas exchange in the tissues. Conversely, a raised Po_2 level promotes unloading of CO_2 from haemoglobin in the lungs (Haldane effect, Figure 13.13).

SUMMARY OF CARBON DIOXIDE TRANSPORT

The fate of CO_2 added to blood from the tissues is summarized in Figure 13.14.

Dissolved CO_2 diffuses from the tissues into the plasma down the partial pressure gradient. Less than 1% of the total CO_2 carried in blood combines with plasma protein to form a carbamino compound (Prot–NHCOO$^-$). One molecule in 1000 of dissolved carbon dioxide in plasma forms carbonic acid (H_2CO_3). As the Po_2 in plasma rises, the gas is driven into the erythrocyte, where some molecules are converted into carbamino haemoglobin (HbNHCOO$^-$) while others are converted into carbonic acid and thence to bicarbonate ions. Most of the latter then return to the plasma by diffusion down a concentration gradient in exchange for chloride ions.

The conversion of CO_2 to bicarbonate and carbamino haemoglobin produces free H^+ in each case. These are buffered by oxyhaemoglobin,

Figure 13.14 Carbon dioxide transport from the tissues into the blood (see Summary of carbon dioxide transport, below).

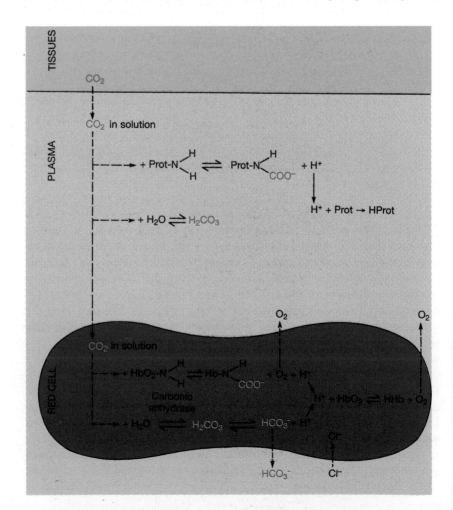

which then releases its O_2 (Bohr effect). The dissolved O_2 then diffuses out of the erythrocyte down the partial pressure gradient between erythrocyte and plasma and into the cells of the tissues down the partial pressure gradient between plasma and intracellular fluid (via interstitial fluid).

When venous blood arrives in the pulmonary capillaries the P_{O_2} gradient between the plasma and alveolar gas results in diffusion of dissolved CO_2 from the plasma into the alveoli. Plasma P_{O_2} therefore falls and causes CO_2 to diffuse out of the erythrocyte into the plasma.

The removal of dissolved CO_2 from the erythrocyte causes the various chemical reactions shown in Figure 13.13 to be reversed (e.g. reduced haemoglobin combines with O_2 to give oxyhaemoglobin and free H^+, which then combines with carbamino haemoglobin to give oxyhaemoglobin and dissolved CO_2).

Arterial blood contains a considerable amount of CO_2; only about 11% of the total gas carried in venous blood is eliminated during its passage through the pulmonary capillaries.

Control of respiration

The respiratory muscles do not possess inherent rhythmicity like the heart. These muscles are composed of skeletal muscle fibres and are activated by impulses transmitted along somatic motor pathways from the respiratory 'centre' in the brain stem, via the ventral columns of the white matter in the spinal cord. In quiet breathing respiratory activity is regular and controlled by reflex activity integrated by the brain stem.

The respiratory centre can be stimulated by other areas of the brain in situations such as emotional states, increased body temperature and physical exercise. Stimulation of ventilation occurs directly from the higher centres in voluntary activities such as speech.

The respiratory system contributes to homoeostasis by maintaining relatively constant concentrations of oxygen, carbon dioxide and hydrogen ions in arterial blood. It is therefore understandable that the arterial concentrations of these substances can alter respiration by influencing the activity of the respiratory centres in the brain.

The respiratory centres

Two of the lower portions of the brain, the medulla and pons, contain groups of neurones that regulate respiratory activity, although the exact arrangement and function of these neurones is controversial. The medulla is regarded as the site of the main respiratory 'centre' that generates the basic rhythm of breathing. The precise nature of this rhythm generation process is unknown, but certain features can be described.

The medulla contains two functional groups of neurones, which can be called the '**inspiratory centre**' (in the dorsal medulla) and the '**expiratory centre**' (in the ventral medulla). Each 'centre' contains neurones which are interconnected, forming a circuit.

Inspiration occurs as a result of nerve impulses that arise spontaneously and pass around the neuronal circuit of the inspiratory centre, and from there to the inspiratory muscles. The centre is only active for a short while and when its activity ceases the inspiratory muscles relax and quiet expiration occurs.

The expiratory centre is not involved in quiet breathing, but in forced expiration impulses are generated and transmitted to the expiratory muscles.

If the medullary centres are isolated from other areas in the brain, gasping respirations are observed. This is because areas in the pons, immediately above the medulla, act to produce a smooth respiratory cycle.

The **pneumotaxic centre**, located in the upper pons, has nerve connections with the inspiratory centre, which it periodically inhibits. It may be that the pneumotaxic centre is itself stimulated by the inspiratory centre. The pneumotaxic centre primarily controls the rate of breathing, so that when the centre's activity is high it increases breathing rate, whereas low activity reduces the rate.

Another area in the pons, the **apneustic centre**, which has tradition-

Figure 13.15 A summary of the respiratory control centres in the brain stem and the major influences on their activity. The basic rhythm of breathing is generated in the medulla oblongata, and modified by the pneumotaxic centre in the pons, as well as by impulses from chemoreceptors and mechano-receptors. The pneumotaxic centre is influenced by the hypothalamus and cerebral cortex. Involuntary breathing is effected by somatic motor neurone pathways from the medulla to the respiratory muscles in the anterior white matter of the spinal cord. The pathway for voluntary activity (pyramidal tract) bypasses the respiratory centres and descends in the corticospinal tract in the lateral white matter of the spinal cord.

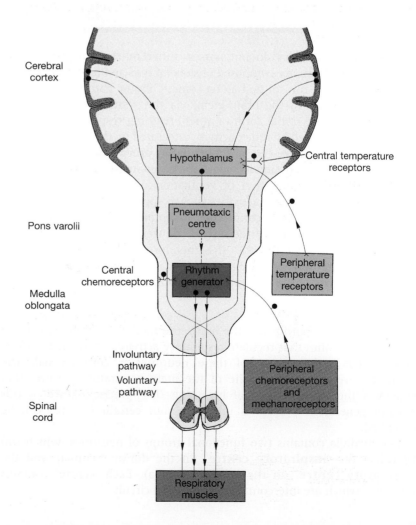

ally been described as important in the control of respiration, has nerve connections with the inspiratory centre. 'Apneusis' means 'sustained inspiration', and experimental evidence has suggested that, when the centre is active, it stimulates the inspiratory centre and prolongs inspiration. However, its role in respiration is now regarded as relatively unimportant.

The precise organization and activities of the neurones in the respiratory 'centre' are not known. The essential features are, however, that the **'rhythm generator'** is located in the medulla and is subject to control by the pneumotaxic centre in the upper pons, as well as by other areas of the brain. In addition, sensory information from the brain itself as well as from many other sites of the body, influences the rhythm generator continuously (Figure 13.15).

Reflex control of ventilation

The sensory receptors that influence the rate and depth of ventilation fall into two main groups: chemoreceptors, which respond to chemical changes in the internal environment, and mechanoreceptors, which respond to pressure and tissue deformation. When stimulated, these receptors initiate various chemoreceptor or mechanoreceptor reflexes.

CHEMORECEPTOR REFLEXES

Chemoreceptors are located centrally in the medulla, just below the ventral surface, and peripherally in the carotid and aortic bodies (Figure 13.16).

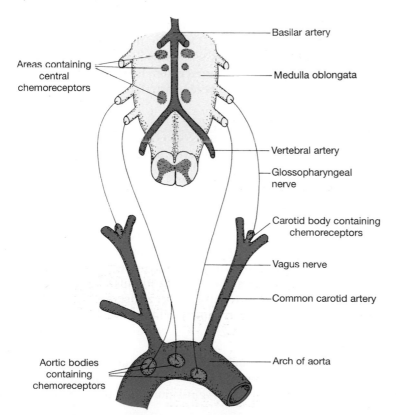

Areas containing central chemoreceptors

Basilar artery

Medulla oblongata

Vertebral artery

Glossopharyngeal nerve

Carotid body containing chemoreceptors

Vagus nerve

Common carotid artery

Aortic bodies containing chemoreceptors

Arch of aorta

Figure 13.16 Central and peripheral chemoreceptors and their nerve connections with the medulla oblongata. The central chemoreceptors lie within the areas coloured purple, just below the anterior surface of the medulla oblongata. The peripheral chemoreceptors are located within the carotid and aortic bodies.

The aortic bodies atrophy with age, so that the carotid bodies are functionally more important. Ventilation is stimulated by an increase in arterial P_{CO_2}, a fall in arterial pH (increase in H^+ concentration) and, to a lesser extent, to a fall in arterial P_{O_2}. Increased ventilation will then tend to reduce the changes back towards normal. The central and peripheral chemoreceptors act in different ways.

Increased arterial P_{CO_2}

An increase in arterial P_{CO_2} results in hyperventilation; for example, a rise of 0.13 kPa in arterial P_{CO_2} can cause a 2.5 L increase in the minute volume. Breathing CO_2-enriched air increases the rate and depth of breathing, but only up to a point; above about 10%, the CO_2-sensitive areas of the brain become depressed.

Both peripheral and central chemoreceptors respond to changes in arterial P_{CO_2}. However, those situated in the carotid and aortic bodies, while they exhibit a rapid response, are considerably less sensitive than those of the medulla. The central receptors actually respond to an increase in H^+ in the cerebrospinal fluid (CSF) and interstitial fluid, although this is linked to changes in arterial P_{CO_2}. Should arterial P_{CO_2} rise, the CO_2 crosses the blood–brain and blood–CSF barriers. Some of the CO_2 in the interstitial fluid and CSF combines with water to form H^+ and HCO_3^-. Since there is a relatively small amount of protein in the interstitial fluid and CSF to act as a buffer for the H^+, free ions remain in solution, stimulate the medullary receptors and increase ventilation.

Increased arterial H^+ concentration

A rise in arterial H^+ concentration stimulates the peripheral chemoreceptors and increases ventilation. H^+ ions in the blood only cross the blood–brain or blood–CSF barriers with difficulty, however, so that they do not stimulate the central chemoreceptors for some time. The buffers in plasma, however, normally prevent arterial H^+ concentration from changing.

Decreased arterial P_{O_2}

A fall in arterial P_{O_2} results in hyperventilation. However, the mechanisms which detect changes in blood O_2 are relatively insensitive. Only when the O_2 content of inspired air is decreased below about 8% is there a significant increase in the rate and depth of ventilation.

The receptors which are sensitive to O_2 deficiency are contained within the carotid and aortic bodies. These structures have a relatively large blood supply (20 mL/g/min), thereby supplying the receptors with plenty of O_2. A decrease in the amount of O_2 presented to these cells in a given time period stimulates them. Thus stimulation can arise either from a lowering of the arterial P_{O_2} or a decrease in blood flow. Haemorrhage can induce hyperventilation in this way.

Cheyne–Stokes breathing

There is a pattern of breathing in which a few deep breaths are taken, followed by very shallow or no breaths. This type of breathing exaggerates the normal pattern of events: ventilation tends to lower arterial P_{CO_2}

and, after a delay, this change reaches the brain and ventilation is inhibited (negative feedback). Following the period of hypoventilation, P_{CO_2} rises and stimulates ventilation.

If there is an increase in the time taken for blood to reach the brain from the lungs (e.g. in left-sided heart failure), feedback is delayed and Cheyne–Stokes breathing can develop.

Another cause of Cheyne–Stokes breathing is brain damage in which there is an increased responsiveness to a rise in P_{CO_2}. The resultant strong hyperventilation causes a sharp fall in P_{CO_2}, which in turn results in apnoea. During the period of apnoea, the blood P_{CO_2} rises again and the cycle then repeats itself. Cheyne–Stokes breathing in this situation often occurs before death.

MECHANORECEPTOR REFLEXES

Several types of receptor that influence ventilation are present in the tracheobronchial tree and alveolar walls, as well as in and around joints.

Pulmonary stretch receptors are found in the smooth muscle walls of the bronchi and bronchioles; lung irritant receptors are found in the epithelial lining of the tracheobronchial tree. There are proprioceptors in and around the limb joints that are stimulated by movement.

Hering–Breuer reflex

During inflation of the lungs, the **pulmonary stretch receptors** are stimulated and a stream of impulses pass to the inspiratory centre in the medulla, where they have an inhibitory action. This reflex, therefore, acts like the pneumotaxic centre and reduces both the rate and depth of breathing. As the reflex does not operate below a tidal volume of 1 litre, its main action is protection of the lungs from overinflation. Some physiologists regard this reflex as relatively unimportant in humans.

Cough reflex

The presence of chemical substances such as cigarette smoke or ammonia, or accumulation of bronchial secretions, brings about excitation of the **lung irritant receptors**, which stimulate the respiratory centres and cause coughing. Following inspiration of around 2.5 L of air, the glottis closes and the epiglottis reflects back over it. The expiratory muscles then contract strongly so that intrathoracic pressure rises to 13 kPa or more. This high pressure partially collapses the respiratory tract and causes the epiglottis and vocal cords to open suddenly and expel the air very rapidly. The action can expel mucus containing the irritants, at maximum speeds estimated as between 100 and 500 mph! Clearly, this can be an effective way of eliminating toxins from the body.

Sneeze reflex

The mechanism of sneezing is analogous to coughing, but the stimulus is irritation of the walls of the nasal cavity. Impulses travel along the trigeminal (Vth) cranial nerves to the medulla. Similar responses to coughing are initiated, but the uvula at the back of the soft palate is depressed, which closes the oral cavity off from pharynx, so the air from the lungs is directed through the nose. The process can reduce the amount of infective or irritating substances in the nasal cavity by forcefully expelling the secretions that contain them.

Limb proprioceptor reflex
Movement of joints in activities such as walking, cycling or running stimulates the **limb proprioceptors** which, by means of their neural connections with the brain stem, stimulate ventilation. It is thought that they are particularly important in stimulating ventilation at the beginning of exercise.

Temperature

A rise in body temperature initiates an increase in the rate of respiration by means of nerve connections between the hypothalamus and the respiratory centre. This can be caused both by a rise in the temperature of the blood and by warming the skin. Sudden cooling of the skin, on the other hand, induces a sudden inspiration, followed by hyperventilation.

Control of ventilation by the higher centres of the brain

Although breathing is usually an involuntary activity, it is evident that some conscious control can be exerted over the process. For example, in talking, irregular breaths are taken, which are then exhaled slowly as the sound is made. Such activities are mediated by descending pathways from the cerebral cortex, which bypass the respiratory centres in the brain stem and innervate the respiratory muscles via neurones in the lateral corticospinal (pyramidal) tract (Figure 13.15).

Neural information can also be passed to the respiratory centres from the higher centres of the brain. The immediate increase in ventilation at the onset of exercise is thought to be partly due to stimulation of respiratory centres by the motor cortex. Emotional states, pain, adrenaline and noradrenaline have all been shown to stimulate ventilation via the respiratory centres.

Control of ventilation in exercise

The increased metabolic rate incurred by a period of physical exercise is accompanied by an increase in ventilation during the exercise as well as during the subsequent period of recovery. Overall, the increased ventilation matches the increased metabolic activity. It is still far from clear which control mechanisms are responsible.

Given that ventilation is stimulated primarily by CO_2, and that metabolism produces CO_2 at an increased rate, it might be expected that this would account for the increased ventilation incurred by exercise. Changes in arterial blood P_{CO_2}, even in very severe exercise, are, however, extremely small and are generally regarded as insufficient to stimulate the increased ventilation. A similar argument is used with regard to a rise in arterial H^+ concentration due to increased lactic acid production in the active muscles. It is possible, however, that the sensitivity of the chemoreceptors changes during exercise. Sympathetic stimulation of the chemoreceptors has been shown to increase their sensitivity to O_2 lack so that the threshold for the detection of hypoxia is lowered. Thus if the O_2 level of the blood should drop by even a very small amount it might augment the other mechanisms which are stimulating the respiratory centres.

Other probable stimuli include the cerebral cortex, raised temperature and limb proprioceptors. It is also possible that there are receptors in the muscle which respond to a change in the local environment, such as a drop in Po_2.

OXYGEN DEBT

During a period of steady work, O_2 uptake increases over the first few minutes, then reaches a steady level, and then declines after the work finishes (Figure 13.17).

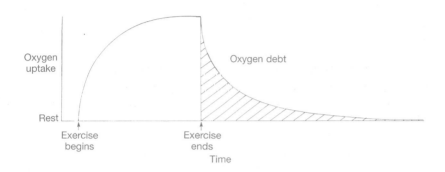

Figure 13.17 The pattern of oxygen uptake during exercise and recovery. Oxygen uptake rises over the first few minutes of exercise before reaching a plateau during which oxygen usage in the tissues is matched by oxygen uptake. After exercise, oxygen uptake falls as the 'oxygen debt' incurred at the beginning of exercise is paid off. Oxygen uptake falls rapidly during the first 30 s of recovery. Complete return to the pre-exercise oxygen uptake level can take several hours. (Redrawn from Astrand, P.-O. and Rodahl, K. (1986) *Textbook of Work Physiology*, 3rd edn, McGraw-Hill, New York.)

Initially, O_2 uptake lags behind the amount required to meet the energy being used by the body. This is followed by a steady-state period during which O_2 uptake matches energy usage. After exercise, O_2 uptake remains raised above the resting value. This is known as the **oxygen debt**, and represents the amount of O_2 used over and above that used at rest after the exercise has stopped, until the pre-exercise state is restored. The heavier the work, the larger the O_2 debt incurred; it may reach 40 L following a few minutes of maximal exercise.

The oxygen debt is used for the following:

- refilling O_2 stores in haemoglobin and myoglobin;
- meeting the increased metabolic rate incurred by the rise in body temperature and adrenaline release during exercise;
- fuelling the increase in heart and respiratory functions that occurred during exercise;
- replacing stores of glycogen, ATP and creatine phosphate;
- converting the lactic acid produced during anaerobic oxidation to pyruvic acid, glucose or glycogen.

Training improves the ability to use oxidative processes during exercise and therefore reduces the volume of the O_2 debt.

Sources of energy for muscle contraction are discussed on page 296, in Ch. 9, Autonomic and Somatic Motor Activity.

Causes of respiratory hypofunction

Overall, the delivery of O_2 to and removal of CO_2 from the tissues depends upon an adequate supply of O_2 from atmospheric air as well as effective respiratory and circulatory systems. As a consequence, impaired function of either of these systems can lead to respiratory insufficiency.

Impaired functions of the respiratory system can be classified as hypoventilation, uneven distribution of air and blood within the lungs or a reduced or thickened pulmonary membrane. All of these changes can impede the process of gas exchange in the lungs, as indeed can a reduced atmospheric Po_2.

Various changes in the cardiovascular system can cause respiratory deficiency. The O_2 content in the blood can be lowered by venous and arterial bloods mixing together (**venous-to-arterial shunt**) or by a reduced number of erythrocytes in the blood (**anaemia**). Reduced circulation to the tissues is a further cause of respiratory deficiency.

Even if gas exchange in the lungs is adequate and blood with adequate O_2 is supplied to the tissues, the cells must be able to use the O_2 for respiration to occur. Any interference with the cellular use of O_2, therefore, is a cause of respiratory hypofunction.

Causes of reduced gas exchange in the lungs

REDUCED ATMOSPHERIC Po_2

Atmospheric Po_2 falls with increasing height above sea level, so that at 3000 m Po_2 in air has fallen from 21.2 kPa to 14.7 kPa, which results in alveolar Po_2 falling to 4.8 kPa. At 15 150 m, Po_2 in air is only 2.4 kPa, and in alveolar gas it is a mere 0.27 kPa.

Mountain sickness begins to manifest itself at heights of some 730 m and above. The chemoreceptor reflex, stimulated by a low Po_2, results in hyperventilation. At altitudes of about 1100 m and above, the increasing hypoxia results in the general symptoms of lack of energy mentioned above.

HYPOVENTILATION

Effective ventilation requires a functional respiratory centre, nerve connections to the respiratory muscles and effective muscle contraction, as well as a patent airway. Table 13.7 lists examples of conditions that lead to hypoventilation by impairment of these functions.

Suppression of the respiratory centre reduces the ability of the medulla both to generate the basic rhythm of breathing, and to respond to sensory inputs such as raised arterial Pco_2.

Functional disconnection of the respiratory muscles from the respiratory centre by section of the nerves or impaired conduction along them will suppress or totally inhibit ventilation. A range of muscle diseases (myopathies) result in the respiratory muscles being unable to contract effectively in response to nerve stimulation.

Inflation of the lungs is impaired if the compliance of the lungs or chest wall is reduced. Lung compliance falls if lung elasticity is reduced by a lack of surfactant or loss of elastic tissue. Compliance is also reduced if the lungs become heavier with fluid congestion or fibrosis (Table 13.7).

Chest wall compliance is reduced by conditions in which movement of the chest wall is restricted, such as curvature of the spine posteriorly (kyphosis) or laterally (scoliosis). Chest wall movements are also restricted by pain induced, for example, by pleurisy or broken ribs.

Airflow, particularly during expiration, is impaired by an increase in airway resistance due to a blockage or narrowing of some part of the conducting airways (Table 13.7).

The intense bronchoconstriction that characterizes **asthma** has a variety of causes. Foreign substances in the air can cause asthma, either

---

Table 13.7 Causes of hypoventilation

Reduced activity of respiratory centres in the brain stem

Drugs
Morphine
Some anaesthetics in high doses

Cerebral ischaemia
Cerebrovascular disease, especially following a stroke,
Cerebral oedema, e.g. following a head injury, results in a reduction in
   blood flow in the arteries supplying the brain

Reduced nerve and respiratory muscle activity

Impaired nerve impulse conduction
Cervical transection of the spinal cord (broken neck)
Poliomyelitis
Polyneuritis
Motor neurone disease

Impaired respiratory muscle contraction
Myopathies

Reduced inflow of air and outflow of expired gas

Reduced lung compliance
↓Production of surfactant (e.g. respiratory distress syndrome)
Pulmonary congestion and/or oedema (e.g. left-sided heart failure)
Fibrosis (e.g. pneumoconiosis)
↓Elastic tissue (e.g. emphysema)
Collapsed lung

Reduced chest wall compliance
Restricted rib cage movement (e.g. kyphosis, scoliosis; pain)

Increased airway resistance
Blockage by a tumour or foreign body
Narrowing by: – bronchoconstriction (e.g. asthma)
                – mucus or swelling (e.g. chronic obstructive airways
                   disease, bronchitis, emphysema)
                – scarring

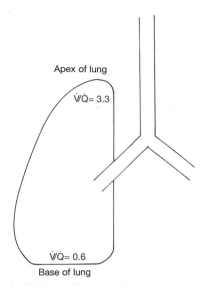

$\dot{V}/\dot{Q}= 3.3$

Apex of lung

$\dot{V}/\dot{Q}= 0.6$

Base of lung

Figure 13.18 Typical ventilation/perfusion ratios in different parts of a healthy lung. Values near the apex of the lung are raised by relatively high ventilation compared with the base, and values near the base are lowered by the higher perfusion rate due to gravity.

due to hypersensitivity of the bronchioles or through allergic hypersensitivity. When an allergic reaction to foreign substances is involved, a number of chemicals are released including histamine from mast cells and a mixture of leukotrienes called slow-reacting substance of anaphylaxis. These cause oedema of the bronchiolar walls and bronchoconstriction. Both of these effects increase airway resistance.

If the airflow is impaired, **wheezing** occurs, usually on expiration when the bronchi narrow. **Stridor** is a high-pitched sound that occurs if there is an obstruction high in the respiratory tract, in the trachea or larynx.

UNEVEN RATES OF VENTILATION AND PERFUSION

Optimal gas exchange occurs when the rates of lung ventilation ($\dot{V}$) and blood flow (perfusion, $\dot{Q}$) are equal, so that the $\dot{V}/\dot{Q}$ ratio is 1. There is always some variation in $\dot{V}/\dot{Q}$ in different parts of the lung because the apex is better ventilated than the base, and perfusion of the base is higher than the apex because of gravity (Figure 13.18).

If an area in the lung had no ventilation at all, but the perfusion was normal, then $\dot{V}/\dot{Q}$ would be zero and the blood leaving the area would have the same respiratory gas composition as mixed venous blood. At the other extreme, alveoli that were ventilated but not perfused at all would have a $\dot{V}/\dot{Q}$ of infinity; there would be no gas exchange so that the alveolar gas composition would be the same as saturated inspired air. Figure 13.19 shows how independent variations in $\dot{V}$ or $\dot{Q}$ affect the $\dot{V}/\dot{Q}$ ratio.

Figure 13.19 Diagrammatic representation of an alveolus and its blood supply, to show possible regional variations in ventilation/perfusion ratio $\dot{V}/\dot{Q}$
(a) Optimal $\dot{V}/\dot{Q}$– balanced ventilation and perfusion.
(b) Increased $\dot{V}$, raised $\dot{V}/\dot{Q}$
(c) Increased $\dot{Q}$ lowered $\dot{V}/\dot{Q}$
(d) Reduced $\dot{Q}$ raised $\dot{V}/\dot{Q}$
(e) Reduced $\dot{V}$, lowered $\dot{V}/\dot{Q}$. A lowered $\dot{V}/\dot{Q}$ ((c) and (e)) causes poor gas exchange and results in blood leaving these alveoli with respiratory gas composition nearer to that in mixed venous blood. A raised $\dot{V}/\dot{Q}$ ((b) and (d)) results in increased gas exchange so that the blood draining these alveoli has a lower Pco_2 and a higher Po_2 than normal arterial blood.

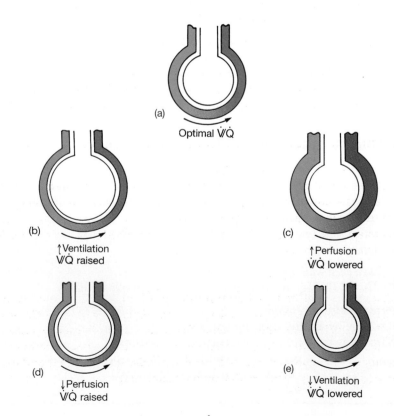

(a) Optimal $\dot{V}/\dot{Q}$

(b) ↑Ventilation $\dot{V}/\dot{Q}$ raised

(c) ↑Perfusion $\dot{V}/\dot{Q}$ lowered

(d) ↓Perfusion $\dot{V}/\dot{Q}$ raised

(e) ↓Ventilation $\dot{V}/\dot{Q}$ lowered

Uneven ventilation can be increased by conditions that affect lung compliance or airway resistance in some parts of the lungs more than others.

Uneven perfusion can be caused by blood vessels being destroyed, externally compressed (by a tumour) or internally occluded (e.g. thrombosis)

There are some local physiological mechanisms that bring the $\dot{V}/\dot{Q}$ ratio nearer to 1 if ventilation or perfusion are uneven.

If underventilation occurs in a local section of the lung, then the local P_{O_2} will drop. This causes vasoconstriction so that perfusion will drop in that area, thereby matching $\dot{V}$ with $\dot{Q}$. (It may be noted that in most tissues, a fall in P_{O_2} causes vasodilation, thereby increasing blood flow and reversing the stimulus.)

If an area of the lung is underperfused, then the local P_{CO_2} falls and results in local bronchoconstriction, again resulting in the $\dot{V}/\dot{Q}$ ratio becoming closer to 1.

The effect of mixing blood from areas of low $\dot{V}/\dot{Q}$ with that from areas of high $\dot{V}/\dot{Q}$ as it flows into the pulmonary veins, therefore, is mainly that the O_2 content is reduced. Because of the shape of the oxyhaemoglobin dissociation curve, areas of high $\dot{V}/\dot{Q}$ cannot add sufficient O_2 to the blood to compensate for areas of low $\dot{V}/\dot{Q}$. Blood draining lungs that have an uneven $\dot{V}/\dot{Q}$, therefore, always has a reduced P_{O_2}.

The CO_2 dissociation curve, on the other hand, is relatively linear, compensation can occur and so P_{CO_2} may not rise (Figure 13.20).

REDUCED SURFACE AREA AND INCREASED THICKNESS OF THE PULMONARY MEMBRANE

The process of gas exchange involves diffusion of O_2 and CO_2 in solution through two layers of simple squamous epithelium supported by basement membranes. Any conditions that increase the thickness or reduce the surface area of the pulmonary membrane will reduce gas exchange and thereby reduce the oxygenation of arterial blood (Table 13.8).

Circulatory causes of respiratory hypofunction

VENOUS-TO-ARTERIAL SHUNT

If there is a connection between the right and left sides of the heart (a hole in the atrial or ventricular septum), coupled with high pressure on the right side (such as in pulmonary stenosis or hypertension), then venous blood from the right side flows into arterial blood on the left, reducing its O_2 content.

ANAEMIA

Anaemia is a deficiency of erythrocytes or of their haemoglobin content whereby the O_2-carrying capacity of the blood is reduced. Causes of anaemia include nutritional deficiencies (e.g. iron-deficiency anaemia, pernicious anaemia – lack of vitamin B_{12}), defective enzyme systems for haemoglobin synthesis (e.g. sickle cell anaemia, thalassaemia) and excess breakdown of erythrocytes (haemolytic anaemia).

Table 13.8 Causes of impaired gas exchange in the lungs

Increased thickness of respiratory membrane

Fibrosis
Silicosis
Tuberculosis

Accumulation of fluid in alveoli
Pneumonia
Pulmonary oedema

Reduction in surface area of respiratory membrane

Collapse of alveoli
Atelectasis

Destruction of lung tissue
Tuberculosis
Cancer
Emphysema

Uneven ventilation–perfusion ratio

↓$\dot{V}$
Uneven reduction in compliance or airway resistance

↓$\dot{Q}$
Regional reduction in blood flow (e.g. tumour or thrombosis)

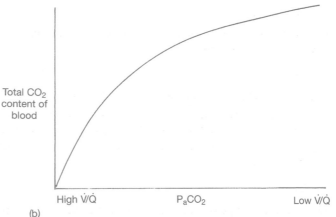

(a)

(b)

Figure 13.20 **(a)** Oxyhaemoglobin dissociation curve showing the relationship between percentage saturation of haemoglobin and P_{O_2} in arterial blood. A low $\dot{V}/\dot{Q}$ lowers gas exchange, arterial P_{O_2} and total oxygen content. A high $\dot{V}/\dot{Q}$ increases gas exchange, arterial P_{O_2}, but this has little effect on oxygen saturation and therefore the total oxygen content. **(b)** Carbon dioxide dissociation curve, showing the relationship between total carbon dioxide content and P_{CO_2} in arterial blood. A low $\dot{V}/\dot{Q}$ lowers gas exchange and raises arterial P_{CO_2}. A high $\dot{V}/\dot{Q}$ increases gas exchange and lowers arterial P_{CO_2}.

See also **Effects of nutritional deficiencies on erythropoiesis (anaemias)** (page 336) and **Other forms of haemoglobin in sickle cell anaemia and thalassaemia** (page 334), in Ch. 11, Blood, Lymphoid Tissue and Immunity.

CIRCULATORY DEFICIENCY

Factors that reduce the circulation of arterial blood to the tissues can result in inadequate oxygenation of the cells. Causes include: left ventricular failure; arteriosclerosis or an embolism causing local ischaemia; and tissue oedema which impairs blood flow.

Inadequate use of oxygen by the tissues

Even if ventilation, gas exchange and circulation are all adequate, tissues may be unable to use the O_2 that is delivered to them. Examples of this include poisoning with cyanide, or thiamine deficiency, as in beri-beri.

Effects of respiratory hypofunction

The various processes that constitute respiration enable O_2 to enter the blood, circulate to and be used by the tissues, and CO_2 to be removed. Respiratory hypofunction can therefore result in O_2 deficiency (**hypoxia**) and CO_2 excess (**hypercapnia**), which in turn raises H^+ concentration (**acidosis**). If these changes are sufficiently great, then they constitute **respiratory failure**.

Hypoxia

Anything that impedes the process of O_2 transfer from atmospheric air to the tissues is a possible cause of O_2 deficiency at the cellular level (hypoxia). Table 13.9 lists such causes, stage by stage, from a reduced Po_2 in the air through to reduced O_2 uptake by the tissues.

Hypoxia results in a reduction in cellular oxidation and therefore a reduction in ATP synthesis, and so activity is depressed. Hypoxia is manifested by mental fatigue, drowsiness and general weakness. Sometimes there is nausea, euphoria and/or headaches. Severe hypoxia to the brain results in muscle twitching, convulsions and eventually coma and death.

CLASSIFICATION OF HYPOXIA

The causes of hypoxia can be classified into four main types: hypoxic, anaemic, stagnant and histotoxic.

Hypoxic hypoxia

Hypoxic hypoxia is characterized by a reduced arterial Po_2, so that the problem is an inadequate amount of O_2 in solution in the blood. The cause of this may be a reduced inspired Po_2, reduced alveolar ventilation, reduced uptake of O_2 in the lungs or mixing of venous blood with arterial blood.

Anaemic hypoxia

The cause of anaemic hypoxia is a lack of haemoglobin, so that the Po_2 is unchanged but the total O_2 content is reduced. The main manifestations are therefore to be seen during exercise, in which the replenishment of the dissolved O_2 from the oxyhaemoglobin is impaired.

Stagnant hypoxia

In stagnant hypoxia, the tissues are deficient in O_2 not because the blood O_2 content is deficient but rather because the rate of blood flow through the tissues is reduced as a result of some type of circulatory deficiency, and so the rate of supply of O_2 to the tissues is insufficient to maintain the Po_2.

Histotoxic hypoxia

The cause of O_2 deficiency in histotoxic hypoxia is an inability of the tissues to use O_2 because of enzyme deficiency (e.g. in beri-beri due to vitamin B_1 deficiency) or poisoning (e.g. by cyanide).

Table 13.9 Causes of hypoxia

Hypoxic hypoxia

↓Po_2 in atmospheric air

↓Activity of respiratory centres in brain stem

↓Nerve and respiratory muscle activity

↓Inflow of air and outflow of expired gas

Regional imbalance between the ventilation of the lungs (V̇) and pulmonary blood flow (perfusion) (Q̇)

↑Thickness or ↓surface area of pulmonary membrane

Venous-to-arterial shunt

Anaemic hypoxia

↓Haemoglobin concentration in blood

Stagnant hypoxia

↓Circulation of blood

Histotoxic hypoxia

↓Oxygen uptake by the tissues

CYANOSIS

'Cyan' means 'blue', and the term 'cyanosis' refers to the blue tinge that pink skin or mucous membranes take on if there is an increase in the concentration of reduced haemoglobin (HHb) in the blood. HHb is dark red, whereas oxyhaemoglobin (HbO_2) is bright red.

Cyanosis can be classified by its cause as either central or peripheral.

Central cyanosis is characterized by a reduction in HbO_2 (hypoxic hypoxia) and an increase in HHb in the arterial blood leaving the heart. It may be due to inadequate oxygenation in the lungs or venous-to-arterial shunts.

Peripheral cyanosis results from poor blood flow to the tissues, so that the blood becomes cyanotic peripherally rather than centrally, and causes stagnant hypoxia. Examples of causes of this include severe cold and reduced cardiac output.

Hypercapnia

CO_2 excess (hypercapnia) can be caused by many of the same factors that cause hypoxia, principally hypoventilation or circulatory deficiency. Uneven $\dot{V}/\dot{Q}$ however, affects arterial O_2 content much more than CO_2 (see *Uneven rates of ventilation and perfusion*, above), and an altered pulmonary membrane has a much greater effect on O_2 diffusion than it does on CO_2, because the latter is so much more soluble and diffuses very much faster.

Hypercapnia stimulates the medullary respiratory centre but if the increased ventilation does not reverse the stimulus the effort of breathing becomes distressing and disproportionate to the volume of air breathed. This is 'air hunger' or dyspnoea. Sustained hypercapnia results in the respiratory centre 'adapting' to the stimulus, and it shows a diminished ventilatory response. In this situation, if there is also reduced P_{O_2}, then this becomes the chief chemical stimulus for breathing. If O_2 is administered, extreme caution is required to avoid underventilation, a rise in P_{CO_2} and unconsciousness. Alveolar or arterial levels of P_{CO_2} between 10.7 and 13.3 kPa induce lethargy. Coma and death can result from P_{CO_2} levels between 13.3 and 20 kPa.

Respiratory acidosis

If CO_2 levels in blood rise, then the concentration of H^+ also rises because of the production of carbonic acid in plasma and erythrocytes. The formation of carbamino haemoglobin displaces H^+ from haemoglobin. Acidosis depresses the central nervous system, causing firstly disorientation and eventually coma.

Hyperventilation

The term 'hyperventilation' means an increase in minute volume ($\dot{V}$), which could be caused by an increase in rate or depth of breathing, or both.

Hyperventilation can be voluntary. Snorkellers have been known to do this in order to increase breath-holding time underwater. The process of hyperventilation eliminates excessive amounts of CO_2 from the blood, so that the principal stimulus for ventilation is reduced and the breath-holding time is prolonged. The danger of this procedure lies in the hypoxia which results from reduced ventilation. This can lead to a loss of consciousness, which, if it occurs under water, is clearly highly dangerous.

Hyperventilation can also occur if someone becomes hysterical.

The reduced arterial P_{CO_2} increases pH (lower H^+ concentration). This condition is called respiratory alkalosis.

Respiratory alkalosis

An increase in pH changes the equilibrium between free Ca^{2+} and its bound form attached to plasma protein, with the result that more Ca^{2+} becomes attached to protein and so free Ca^{2+} concentration is reduced. Ca^{2+} has the effect of stabilizing cell membranes, so that neurones and muscle cells are less excitable. If the Ca^{2+} concentration of the fluid bathing such cells is reduced, then their excitability is increased and the result is increased nerve and muscle activity, muscle twitching, developing into tetany (sustained muscular contraction). A rapid treatment for hyperventilation of this type is for the person to raise their arterial P_{CO_2} level by rebreathing their expired air.

Effects of smoking on respiratory functions

If tobacco smoke is condensed using a filter or by cooling, a dark brown tar is formed which contains about 1000 different substances. These include nicotine and carbon monoxide, irritants and substances that either cause cancer (carcinogens) or accelerate the growth of established cancers (cancer promoters).

The **nicotine** in cigarette smoke is absorbed from the lungs and creates dependency on the part of the smoker. Its main effects are not on the respiratory system but on 'nicotinic receptors' to which acetylcholine binds in autonomic ganglia and motor end-plates in skeletal muscle. The effects of nicotine, therefore, exaggerate the normal effects of acetylcholine in these sites. The actions are complex, however, because in low doses nicotine stimulates activity whereas in high doses it depresses activity.

The **irritants** in the smoke, such as the compound acrolein, inhibit the action of the cilia, cause bronchoconstriction and stimulate the secretion of mucus. This accumulates in the tract because the propellant action of the cilia is impaired. The irritants also initiate inflammation, so that the tract can become oedematous and has dilated blood vessels and increased leucocyte migration.

These changes in the respiratory tract lead to the condition known as **bronchitis**, the key features of which are wheezing from the increased airway resistance and a cough, particularly in the morning, from the accumulation of mucus, which may contain numerous dead leucocytes (pus).

Acetylcholine receptors are discussed in **Neurotransmitters in the peripheral nervous system** (page 126), in Ch. 4, Cellular Mechanisms of Neural Control.

Irritants, carcinogens and cancer promoters can be retained in the lungs for years. They are initially phagocytosed by macrophages, some of which are walled up by fibroblasts. Long-term irritation of the respiratory tract mucosa can result in a change in the tissue from pseudostratified ciliated epithelium to stratified squamous epithelium, a process known as **metaplasia**. Clearly the loss of cilia exacerbates the poor clearance of inhaled substances. The metaplastic tissue can develop into invasive cancer (**carcinoma**).

The principal **carcinogens** in tobacco tar are polycyclic aromatic hydrocarbons and N-nitroso compounds. Substances that have been found to act as cancer promoters include phenols, fatty acids and fatty acid esters.

Smoking also has a toxic effect on lung tissue. In the condition known as **emphysema**, respiratory bronchioles and alveolar walls are broken down, leading to impaired gas exchange.

Carboxyhaemoglobin is a compound formed when carbon monoxide and haemoglobin combine. Haemoglobin has a very high affinity for the gas, so when carbon monoxide is inhaled in inspired air, and gains access to arterial blood, it competes successfully with O_2 for haemoglobin and thereby reduces the O_2 content of the blood by as much as 15%. This reduction of O_2 carriage by haemoglobin results in symptoms similar to anaemia, mainly a limited ability to undertake exercise.

A reduction in the O_2 content of the blood stimulates the activation of erythropoietin, so that the long-term effect will be a raised haematocrit. This tends to raise the viscosity of the blood and therefore arterial blood pressure.

Effects of breathing air or gas mixtures at increased pressures

Oxygen

O_2-enriched air or 100% O_2 clearly has a higher Po_2 than air at normal atmospheric pressure. The partial pressure gradient will therefore be greater so that more O_2 will diffuse into the blood in the lungs and raise the Po_2 of the plasma. This is clearly beneficial in the relief of some types of hypoxia.

Breathing O_2 can, however, be hazardous as pioneers in underwater diving discovered when using rebreathing apparatus. Below about 10 m depth underwater, breathing pure O_2 has a toxic effect. At this depth the Po_2 is 10 times higher than it is in air at sea-level pressure. **Oxygen toxicity** causes twitching of the facial muscles, vertigo, nausea, tiredness, dyspnoea, unusual mental states, disturbances of sight, unconsciousness and even convulsions.

Nitrogen

Amateur divers generally breathe compressed air from an aqualung. The air is delivered on demand through a valve, at the same pressure as the surrounding water. The deeper the dive, the greater the pressure of the air mixture and therefore the greater the partial pressure of the constituent gases. Since N_2 comprises about 80% of atmospheric air, clearly an increase in its partial pressure can cause a large amount of the gas to enter the body by diffusion in the lungs.

NITROGEN NARCOSIS

Typically, at about 30 m depth (four times sea-level pressure), the partial pressure of N_2 in the air is sufficient to causes symptoms of N_2 narcosis, sometimes known as '**rapture of the deep**'. This condition is similar in its manifestations to alcohol intoxication and the early stages of hypoxia, so that the person may be euphoric, overconfident and detached from reality, displaying impaired manual dexterity and intellectual functions.

Commercial divers who work at depths exceeding 30 m breathe a mixture of O_2 and helium, and this has a greatly reduced narcotic action. The lightness of helium, however, affects the vibration of the vocal cords, so that speech in these conditions is much higher-pitched and rather more difficult to understand.

DECOMPRESSION SICKNESS

Another hazard of breathing N_2 under pressure occurs when returning to normal atmospheric pressure.

N_2 is slow to dissolve and diffuse to every part of the body. This means that the longer a diver stays underwater, the greater the amount of N_2 that dissolves in the tissues. Also, the deeper the dive, the greater the P_{N_2} inhaled, which increases the amount of N_2 dissolving in the tissues.

If an ascent from a long, deep dive is made rapidly, then the N_2 comes out of solution and forms bubbles of gas in the tissues or the blood. This is decompression sickness and causes a variety of symptoms depending on the site of the bubble formation. In joints, they cause '**the bends**', which consists of limb pain and bubbles in the skin, causing itching; if bubbles form in the spinal cord, weakness or paralysis can result.

Decompression sickness is avoided by divers adhering closely to decompression tables which indicate the upper time limit at each depth at which it is safe to dive and then ascend at a controlled rate. Exceeding the 'no stop time' involves a programme of staged decompression stops at various depths to allow time for the N_2 to come out of the tissues, into the blood and out of the lungs.

Renal control of body fluid volume and composition

14

The kidneys regulate the rates of elimination of water and electrolytes from the body and contribute to the maintenance of a constant blood pH. They eliminate waste and toxic substances, and retain nutrients. Red blood cell production in the bone marrow is stimulated by the hormone erythropoietin, secreted by the kidneys. They also play a role in the activation of vitamin D, which stimulates the absorption of dietary Ca^{2+} and PO_4^{3-} by the small intestine.

Approximately one-fifth of the plasma (one-ninth of the blood) is filtered each time it flows through the kidneys. The filtrate is modified by the processes of reabsorption and secretion in the kidneys and emerges as urine.

Typically, 1.5 L of urine is produced daily (roughly 1 mL/min), but the range of volumes that can be produced is considerable (between 400 mL and 23 L/d.

Structure of the urinary tract

The urinary tract comprises the ureters, bladder and urethra.

Ureters

The ureters are two narrow, thick-walled muscular tubes, 25–30 cm long, which originate in the pelves of the two kidneys (Figure 14.1). They pass down through the abdomen and open into the base of the bladder. Each tube is lined by transitional epithelium, around which lie two layers of smooth muscle. The inner layer has fibres orientated longitudinally, whereas the outer layer has circular fibres. The lower third of the ureter has an additional external layer of longitudinal muscle fibres. A fibrous coat or adventitia, continuous with the renal capsule, forms the outermost layer of the ureter.

Bladder

The ureters enter the bladder at an oblique angle, so that as the bladder fills or contracts, reflux of urine is prevented.

The bladder itself is a hollow muscular organ with a four-sided (tetra-hedral) appearance when empty, becoming oval as it fills with urine. The bladder is held in position by various ligaments, which attach it to the pelvic floor, the umbilicus and, in men, the prostate gland. A serosal coat, which is part of the peritoneum, covers its superior surface. Underneath this lies the **detrusor muscle**, which consists of three layers of smooth muscle: a layer of circular fibres sandwiched between two layers of longitudinal fibres. A triangular area, connecting the openings of the two ureters and the urethra, is known as the **trigone**. Internally the bladder is lined with mucous membrane, consisting of transitional epithelium, and connective tissue (lamina propria). When the bladder is empty, the mucous membrane is thrown into folds or **rugae**, except in the region of the trigone, where it remains flat.

Below the neck of the bladder the smooth muscle layer is modified to form an **internal sphincter**. An **external sphincter** composed of skeletal muscle surrounds the urethra. In men, this is located surrounding the membranous urethra, whereas in women it lies just above the external urethral orifice.

Urethra

The urethra extends from the neck of the bladder to the external meatus. In men it travels the length of the penis and is typically about 20 cm long, while in women it is around 4 cm long. In both sexes it is lined by transitional epithelium near the bladder and stratified squamous epithelium distally. Smooth muscle is also present. The urethra proximal to the external sphincter is normally closed by tension in the elastic fibres of the urethral wall.

The male urethra runs from the bladder through the prostate gland; a short membranous section (surrounded by the external sphincter) connects the prostatic part of the urethra with the most distal section, the spongiose part, which runs through the corpus spongiosum of the penis (see Figure 17.12). The external urethral orifice is a sagittal slit, about 6 mm long, at the end of the penis.

The female urethra is embedded in the anterior wall of the vagina. The external urethral orifice is an anteroposterior slit located immediately in front of the vaginal opening and some 2.5 cm behind the clitoris (glans clitoridis).

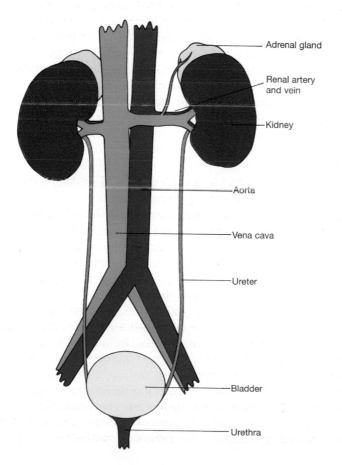

Figure 14.1 General plan of the kidneys and urinary tract viewed from the front.

Micturition

Urine is carried down the ureters by peristaltic waves, which occur approximately every 10 seconds, travelling down at 2–3 cm/s. Each wave sends a spurt of urine into the bladder. The bladder fills slowly over a long period of time, but is evacuated relatively quickly by the micturition reflex.

Micturition is a complex act involving sensory, and autonomic and somatic motor, nerve pathways. The reflex is coordinated by centres in the cerebral cortex and the spinal cord.

Two types of motor neurone are involved: parasympathetic fibres from the spinal cord travel to the bladder wall in the **pelvic splanchnic nerves**, while somatic fibres are carried in the **pudendal nerves** from the spinal cord to the external sphincter.

The pelvic splanchnic nerves also carry sensory fibres to the spinal cord from stretch receptors in the bladder wall and posterior urethra.

The process of micturition is regulated by a reflex initiated by impulses from **stretch receptors** in the bladder wall when the bladder contains about 300 mL of urine. The sensory neurones transmit the impulses to the spinal cord where they are relayed to the parasympathetic neurones that innervate the detrusor muscle in the bladder wall and cause it to contract. Simultaneously, impulses travelling down the pudendal nerve to the external sphincter are inhibited in the spinal cord, so that the sphincter relaxes and urine can be voided. The reflex pathways for this are shown in Figure 14.2.

Voluntary delay of micturition is achieved via descending pathways from the brain, which inhibit the parasympathetic fibres to the bladder and stimulate the somatic fibres to the external sphincter.

Alternatively, micturition can be initiated voluntarily via descending pathways from the brain to the spinal centre whereby the parasympathetic neurones are further stimulated and the somatic neurones inhibited. Urine is thus forced into the neck of the bladder. This results in a volley of impulses in the pelvic splanchnic nerves passing to the spinal cord and subsequently inhibiting impulses to the external sphincter.

Muscle tone in the **pelvic floor** causes pressure on the neck of the bladder and effectively closes the outflow of urine from it. Micturition is thus aided by relaxation of the pelvic floor, including the internal sphincter.

Incontinence

Incontinence is the inability to control the flow of urine from the bladder. In young children, who have not yet learned to control micturition, when the bladder fills the micturition reflex is initiated and the external sphincter remains relaxed. The internal sphincter remains closed between episodes of micturition.

In adults, incontinence is commonly relatively mild. One form, known as **stress incontinence**, involves the expulsion of small amounts of urine when intra-abdominal pressure rises, e.g. when coughing or laughing. Pregnancy can cause this by stretching the pelvic

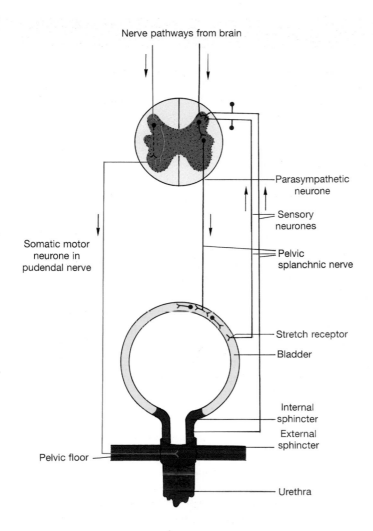

Nerve pathways from brain

Parasympathetic neurone

Sensory neurones

Pelvic splanchnic nerve

Somatic motor neurone in pudendal nerve

Stretch receptor

Bladder

Internal sphincter

External sphincter

Pelvic floor

Urethra

Figure 14.2 Nerve pathways involved in the micturition reflex (the pelvic splanchnic and pudendal nerves are shown on one side only). As the bladder fills, sensory neurones from stretch receptors in the wall transmit impulses to the spinal cord in the pelvic splanchnic nerves. The impulses are relayed to the parasympathetic neurones in the pelvic splanchnic nerves which innervate the detrusor muscle in the bladder wall and cause it to contract. Simultaneously, impulses travelling down the pudendal nerve in somatic motor neurones to the external sphincter are inhibited by interneurones in the spinal cord (dotted line), so that the sphincter relaxes and urine can be voided.

floor through which the urethra passes. Exercises that strengthen the pelvic floor muscles can increase external pressure on the neck of the bladder and prevent urine leakage.

Damage to components of the micturition reflex or pathways from the brain affecting micturition can result in an inability to evacuate the bladder and/or control the process.

If the sensory input from the bladder to the spinal cord is impaired, then not only will the person be unaware of the sensation of a full bladder, but also the reflex will not be initiated, so that the full bladder simply overflows (**outflow incontinence**).

Should spinal cord damage occur above the sacral region, the micturition reflex will be intact but micturition will not be subject to voluntary control, as descending pathways from the brain will be interrupted. Initially after a spinal injury (days or weeks), a period of spinal shock occurs in which the micturition reflex (along with other reflexes) is absent. During this period, the bladder has to be emptied by catheterization.

Spinal shock is discussed on page 207 in Ch. 6, The Spinal Cord.

If the pathway from the brain to the spinal cord which inhibits micturition is damaged, then the micturition reflex is subject only to the stimulatory influences which pass down the cord, so that the micturition reflex is exaggerated, resulting in frequent and relatively uncontrollable micturition.

Structure of the kidneys

The two kidneys are bean-shaped organs situated behind the peritoneum on the posterior wall of the abdominal cavity on either side of the vertebral column, extending from the 12th thoracic to the third lumbar vertebrae. They each weigh between 120 and 170 g; and are 10–13 cm in length, 5–6 cm wide and 3–4 cm in thickness. A deep indentation, the **hilus**, is found on the medial border, from which the ureter emerges. The renal artery and renal vein both pass through the hilus.

A section through the kidney (Figure 14.3) shows three distinct anatomical regions: the cortex, the medulla and the pelvis.

The outer **cortex**, which is covered on its outer edge by a dense connective tissue capsule, is easily distinguishable from the inner **medulla**. The latter is made up of a variable number (5–14), of **renal pyramids** whose apices (**papillae**) protrude into the innermost region, the **pelvis**. This is a funnel-like expansion of the upper end of the ureter, which possesses two or three outgrowths or **major calyces**.

Figure 14.3 Vertical section through the kidney to show the major areas and blood vessels. The upper part of the pelvis is cut open to show the insides of the calyces.

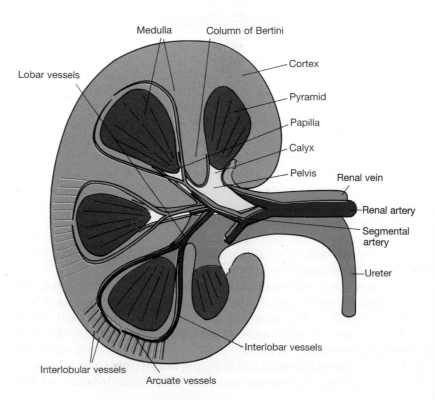

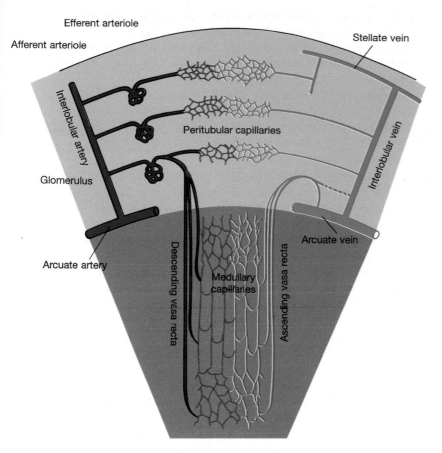

Figure 14.4 Blood vessels of the cortex and a medullary pyramid. Blood flows from the glomeruli into efferent arterioles, which then lead into peritubular capillary networks before draining into the venous system. In the inner medulla the descending vasa recta give rise to a number of parallel capillaries, which lie close to the long loops of Henle of the juxtamedullary nephrons.

These, in turn, have a number of smaller pockets, the **minor calyces**. Each papilla protrudes into the lumen of a minor calyx.

The medullary pyramids are separated from one another by ingrowth of cortical tissue, the renal columns (**columns of Bertini**). Each medullary pyramid and its cap of cortical tissue constitutes a **lobe** of the kidney.

Each kidney contains at least 1 million **nephrons** (some estimates are as high as 3 million per kidney). The nephron is the functional unit of the kidney, which filters plasma at one end, modifies the fluid as it flows through and then drains into a collecting duct, which receives fluid from several nephrons. The fluid emerging from the collecting ducts is **urine**.

The collecting ducts run from the renal cortex into the medulla, pointing towards the pelvis of the kidney, like spokes in a bicycle wheel.

Renal circulation

Blood enters the kidney in the **renal artery**; the latter divides into two main branches, which give rise to several **segmental arteries** (Figure 14.3). Each lobe of the kidney is supplied by a **lobar artery**, which divides into two or three **interlobar arteries**. These lie in the renal columns between the pyramids. At the junction of the cortex and medulla, the interlobar vessels arch over and run parallel to the organ's surface, becoming the **arcuate arteries**. Small **interlobular arteries** radiate towards the periphery from the arcuate arteries. (A kidney **lobule** comprises a central collecting duct, together with parts of the nephrons which drain into it.) The interlobular arteries give off numerous **afferent arterioles** which lead into capillaries (glomeruli) from which fluid is filtered into the nephrons.

The drainage of blood from the glomeruli is unusual because it flows into a second set of arterioles (**efferent arterioles**, Figure 14.4). The effect of this arrangement is that the blood pressure (hydrostatic pressure) within the glomerular capillaries is higher than it would be if drainage into low-resistance venules occurred.

Efferent arterioles supply blood to the cortical **peritubular capillary network**. Blood from peritubular capillaries close to the kidney surface drains into **stellate veins** and then into **interlobular veins**. Most, however, pass their blood directly into the interlobular veins. These drain into **arcuate veins** and then **interlobar veins**, which converge and drain into the **renal vein**.

The efferent vessels of glomeruli situated deep in the cortex (the juxtamedullary glomeruli) not only supply the cortical peritubular capillaries, but they also enter the medulla and give rise to bundles of between 12 and 25 large, thin-walled vessels, the **descending vasa**

Figure 14.5 General structure of the nephron with details of the cell types in the various sections of the tubule. **(a)** Malpighian corpuscle. **(b)** Proximal convoluted tubule. **(c)** Loop of Henle. **(d)** Distal convoluted tubule.

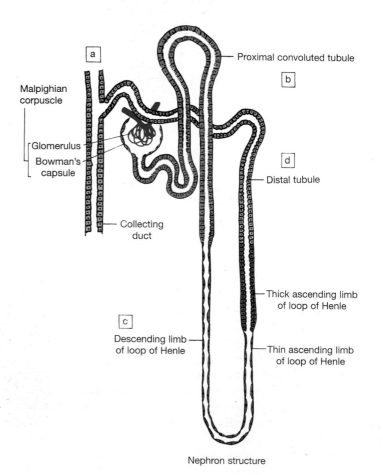

Nephron structure

recta. These form hairpin loops at various levels in the medulla and supply an elongated capillary bed that surrounds parts of the juxtamedullary nephrons. The capillaries then drain into the **ascending vasa recta**, which return blood either to the interlobular or arcuate veins (Figure 14.4).

Nerve supply of the kidneys

Sympathetic fibres enter the kidney from the coeliac plexus. They course alongside some of the major blood vessels and innervate the small arteries and afferent arterioles. Stimulation causes vasoconstriction and a

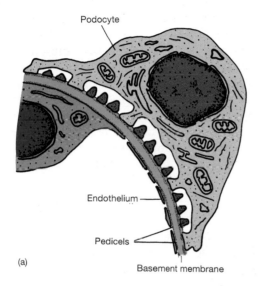

(a)

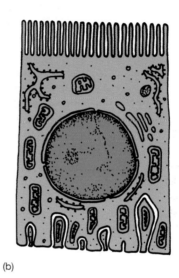

(b)

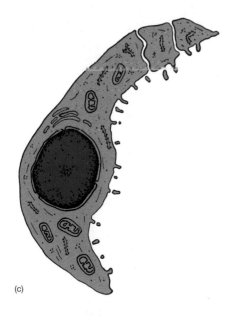

(c)

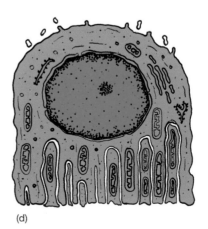

(d)

consequent reduction in blood flow into the glomeruli. Sympathetic fibres also innervate the juxtaglomerular cells and stimulate the release of renin (see *Juxtaglomerular apparatus*, below).

Structure of the nephrons

Each nephron consists of five sections; the Malpighian corpuscle, proximal tubule, loop of Henle, distal tubule and a collecting duct shared by several nephrons (Figure 14.5).

MALPIGHIAN CORPUSCLE

The Malpighian or renal corpuscles are distributed throughout the cortex. Each corpuscle is composed of a tuft of capillaries, the **glomerulus**, which is inserted into the dilated, blind end of the renal tubule, the **Bowman's capsule**.

The outer wall (parietal layer) of the Bowman's capsule is composed of extremely flattened squamous epithelium. At the point where the afferent and efferent arterioles join the glomerulus (the vascular pole), the parietal layer of Bowman's capsule is reflected inwards to join the inner visceral layer, which is very closely applied to the glomerular capillaries (Figure 14.6).

The cells of the visceral layer (**podocytes**) are a type of epithelium unique to the kidney. Podocytes have a small cell body (perikaryon)

Figure 14.6 Vertical section through a Malpighian corpuscle. Only a few capillaries are drawn.

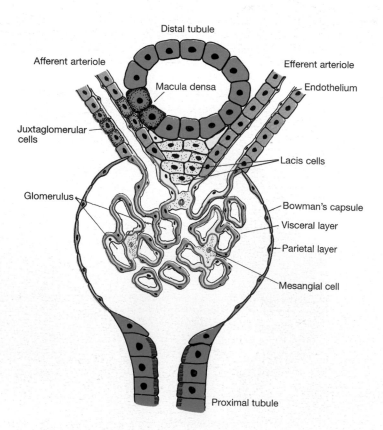

from which radiate a number of major processes (Figures 14.7, 14.8). These, in turn, give rise to a large number of thin secondary processes (**pedicels**) which interdigitate with those of other podocytes. In section, pedicels from adjacent podocytes may be seen in contact with the basement membrane (basal lamina). (Figures 14.5, 14.9, 14.10).

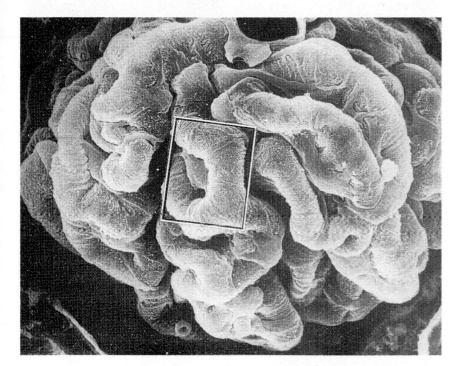

Figure 14.7 Scanning micrograph of a renal glomerulus. The area enclosed in the rectangle is shown at higher magnification in Figure 14.8. (Reproduced from Andrews, P. (1988) *Journal of Electron Microscope Technology*, **9**, 115, by permission of the publishers.)

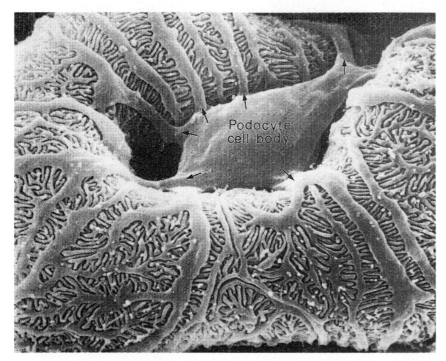

Figure 14.8 Higher magnification of the area in the rectangle on Figure 14.7, which includes a glomerular capillary loop and a podocyte cell body, its primary processes (indicated by arrows) and the interdigitating pedicels that bound the filtration slits. (Reproduced from Andrews, P. (1988) *Journal of Electron Microscopy Technique*, **9**, 115, by permission of the publishers.)

Figure 14.9 Electron micrograph of a transverse section through a glomerular capillary showing the basal lamina interposed between the fenestrated endothelium and the slit pores between pedicels of the visceral epithelium of Bowman's capsule. An area comparable to that in the rectangle is shown at higher magnification in Figure 14.10. (Reproduced from Tyson, G. and Bulger, R. (1972) *Anatomical Record*, **172**, 669, by permission of the publishers.)

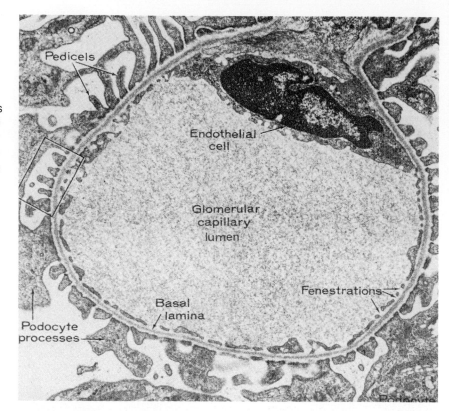

Figure 14.10 Electron micrograph of a portion of the wall of a glomerular capillary showing the foot processes of a podocyte on the outer surface of the basement lamina and the fenestrated endothelium on its inner aspect. (Reproduced with permission from Fawcett, D. W. (1993) *Bloom and Fawcett: A Textbook of Histology*, Chapman & Hall, London, by courtesy of Dr Daniel Friend.)

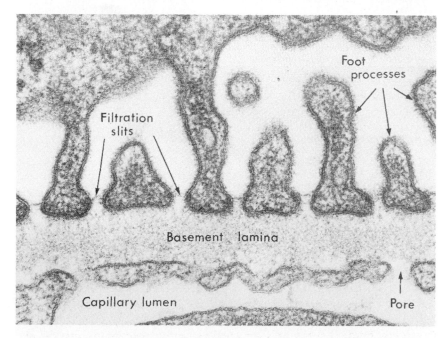

The pedicels lie on a continuous basal lamina that is fused with the basal lamina surrounding the glomerular endothelium. Adjacent pedicels are separated by gaps or **filtration slits** approximately 25 nm wide and bridged by a fine slit membrane.

The glomerular endothelium is very thin and is perforated by circular pores or **fenestrations** 50–100 nm in diameter.

Fluid filtered from the glomerulus into the cavity of Bowman's capsule passes between the cells of the visceral layer, through the filtration slits, and not through the podocytes themselves.

JUXTAGLOMERULAR APPARATUS

In the wall of the afferent arteriole, immediately before its entry into the glomerulus, there is a group of modified smooth muscle cells, the **juxtaglomerular cells** (Figure 14.6). These cells contain a large number of crystalline granules that contain the enzyme **renin**. Renin secretion is increased when renal blood flow is decreased.

The distal tubule passes between the glomerular arterioles. At the point where the tubule and the afferent arteriole are closest, the tubular cells are slightly modified, being taller with more prominent nuclei than the other cells of the distal tubule. This structure constitutes the **macula densa** which acts as a sensor of tubular fluid composition or flow.

The juxtaglomerular cells, together with the macula densa, comprise the juxtaglomerular apparatus, a regulator of the secretion of the hormone aldosterone.

MESANGIAL CELLS

Mesangial cells are found in two sites: packed between the afferent and efferent arterioles outside the glomerulus, where they are known as **lacis cells**; and also between the glomerular capillaries within Bowman's capsule (Figure 14.6). The cells are irregularly shaped and contain filaments of contractile proteins.

Lacis cells are thought to produce the hormone **erythropoietin**, which stimulates red blood cell production in bone marrow.

The other mesangial cells appear to hold the glomerular capillaries in position, and remove macromolecules which have been caught on the glomerular membrane, by phagocytosis.

See also **Hormonal control of erythropoiesis** (page 335), in Ch. 11, Blood, Lymphoid Tissue and Immunity.

PROXIMAL TUBULE

The Malpighian corpuscle tapers into the proximal tubule, which is about 14 mm long. The first two-thirds constitutes the proximal convoluted tubule, whereas the last third is straight. The convoluted section follows a tortuous route through the cortex as a number of small loops, and normally one larger loop is directed out towards the periphery. From here the straight part of the tubule courses inwards into the outer zone of the medulla, where it tapers into the loop of Henle.

The epithelial cells of the proximal tubule have pronounced, closely packed microvilli on their apical surfaces. A large number of slender, lateral processes at the cell base extend under adjacent cells and occupy deep recesses in their bases, thereby attaching adjacent cells together. The lateral borders of the cells are attached only at one point, just below the microvilli. Below this there is a gap between the cells, forming a lateral channel through which water and some reabsorbed solutes flow.

Large numbers of mitochondria and the large surface area afforded by the microvilli reflect the intense reabsorptive activity taking place in the convoluted section. The cells in the straight part of the tubule have fewer microvilli and are less active.

LOOP OF HENLE

The loop of Henle consists of a descending and an ascending limb. Loops of Henle vary in length depending upon the position of their Malpighian corpuscles in the cortex.

In the majority of nephrons (about 85% of the total) which originate from corpuscles situated in the outermost parts of the cortex, the bend is formed from the thick ascending limb and lies in the outer part of the medulla. The thin section is restricted to a very short section of the descending limb.

About 15% of nephrons have their corpuscles in the inner cortex. These juxtamedullary nephrons have long loops of Henle that pass deep into the medullary tissue and here it is the thin limb that actually makes the loop. It is these nephrons that contribute to the formation of hypertonic urine.

The descending limb is thin-walled and consists of simple squamous epithelium with elaborate interdigitations; thus in section small membrane-bound areas of cytoplasm may be seen (Figure 14.5).

The first part of the ascending limb is also thin and structurally similar to the descending limb, but distally the ascending limb has a thick section consisting of cuboidal epithelium.

DISTAL TUBULE

Functionally, the distal tubule is that section lying in the cortex between the loop of Henle and the collecting duct. The tubule follows a tortuous route back to the Malpighian corpuscle, where it passes between the afferent and efferent arterioles before joining the collecting duct.

The cells are slightly flatter than those in the proximal tubule and lack well-developed microvilli. The basal portions of the cells are compartmentalized by interdigitating lateral processes (as in the proximal tubule).

COLLECTING DUCT

Typically, six distal tubules lead into each straight collecting duct in the cortex. Pairs of ducts fuse in the medulla and the new ones then fuse several times and eventually form the large **papillary ducts** or ducts of Bellini, which open into the calyces.

The cells of the collecting ducts are cuboidal, becoming progressively taller in the larger ducts.

Glomerular filtration

The kidneys receive about one-fifth of the cardiac output per minute, 1000–1200 mL/min, when the body is at rest. About one-fifth of the plasma is filtered as it flows through the glomeruli to produce glomerular filtrate at the rate of about 125 mL/min (180 L/d).

Blood is filtered in the glomerulus and the filtrate flows into the space between the visceral and parietal layers of Bowman's capsule. The process is driven by Starling's pressures, principally the hydrostatic pressure of the blood in the glomerulus.

The glomerular hydrostatic pressure is higher than the average pressure found in capillaries. This is because of the relatively short distance from the high pressure blood in the aorta, and because the glomerulus is drained by an arteriole rather than a venule, so that the pressure drops very little as it flows through the capillaries of the glomerulus. Furthermore, in the outer cortex, efferent arterioles are narrower than afferent ones. The resultant increased resistance of the efferent arterioles also helps to keep glomerular hydrostatic pressure relatively high.

The **glomerular hydrostatic pressure** (60 mmHg) is opposed by the plasma colloid osmotic pressure exerted by the plasma proteins (32 mmHg) and by the hydrostatic pressure exerted by the filtered fluid in the capsule (18 mmHg). The net pressure which causes filtration then is

glomerular capillary hydrostatic pressure – plasma colloid osmotic pressure – Bowman's capsule hydrostatic pressure = filtration pressure

$$60 \, mmHg - 32 \, mmHg - 18 \, mmHg = 10 \, mmHg.$$

> Starling's pressures are discussed in **Formation and reabsorption of interstitial fluid** (page 409), in Ch. 12, Circulation of Blood and Lymph.

Experiments have shown that molecules of molecular weight less than 7000 can pass freely through the glomerular filter. The filter is less permeable to larger molecules and those above molecular weight 70 000 cross hardly at all. Albumin has a molecular weight of 69 000 so that it does pass across the filter, though in very small quantities.

The exact nature of the glomerular filtering membrane is not clear, although it is probable that the fenestrations in the capillary endothelium allow free passage of molecules whereas the basement membrane is a more selective filter, which has a strong negative charge that repels proteins, which also have a strong negative charge. The podocytes produce and maintain the basement membrane. The slit membranes between the pedicels may act as the finest filters (Figures 14.9, 14.10).

Because cells and protein molecules do not generally filter through into Bowman's capsule, **glomerular filtrate** is essentially protein-free plasma.

Factors affecting glomerular filtration rate

The glomerular filtration rate (GFR) averages 125 mL/min but it can vary from a few millilitres up to about 200 mL/min. The major factor affecting GFR is glomerular hydrostatic pressure, which in turn is affected by the rates of blood flow into and out of the glomerulus.

Should renal blood flow into the kidney increase, then GFR also increases. A rise in arterial blood pressure results in some increase in GFR, but the extent of the rise is limited by the phenomenon of **autoregulation**. When systemic blood pressure rises, the afferent arterioles constrict, reducing blood flow into the glomeruli and limiting the resultant rise in glomerular hydrostatic pressure.

The degree of constriction of afferent and efferent arterioles will affect the hydrostatic pressure of blood within the glomerulus and therefore GFR. Constriction of the afferent arterioles reduces blood flow into the glomeruli, reducing glomerular hydrostatic pressure and therefore GFR. Constriction of the efferent arterioles, on the other hand, reduces blood flow out of the kidney, raises glomerular hydrostatic pressure and therefore GFR.

Research into the effects of specific substances on afferent and efferent arteriolar resistance has produced rather conflicting results depending on the methods used and the animals studied.

Adrenaline and noradrenaline can potentially constrict or dilate both vessels as there are both alpha- and beta-adrenoceptors present. There is some evidence that there is a stronger constrictor (alpha) effect on the efferent arterioles compared with the afferent ones.

ADH and angiotensin II constrict efferent arterioles, whereas it is likely that atrial natriuretic peptide preferentially dilates afferent arterioles.

Tubular function

Filtration is a relatively non-selective process and therefore the fluid entering the tubule contains all the constituents of plasma except protein.

Tubular activity involves the return of nutritionally useful substances to the blood and the elimination of the waste products of metabolism from the body. In addition, the tubule makes a major contribution to homoeostasis by its ability to vary the elimination of physiologically important substances such as acid, salts and water according to their levels in the body fluids.

Therefore the volume and composition of glomerular filtrate and urine are substantially different (see Table 14.2). The changes are brought about by two processes, reabsorption and secretion.

Reabsorption

Reabsorption is the net transfer of solute or water from the tubular fluid back into the blood (Figure 14.11). Such substances travel through the tubular epithelium into the interstitial spaces and from there into the peritubular capillary network.

Any substances which are filtered, but which do not appear in the urine at all, are reabsorbed completely in their passage through the tubules. They include substances of particular nutritional value such as amino acids, acetoacetate, vitamins and glucose.

Most of the substances in the glomerular filtrate are only partially reabsorbed and therefore appear in the urine. In some instances the amount reabsorbed is under hormonal control. Table 14.1 shows some constituents of glomerular filtrate and the amounts typically reabsorbed from the tubules.

Uptake of material by the tubular cells may either be a passive or an active process.

Passive transport of solutes (diffusion) requires a favourable

See also **Diffusion** and **Osmosis** (page 13), in Ch. 1, Molecules, Ions and Unit and **Movement of substances across the cell membrane** (page 48), in Ch. 2, Cells and the Internal Environment.

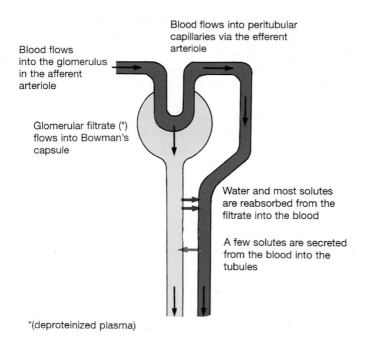

Blood flows into the glomerulus in the afferent arteriole

Blood flows into peritubular capillaries via the efferent arteriole

Glomerular filtrate (*) flows into Bowman's capsule

Water and most solutes are reabsorbed from the filtrate into the blood

A few solutes are secreted from the blood into the tubules

*(deproteinized plasma)

Figure 14.11 The three major processes occurring in the nephron: glomerular filtration, tubular reabsorption and secretion.

concentration or electrochemical gradient. However, only a minority of substances are carried by this method (e.g. urea, and some ions 'follow' ions of the opposite charge that are transported actively). Water is also reabsorbed passively (**osmosis**) as it moves down the osmotic gradients created by reabsorption of solutes.

Active transport, the method by which most substances are reabsorbed, involves the movement of solutes across a cell membrane by carrier molecules. For most solutes moved by active transport there is a point at which all of the carrier molecules are saturated and, therefore, a maximum number of molecules that can be transported at any one

Table 14.1 Typical values for renal reabsorption and secretion of some plasma constituents (modified from Ganong, W.F. (1995) *Review of Medical Physiology*, 17th edn, Appleton & Lange, New York). P = proximal tubule; L = loop of Henle; D = distal tubule; C = collecting duct

Substance	% secreted	% reabsorbed	Location
Na^+		99.4	P, L, D, C
K^+	8 (D)	93.3	P, L, D, C
Cl^-		99.2	P, L, D, C
HCO_3^-		100	P, D
Urea		53	P, L, D, C
Urate	8 (P)	98	P
Glucose		100	P
Water		99.4	P, L, D, C

instant. This maximum rate of solute transfer is known as the **tubular maximum** or **Tm** for that particular substance, e.g. the Tm value for glucose is about 380 mg/min.

For a typical blood glucose concentration of 100 mg/100 mL and a glomerular filtration rate of 125 ml/min all the glucose is reabsorbed at a rate of 125 mg/min.

A glucose concentration above about 200 mg/100 mL plasma exceeds the transport capacity of some nephrons, whereas a concentration above about 400 mg/100 mL plasma exceeds the transport capacity of all nephrons. Glucose starts to appear in the urine (glycosuria), therefore, if its plasma concentration exceeds about 200 mg/100 mL, e.g. in diabetes mellitus.

See also **Effects of insulin deficiency (diabetes mellitus)** (page 634), in Ch. 16, Endocrine Physiology.

Secretion

The process of secretion involves the net transfer of solute from the peritubular capillaries through the tubular cells and into the tubular fluid (Figure 14.11). It is therefore an additional, albeit minor route whereby substances can enter the urine.

Secretion is generally an active process. The major endogenous substances secreted by the tubular cells are potassium and hydrogen ions (both of which are secreted in exchange for sodium). In addition, the bases thiamine, guanidine, histamine and choline are secreted in the proximal tubule.

Foreign substances such as penicillin, and para-amino hippuric acid (PAH) are also actively secreted. PAH is in fact secreted so strongly by the tubular cells that it is completely removed from the blood. PAH clearance is used clinically to estimate renal plasma flow (see *Renal clearance*, below).

Renal clearance

The clearance rate of a substance is defined as that volume of plasma completely cleared of a given substance in 1 minute. Alternatively, it is that volume of plasma which contains the amount of a substance that is excreted in the urine in one minute.

The measurement of inulin or creatinine clearance is used to measure glomerular filtration rate. Para-amino hippuric acid (PAH) clearance is used in the measurement of renal blood flow.

MEASUREMENT OF GLOMERULAR FILTRATION RATE

By choosing a substance which filters freely but is neither reabsorbed nor secreted in the tubule the clearance value is found to correspond to the rate of filtration; such a substance is the polysaccharide inulin.

A large dose of inulin is given intravenously, and the following values are measured:

Rate of urine production (V mL/min)
Inulin concentration in plasma (P g/100 mL)
Inulin concentration in urine (U g/100 mL)

Amount of inulin excreted per minute = UV/100 g

Each millilitre of plasma contains P/100 g of inulin

If z mol of filtrate is formed per minute
then $zP/100$ g of inulin is filtered per minute.

Since inulin is neither secreted nor reabsorbed in the tubule, then:
$UV/100 = zP/100$

and $UV/P = z$ mL/min = filtrate formed/min = inulin clearance.

Typical values might be:
V = 1 mL/min
P = 0.05 g/100 mL
U = 6.25 g/100 mL.

$z = UV/P = (6.25 \times 1)/0.05 = 125$ mL/min.

Thus the clearance/filtration value for inulin is 125 mL/min. A clearance value of less than 125 mL/min indicates that the substance is reabsorbed in the tubule, e.g. glucose = 0 mL/min (total reabsorption) and urea = 70 mL/min (partial reabsorption). Table 14.2 gives typical clearance values for the major substances in glomerular filtrate.

Table 14.2 Concentrations of substances in glomerular filtrate (125 mL/min) and in urine (1 mL/min) (modified from Guyton, A.C. (1991) *Textbook of Medical Physiology*, 8th edn, W.B. Saunders, Philadelphia)

Substance	Concentration in glomerular filtrate (meq/L)	Concentration in urine (meq/L)	Concentration in urine/Concentration in plasma (plasma clearance/min)
Na^+	142	128	0.9
K^+	5	60	12
Ca^{2+}	4	4.8	1.2
Mg^{2+}	3	15	5
Cl^-	103	134	1.3
HCO_3^-	28	0	0
HPO_4^{2-}	2	50	25
SO_4^{2-}	0.7	33	47
	(mg/dL)	*(mg/dL)*	
Glucose	100	0	0
Urea	26	1820	70
Uric acid	3	42	14
Inulin			125
PAH			585

Creatinine clearance can be used to estimate glomerular filtration rate. Creatinine is filtered completely and a very small amount is secreted into the tubules. However, since the plasma creatinine level usually appears to have a higher value than it should (because plasma chromogens have a similar reaction) the clearance value is approximately 125 mL/min.

MEASUREMENT OF RENAL BLOOD FLOW

A clearance value greater than 125 mL/min indicates tubular secretion, e.g. PAH = 585 mL/min. PAH filters freely at the glomerulus and about 91% is then removed by the tubular cells. If 100% of the PAH were cleared from the plasma, then the clearance value for PAH would be equal to total renal plasma flow. As the clearance is actually nearer 91%, then

total renal plasma flow = 585 × 100/91 = 643 mL/min.

To convert plasma flow to blood flow requires a knowledge of the percentage of plasma in whole blood (about 55%).

Total renal blood flow = 643 × 100/55 = 1170 mL/min.

Proximal tubule

About 70% of all reabsorptive and secretory activity takes place in the proximal tubule, with water following the reabsorption of solutes, thereby maintaining isotonicity. The fluid leaving the proximal tubule and entering the loop of Henle is therefore still isotonic with plasma but is reduced to some 30% of its original volume.

The structure of the proximal tubular cells reflects their reabsorptive role. The surface exposed to the tubular lumen has its area increased 20-fold by microvilli and the lateral channels receive solutes and water, which then move by bulk flow into the low-pressure peritubular capillaries.

Nutrients such as glucose, amino acids, acetoacetate and vitamins are normally completely reabsorbed from the filtrate. All these substances are reabsorbed in the proximal convoluted tubule by active transport mechanisms; much of the filtered potassium is also reabsorbed here. Any protein which has leaked through the glomerular membrane is completely reabsorbed by pinocytosis and is therefore normally absent from the urine.

Many substances are incompletely reabsorbed in the proximal tubule. These include Na^+, Cl^-, PO_4^{3-}, NO_3^{2-}, urate and urea.

HCO_3^- is normally completely reabsorbed in the form of carbon dioxide (see *Renal regulation of pH of body fluids*, below).

The cells of the proximal tubule also actively secrete the bases thiamine, guanidine, choline and histamine, and the acids penicillin, PAH, and uric acid. The proximal tubule is also the major site of hydrogen ion secretion (see *Renal regulation of pH of body fluids*, below).

REABSORPTION OF SPECIFIC SUBSTANCES IN THE PROXIMAL TUBULE

Sodium ions

The reabsorption of Na^+ is particularly important, not only because it is present in relatively large quantities in blood and therefore glomerular filtrate but also because its reabsorption is linked to that of Cl^-, glucose, amino acids and water.

Generally about 99% of the filtered Na^+ is reabsorbed by the tubular cells, most of this occurring in the proximal tubule. Na^+ is actively transported out of the basal and lateral surfaces of the cell by the **sodium–potassium pump** (**Na^+-K^+-ATPase**). The low intracellular concentration of Na^+, together with the negative intracellular potential of about $-70\,mV$ creates a large electrochemical gradient, so that Na^+ diffuses into the cell across the luminal cell membrane (Figure 14.12).

The entry of the positively charged Na^+ is almost (80%) matched by the diffusion of Cl^- into the cell, which maintains the membrane potential. The remaining 20% of Na^+ entry is 'exchanged' for H^+.

Glucose

The diffusion of Na^+ into the tubular cells is accompanied by glucose. Na^+ diffuses down its concentration gradient (maintained by the Na^+-K^+-ATPase) and 'drags' glucose with it, even though it is moving against its concentration gradient. The reabsorption of glucose is, therefore, a form of secondary active transport (**cotransport**), whereby the Na^+-K^+-

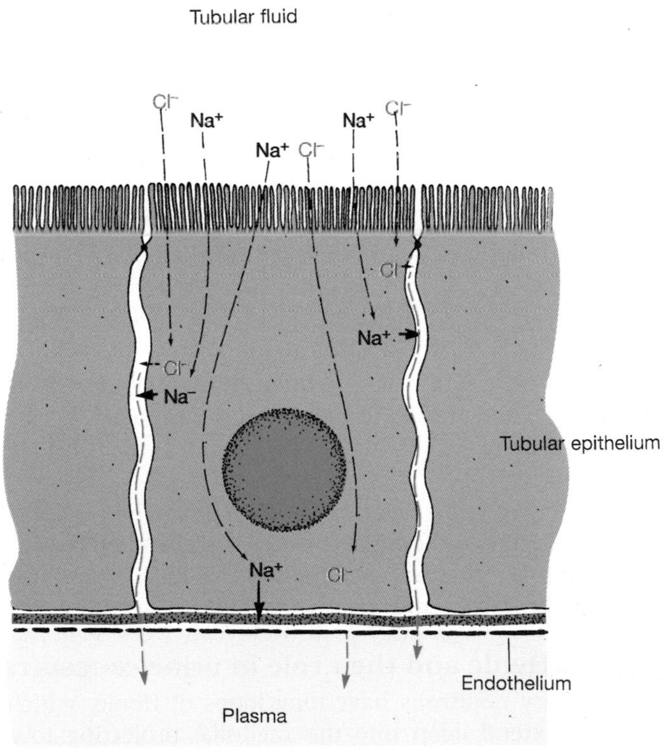

Figure 14.12 Mechanism of Na^+ reabsorption in the proximal tubule. The active transport of Na^+ (Na^+–K^+ pump) creates a low intracellular concentration of Na^+, which promotes the diffusion of Na^+ into the cell from the tubular fluid. Na^+ diffuses through the brush border attached to several different carrier proteins, which carry glucose or amino acids as well as Na^+ into the cell. Cl^- is reabsorbed by diffusion, attracted by the reabsorption of Na^+. Solid arrows = active transport; broken arrows = diffusion. Green broken arrow = bulk flow.

ATPase is creating the conditions under which glucose is reabsorbed along with Na^+.

Amino acids

The reabsorption of amino acids by the proximal tubular cells is essentially the same as that for glucose, i.e. a cotransport system with Na^+. There are several different carriers for different amino acids.

Phosphate ions

Phosphate reabsorption is coupled to Na^+ reabsorption in the same way as that of glucose and amino acids.

Chloride ions

In the first part of the proximal tubule, the reabsorption of Cl^- passively follows the active reabsorption of Na^+, attracted by its positive charge.

In the distal two-thirds of the proximal convoluted tubule in all but the juxtamedullary nephrons, the permeability to Cl^- is higher than for other anions and it diffuses down its concentration gradient, followed by the passive diffusion of Na^+

Bicarbonate (hydrogen carbonate) ions

Bicarbonate ions are not reabsorbed as such, rather as dissolved carbon dioxide. Filtered HCO_3^- combines with H^+ that has been secreted into the tubular lumen, forming carbonic acid (see Figure 14.20). The acid dissociates into carbon dioxide and water. Carbon dioxide diffuses easily into the tubular cells where, in a reaction catalysed by the enzyme carbonic anhydrase, it combines with water, forming carbonic acid which dissociates into HCO_3^- and H^+. HCO_3^- then diffuses out of the cell into the peritubular capillaries.

Potassium ions

About 80% of filtered K^+ is reabsorbed in the proximal tubule, mainly by passive transport through the tight junctions between the cells. The Na^+-K^+-ATPase causes K^+ to enter the cells, but it rapidly diffuses out again down its concentration gradient. There is some active reabsorption of K^+ too.

Hydrogen ions

Secretion of H^+ occurs in the proximal tubule, where it is mainly exchanged for Na^+, and results in the reabsorption of HCO_3^- (see Figure 14.20).

Water

Typically, around 70% of the filtered water is reabsorbed passively down an osmotic gradient in the proximal tubule; this reabsorption is independent of hormonal control and is relatively constant in volume.

Long loops of Henle and their role in urine concentration

The juxtamedullary nephrons have long loops of Henle, which start in the cortex and extend deep into the medulla, projecting towards the pelvis of the kidney. These loops create an osmotic gradient in the medulla that enables water to be reabsorbed from the collecting ducts and produce hypertonic urine (typically 300–500 mosmol/kg H_2O, but it can be as high as 1400 mosmol/kg H_2O).

The tubular fluid leaving the proximal tubule passes down through the descending limb of the loop of Henle deep into the medulla, round the hairpin loop and then back to the cortex in the ascending limb. When it enters the loop of Henle the fluid is isotonic with plasma, but when it leaves it and flows into the distal tubule it has become hypotonic.

The fluid surrounding the loop of Henle has an osmotic pressure that increases between the outer and inner medulla (Figure 14.13). This gradient is created by the '**countercurrent mechanism**' operating in the long loops of Henle (Figure 14.14).

As fluid passes up the thick ascending limb of the loop of Henle in the outer medulla, Na^+ is actively transported out of the cells into the medullary interstitium. Cl^- follows, attracted by its positive charge. The ascending limb is unusual in that it is impermeable to water, so that the movement of Na^+ and Cl^- is not followed by an equivalent amount of water. As the fluid passes up the ascending limb, therefore, it becomes progressively less concentrated, so that by the time it reaches the distal tubule it is hypotonic to plasma.

The presence of increasing amounts of Na^+ and Cl^- in the interstitial fluid of the outer medulla causes the removal of water from and the addition of Na^+ and Cl^- to the descending loop of Henle. This passive diffusion and osmosis results in the equilibration of the tubular fluid in the descending limb and the medullary interstitium at each level (Figure 14.14). As the fluid flows towards the tip of the loop, therefore, it and

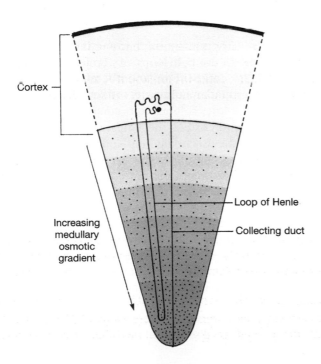

Figure 14.13 A juxtamedullary nephron and the medullary osmotic gradient created by the long loops of Henle of such nephrons.

Cortex

Increasing medullary osmotic gradient

Loop of Henle

Collecting duct

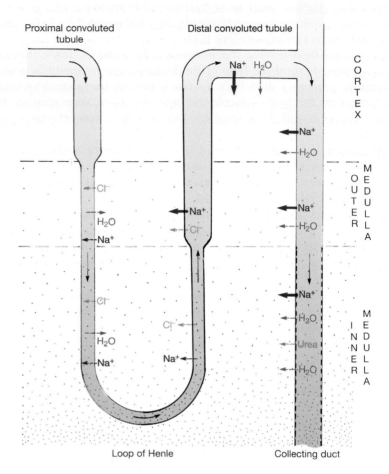

Figure 14.14 Countercurrent mechanism. The long loops of Henle generate a hypertonic interstitial fluid, which increases from the outer to the inner medulla This enables water to be reabsorbed from the collecting duct, producing a hypertonic urine. Thick horizontal arrows – active transport.

the surrounding medullary interstitium become increasingly hypertonic. Indeed, animals with the longest loops of Henle can create the most concentrated medullary interstitium and therefore the most concentrated urine. Once the tubular fluid enters the ascending limb, which is impermeable to water, it loses solute and becomes hypotonic.

The key to the countercurrent mechanism, therefore, is the active transport of Na^+ out of the ascending limb and into the medullary interstitium, a process which is not followed by a corresponding movement of water because this section of the nephron is impermeable to water. This process, coupled with the contraflow of fluid in the two limbs, results in an osmotic pressure gradient between the outer and inner medulla.

In the distal tubule, further solute and an equivalent amount of water is reabsorbed, but the tubular fluid remains hypotonic.

As the filtrate passes down the collecting duct, the reabsorption of water occurs by osmosis into the increasingly hypertonic interstitial fluid. Therefore, as the tubular fluid flows deeper into the medulla it becomes hypertonic urine.

In the inner medulla, the cells of the collecting duct are permeable to urea, whereas those of the distal tubule and the cortical collecting duct are not. As a consequence, urea concentration rises as tubular fluid flows through the cortical and outer medullary sections, as a result of the reabsorption of water. In the inner medulla, however, urea diffuses from the tubular fluid into the interstitium, further raising the osmotic pressure and drawing water out of the thin descending limb of the loop of Henle. Immediately after the loop turns back towards the cortex, the high concentrations of Na$^+$ and Cl$^-$ in the tubular fluid cause them to diffuse passively out of the thin medullary portion into the surrounding environment. The presence of urea, Na$^+$ and Cl$^-$ serves to make the interstitium of the inner medulla extremely hypertonic.

Antidiuretic hormone (ADH) influences the countercurrent mechanism in two ways. It increases the permeability of the inner medullary collecting duct to urea, and increases the permeability of both the cortical and medullary sections of the collecting duct to water.

In conditions of **dehydration**, more ADH is released by the posterior pituitary gland (see *Regulation of osmotic pressure by antidiuretic hormone*, below). More urea is therefore able to leave the medullary collecting duct and raise the osmotic pressure of the medullary interstitium (Figure 14.15).

Also, the high ADH level enables more water to be drawn out along the length of the collecting duct. A smaller volume of more hypertonic urine is, therefore, produced during dehydration compared with normal hydration levels.

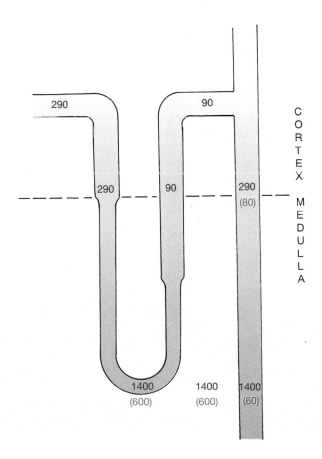

Figure 14.15 Typical values for osmotic pressure (mosmol/kg H$_2$O) at various points along the long loops of Henle in the presence of maximal ADH concentration (e.g. in dehydration). Values found in the absence of ADH (e.g. in overhydration or diabetes inspidus) are given in brackets. The resultant urine produced at the end of the collecting duct can thereby vary from 60 mosmol/kg H$_2$O to 1400 mosmol/kg H$_2$O.

Conversely, in conditions of overhydration, ADH concentration in the blood falls, with subsequent reduction in the tonicity of the medullary interstitium and less water reabsorption from the collecting duct; therefore a larger volume of more dilute urine ensues (Figure 14.15).

It is evident that the entry of water into the interstitial fluid of the medulla from the loops of Henle and collecting duct would cause a decrease in the osmotic concentration. This decrease is prevented by the hairpin capillary loops, the vasa recta, which abound in the medulla. The vasa recta act as 'countercurrent diffusion exchangers'. As blood passes down the descending limb of a vessel, water diffuses out and osmotically active particles (Na^+, Cl^- and urea) diffuse in (Figure 14.16).

As blood flows towards the cortex, water enters and osmotically active particles pass out. The net effect is therefore to trap solutes in the tip of the loop, in equilibrium with the medullary interstitium and the loop of Henle.

Water that has entered the interstitium from both the loops of Henle and the collecting ducts dilutes it to a level just below that in the vasa recta. This water therefore moves into the ascending limbs of the vasa recta by osmosis and is reabsorbed into the blood.

Figure 14.16 Countercurrent diffusion exchange in the vasa recta. Water diffuses out of the descending vasa recta and into the ascending vessel. Solutes diffuse into the descending vessel and out of the ascending vessel. Water reabsorbed from the collecting duct diffuses into the ascending vasa recta.

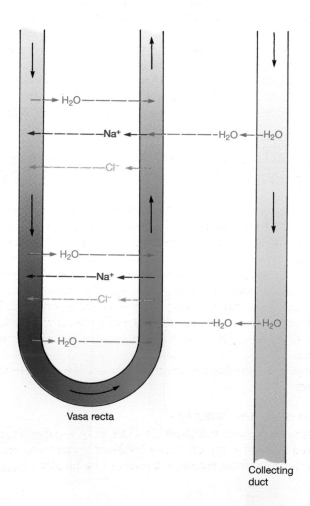

Distal nephron

The distal tubule of the nephron is not really a distinct physiological unit. Proximally it consists of an extension of the ascending limb of the loop of Henle, consisting of cells that are essentially impermeable to water, and distally the cells become like those of the cortical collecting duct. Physiologically, the collective term 'distal nephron' is used to describe the functional unit of distal tubule and collecting duct.

The fluid entering the distal tubule is hypotonic to the surrounding interstitial fluid. Na^+ is reabsorbed from the tubule along with Cl^- and HCO_3^-, while H^+ and K^+ are secreted into the tubular fluid. A further 10% of the glomerular filtrate is reabsorbed by osmosis, following the reabsorption of solute. The tubular fluid remains, however, hypotonic at about 90 mosmol/kg H_2O.

The collecting duct is a particularly important structure (shared by several nephrons) because the reabsorption of water, Na^+, Cl^- and the secretion of H^+ and K^+ vary according to their levels in the blood. This section, then, is demonstrably active in the maintenance of homoeostasis with regard to some key constituents of body fluids.

The reabsorption of water by osmosis in the collecting duct is made possible by the high osmotic pressure in the medulla and controlled by the hormone **ADH** (see *Regulation of water balance*, below).

The hormone **aldosterone** affects the quantities of Na^+, Cl^- and water reabsorbed as well as the amount of K^+ secreted (see *Role of aldosterone in the regulation of sodium and potassium balance and blood volume*, below).

An important mechanism which maintains a constant H^+ concentration in body fluids occurs in the distal nephron. The amounts of H^+ secreted and HCO_3^- reabsorbed vary according to the state of acid–base balance in the body (see *Renal regulation of pH of body fluids*, below).

Regulation of nephron function

The kidneys play a particularly important role in the maintenance of homoeostasis by varying the rates of reabsorption and secretion of water and solutes according to their concentrations in the blood. An excess of a substance leads to an increase in its elimination by the kidneys, thereby restoring the concentration to its usual level. This process is controlled by hormones, different substances being affected by different hormones. Water reabsorption is controlled by ADH from the neurohypophysis as well as by mineralocorticoids from the adrenal cortices, which also regulate Na^+ and K^+ balance. Ca^{2+} and PO_4^{3-} balance is controlled by parathyroid hormone.

The kidneys also contribute to the maintenance of a constant blood H^+ concentration.

Regulation of water balance

Water is ingested in food and drink in extremely variable amounts. If there is such a thing as a 'typical' water intake, it is said to be around 2 L per day. Oxidation of food produces a further few hundred millilitres of fluid, so that a rough estimate of the total amount of fluid added to the body daily is around 2.5 L.

Whatever the precise volume of fluid taken in daily, the maintenance of a constant body fluid volume (and concentration of its solutes) clearly requires an equal amount of water to be lost. Water is continually lost from the lungs on breathing out and through the skin by diffusion and then evaporation from its surface. These two routes normally cause about 400 mL each per day to be lost. A further 100 mL or so is lost in faeces. The remaining 1.5 L of fluid is usually lost in the urine.

Table 14.3 gives some examples of how daily input and output of fluid can vary.

If input should rise or fall, the physiological response is for the kidneys to vary the amount of water reabsorbed in the distal nephrons. An increase in fluid intake results in less reabsorption and a greater volume of urine; whereas a reduced fluid intake is followed by more water reabsorption and a smaller volume of urine.

Table 14.3 Examples of ways of varying fluid intake and output

Increased intake
Larger meals
More drink

Reduced intake
Limited access to food/drink or dieting
Feeling unwell and not wanting to eat/drink
Gastrointestinal problems preventing adequate intake

Increased output
Sweating – due to exercise, high ambient temperature or fever
Hyperventilation
Loss of body fluids, e.g. haemorrhage, burns, vomiting, diarrhoea

---

Table 14.4 Water reabsorption in different parts of the nephron under varying conditions of hydration (expressed as a percentage of the glomerular filtrate)

	Overhydration (%)	Typical (%)	Dehydration (%)
Proximal tubule	70	70	70
Loop of Henle	5	5	5
Distal nephron	12	24	24.8
Volume of urine	13	1	0.2
mL/min	16	1	0.25
L/d	23	1.5	0.4

The amount of water reabsorbed from the proximal tubule and the descending limb of the loop of Henle is relatively constant from day to day and represents about 75% of the glomerular filtrate. The amount of water reabsorbed by the distal nephron can vary from 13– 24.8% of the glomerular filtrate, which would produce a urine volume ranging from 23 L down to 400 mL per day (Table 14.4).

Control of water reabsorption in the distal nephron is regulated primarily by ADH, which is released by the neurohypophysis. The hormone is actually synthesized within the cell bodies of the supraoptic (SO) nucleus, and to a lesser extent the paraventricular nucleus, both of which lie within the hypothalamus (see Figure 16.5). Following synthesis, the neurosecretory material is transported along the axons to their terminals in the neurohypophysis by a rapid transport system involving the microtubules. It is this stored hormone that is released directly into the blood stream. The mechanism is essentially the same as that found in synapses or neuroeffector junctions, in which the arrival of an action potential at the axon ending results in a small amount of chemical being released by exocytosis.

Usually, a small amount of ADH is constantly being released into the blood in response to a tonic discharge of action potentials from the cell bodies in the SO nucleus down the axons to the neurohypophysis. The rate of secretion of ADH can therefore either increase as a result of an increased rate of firing of the SO nucleus, or decrease if it fires at a slower frequency.

There are cells termed **osmoreceptors** in the vicinity of the SO nucleus in the hypothalamus, which respond to a change in osmotic pressure of the fluid bathing them. An increase in osmotic pressure stimulates the osmoreceptors, which in turn increases the rate of firing of the SO nucleus.

REGULATION OF OSMOTIC PRESSURE BY ANTIDIURETIC HORMONE

Dehydration (negative water balance) causes a rise in osmotic pressure of the plasma flowing to the brain and increases the release of ADH (Figure 14.17). As a result of stimulation of the osmoreceptors, nerve impulses pass down the axons of the hypothalamo-hypophysial tract with increased frequency and cause a more rapid release of ADH into the blood stream.

ADH passes to the kidneys, where it increases the permeability of the collecting ducts to both water and urea. An increased amount of water is then drawn back from the tubules into the medullary interstitium, where the osmotic pressure is raised further by the addition of urea (see also *Long loops of Henle and their role in urine concentration*, above). Water diffuses from the medullary interstitium into the vasa recta and is reabsorbed into the blood. As a result the osmotic pressure of the plasma is reduced and the stimulus removed, or at least reduced. This is an example of negative feedback, whereby the physiological response (reduced osmotic pressure) inhibits further change (reduces ADH secretion rate).

Typically, the daily output of urine is about 1.5 L, with an osmolality of 300–500 mosmol/kg H_2O. In conditions of dehydration a reduced

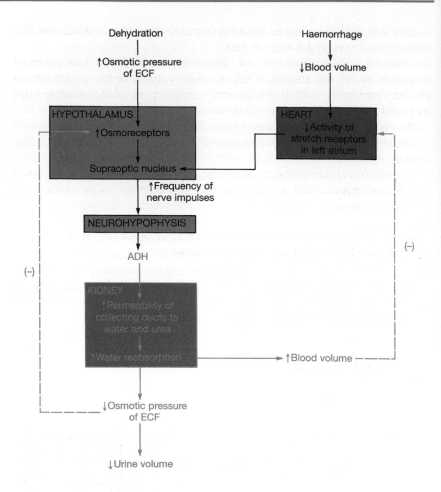

Figure 14.17 Role of ADH in the regulation of water loss by the kidneys.

volume (down to 400 mL) of hypertonic urine (up to about 1400 mosmol/kg H_2O), is produced. A small urine output is known as **oliguria**.

Overhydration (positive water balance) causes a reduction in the osmotic pressure of the blood and reduces ADH release below the basal level. A larger volume (up to 23 L) of more dilute urine (down to 30 mosmol/kg H_2O), i.e. a **diuresis**, is produced, bringing the body back into water balance.

As Na^+ is the major cation in extracellular fluid, this system of osmoregulation is also a major controller of plasma Na^+ concentration. Should the ingestion of Na^+ increase, the resultant rise in osmotic pressure of the blood stimulates increased ADH secretion and dilutes the plasma by increasing the reabsorption of water. The osmoreceptors also initiate the sensation of thirst, which, if it results in drinking water, will clearly lower plasma Na^+ concentration.

REGULATION OF BLOOD VOLUME BY ANTIDIURETIC HORMONE
ADH release is also affected by changes in blood volume, and the hormone in turn contributes to the maintenance of a constant blood volume, particularly in an 'emergency' such as a sudden haemorrhage.

Such a fall in blood volume would result in an increase in ADH concentration, water retention and oliguria.

Changes in blood volume are detected principally by low-pressure receptors in the left atrium. A fall in blood volume reduces stimulation of the receptors in the left atrium, resulting in a decrease in the frequency of action potentials transmitted along the vagus nerve to the brain. ADH secretion is increased and a fall in urine output results.

Conversely, a rise in blood volume results in a decrease in ADH secretion, resulting in diuresis.

The high-pressure baroreceptors in the carotid sinuses and aortic arch can also influence ADH secretion rate in an analogous way to the low-pressure receptors.

Role of aldosterone in the regulation of sodium and potassium balance and blood volume

The hormone aldosterone is synthesized and released by the adrenal cortices. Aldosterone acts on the distal nephron, particularly the cortical section of the collecting duct, and has two separate primary actions, Na⁺ reabsorption and K⁺ secretion (Figure 14.18).

Figure 14.18 Actions of aldosterone on the kidney in response to low blood volume/pressure, raised blood K⁺ concentration or reduced blood Na⁺ concentration.

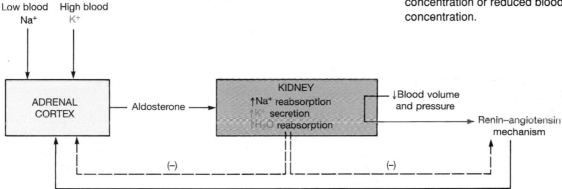

Under the action of aldosterone there is more Na⁺ reabsorbed than K⁺ secreted. This creates a charge difference, which promotes the reabsorption of anions such as Cl⁻. The net reabsorption of solutes in turn causes the osmotic reabsorption of water. Aldosterone, then, indirectly causes an increase in water reabsorption and therefore an increase in blood volume.

The stimuli that increase the secretion rate of aldosterone are the converse of its actions: a drop in plasma Na⁺ concentration, a rise in plasma K⁺ concentration or a fall in blood volume or blood pressure.

Altered concentrations of Na⁺ or K⁺ act directly on the zona glomerulosa and influence aldosterone secretion rates. The effect of K⁺ is much more powerful than that of Na⁺.

A fall in blood volume and/or arterial blood pressure results in an increased release of aldosterone by a chain of events known as the **renin–angiotensin mechanism** (Figure 14.19).

See also **The adrenal cortices** (page 637), in Ch. 16, Endocrine Physiology.

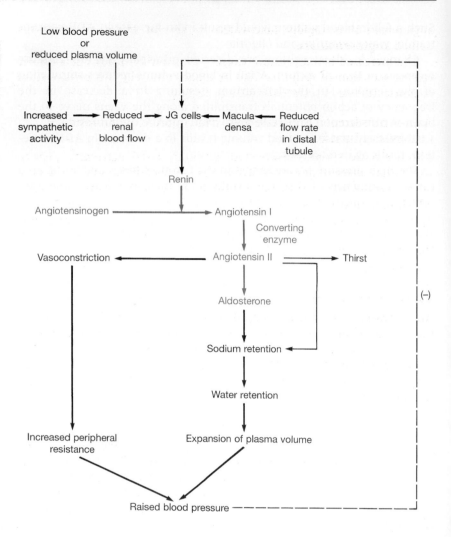

Figure 14.19 Role of the renin–angiotensin mechanism in the regulation of aldosterone secretion.

A drop in blood volume or arterial blood pressure leads to a drop in blood flow through the afferent arterioles leading to the glomeruli. This occurs both directly, due to the low blood pressure driving the blood, but also as a consequence of arteriolar vasoconstriction resulting from the baroreceptor reflex initiated by the low blood pressure.

In response to reduced perfusion, the juxtaglomerular cells increase their rate of secretion of the enzyme **renin** into the blood. This enzyme catalyses the conversion of a plasma protein, **angiotensinogen**, into **angiotensin I**. A converting enzyme in the endothelial lining of lung blood vessels then converts angiotensin I to **angiotensin II**, a process that involves splitting off two amino acids.

Angiotensin II is a pivotal substance because of its variety of actions: vasoconstriction, which leads to a rise in blood pressure; stimulation of aldosterone secretion, which leads to an increase in water reabsorption and blood volume; stimulation of thirst, which leads to an increase in blood volume by fluid ingestion; direct Na⁺-retaining action on the distal nephron. In view of its powerful actions, it is understandable that angiotensin II is rapidly inactivated by several enzymes collectively named **angiotensinase**.

The increased blood pressure exerts a negative feedback effect on the rate of secretion of renin, so that as aldosterone elicits a physiological response, its rate of secretion begins to decline.

See also **Neurohypophysis** (page 621), in Ch. 16, Endocrine Physiology.

Atrial natriuretic peptide and the regulation of sodium and potassium balance

Another more recently discovered hormone, atrial natriuretic peptide (ANP), has effects that may contribute to the overall Na^+ and K^+ balance of the body. ANP is secreted by cardiac atrial cells in response to stretch, which in turn could be caused by increased venous return due to a rise in blood volume. It appears to have several different actions, including the inhibition of aldosterone secretion. This action is natriuretic in that there is less Na^+ reabsorption in the distal nephron and therefore more Na^+ in the urine.

Causes of diuresis

An increased rate of urine output (diuresis) can result from either an increase in glomerular filtration rate or a reduction in the reabsorption of water from the tubule. Reduced water reabsorption has several causes: a fall in blood ADH concentration; a rise in osmotically active substances in the glomerular filtrate; or drug-induced inhibition of solute reabsorption.

INCREASED GLOMERULAR FILTRATION RATE

Autoregulation of renal blood flow results in a relatively constant GFR when mean arterial blood pressure is between about 75 and 160 mmHg. Above this level, however, the resultant increase in GFR causes the tubular fluid to flow through the nephron at a faster rate, producing a greater urine volume. This phenomenon is known as **pressure diuresis**.

GFR can also be increased by afferent arteriolar dilation caused, for example, by **caffeine** or **ANP**.

REDUCED ANTIDIURETIC HORMONE CONCENTRATION

If ADH concentration in the blood falls, water reabsorption from the collecting ducts is consequently reduced and a diuresis ensues. Ingestion of large amounts of water lowers the osmotic pressure of the blood and leads to such a fall in ADH concentration.

Diabetes insipidus is a rare condition in which the synthesis or secretion of ADH from the neurohypophysis is impaired. The resultant diuresis can reach 15 L/d.

Alcohol inhibits the release of ADH from the neurohypophysis, thereby inducing diuresis. This effect explains the dehydrating effect of drinking alcohol.

OSMOTIC DIURESIS

Osmotic diuresis is caused by increasing the load of osmotically active substances in the glomerular filtrate. If excess solute is filtered and cannot be reabsorbed, it will retain water in the kidney tubules and be passed as urine. This can occur as a result of hyperglycaemia in, for instance, **diabetes mellitus**. It can also be induced by an intravenous infusion of **mannitol**, a monosaccharide that is filtered but not absorbed in the tubules

DRUG-INDUCED DIURESIS

Drug-induced diuresis can be caused by inhibition of solute reabsorption at various points along the nephron; a few examples are given here to illustrate the modes of action. **Loop diuretics** (e.g. frusemide and ethacrynic acid) act on the ascending limb of the loop of Henle and inhibit the extrusion of Na^+ and Cl^-. This reduces the osmotic gradient in the medullary interstitium and thereby reduces water reabsorption from the collecting duct. **Thiazide diuretics** inhibit Na^+ reabsorption in the distal tubule. **Aldosterone antagonists**, such as spironolactone, compete with aldosterone for receptor sites in the distal nephron, thereby inhibiting the action of aldosterone in these areas. This action results in diuresis by blocking Na^+ reabsorption.

Renal regulation of calcium and phosphate balance

About half of the calcium in the blood is carried bound to plasma protein, and most of the remainder circulates as Ca^{2+}. Phosphate is carried in the blood as HPO_4^{2-} and $H_2PO_4^-$, important buffers for H^+.

Ca^{2+}, HPO_4^{2-} and $H_2PO_4^-$ are filtered freely at the glomeruli and reabsorbed by active transport from the tubules. The amount filtered, as for all ions, depends upon the plasma concentration and the glomerular filtration rate.

Ca^{2+} is reabsorbed in the proximal tubule, the ascending limb of the loop of Henle, as well as the distal tubules and collecting ducts. HPO_4^{2-} and $H_2PO_4^-$ are actively reabsorbed in the proximal tubule. The amounts reabsorbed depend upon the plasma level of **parathyroid hormone (PTH)**.

Low levels of Ca^{2+} in the blood stimulate the parathyroid glands to increase the secretion rate of PTH. This then acts rapidly on the kidney tubules and reduces the reabsorption of phosphate and increases the reabsorption of Ca^{2+}. It should be noted that, in addition to the effects upon the kidney, PTH also controls bone metabolism by promoting the removal of Ca^{2+} and phosphate from bone. Under the influence of PTH there is a net rise in blood Ca^{2+}, but a drop in blood phosphate.

The proximal tubules convert 25-hydroxycholecalciferol (produced in the liver from calciferol or cholecalciferol) to 1,25-dihydroxycholecalciferol, the active form of **vitamin D**. The principal action of vitamin D is to stimulate the absorption of dietary Ca^{2+} and PO_4^{3-} from the small intestine.

Renal regulation of pH of body fluids (acid–base balance)

The blood pH is typically about 7.4 ($10^{-7.4}$ mol/L, 40 nmol/L), and it is maintained within the pH range 7.35–7.45. Venous blood pH is about 0.03 units less than that of arterial blood. The maintenance of a constant pH is important because of the sensitivity of enzymes to the concentra-

The pH scale is explained on page 15 in Ch. 1, Molecules, Ions and Units.

tion of acid. If the acidity of body fluids changes, then some chemical reactions are stimulated, others are depressed, so that homoeostasis is disturbed.

Acid is constantly being produced by metabolic activity and there is therefore a continuous loss of it from the body. Base is also continuously conserved.

Metabolism produces several acids (principally sulphuric and phosphoric), but the major source of acid is carbon dioxide which forms carbonic acid in water.

$$H_2O + CO_2 \longrightarrow H_2CO_3$$

As pH is a measure of the concentration of free H^+, then, provided that the H^+ ions produced by metabolism are effectively removed by chemical combination with other substances (buffers), the pH will be unaffected.

H^+ may be buffered by the blood (both in the plasma and in the red cells), by interstitial fluid and by intracellular fluid. When H^+ ions enter cells, electrical neutrality is maintained by K^+ leaving the cells in exchange. Such buffering is obviously only a temporary solution to the accumulation of acid and ultimately it must be excreted.

The bicarbonate buffer system involves two consecutive reversible reactions.

1. When carbon dioxide is dissolved in water some of it forms carbonic acid.
2. Some carbonic acid dissociates into hydrogen ions and bicarbonate ions.

$$\underset{(1)}{H_2O + CO_2} \rightleftharpoons H_2CO_3 \underset{(2)}{\rightleftharpoons} H^+ + HCO_3^-$$

Thus if acid is added to the blood it will 'push' the above reactions to the left using up HCO_3^- and increasing the concentrations of H_2CO_3 and CO_2. The particular importance of the bicarbonate buffer system is that the CO_2 can be eliminated from the body relatively easily and continuously by breathing it out.

The relationships between pH, HCO_3^- and CO_2 concentrations at any one instant are summarized by the Henderson–Hasselbalch equation:

$$pH \propto \frac{HCO_3^- \text{ concentration}}{\text{dissolved } CO_2 \text{ concentration}}$$

It follows then that a rise in pH (less acid) could be achieved by an increase in HCO_3^-, a fall in CO_2 and, of course, a fall in H^+.

All three factors are subject to physiological regulation. Plasma pH ($-\log_{10} H^+$ concentration) is regulated by the amount secreted into urine; plasma HCO_3^- concentration is regulated by the degree of its renal reabsorption, and dissolved plasma CO_2 concentration is regulated by the rate of ventilation.

BICARBONATE REABSORPTION

HCO_3^- reabsorption has a threshold value of around 28 mmol/L. Below this plasma concentration, practically all filtered HCO_3^- is reabsorbed.

> See also **Buffers** (page 15), in Ch. 1, Molecules, Ions and Units.

Above the threshold value the excess HCO_3^- that is not absorbed appears in the urine.

HCO_3^- is reabsorbed indirectly as CO_2 and this is linked to Na^+ reabsorption and H^+ secretion, as shown in Figure 14.20(a).

The Na^+ pump (1) actively extrudes Na^+ from the basal and lateral surfaces of the tubular cell into the interstitial fluid, and Na^+ diffuses from the luminal surface of the tubular fluid into the cell. H^+ ions are actively secreted into the tubular fluid (2), where they combine with the filtered HCO_3^- to form H_2CO_3.

H_2CO_3 then splits to form CO_2 and water by the catalytic action of the enzyme carbonic anhydrase (3), which is present on the cell membrane of the proximal tubule cell.

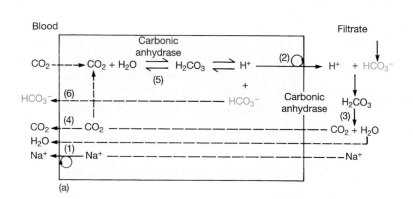

(a)

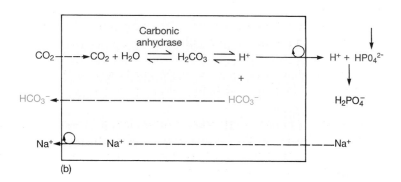

(b)

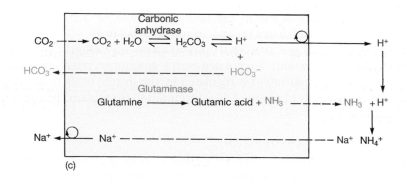

(c)

See also **Enzymes** (page 23), in Ch. 1, Molecules, Ions and Units.

Figure 14.20 Bicarbonate reabsorption and hydrogen ion secretion in the nephron. CO_2 diffuses into the cell, combines with water and, catalysed by the enzyme carbonic anhydrase, forms carbonic acid. This dissociates into H^+ and HCO_3^-. H^+ is actively transported into the tubular fluid across the luminal membrane in exchange for Na^+, which is actively transported out of the basal and lateral margins of the cell. HCO_3^- diffuses out of the cell and is reabsorbed into the blood. **Buffering of H^+ in tubular fluid: (a) Bicarbonate buffer.** HCO_3^- in the glomerular filtrate combines with H^+ secreted mainly by the proximal tubular cells to form H_2CO_3, which then dissociates into CO_2 and H_2O. The CO_2 is reabsorbed. **(b) Phosphate buffer.** HPO_4^{2-} combines with H^+ secreted by the proximal and distal tubular cells to form $H_2PO_4^-$.
(c) Ammonia. NH_3 is synthesized in the proximal and distal tubular cells from the amino acid glutamine, and secreted into the tubular lumen, where it combines with H^+ secreted by the proximal and distal tubular cells.

The CO_2 then diffuses into the cell to join the 'pool' of dissolved gas which may diffuse out (4) or combine with water to form H_2CO_3 under the influence of carbonic anhydrase in the cytoplasm (5). The intracellular dissociation of H_2CO_3 provides the H^+ for secretion (2); the HCO_3^- is reabsorbed by diffusion (6).

These events occur mainly in the proximal convoluted tubule where about 90% of the filtered HCO_3^- is normally reabsorbed.

HYDROGEN ION SECRETION

The amount of H^+ secreted is much higher in the proximal convoluted tubule than in the distal nephron. These H^+ ions are immediately reabsorbed as H_2O so that there is no net loss of acid from this site (Figure 14.20). The proximal tubule, therefore, reduces acidity by conserving base (HCO_3^-) rather than by eliminating acid.

Acidification of the urine is limited to a minimum pH of 4.5. Elimination of acid occurs by the secreted H^+ being buffered in the tubular fluid and subsequently excreted in the urine. The two principal buffers are hydrogen phosphate (HPO_4^{2-}) (Figure 14.20(b)) and ammonia (NH_3) (Figure 14.20(c)).

The phosphate buffer is filtered at the glomerulus and is therefore available in the tubular fluid to accept H^+. If, however, the amount of HPO_4^{2-} is small because it has already buffered H^+ in the blood, H^+ accumulates in the tubular cells because of the build-up of unbuffered H^+ in the tubular fluid.

The accumulation of acid within the tubular cells stimulates the production of NH_3 from the amino acid glutamine (Figure 14.20(c)). The NH_3 can then act as a H^+ acceptor, converting it to NH_4 and thereby enabling the elimination of acid to take place. This process occurs in the proximal convoluted tubule and the collecting duct.

EFFECTS OF BLOOD POTASSIUM ION CONCENTRATION ON HYDROGEN ION SECRETION AND BICARBONATE ION REABSORPTION

If blood K^+ levels are raised (**hyperkalaemia**) then K^+ enters the body cells in exchange for H^+. In the kidney the loss of H^+ into the interstitial fluid results in less H^+ being available for secretion into the tubular lumen so that less HCO_3^- reabsorption can occur.

Thus hyperkalaemia results in reduced H^+ secretion and reduced HCO_3^- reabsorption, while **hypokalaemia** results in increased H^+ secretion and increased HCO_3^- reabsorption.

Respiratory and renal regulation of pH in acidosis and alkalosis

It may be recalled from the Henderson–Hasselbalch equation that pH is directly proportional to HCO_3^- and inversely proportional to the amount of dissolved CO_2.

$$pH \propto \frac{HCO_3^-}{CO_2}$$

The kidneys prevent acidosis by the constant reabsorption of HCO_3^- and secretion of H^+, while the lungs eliminate CO_2 thereby effectively removing acid.

The interplay between the lungs and the kidneys in the maintenance of a constant pH may be illustrated by a brief consideration of altered acid–base states.

Acidosis is a condition in which a raised concentration of H^+ (fall in pH) in body fluids would occur if no compensatory mechanisms occurred. **Alkalosis**, on the other hand, would involve a rise in pH and a fall in H^+ concentration. Each condition is classified by cause as either 'respiratory' or 'metabolic'.

In each of these cases, the physiological responses to a change in body fluid pH act to reverse the change, maintaining the pH within a narrow range. The total amount of CO_2 and HCO_3^- in the body, however, may well have altered as a result of the responses. From a homoeostatic point of view, therefore, it is pH that is maintained and not total acid or base.

METABOLIC ACIDOSIS

Metabolic acidosis may arise: from an excessive production of H^+, e.g. in **diabetes mellitus**; from excessive ingestion of acid; by a loss of alkaline fluids such as occurs in **diarrhoea**; or by a failure to excrete H^+, e.g. in **renal failure**.

The fall in pH stimulates ventilation thereby eliminating CO_2 and tending therefore to reduce the acidity. Respiratory compensation, however, also lowers the plasma HCO_3^- concentration, so that restoration of the normal pH requires conservation of all the filtered HCO_3^- as well as increased elimination of H^+. The increased secretion of H^+ into the tubular lumen is followed by increased buffering by HPO_4^{2-} and NH_3. If there is increased acidity in the tubular fluid over some days, it induces an increased production of the enzyme glutaminase by the tubular cells and a consequent increase in the quantity of NH_3.

METABOLIC ALKALOSIS

Metabolic alkalosis can arise from persistent **vomiting**, whereby hydrochloric acid is lost from the stomach, or from infusion of **excessive amounts of HCO_3^-**.

The immediate effects are that blood pH and HCO_3^- concentration increase. The increased pH may reduce ventilation, thereby raising blood CO_2 and acidity so that the pH will tend to fall. The renal compensation is that the excess HCO_3^- is lost in the urine.

RESPIRATORY ACIDOSIS

Respiratory acidosis results from impaired elimination of carbon dioxide from the lungs, typically in conditions such as **chronic obstructive airways disease**, but also in any condition in which ventilation is reduced.

The primary effect is raised blood carbon dioxide level (**hypercapnia**). This leads to raised carbonic acid levels and a fall in the pH of the blood. The kidneys compensate for the change in acidity in the following manner. An increased amount of CO_2 diffuses into the tubular

See also **Hypoventilation** (page 464), in Ch. 13, Respiration.

cells, resulting in increased H^+ secretion and HCO_3^- reabsorption (Figure 14.20). Both these effects will tend to reduce the acidosis. Any excess H^+ will combine with HPO_4^{2-} and NH_3 in the same way as in metabolic acidosis. Respiratory compensation, of course, is lacking.

RESPIRATORY ALKALOSIS

Respiratory alkalosis is caused by **chronic hyperventilation**. This has a variety of causes, including anxiety, brain stem damage, increased respiratory stimuli such as hypoxia, fever (pyrexia), drugs such as salicylates and analeptics, adrenaline, pain.

Hyperventilation reduces blood CO_2 and H_2CO_3 levels. Renal compensatory mechanisms are the reverse of those operating in response to respiratory acidosis. Less CO_2 enters the tubular cells from the blood, and therefore less H^+ is secreted and fewer HCO_3^- ions are reabsorbed. The effect of the reduced tubular activity is to conserve more acid and eliminate more base, thereby counteracting the alkalosis.

Summary of renal handling of individual substances

Amino acids

Amino acids are usually completely reabsorbed in the proximal tubule by active transport. The mechanism is a cotransport system with Na^+. There are several different carriers for different amino acids.

Bicarbonate (hydrogen carbonate) ions

Bicarbonate ions are not reabsorbed as such, rather as dissolved carbon dioxide. Filtered HCO_3^- combines with H^+ that has been secreted into the tubular lumen, forming carbonic acid (Figure 14.20). The acid dissociates into carbon dioxide and water. Carbon dioxide diffuses easily into the tubular cells where, in a reaction catalysed by the enzyme carbonic anhydrase, it combines with water and forms carbonic acid, which dissociates into HCO_3^- and H^+. HCO_3^- then diffuses out of the cell into the peritubular capillaries.

About 90% of the filtered HCO_3^- is reabsorbed in this way from the proximal tubule, the remaining 10% from the distal tubule and collecting duct. In alkalosis, when there is a high concentration of HCO_3^- in the blood and therefore glomerular filtrate, the excess is not reabsorbed and appears in the urine.

Calcium ions

Ca^{2+} ions are actively reabsorbed in the ascending limb of the loop of Henle, the distal tubule and collecting duct. Parathyroid hormone stimulates this process.

Chloride ions

In the first part of the proximal tubule, the reabsorption of Cl^- passively follows the active reabsorption of Na^+.

In the distal two-thirds of the proximal convoluted tubule, in all but the juxtamedullary nephrons, the permeability to Cl⁻ is higher than for other anions and it diffuses down its concentration gradient, followed by the passive diffusion of Na⁺. Generally, the reabsorption of Cl⁻ follows that of Na⁺ in the loop of Henle, distal tubule and collecting duct.

Creatinine

Creatinine is derived from the breakdown of muscle creatine and creatine phosphate and over a period of hours excretion is relatively constant.

Creatinine is filtered freely; it is not reabsorbed at all by the tubules but is actively secreted to a small extent by the proximal tubule. The clearance value for creatinine is used to estimate the glomerular filtration rate.

Glucose

Glucose is normally completely reabsorbed in the proximal tubule by an active transport system linked to Na⁺. The diffusion of Na⁺ into the tubular cells is accompanied by glucose. Na⁺ diffuses down its concentration gradient (maintained by the Na^+-K^+-ATPase) and 'drags' glucose with it, even though it is moving against its concentration gradient. The reabsorption of glucose is, therefore, a form of secondary active transport (cotransport), in which the Na^+-K^+-ATPase is creating the conditions whereby glucose is reabsorbed along with Na⁺.

Hydrogen ions

H⁺ is actively secreted in the proximal tubule, where it is mainly exchanged for Na⁺ and results in the reabsorption of HCO_3^-. In the distal tubule and collecting duct, the secretion of H⁺ is active and can produce urine with a pH as low as 4.5 ($10^{-4.5}$ mmol/L).

Phosphate

The term 'phosphate' in physiology covers the two forms in which the phosphate group is carried in body fluids: dihydrogen or acid phosphate ($H_2PO_4^-$) and hydrogen or alkaline phosphate (HPO_4^{2-}). As these ions buffer H⁺, the proportion of each ion carried in the blood is variable.

$$HPO_4^{2-} + H^+ \rightleftharpoons H_2PO_4^-$$

Phosphate reabsorption in the proximal convoluted tubule is coupled to Na⁺ reabsorption in the same way as that of glucose and amino acids. Its reabsorption is reduced by parathyroid hormone.

Potassium ions

About 80% of filtered K⁺ is reabsorbed in the proximal tubule, probably by passive transport through the tight junctions between the cells. The Na^+-K^+-ATPase causes K⁺ to enter the cells, but it rapidly diffuses out again down its concentration gradient. There is some active reabsorption of K⁺ too.

K⁺ is secreted in the late distal tubule and the collecting duct, and again the mechanism is passive. Aldosterone stimulates K⁺ secretion.

Sodium ions

The reabsorption of Na^+ is particularly important, not only because it is present in relatively large quantities in blood and therefore glomerular filtrate, but also because its reabsorption is linked to that of Cl^-, glucose, amino acids and water.

Generally about 99% of the filtered Na^+ is reabsorbed by the tubular cells, most of this occurring in the proximal tubule. Na^+ is actively transported out of the basal and lateral surfaces of the cell by the sodium–potassium pump (Na^+-K^+-ATPase). The low intracellular concentration of Na^+, together with the negative intracellular potential of about -70 mV creates a large electrochemical gradient, so that Na^+ diffuses into the cell across the luminal cell membrane (Figure 14.12).

The entry of the positively charged Na^+ is almost (80%) matched by the diffusion of Cl^- into the cell, which maintains the membrane potential. The remaining 20% of Na^+ entry is 'exchanged' for H^+.

A further 20% of the filtered Na^+ is reabsorbed from the ascending limb of the loop of Henle by the Na^+-K^+-ATPase system.

The distal nephron (principally the collecting duct) usually reabsorbs a further 9% of the filtered Na^+, although this amount varies according to the state of Na^+ balance, fluid balance and K^+ balance in the body. The hormone aldosterone, whose secretion rate is controlled by these factors, causes an increased reabsorption of Na^+ in the collecting duct. The probable mechanism is that aldosterone increases the permeability of the luminal membrane to Na^+. The resultant increased influx of Na^+ then stimulates the Na^+-K^+-ATPase, which in turn increases Na^+ reabsorption.

Urate ions

Urate is formed in the liver as a breakdown product of nucleic acids. Approximately 90% of the filtered urate is reabsorbed in the proximal tubule and loop of Henle. Urate is also secreted in the proximal tubule.

Urea

Urea is a breakdown product of proteins and nucleic acids. Its toxicity level is, however, relatively low, and there is no active transport system involved in its elimination.

Cell membranes have a very high permeability to urea, and it generally diffuses with ease down its concentration gradient. In the proximal tubule, as water follows the reabsorption of solutes, it creates a concentration gradient for urea, and therefore urea is reabsorbed.

The cortical collecting duct is impermeable to urea, and the permeability of the medullary collecting duct varies according to the amount of circulating ADH. In conditions of dehydration, when ADH levels are high, more urea is reabsorbed from the medullary collecting duct. This raises the osmolarity of the medullary interstitium and contributes to the formation of a hypertonic urine. Under these conditions, therefore, less urea is eliminated from the body. Conversely, in conditions of overhydration when the urine produced is hypotonic, less urea is reabsorbed and more is excreted.

Water

Water is reabsorbed passively down an osmotic gradient from the proximal tubule, the descending limb of the loop of Henle, the distal tubule and the collecting duct.

Typically, around 70% of the filtered water is reabsorbed in the proximal tubule; this reabsorption is independent of hormonal control and is relatively constant (**obligatory reabsorption**). About 5% is usually reabsorbed from the descending limb of the loop of Henle (less if ADH is low).

Reabsorption from the distal tubule and collecting duct together is normally about 24% It may, however, vary from about 12% to 24.8% This **facultative reabsorption** is controlled by aldosterone and ADH. Aldosterone stimulates Na^+ reabsorption which is followed by water in the distal tubule and collecting duct, and ADH promotes water reabsorption from the collecting duct. Depending on the concentrations of these hormones in the blood, therefore, urine production can vary from less than half a millilitre per minute to about 16 mL/min.

Renal failure

If the activity of the kidneys becomes impaired, then the physiological consequences are a reversal of the usual kidney functions. The main features are the accumulation of nitrogenous waste, impaired electrolyte and water balance and proteinuria.

Acute renal failure

Acute renal failure (ARF) is a rapid deterioration in kidney function over a period of some 12–72 h, commonly caused by renal hypoxia.

A range of conditions can deprive the kidneys of adequate oxygen, including haemorrhage, cardiac failure, postoperative shock and respiratory insufficiency. These are examples of **prerenal ARF**. Kidney disease, such a glomerulonephritis, and poisoning of the nephrons by substances such as heavy metals, carbon tetrachloride and some weedkillers, can lead to **renal ARF**. **Postrenal ARF** is caused by urinary tract obstruction.

Urine production of less than 20 mL/h (**oliguria**) occurs in some 70% of people with ARF. The oliguria is accompanied by salt and water retention. The reduced urine volume is a direct result of a reduction in GFR, which can have several causes. GFR falls if renal perfusion is reduced, if the glomerular membrane is damaged or if there is urinary tract obstruction.

Nephrons can recover from acute renal hypoxia, usually after about 4 weeks. Urine output improves and becomes high (2–6 L/d) and dilute. Usually this represents the physiological responses to the fluid retention occurring in the initial phase of ARF.

The presence of protein, particularly albumin, in the urine (**albumin-uria**) is a consistent finding in ARF. Damage to the glomerular membrane results in plasma proteins leaking through, particularly albumin, which is the smallest of the plasma proteins. The consequence of losses above about 5 g/d is that plasma colloid osmotic pressure falls and causes oedema. This is caused by a reduction in reabsorption of interstitial fluid in the tissues. Renal failure involving protein loss of this severity is known as the **nephrotic syndrome**.

If the glomerular membrane has been damaged, bleeding occurs and blood appears in the urine (**haematuria**).

Nitrogenous substances such as creatinine and urea, which are normally excreted in the urine, are retained and therefore their concentrations in blood rise.

In ARF, the nephrons' ability to secrete both H^+ and K^+ is impaired. This means that H^+ concentration in blood rises (**acidosis**) and K^+ also rises (hyperkalaemia). Acidosis can cause coma.

Chronic renal failure (CRF)

This type of failure progresses over many years. Although CRF may follow ARF or the nephrotic syndrome, it is generally caused by specific kidney diseases, principally glomerulonephritis, pyelonephritis and congenital renal abnormalities.

Generally, the changes in blood electrolyte levels are qualitatively similar to those seen in ARF, but slower to change.

In CRF, as the destruction of nephrons increases, the solute load on the remaining functioning nephrons increases. There is, therefore, an **osmotic diuresis**, resulting in an increase in urine output of 2 L/d or more, which can cause dehydration

Hypertension is common in CRF. It may result from increased renin production, which would increase circulating angiotensin, resulting in vasoconstriction.

Impairment of the kidneys' role in activating vitamin D can lead to alterations to bone structure (**osteodystrophy**). The probable sequence of events is that the lack of vitamin D leads to reduced absorption of Ca^{2+}, resulting in a fall in plasma Ca^{2+}, which in turn stimulates an increased release of PTH. Increased resorption of bone follows, so that 'holes' appear in it and it becomes very fragile.

The kidney normally produces erythropoietin. In CRF this function can be depressed sufficiently to cause severe **anaemia**.

End-stage renal disease is characterized by very high blood urea levels (the **uraemic syndrome**). It is not clear which of the many symptoms exhibited by people with such a condition are attributable specifically to urea, because so many other changes in the blood occur at the same time.

See also **Regulation of blood calcium and phosphate concentrations** (page 630), in Ch. 16, Endocrine Physiology.

DIALYSIS

The process of dialysis, which 'cleans' the blood, can be used as a temporary measure during the period when the nephrons are recovering in ARF. In CRF, regular dialysis keeps patients alive. There are two types of dialysis: haemodialysis and continuous ambulatory peritoneal dialysis.

In **haemodialysis**, the patient's arterial blood is passed over an artificial membrane, some $1-1.5 m^2$ in surface area. The aim of the process is to lose unwanted solutes out of the blood across the membrane into the dialysing fluid. This does not contain any nitrogenous compounds and it has less K^+ than normal plasma, so that these substances diffuse into it and are thereby lost from uraemic plasma. HCO_3^- on the other hand is higher in dialysing fluid than normal plasma, which will promote diffusion of HCO_3^- into the blood and combat the acidosis. Glucose can also be added to the blood as it flows through the dialysing unit.

In **CAPD** the dialysing fluid is introduced into the peritoneal cavity and the peritoneal membrane acts as a dialysing membrane. The fluid is later withdrawn from the peritoneal cavity and the procedure repeated as necessary.

Digestion, absorption and metabolism of food

The process of digestion brings about the breakdown of food into a form in which it can be absorbed. Carbohydrates, lipids and proteins are split into smaller fragments by the addition of water, a chemical reaction known as hydrolysis (Figure 15.1). These substances are then absorbed into the blood and transported to the cells where they are used in a variety of ways.

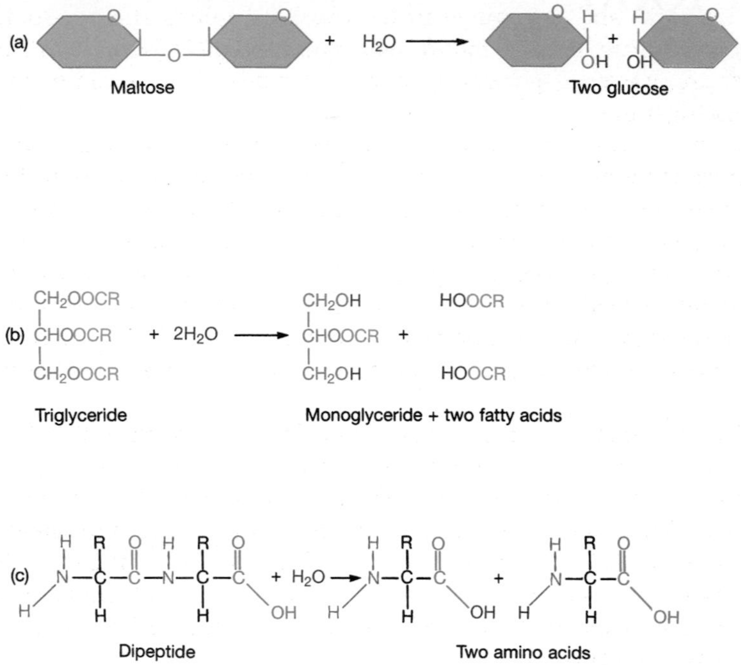

Figure 15.1 Hydrolysis of carbohydrate, lipid and protein molecules. **(a)** Hydrolysis of maltose to form two glucose molecules. **(b)** Hydrolysis of triglyceride to form monoglyceride and two free fatty acids. **(c)** Hydrolysis of a dipeptide to form two amino acids.

(a) Maltose $+ H_2O \longrightarrow$ Two glucose

(b)
$$\begin{array}{c} CH_2OOCR \\ | \\ CHOOCR \\ | \\ CH_2OOCR \end{array} + 2H_2O \longrightarrow \begin{array}{c} CH_2OH \\ | \\ CHOOCR \\ | \\ CH_2OH \end{array} + \begin{array}{c} HOOCR \\ \\ HOOCR \end{array}$$

Triglyceride   Monoglyceride + two fatty acids

(c) Dipeptide $+ H_2O \longrightarrow$ Two amino acids

Food and diet

Food contains a variety of different molecules, most of which are used by the body for the growth and replenishment of its tissues; these substances are defined as **nutrients**. Most foods contain a variety of nutrients, but no single food contains all of them. It is therefore necessary that a variety of different foods are eaten in order to maintain optimal health.

The human diet contains five groups of nutrients: carbohydrates, lipids, proteins, vitamins and minerals. Water and dietary fibre (roughage), though not usually classed as nutrients, are also required.

The structures of carbohydrates, fats and proteins are described in **Biological molecules** (page 16), in Ch. 1, Molecules, Ions and Units.

Carbohydrates

Carbohydrates have simpler chemical structures than proteins, although some are still quite large. Carbohydrates are major sources of energy in animals and plants: 1 g of carbohydrate yields 17.22 kJ of energy when it is oxidized to carbon dioxide and water. Excess carbohydrate in the diet is converted into glycogen and stored in the liver or converted to fat and stored under the skin. In plants carbohydrate is stored as starch. The polysaccharide cellulose is the major component of plant cell walls, to which it confers strength and shape.

Three principal types of sugar are found in the diet: monosaccharides, disaccharides and polysaccharides.

The common dietary **monosaccharides** are **glucose**, which is found in ripe fruits and in some vegetables such as onions and beetroot, and **fructose** ('fruit sugar'), found in fruit and in plant juices. Both molecules are, however, present in much larger quantities as components of larger sugar units.

There are two principal dietary **disaccharides: sucrose** and **lactose**. Sucrose is found in sugar cane and some fruits, and in its pure form is the main type of 'sugar' included in the diet. Each sucrose molecule is made from one glucose and one fructose molecule. Lactose is made from glucose and galactose and is found in milk. A third disaccharide, **maltose**, is made from two glucose molecules and is found in cereals such as barley; it is also a breakdown product of starch. All disaccharides are broken down into monosaccharides prior to absorption into the blood.

The two major dietary **polysaccharides** are **starch** and **cellulose**. Starch is the major food reserve of plants; it is found in root vegetables, cereals and pulses. Its presence in cereals means that it is a major component of flour and its products, including pastry, bread and cakes. The cellulose in plants cannot be digested by humans, but is of great value as dietary fibre. It can, however, be digested by many food animals such as cattle and sheep, so that it is of indirect nutritional benefit to those humans who eat meat.

Lipids

Lipids, like carbohydrates, are sources of energy and, in fact, supply more energy than a comparable amount of carbohydrate (1 g liberates 39.06 kJ of energy).

Fat is eaten primarily in the form of **triglycerides**, which comprise **glycerol** and three fatty acid residues. The commonest fatty acids are **stearic, oleic** and **palmitic**.

The liver can synthesize all but two fatty acids: **linoleic** and **linolenic acids**, which are therefore **essential nutrients**. Linoleic acid is a component of the phospholipid lecithin and a precursor of prostaglandins.

Fatty acids are described as either **saturated**, in which case all carbon atoms are saturated with hydrogen, or **unsaturated**, when double bonds are present and there is less hydrogen. It is widely held that **polyunsaturated** fats (which have more than one double bond) are beneficial in that they depress the level of cholesterol in the blood and therefore help to reduce the incidence of arteriosclerosis.

Meat and animal fat products contain a large proportion of saturated fats, while dairy products (milk, butter, cream, cheese and eggs) have a mixture of saturated and unsaturated fats. Oily fish (tuna, herring,

Table 15.1 Amino acids in food – essential amino acids must be eaten as constituents of dietary proteins; non-essential amino acids can be synthesized in the tissues, as well as eaten as constituents of dietary proteins.

Essential amino acids
Cysteine
Histidine
Isoleucine
Leucine
Lysine
Methionine
Phenylalanine
Threonine
Tryptophan
Tyrosine
Valine

Non-essential amino acids
Alanine
Arginine
Aspartic acid
Glutamic acid
Glycine
Hydroxyproline
Ornithine
Proline
Serine

salmon and pilchard) and fish liver oils contain largely unsaturated fats, as do most plant oils (olive, sunflower and maize), although coconut oil contains saturated fat.

Proteins

Proteins are the largest and most complicated molecules found in the diet and are composed of 20 amino acids. Nine of these can be synthesized in the body and are therefore not essential constituents of the diet; the remaining 11 cannot be synthesized, however, and must, therefore, form part of the diet. All the amino acids are required to build proteins within the body, but because of the particular dietary requirement for some of them, they are known as '**essential amino acids**'; those that can be synthesized are therefore described as '**non-essential amino acids**' (Table 15.1).

Protein that contains all the essential amino acids is said to have 'high biological value' (HBV) and is sometimes known as 'complete' protein. This is characteristic of animal products such as meat, eggs, milk, cheese and fish. Protein that lacks one or more of the essential amino acids is known as 'incomplete' protein and has 'low biological value' (LBV). LBV protein is generally found in plant products, including cereals, pulses (peas, etc.), some nuts and vegetables. Exceptions to this general trend are soya beans, in that they are plants which have HBV protein, and gelatin (collagen from animal tissue), which contains LBV protein.

Demand for protein varies with age and is highest in adolescence, the time of life when the most rapid growth and development is taking place. The average minimum daily requirement for protein ranges from about 30 to about 60 g, depending upon age, size and level of activity.

Nutritional deficiency

Primary nutritional deficiency results from inadequate food intake. Malnutrition can also result from the body's failure to absorb food from the gut (see *The malabsorption syndrome*, below), or from increased metabolic rate caused, for example, by hyperthyroidism.

Patients with cancer secrete the chemical **cachexin** (tumour necrosis factor), which increases metabolic rate. Cachexin increases the breakdown of muscle protein, which gives rise to **cachexia** (Greek, 'in poor condition').

A chronic shortage of food, or a refusal to eat, as in **anorexia nervosa**, leads to **starvation**. Lack of protein and energy sources leads to growth retardation in children, emaciation and immunological deficiency.

Starvation leads to the compensatory breakdown of the body's 'expendable' tissues leading to a wasted state known as **marasmus**. Lack of carbohydrate intake rapidly leads to depletion of glycogen in the liver and muscles as it is broken down to release glucose which is oxidized and provides energy. Fat is then mobilized and continues to be metabolized until the body's fat stores have been exhausted. Breakdown of easily mobilized protein provides glucose, by gluconeogenesis; this supply of glucose is particularly important in the maintenance of brain function.

Reduced protein synthesis results in impaired immunity and therefore an increased risk of infection. Signs of vitamin A deficiency result from a reduction in plasma retinol binding protein which transports vitamin A from the liver to the tissues.

Severe malnutrition reduces enzyme production, including digestive enzymes, so that food is digested poorly. Also, the lining of the intestinal tract is poorly replenished, so that absorption is impaired. Food replacement therapy has therefore to be cautious and progressive, otherwise it results in gastrointestinal disturbance.

Whereas marasmus can occur in both children and adults another deficiency disease, **kwashiorkor**, only affects children. Marasmus and kwashiorkor both show muscle wasting, loss of intestinal mucosa and reduced immunity. Kwashiorkor is characterized, in addition, by fluid retention and oedema, an enlarged liver due to the accumulation of fat, and sparse, wispy hair. Originally, kwashiorkor was thought to be a disease of protein deficiency, leading to reduced plasma protein synthesis and resultant oedema. Kwashiorkor is now regarded as another manifestation of general malnutrition, the plasma protein being lowered because protein is being used for energy production in place of adequate supplies of carbohydrate and fat. It is not clear why some children develop kwashiorkor rather than marasmus.

> The causes of oedema are explained in **Physiological causes of oedema** (page 412), in Ch. 12, Circulation of Blood and Lymph.

Excess food intake

Excessive intake of food leads to a metabolic imbalance so that energy intake is greater than output. The result of this is that fat is deposited in the body's stores and the person is said to be **obese**. Studies have shown that, once the fat stores are filled, energy input once again equals output. Obviously, if the excess weight is to be shed then input has to be reduced and/or output increased. This can be achieved by restricting the diet and increasing the level of exercise.

Since food intake is apparently regulated by the levels of nutrients in the body's stores, it is evident that in the obese person there is a breakdown in the regulatory mechanism. Obesity is often due to psychogenic factors, but a genetic predisposition is also known to exist. Hypothalamic disorders have also been shown lead to obesity.

Obesity is associated with hypertension and arterial disease, but the precise mechanisms of these associations are unknown.

Vitamins

Vitamins are substances that are required in varying, though small, amounts in the diet because most of them cannot be synthesized in the body. They are not digested, but are absorbed intact and each is required for a specific metabolic function. Many vitamins are employed as coenzymes and help catalyse metabolic reactions taking place within cells; others have more particular functions – for example, vitamin A is the precursor of the visual pigments of the retina. Vitamin E, working with vitamin C, has been shown to be an antioxidant that removes intracellular 'free radicals', which damage lipids in cell membranes and lipoproteins. Free radicals are formed when oxygen is reduced to water in the electron transport chain. They are characterized by the possession of unpaired electrons. A particularly damaging free radical is the hydroxyl radical.

Lack of vitamins in the diet usually leads to a deficiency disease. Vitamin supplements are readily available in chemists' and health food shops but their benefits, when they are taken in conjunction with a reasonably balanced diet, are somewhat questionable. Excessive doses of some vitamins apparently have no effect at all, while others, such as vitamins A, C, D and K, have been shown to be toxic.

Vitamins are classified according to their solubilities as **fat-soluble** or **water-soluble**. The former category includes vitamins A, D, E and K while the latter includes several vitamin B compounds (B_1, B_2, nicotinic acid, B_6, B_{12} and folic acid) and vitamin C.

Details of vitamin function, their sources and the effects of deficiency are given in Table 15.2.

Minerals

In addition to vitamins, the body also uses varying amounts of about 20 different mineral ions. Eight are needed in relatively large amounts in order to maintain optimal body function; they are **calcium, iron, magnesium, phosphorus, potassium, sodium, chloride** and **sulphur**. Much smaller quantities of a number of others are also required. These 'trace' elements include chromium, cobalt, copper, fluorine, iodine, manganese, nickel and zinc.

Since many of the major ions and most trace elements are present in a wide variety of foods they are unlikely to be deficient. Some of the elements can, however, be in short supply or may be lost from the body in excessive amounts, thus leading to specific deficiency states.

Details of mineral function, their sources and the effects of deficiency are given in Table 15.3.

Dietary fibre

Dietary fibre ('roughage') consists largely of indigestible material derived from the cellulose cell walls of plants. It is found particularly as bran which is derived from cereals, as fruit skins, potato skins and leafy vegetables.

Dietary fibre gives bulk to the food in the gut. This promotes peristaltic contraction in the gut wall which causes the material to be moved through the gut. In the small intestine this tends to restrict the absorption of, particularly, fats. In the large intestine it retains water and food residues and metabolic wastes and gives bulk to the faeces.

DEFICIENCY

Lack of roughage slows down the passage of material through the large intestine so that large amounts of water are reabsorbed and the faeces become hard and difficult to pass (**constipation**). Excessive constipation may lead to diverticulitis, in which small pouches (diverticula) appear in the large intestinal wall. The increased effort required by people with constipation to expel their faeces can lead to hernia and **haemorrhoids**.

It is further believed that lack of roughage in the intestine allows excessive absorption of fats and harmful metabolites. This is supported

Table 15.2 Vitamins

Functions	Sources	Deficiency
Fat soluble vitamins		
Vitamin A Vitamin A (retinol) is used in the synthesis of the visual pigment rhodopsin and is therefore required so that vision can occur in dim light. It is also required to maintain mucous membranes and the skin and for growth of bones and teeth.	Found as carotene in plant foods, particularly carrots, watercress, cabbage, prunes and tomatoes. In animal foods, found as retinol, especial in dairy products and oily fish. Both retinol and carotene are unaffected by heat and so are not destroyed during food preparation.	Deficiency in the diet leads to failure to synthesize rhodopsin and therefore to **night blindness**. In severe cases it may lead to total blindness. Resistance to disease may be reduced and growth retarded. In addition, the skin and mucous membranes may dry up and become infected.
Vitamin D Vitamin D promotes the absorption of Ca^{2+} and phosphate, the two major components of bone, from the gut and into the blood. Vitamin D promotes Ca^{2+} absorption in the small intestine by increasing the synthesis of Ca^{2+}-binding protein and enzymes, which pump Ca^{2+} through the intestinal cell membranes. It also mobilizes Ca^{2+} from bone. The vitamin is therefore needed for the formation and maintenance of bone.	Found in liver, fish liver oils and all oily fish, as well as eggs and dairy products. In addition, it is formed in the skin upon exposure to sunlight. Unaffected by cooking.	Dietary deficiency, particularly when coupled with a lack of exposure to sunlight, leads to a reduction in the absorption of Ca^{2+} and phosphate from the gut, which results in weakness in the bones and teeth. Since vitamin D is fat-soluble, malabsorption of fat can also lead to deficiency, particularly in adults. In children, deficiency gives rise to rickets, characterized by bow legs and generally fragile bones. In adults, particularly the elderly, it gives rise to osteomalacia, in which the bones become weakened so that a minor fall may result in a bone fracture.
Vitamin E Vitamin E helps to prevent the oxidation of unsaturated fatty acids within cells, which helps in the maintenance of cell membranes. It also helps to prevent the oxidation of vitamins A and C in the intestine. It has been shown to prevent sterility in male rats, but this role in humans is uncertain.	The best sources are vegetable oils, whole grain cereals and wheatgerm.	Very rare, and its effects would usually be masked by deficiency of other fat-soluble vitamins. By itself, vitamin E deficiency may result in infertility and increase the fragility of capillaries and red blood cells.
Vitamin K Vitamin K assists in the production of blood clotting factors II, VII, IX and X by the liver.	Widely distributed in a variety of leafy vegetables (e.g. spinach). It is also produced by the bacterial flora in the large intestine.	Rare, although it sometimes occurs in the newborn, in which case the blood does not clot following an injury.

Table 15.2 Continued

Functions	Sources	Deficiency

Water-soluble vitamins

Vitamin B compounds

At least 13 different substances are included in the group of vitamin B compounds, but not all seem to be of particular physiological importance. Only the major ones are described here.

Vitamin B$_1$ Vitamin B$_1$ (thiamine) is involved in the metabolism of carbohydrates and some amino acids. It is required for growth in children and for the maintenance of nerve and heart function.	Since vitamin B$_1$ cannot be stored, a regular daily supply is required. The amount required is larger in those who are particularly active, pregnant women and lactating mothers. It is very soluble in water and a proportion is destroyed by the high temperatures used in cooking. It is found in lean meat, liver, eggs, whole grains and leafy green vegetables.	Caused by a lack of suitable foods, as well as disorders which lead to a reduction in its absorption, including persistent vomiting and alcoholism. The nervous system is affected, so that there may be depression, irritability, defective memory, etc., and also be inflammation of the nerves (**neuritis**), leading to pain and weakness. Heart weakness may lead to **heart failure**, with consequent oedema. Growth in children is retarded. In severe deficiency, called **beriberi**, there is gastrointestinal hypofunction as well as polyneuritis and heart failure.
Vitamin B$_2$ Vitamin B$_2$ (riboflavin) is used in the process of oxidation of food substances. It is therefore involved in energy production in the cells and consequently in a whole range of functions.	Even though small amounts of the vitamin can be stored in the body and a little is produced by bacterial action in the large intestine, a daily intake is required. Like thiamine, it is destroyed in cooking, but, unlike thiamine, it is also denatured by light.	Rarely severe in humans but it can nevertheless lead to digestive and mental disturbances and **dermatitis**.
Nicotinic acid Nicotinic acid (niacin) is involved in the process of oxidation and, like the other B vitamins, it influences a range of cellular activities, particularly in neurones.	The vitamin is not stored and is therefore required on a daily basis. Apart from the foods that contain all B vitamins, nicotinic acid may also be synthesized from the amino acid tryptophan. Thus, foods that contain large amounts of tryptophan (e.g. eggs and milk) may be an indirect source of the vitamin. Nicotinic acid is the most stable B vitamin and is relatively unaffected by cooking.	**Pellagra** occurs as a result of nicotinic acid deficiency. It is characterized by dermatitis, particularly around the neck, loss of memory and depression and inflammation of the gastrointestinal tract.
Vitamin B$_6$ Vitamin B$_6$ (pyridoxine) functions as a coenzyme in amino acid and protein metabolism. It may also act as a carrier for the transport of some amino acids across cell membranes.	Found in red meat, liver and poultry, eggs, fish and whole-grain cereals.	Occurs rarely in children, but effects are pronounced. They include convulsions, nausea and vomiting, and dermatitis.

Table 15.2 Continued

Functions	Sources	Deficiency
Vitamin B₁₂ Vitamin B_{12} (cobalamin) is required for DNA synthesis. It is therefore a promoter of growth and its presence is required for the formation of red blood cells.	Only found in animal foods, but is also synthesized by intestinal bacteria.	Normally occurs as a result of lack of intrinsic factor, which is secreted by the gastric glands and is required for the absorption of the vitamin in the small intestine. Deficiency results in **pernicious anaemia**, in which red blood cells are not able to mature. The immature cells easily rupture, thereby reducing the total number of red blood cells. During exercise, therefore, dissolved oxygen is poorly replenished from the low oxyhaemoglobin stores and the person feels tired. Sometimes there is a loss of peripheral sensation, because some spinal nerve fibres become demyelinated.
Folic acid Folic acid is required in the synthesis of DNA and is thus a potent promoter of growth; like vitamin B_{12}, it is necessary for the formation of red blood cells.	Found in lean meat, liver, eggs, yeast, whole grains and leafy vegetables. It is also synthesized by bacteria in the large intestine.	Leads to **megaloblastic anaemia**, which is essentially the same as pernicious anaemia in its manifestations.
Vitamin C Vitamin C (ascorbic acid) has a number of important functions. It is required for the synthesis of collagen and therefore has an essential role in connective tissue formation. As a result, vitamin C is required for the maintenance of the skin and the lining of the gut. It is also used in the growth of bone. Iron absorption in the small intestine, and therefore the formation of red blood cells, also occurs with the aid of vitamin C. Functions (with vitamin E) as an antioxidant.	Found in fresh fruit and vegetables, rosehips, blackcurrants and green peppers being the best sources. It is relatively easily destroyed in cooking, especially slow cooking.	Chronic lack of vitamin C produces a number of symptoms, including general weakness and pain in muscles and joints; breakdown of connective tissue; weakness in the walls of blood vessels so that minor haemorrhages occur; bleeding gums and loose teeth. Acute lack of the vitamin leads to **scurvy**, a condition that used to be common among sailors who undertook long sea voyages without sufficient fresh fruit and vegetables. Additional symptoms of scurvy include anaemia, brought on by lack of iron; failure of cuts and scratches to heal properly and breakdown of scar tissue.

Table 15.3 Major dietary minerals

Functions	Sources	Deficiency
Calcium Calcium is a component of bone salt and is therefore necessary for the formation and maintenance of bones and teeth. Calcium is also a blood clotting agent and is involved in the release of neurotransmitters from nerve terminals and in muscle contraction.	Found in dairy products, bread (to which it is added during manufacture) and hard water.	In children, leads to soft bones which, because of the body's weight, tend to bend. Thus bow legs are common in such children, who are said to have **rickets**. In adults the bones and teeth are very weak in the condition known as **osteomalacia**. Calcium deficiency also results in changes in the functions of muscles and nerves. It normally suppresses the excitability of nerve and muscle cell membranes, so that deficiency can lead to spontaneous, prolonged muscle contractions (**tetany**).
Iron Iron is a component of haemoglobin, the oxygen-carrying molecule found in red blood cells. It is therefore required for the formation of red blood cells and, since the latter only live about 120 days and new ones are constantly being formed, there is a constant demand for iron. This demand is slightly greater in women of child-bearing age than in men, since they lose a small amount of blood each month during the menstrual period.	Found in liver and kidney, cocoa and plain chocolate and in smaller amounts in bread, to which it is added during manufacture. The absorption of iron from the gut is aided by vitamin C and by the acid in the stomach, which converts it from the ferric form, in which it usually exists in the diet, to the more soluble ferrous form.	Leads to **iron-deficiency anaemia**. In this condition there is a lack of haemoglobin and a consequent reduction in the blood's oxygen carrying capacity. This leads to the general consequences of anaemia: increased cardiac output and fatigue due to tissue hypoxia on exercise. In addition, lack of iron leads to gastrointestinal disturbance, including anorexia and constipation.
Magnesium Magnesium is a constituent of a number of coenzymes concerned with carbohydrate metabolism.	Found in milk and dairy products as well as a variety of cereals and green vegetables.	Leads to an increased irritability of the nervous system, muscle tremors, peripheral vasodilation and tachycardia.
Phosphorus Phosphorus is a component of bone salt and is also found in nucleic acids, adenosine triphosphate and other 'high-energy' nucleotides used in the provision of the energy that drives bodily processes.	Widely distributed within plant and animal cells.	Dietary deficiency is unknown. Rickets can result from renal disease when phosphates are poorly reabsorbed from the nephrons.

Potassium
Potassium is the main intracellular cation and thus helps to maintain intracellular osmotic pressure. It is of major importance in the maintenance of ionic potentials across cell membranes, the generation of action potentials in nerve fibres and in muscle contraction.

Widely distributed but particularly good sources include meat, fish, fruit and cereals.

Very rare, but may occur following diarrhoea or vomiting; potassium loss is also a side-effect of some diuretic drugs, so that their use is accompanied by potassium supplements. Potassium deficiency leads to muscle weakness, nausea, cardiac arrhythmia, possibly heart failure, and confusion, particularly in the elderly.

Sodium and chloride
Sodium and chloride ions are found in relatively high concentrations in extracellular fluids so that they play a major role in maintaining osmotic pressure. Sodium is also of major importance in the generation and transmission of nerve impulses.

Found in most foods, particularly in fish and meat. Sodium chloride (common salt) is also added to food.

May occur due to excessive sweating or vomiting or diarrhoea; not usually because of lack of sodium chloride in diet. Lost salt can be replaced by taking salt tablets. Should there be a low sodium ion concentration in extracellular fluid, then a salt appetite mechanism, located within the hypothalamus, causes a craving for salt. Excessive salt loss leads to **dehydration** and perhaps a reduction in blood volume, which may result in hypovolaemic shock.

Sulphur
Sulphur is a constituent of many proteins, including antibodies, some vitamins and mucopolysaccharides such as those found in cartilage, tendons and bone.

Found in proteins and is thus abundant in eggs, milk and meat.

No known deficiency.

Trace elements
Iodine
Iodine is required for the formation of the hormones thyroxine and tri-iodothyronine by the thyroid gland. These are largely responsible for the control of the metabolic rate and therefore exert a very strong influence over most bodily functions.

Found in seafood, milk and green vegetables. It is also added to table salt.

One of the best known mineral deficiencies. Prevents the formation of thyroid hormones, but not of the colloid thyroglobulin, which continues to be synthesized under the influence of the pituitary. Since there is a lack of thyroid hormones suppressing the anterior pituitary gland, its stimulation of the thyroid gland continues, leading to swelling of the thyroid (**goitre**). Lack of hormone depresses the metabolic rate.

Zinc
Zinc is an important component of many enzymes, including carbonic anhydrase, which catalyses the formation of carbonic acid from carbon dioxide and water. It is also part of some peptidases and thus contributes to protein digestion.

Found in red meat, fish, cereals and legumes.

Results in a variety of consequences, including retardation of growth, learning difficulties and a depressed immune response.

by evidence that people who have a diet low in roughage have a much higher incidence of ischaemic heart disease and cancer of the colon than those who have high roughage diets.

Water

Water constitutes approximately 60% of body weight. It is the solvent within which all of the chemical reactions that determine body function take place. It is therefore essential that the body receives an adequate supply. In order to maintain a constant osmotic pressure and body fluid volume, water intake must balance total output. Water is taken into the body in fluids, i.e. 'drinks', and in food: many foods consist largely of water; for example, lettuce contains 95% water, potatoes 90% and even butter contains about 16%!

DEFICIENCY

Loss of water from the fluid compartments of the body results in **dehydration**. This may occur due to a number of reasons: either lack of water intake or excessive fluid loss due, for example, to excessive sweating, diarrhoea, vomiting, burns to the skin, haemorrhage or diuresis.

A reduction in the volume of blood in the cardiovascular system may lead to hypovolaemic shock. Symptoms of dehydration include a dry or 'sticky' oral mucosa, dry, pale skin, decreased urine output (oliguria) and thirst. If dehydration is prolonged it results in weight loss and possibly fever and mental imbalance.

The hypothalamus contains a **'thirst' centre** which promotes water uptake. This response is elicited by a rise in plasma osmotic pressure and it is believed that the receptors are the same ones whose stimulation leads to the secretion of antidiuretic hormone.

The regulation of water balance is discussed in **Regulation of nephron function** (page 501), in Ch. 14, Renal Control of Body Fluid Volume and Composition.

Hypovolaemic shock is discussed on page 421, in Ch. 12, Circulation of Blood and Lymph.

The regulation of ADH secretion is described in **Regulation of water balance** (page 501), in Ch. 14, Renal Control of Body Fluid Volume and Composition.

General features of the alimentary canal

Also known as the digestive or gastrointestinal tract, or gut, the alimentary canal extends from the mouth to the anus and has several associated glands (Figure 15.2).

At the top (anterior end) is the **oral cavity** which opens into the **pharynx**, a cavity that is shared with the upper airways. The pharynx then leads into the **oesophagus**, a narrow muscular tube that conveys food to the **stomach**. The process of digestion continues in the **small intestine**, which receives pancreatic juice from the pancreas and bile from the liver. It is in the small intestine that most of the digested food is absorbed. Lastly, the **large intestine** completes the absorption of water and digested food, and conveys the residue to the opening to the exterior, the anus.

The alimentary canal is essentially a tube that carries material from the mouth to the anus. Anything that is not absorbed through the wall of this tube into the blood or lymph is passed out through the anus by the process of defaecation. If the true 'inside' of the body is considered to

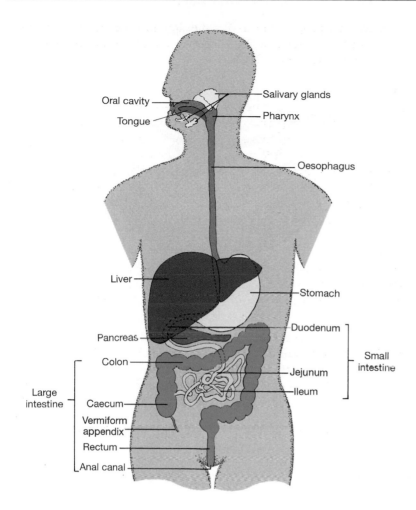

Figure 15.2 General plan of the alimentary canal and associated glands.

be the body cavities and their contents (the **viscera**) then the alimentary tract is effectively an extension of the outer surface of the body.

Layers of the alimentary canal wall

The wall of the alimentary canal consists of four principal layers: the inner mucosa, the submucosa, the muscularis externa and the outer serosa (Figure 15.3). The detailed structure of each layer varies somewhat in the different regions of the canal according to the specialized function of each section.

The **mucosa**, whose surface is folded extensively, consists of an **epithelial lining** enclosing a **lamina propria** of loose connective tissue that is especially rich in blood and lymphatic capillaries and sometimes contains glands. Smooth muscle cells and lymphoid tissues are also present. A thin layer of smooth muscle, the **muscularis mucosae**, constitutes the deepest layer of the mucosa and separates it from the submucosa. The mucosa provides enzymes for the final stages of digestion and absorbs the products of that digestion.

The **submucosa** is composed of connective tissue and contains many large blood and lymph vessels, which supply those of the mucosa and

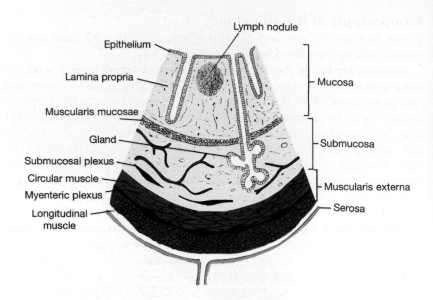

Figure 15.3   General structure of the alimentary canal wall.

the muscularis externa. An extensive network of nerve fibres and ganglia, the **submucosal plexus**, is also present.

The **muscularis externa** comprises an inner circular layer and an outer longitudinal layer of smooth muscle. Between the two layers blood vessels and lymphatics are found, together with a network of nerve fibres and ganglia, the **myenteric plexus**. The muscle layer enables a variety of movements to occur in the gut wall; these movements contribute to the breakdown of food and its passage along the digestive tube.

The outer **serosa** consists of loose connective tissue, rich in blood and lymph vessels and adipose tissue, covered by a layer of simple squamous epithelium (mesothelium). The moist, smooth mesothelium covering the viscera also lines the abdominal cavity. This enables the viscera to glide over one another as well as against the abdominal wall.

Peritoneum

The peritoneum is a serous membrane lining the abdominal wall (**parietal pleura**) and covering the organs contained within the abdomen (**visceral pleura** or **serosa**). It also extends as sheets, or folds, within the abdominal cavity where it supports the viscera and blood and lymphatic vessels and nerves.

The **lesser omentum** is a double layer of peritoneum connecting the lesser curvature of the stomach with the liver.

The **greater omentum** extends from the greater curvature of the stomach to form an apron-like fold in front of the small intestine. It is reflected backwards and upwards and wraps around the organs of the upper abdomen. As the greater omentum is a double layer folded back on itself, it contains four layers of serous membranes.

The **mesentery** is a fan-shaped fold of peritoneum that supports the jejunum and ileum and connects with the posterior abdominal wall.

Blood supply of the alimentary canal

Blood flow to the gut and associated organs is derived from several vessels, arising from the dorsal aorta (Figure 15.4).

Immediately below the diaphragm the **coeliac trunk** branches off the aorta and shortly divides into three branches. One of these forms the **left gastric artery** to the stomach while a second branch, the **hepatic artery**, takes blood to the liver and part of the stomach wall. The third branch, the **splenic artery**, carries blood to the spleen and pancreas. Also arising from the aorta is the **superior mesenteric artery** to the small intestine and proximal half of the large intestine and the **inferior mesenteric artery** to the lower half of the large intestine.

Venous blood from the alimentary tract drains largely into the **hepatic portal vein** and thence to the liver.

The gut has a relatively high perfusion rate for its percentage body weight (see Table 12.1). Blood flow is unevenly divided between the tissues, however: about two-thirds passes to the mucosa and submucosa and one-third to the muscle layers. Blood flow to the two areas can be altered independently, such that when activity in the muscle layers is increased, blood flow to that area is also increased. Similarly, when glandular activity is increased, blood flow in the mucosa and submucosa also increases.

As in many areas of the body, blood flow appears to be mainly controlled by local factors, mainly a fall in oxygen levels. However the increased blood flow that accompanies glandular secretion may be due to the production of kinins by these glands. The intestinal mucosa releases several hormones during digestion that are vasodilators; they include CCK, VIP, gastrin and secretin. Increased sympathetic activity,

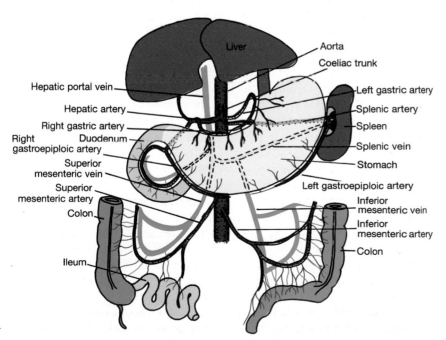

Figure 15.4 Blood vessels of the alimentary canal. Arteries [red], veins [blue]. Gastric and gastroepiploic veins have been omitted.

such as that which occurs in physical exercise, causes an overall vaso-constriction in the gut which may be so intense as to virtually inhibit blood flow completely.

Nerve supply of the alimentary canal

The alimentary canal has both an intrinsic and an extrinsic nerve supply.

The intrinsic or **enteric nervous system** comprises two neural plexuses within the wall of the gut; these are the **myenteric** and **submucosal plexuses**.

The extrinsic nerve supply comprises branches of the sympathetic and parasympathetic systems, both of which innervate the intramural plexuses.

Parasympathetic innervation consists of the **VIIth** and **IXth cranial nerves** to the salivary glands, the two **Xth nerves** as far as the proximal half of the colon, and the **pelvic splanchnic nerves**, which innervate the more distal sections. The preganglionic fibres synapse in the intramural plexuses and the postganglionic neurones supply the muscles and glands in the gut wall. The parasympathetic system, in general, promotes glandular secretion and increases motility in the gut wall together with relaxation of the sphincters.

The **sympathetic** neurones supplying the gut synapse in the coeliac and superior mesenteric ganglia outside the gut wall and then travel in the **splanchnic nerves** to the intramural plexuses, blood vessels and the muscles of the gut wall. Sympathetic stimulation causes reduced muscle and secretory activity and vasoconstriction.

As might be predicted from their relative positions, the myenteric plexus is associated mainly with the control of intestinal movements while the submucosal plexus regulates blood flow and secretion.

Some of the sensory neurones in the gut have their fibres within the plexuses, whereas others run in the autonomic nerves to the coeliac, mesenteric and hypogastric (sympathetic) ganglia. Other fibres travel directly to the spinal cord and thence to the brain.

As a result of the organization of the nerve supply to the alimentary canal, there are two types of reflex pathway, intrinsic and extrinsic. The intrinsic pathway is confined to the wall of the gut itself, whereas the extrinsic reflex pathway includes the spinal cord and brain stem (Figure

Figure 15.5 Intrinsic and extrinsic reflex pathways initiated by stimuli in the alimentary canal.

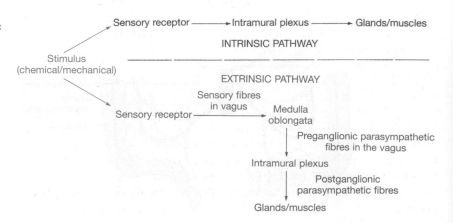

15.5). Pain receptors in the wall of the alimentary canal, for example, initiate impulses that travel up the spinal cord to the brain, where the sensation is experienced. Distension of the gut by, for example, excessive amounts of food is a particularly potent and common stimulus which is perceived as pain.

Neural control of eating

The process of eating is regulated by **hunger** and **satiety 'centres'** in the hypothalamus. A fall in blood glucose, amino acid or lipid break-down products leads to stimulation of the hunger centre, which then promotes feeding. This raises the levels of blood nutrients, which removes the stimuli. It is believed that this is mediated by the satiety centre, which is activated and, in turn, inhibits the hunger centre.

Salivation, chewing and swallowing, all of which are associated with intake of food, are regulated by centres in the brain stem.

Secretions

Digestive enzymes are secreted in digestive juices by a large number of glands associated with the alimentary canal. They include the salivary glands in the mouth, the glands of the stomach and those of the pancreas.

The crypts of Lieberkühn in the wall of the small intestine secrete serous fluid and Brunner's glands in the duodenum secrete an alkaline mucous fluid. There are also millions of goblet cells in the epithelial lining of the gut which secrete mucus.

Bile, which aids the digestion and absorption of fat as well as providing an excretory medium for cholesterol and the breakdown prod-ucts of haemoglobin, is secreted by the liver and stored in the gall bladder before entering the duodenum.

The total daily volume of fluid secreted into the lumen of the alimen-tary canal is around 8 L.

Peristalsis

The main propulsive movement of the gut is peristalsis, which occurs in the **muscularis externa** of the gut wall. Contraction of several centime-tres of longitudinal muscle is followed by contraction of a ring of circular muscle above the point of stimulation and 'receptive relaxation' of the circular layer below. Adjacent sections of circular muscle contract in succession so that the contractile ring appears to move forward for a few centimetres before dying out (Figure 15.6). This activity causes food within the tube to be propelled towards the anus.

The frequency of peristalsis is set by the **basic electrical rhythm (BER)** generated in the longitudinal layer of the wall. This activity occurs all the time, but the depolarizations do not always reach threshold. A number of factors can stimulate peristalsis by increasing depolarization of the cells in the longitudinal muscle layer; they include distension of the wall and increased parasympathetic activity (both of these are mediated via the myenteric plexus). Some hormones and other chemicals can also regulate peristalsis. Further details are given in later sections.

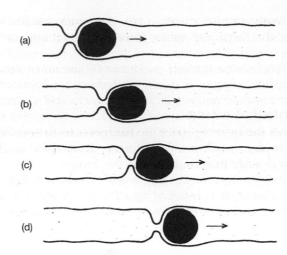

Figure 15.6 A peristaltic wave of contraction moves along the alimentary canal.

The oral cavity and associated structures

In the mouth, food is mixed with saliva and broken down physically by the process of chewing (mastication) to bring about the formation of a moist ball or bolus. By breaking the food up, chewing increases the surface area available to digestive enzymes. It also softens the food so that it passes more easily through the alimentary tract.

The presence of food in the mouth and its taste and smell, apart from producing pleasant sensations, also stimulate the secretion of saliva, as well as gastric and pancreatic juices and bile, by means of parasympathetic pathways.

Figure 15.7 Section through the lower head to show the oral and nasal cavities and neighbouring structures.

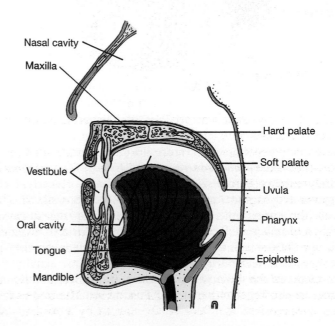

The oral cavity consists of two parts. An outer smaller vestibule is separated by the teeth and gums from the inner oral cavity proper (Figure 15.7).

The outer wall of the vestibule is formed by the inner surfaces of the lips and cheeks. Its superior and inferior surfaces are bounded by reflection of the mucous membrane lining the cheeks and covering the jaw bones. Posteriorly the vestibule communicates with the oral cavity proper through the space between the last molar teeth and the mandible (when the teeth are clamped together). Numerous small, mucus-secreting, glands open into the vestibule.

The lips are formed primarily by the **orbicularis oris muscle** (Figure 15.8) and are covered externally by skin and internally by mucous membrane. They contain many minute blood vessels and nerves.

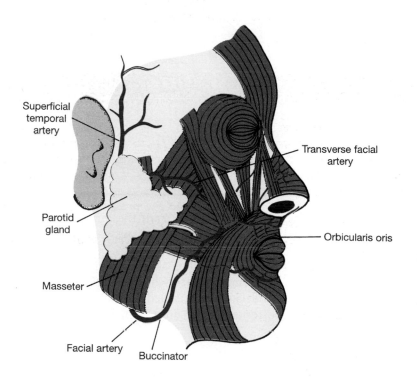

Figure 15.8 Principal muscles and arteries of the face.

Superficial temporal artery

Transverse facial artery

Parotid gland

Orbicularis oris

Masseter

Facial artery   Buccinator

The cheeks are formed principally from the **buccinator muscles**, with variable amounts of adipose tissue.

The jaw movements involved in chewing are brought about primarily by the actions of the **masseter** (Figure 15.8) and the **temporalis** and **pterygoid muscles** (Figure 15.9).

The **gums** or **gingivae** are made of dense fibrous tissue. They are highly vascular and covered by thinly keratinized squamous epithelium. In young people the gums are attached to the enamel covering the teeth, but with age they recede and become attached to the cement covering the root (hence the term 'long in the tooth').

The surface of the floor of the mouth is formed by the mucous membrane connecting the tongue to the mandible. The underside of the tongue is connected to the floor of the mouth by a median fold, the

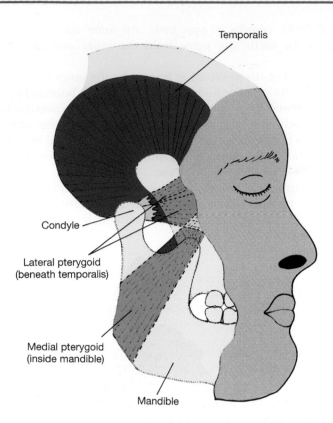

Figure 15.9 The temporalis and pterygoid muscles which, together with the masseter (Figure 15.8), are used in chewing.

frenulum. The sublingual glands lying beneath the mucous membrane form a sublingual fold on each side running backwards and laterally from the frenulum.

The roof of the mouth is formed by the palate. The anterior two-thirds is bony and is known as the **hard palate** while the posterior one-third forms the **soft palate**. The latter is attached to the rear of the hard palate and has a free posterior margin from which the **uvula** hangs down (Figure 15.7).

Teeth

In adults there are up to 16 permanent teeth in each jaw. The teeth lie in sockets in the upper jaw, which comprises the left and right maxillary bones (maxillae), and the lower jaw (mandible). Each half-jaw has two incisors, one canine, two premolars and up to three molars (Figure 15.10). In children, the deciduous (milk) dentition consists of only 10 teeth in each jaw, so that each half jaw has two incisors, one canine and two molar teeth.

All teeth have the same basic structural organization (Figure 15.11) but differ in shape and size. Each tooth has one or more **roots** and a **crown**, which is covered by hard translucent enamel that gives the tooth its cutting or grinding surface.

The bulk of the tooth is constructed of a mineralized, yellow-white substance called **dentine**, which surrounds a central **pulp cavity**. The latter contains nerve fibres and blood and lymphatic vessels, which enter

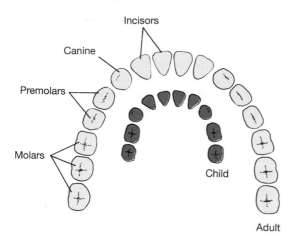

Figure 15.10 Dentition of the upper jaw of an adult (16 teeth) and a child (10 teeth).

through an **apical foramen** at the tip of each root. The root is completely surrounded by a **periodontal ligament**, which anchors the tooth to the bone of the jaw. It is attached to the **cement** that covers the dentine of the root.

The shape of the crown varies depending upon the position of the tooth in the mouth and its function. At the front of the mouth are the **incisors**, chisel-like teeth which cut food. Behind them lie the **canines**, each of which has a single cusp. In carnivorous animals they are often greatly enlarged and are used to tear the animal's food; in humans, however, they are so reduced as to have little specialized function.

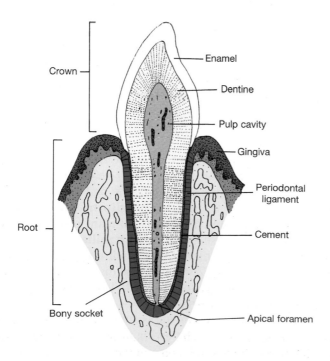

Figure 15.11 Vertical section through an incisor tooth and its socket.

Behind the canines lie the **premolars**, each with two cusps, and behind them the **molars**, which usually have four cusps on their upper (occlusal) surfaces. The premolars and molars are so arranged that when the jaws are clamped together there is maximum contact between the cusps and fissures of the upper and lower molars; this is known as **occlusion**. When food is chewed it is ground between the premolars and molars and reduced to a pulpy consistency.

DENTAL CARIES

If the teeth are not cleaned regularly by brushing and a plentiful flow of saliva, food material accumulates in the fissures of the molars and premolars or may lodge in the spaces between the teeth or at the tooth/gum interface. Bacteria digest this material and produce acids that attack the tooth surface. Once the enamel layer has been penetrated the bacteria are able to enter the dentine and then the pulp cavity. This exposes nerve fibres to the invading organisms and their products, which leads to the pain of toothache. Such holes in the tooth structure are described as **caries**.

Once the infection has entered the pulp cavity it can spread very quickly and perhaps enter the jaw bone, giving rise to an **abscess**.

The addition of fluoride ions to drinking water supplies has been shown to reduce the incidence of dental caries, particularly in children. Fluoride strengthens the enamel covering of the teeth and increases their resistance to bacterial action. Later work has suggested, however, that fluoride is carcinogenic.

Tongue

The tongue is attached to the floor of the mouth. It is covered by stratified squamous epithelium and consists of a mass of striated muscle together with some fat and numerous glands.

The tongue is divided into left and right halves by a median fibrous septum and in each half are two sets of muscles, extrinsic and intrinsic. Extrinsic muscles are attached to structures outside the tongue itself; they include the hyoglossus (attached to the hyoid bone), genioglossus (attached to the mandible), styloglossus (attached to the styloid process), chondroglossus (attached to the hyoid bone) and palatoglossus (attached to the palatine aponeurosis).

The dorsum (upper surface) of the tongue is separated into **palatine** (front) and **pharyngeal** (rear) parts by the V-shaped **sulcus terminalis**. The thick mucous membrane of the palatine part is rough and covered by papillae, two types of which, **fungiform** and **circumvallate papillae**, contain taste buds. The most abundant papillae, however, do not contain taste buds. These are **filiform papillae** and are conical and slender in shape, with keratinized cells at their tips which are continually being lost (see Figure 8.33). Gastrointestinal disturbances may retard the shedding of these cells so that, together with bacteria they accumulate as a grey layer on the tongue's surface, the so-called 'coated tongue'.

The pharyngeal part of the tongue is smoother and thinner than the palatine part, being finely nodular owing to the presence of small lymph follicles in the submucosa.

Taste buds are covered in **Taste** (page 265), in Ch. 8, The Special Senses.

Pharynx

The pharynx forms the passage between the oral cavity and the major parts of the respiratory and digestive tracts. Lined by mucosa, it is a muscular tube about 13 cm long that extends from the base of the skull down behind the larynx to the level of the cricoid cartilage. It is about 3.5 cm wide at the top and 1.5 cm at its junction with the oesophagus.

The submucosa contains numerous pharyngeal mucous glands and nodules of lymph tissue; aggregations of lymph follicles form pharyngeal, tubal and palatine tonsils.

The pharynx contains **three constrictor muscles**, the superior, middle and inferior constrictors (Figure 15.12).

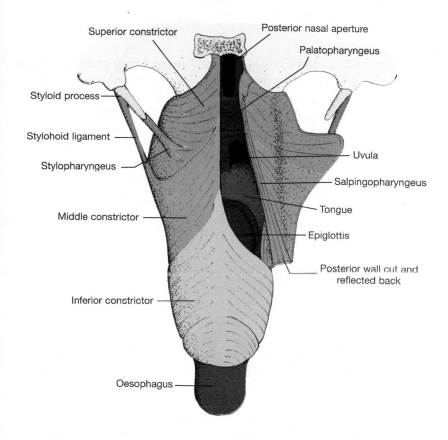

Figure 15.12 Posterior view of the pharynx, opened to show the internal structures.

Three other muscles run longitudinally into the pharyngeal wall, the **stylopharyngeus**, the **salpingopharyngeus** and the **palatopharyngeus**. The last-named forms an arch and extends from the soft palate to form the inner layer of the wall of the pharynx. Between them the pharyngeal muscles constrict and elevate the pharynx during swallowing.

Salivary glands

There are two types of salivary gland associated with the buccal cavity; they are differentiated into major and minor glands. There are three pairs of 'major' glands, the parotid, submandibular (submaxillary) and sublingual glands (Figure 15.13). The 'minor' glands are found within the substance of the lips, the cheeks, the roof of the mouth and the tongue.

Figure 15.13 The location of the salivary glands (right-hand side).

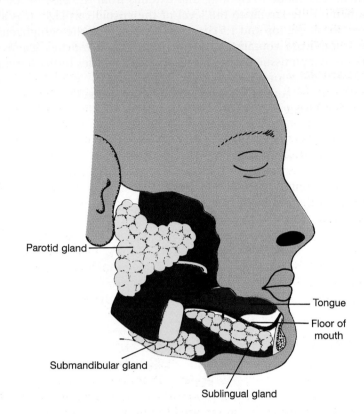

Figure 15.14 Salivary secretory units.

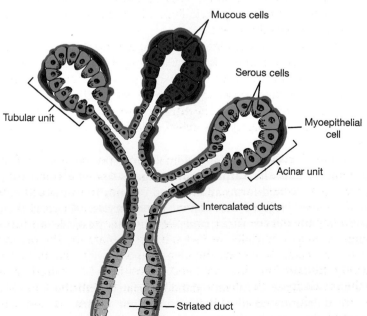

The major glands are composed of secretory units, which may be tubular or acinar. These units are supported by connective tissue and richly supplied with blood and lymph vessels and nerve fibres (Figure 15.14). The secretory units consist of groups of glandular cells of two types; serous and mucous, surrounded by myoepithelial cells. Secretions are conveyed into small (intercalated), ducts which then drain into larger (striated) ducts, which open via secretory ducts into the oral cavity.

The **parotids** are the largest salivary glands, with combined weights of about 50 g. Each gland lies below the ear and between the mandible and the sternocleidomastoid muscle. The glands' secretory cells synthesize the enzyme amylase. Each parotid duct opens through a papilla on the cheek opposite the crown of the second upper molar.

Each **submandibular** gland is about the size of a walnut and lies inside and beneath the mandible, one on each side of the face. The ducts open at the summits of the sublingual papillae which are situated on either side of the frenulum of the tongue. The secretory portions of the glands secrete mucous and small amounts of amylase.

The **sublingual** glands are located beneath the mucous membrane of the floor of the mouth. They are small, with combined weights of only 6–8 g. In spite of its small size, each gland has 8–20 ducts, most of which open on the surface of the sublingual folds on the floor of the mouth. About two-thirds of the cells in these glands are mucus-secreting and the remaining one-third are serous cells.

Oesophagus

The oesophagus is a muscular tube about 25 cm long connecting the pharynx with the stomach. The upper part lies behind the trachea and in front of the vertebral column. Lower down the thorax, below the level of the trachea, it passes behind the right pulmonary artery, the left principal bronchus and the pericardium. It then passes through the diaphragm and joins the stomach.

The **mucosa** of the oesophagus is arranged in folds which disappear when the tube is distended. The inner lining is composed of non-keratinized stratified squamous epithelium. This layer is separated from the submucosa by a typical muscularis mucosae, although the latter is absent at the top of the oesophagus. The **submucosa** contains the oesophageal glands, mucus-secreting glands which open into the lumen by long ducts.

The **muscularis externa** is relatively thick and consists of the typical outer longitudinal and inner circular layers. It may be divided into three roughly equal sections along its length. The upper two-thirds contains striated muscle while the lower third is smooth muscle only. Surrounding the outside of the oesophagus is a layer of fibrous tissue.

There is no anatomically distinct sphincter separating the oesophagus from the stomach. However, the combination of circular muscle fibres adjoining the junction, the shape and disposition of surrounding organs and the proximity of the diaphragm all appear to contribute to the presence of a 'physiological' sphincter. This is known as the **cardiac sphincter**.

Salivation

Saliva is secreted by the paired parotid, sublingual and submandibular glands. It is a watery fluid containing ions, mucin and the digestive enzyme **salivary alpha-amylase** (α-amylase). In addition to its role in digestion, saliva also has several other actions. It lubricates the oral cavity and tongue, which aids speech. This is evident in situations such as fear when saliva flow is reduced and the affected person has difficulty speaking. Saliva also enables molecules to dissolve on the surface of the tongue and stimulate the taste buds. It also washes food particles from the teeth and the enzyme lysozyme has an antibacterial action. In addition, at its normal pH (7.0) it is saturated with Ca^{2+} which prevents calcium from dissolving out of the teeth. Usually a total of between 1000 and 1500 mL of saliva is secreted per day, the rate of secretion varying between about 0.5 mL/min (basal rate) and 4.0 mL/min (during mastication).

The osmolality of saliva varies with its rate of secretion. At low rates it is very hypotonic (about 50 mosm/kg H_2O) compared with plasma (about 300 mosm/kg H_2O), whereas at higher rates of secretion it approaches isotonicity. These differences are largely due to variations in the amounts of Na^+ and Cl^- that are absorbed from the fluid in the tubules of the salivary glands. At faster rates of secretion there is insufficient time for the absorption of these ions so that more remain in the saliva and the tonicity is therefore relatively high.

The formation of saliva is summarized in Figure 15.15.

The acinar cells produce the primary fluid containing enzyme, mucin and ions. This fluid has an ionic composition broadly similar to that of

Figure 15.15 Saliva formation. Primary fluid is produced in the secretory acinus and the secretion is then modified in both the intercalated and striated ducts.

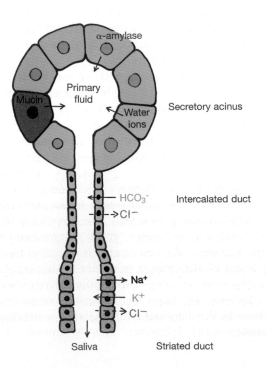

plasma. In the ducts leading from the acini, ionic exchange takes place: Na^+ is actively removed from the fluid while K^+ is added to it, though at a lower rate. Since there is net reabsorption of cation, Cl^- follows Na^+. In addition, HCO_3^- is secreted into the fluid from the cells lining the ducts, at least partly in exchange for Cl^-. As a result of these exchanges the concentrations of Na^+ and Cl^- in saliva are lower than in plasma, whereas those of K^+ and HCO_3^- are higher. The transport of Na^+ and K^+ is stimulated by **aldosterone** in the same way as in the distal nephron of the kidney.

The salivary glands are stimulated by both the sympathetic and parasympathetic divisions of the autonomic nervous system, although the most copious response results from parasympathetic stimulation. Activation of the sympathetic system causes vasoconstriction and a scant, viscous secretion.

Sensory stimuli that initiate salivation include the presence of food in the mouth, taste and smell, although perhaps the most potent stimulus is acid, for example in fruit. Impulses are conveyed to the 'salivary centre' in the medulla oblongata, which initiates reflex secretion of saliva via the parasympathetic fibres in the **glossopharyngeal** and **facial nerves** to the glands. In dogs, the sight and smell of food and conditioned reflexes can evoke secretion, but these effects are relatively slight in man. Salivation may also be induced by the presence of irritating materials in the stomach or small intestine.

Stimulation of the salivary glands releases the enzyme kallikrein into the interstitial fluid, where it activates **bradykinin**. The latter then causes vasodilation which enhances the secretory activity of the glands.

The role of aldosterone is discussed further in: **Role of the renin–angiotensin–aldosterone system in blood volume regulation** (page 421), in Ch. 12, Circulation of Blood and Lymph; **Role of aldosterone in the regulation of sodium and potassium balance and blood volume** (page 505), in Ch. 14, Renal Control of Body Fluid Volume and Composition; and **Aldosterone and deoxycorticosterone (mineralocorticoids)** (page 638), in Ch. 16, Endocrine Physiology.

Chewing (mastication)

Pieces of food are bitten off from the main mass by the incisors and, once inside the mouth, the food is then moved around by the tongue and brought into contact with the occlusal surfaces of the premolars and molars, which crush and grind it into small pieces. This function is particularly important in the breakdown of meat and any other food with a fibrous consistency. It is also a prerequisite for the digestion of plant material because the cellulose walls of plant cells are indigestible and must be ruptured if the nutrients inside are to be released.

Chewing is a reflex activity initiated by the presence of food in the mouth, which stimulates touch receptors in the gums and the front of the hard palate. Sensory information is relayed to the 'chewing centre' in the medulla oblongata of the hindbrain, which brings about reflex inhibition of the masticatory muscles (**masseter** and **temporalis**) and the jaw drops. The subsequent stretching of the muscle fibres then initiates a stretch reflex on the same side, leading to contraction of the muscles which raise the lower jaw and compress the food between the teeth. The **pterygoid muscles** bring about grinding movements and contraction of the muscles in the cheeks and around the lips helps to force the food between the teeth, as does the movement of the tongue. The tongue also rolls the softened food into a bolus, mixing it with saliva before swallowing.

Digestion of starch

During mastication, as the food is ground between the teeth and is mixed with saliva, the water content of the saliva helps to moisten and soften the food, while the mucin acts as a lubricant. Any cooked starch within the food is liable to attack by salivary alpha-amylase. This enzyme catalyses the hydrolysis of starch to maltose, maltotriose and dextrins (which contain two, three and up to nine glucose units respectively) by splitting the α-1,4 links between glucose units (Figure 15.16).

Figure 15.16 Hydrolysis of starch catalysed by the enzyme alpha-amylase.

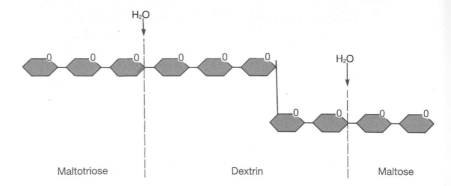

The amount of cooked starch hydrolysed by salivary alpha-amylase depends upon how long it stays in the mouth and how long it takes before the acidity of the gastric juice inhibits the enzyme after the food has been swallowed. The enzyme is active down to a pH of 4, and up to 40% of the starch may have been hydrolysed before inactivation occurs.

Swallowing (deglutition)

Once the food has been formed into a bolus in the mouth it is passed through the pharynx and down the oesophagus to the stomach. This is achieved by the act of swallowing (deglutition).

Deglutition is a complex reflex regulated by a '**swallowing centre**' in the medulla. It is initiated voluntarily (**voluntary stage**) when the tongue muscles contract and push the bolus upwards and backwards into the pharynx. The soft palate is elevated and comes into contact with the posterior wall of the pharynx, thereby closing off the rear openings of the nasal cavities (Figure 15.17).

The **pharyngeal stage** of deglutition is the beginning of involuntary reflex activity and starts when the vocal cords approximate and close the glottis. Respiration is inhibited and the larynx is pulled upwards and forwards by the myohyoid muscles (which run from the tongue to the larynx). These actions prevent food from entering the respiratory tract. The bolus pushes the epiglottis back over the glottis which confers extra protection to the respiratory tract.

The **oesophageal stage** of deglutition commences with contraction of the pharyngeal constrictor muscles; this initiates a peristaltic wave that pushes the bolus into the oesophagus. At rest, the opening to the oesophagus is closed by the **hypopharyngeal sphincter**. This is a 3 cm long segment at the top of the oesophagus within which the muscle fibres are so arranged that when they are relaxed the sphincter is closed.

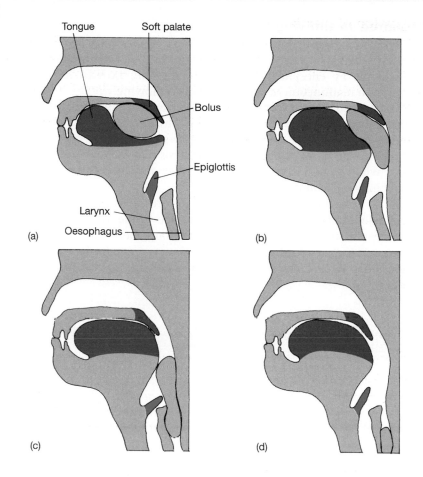

Figure 15.17 Swallowing.
(a) The bolus is propelled towards the pharynx by the tongue.
(b) The soft palate is elevated and closes off the entrance to the nasal passages. **(c)** The glottis (not visible from this angle) closes and the epiglottis reflects back over the entrance to the larynx.
(d) The bolus is propelled down the oesophagus by peristalsis.

During swallowing the muscles contract and cause the sphincter to open, allowing the bolus to pass down into the oesophagus. A wave of contraction in the circular muscle layer then propels the bolus down into the stomach. This peristaltic wave travels at a rate of about 4 cm/s.

Fluids and semi-solid fluids usually pass down the oesophagus ahead of the peristaltic wave in upright subjects simply due to the effect of gravity.

The last 4 cm or so of the oesophagus, though apparently identical to the tissues further up, is normally in a state of tonic contraction and thus forms a functional sphincter. As the peristaltic wave approaches this sphincter, the muscle fibres relax (**receptive relaxation**) and allow the food to enter the stomach. The sphincter then closes again and prevents regurgitation of gastric material back into the oesophagus. Should any such regurgitation occur, sharp pain or '**heartburn**' is felt behind the sternum, due to the irritation of the unprotected oesophageal mucosa by gastric acid.

FLATULENCE

Air may be swallowed along with solid foods and liquids. This gas, primarily nitrogen and oxygen, may be absorbed in the stomach, or may be expelled through the mouth by belching. This is known as flatulence.

Impaired swallowing (dysphagia)

The swallowing mechanism may become paralysed. Such paralysis may be due to: damage to the swallowing centre in the brain, brought about for example by encephalitis; damage to the Vth, IXth or Xth cranial nerves; or a malfunction of the muscles of swallowing.

The consequences of paralysis of swallowing include a complete loss of the ability to swallow, failure of the glottis to close and block off the opening to the larynx and failure of the soft palate to close off the entrance to the nasal passages. Such paralysis may occur in deep anaesthesia, when vomit from the stomach may not be swallowed but is instead inhaled, leading to choking .

Failure of the cardiac sphincter to relax during swallowing (**achalasia**) leads to the accumulation of food in the lower oesophagus. This may, in turn, lead to a permanent enlargement, in the condition known as **megaoesophagus**. The food may remain for such long periods that it becomes infected, causing damage to the oesophageal lining.

The stomach

The stomach stores the food eaten during a meal and later releases it at a rate optimal for digestion. Food is mixed with gastric juice, changing its consistency so that it will be more easily transported to subsequent sections of the gut. In addition, food is exposed to enzymes which begin the digestion of proteins. The acid in gastric juice is bactericidal and also converts ferric iron in the diet to the ferrous form in which it is subsequently absorbed in the intestine. Furthermore, gastric glands produce intrinsic factor which is necessary for the absorption of vitamin B_{12} from the diet.

Figure 15.18 The regions of the stomach.

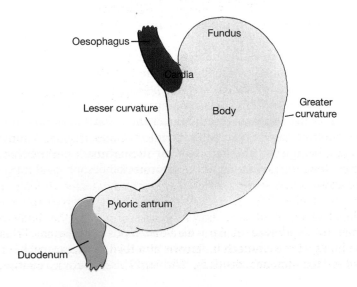

Regions of the stomach

The stomach is a muscular sac divided into four areas, the **fundus, cardia, body** and **pyloric antrum** (Figure 15.18).

Most commonly, the empty stomach is found to be J-shaped, with the pyloric antrum forming the tail. When it fills, the stomach tends to expand downwards and forwards, displacing the intestine. The opening of the oesophagus into the stomach is called the **cardiac orifice**. The **pyloric orifice** connects the pyloric antrum with the duodenum and at the junction is found the **pyloric sphincter** or **pylorus**, which consists of a thickened band of circular muscle.

Layers of the stomach wall

The stomach wall consists of the usual four layers of the gastrointestinal tract (Figure 15.19).

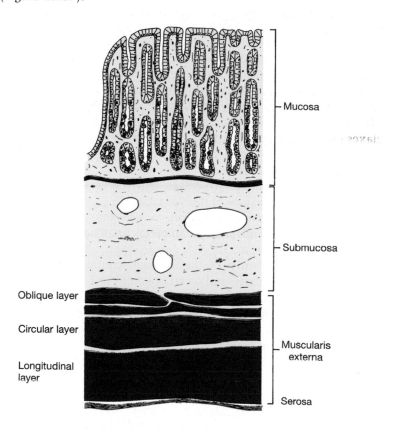

Figure 15.19 The layers of the stomach wall.

The outermost layer, the **serosa**, covers almost the entire surface of the organ, being absent only where the two layers of peritoneum come together along the greater and lesser curvatures.

The **muscularis externa** has the longitudinal and circular muscle layers found elsewhere in the gastrointestinal tract, together with an additional layer of oblique fibres on the inside in the body of the stomach; this layer is particularly well-developed near the cardiac orifice.

The lining of the stomach is thrown into folds or **rugae**, which flatten out when the stomach distends. The surface epithelium consists of a single layer of columnar epithelial cells which continually secrete neutral mucus on to the surface. The **mucosa** is covered by small (0.2 mm diameter) depressions or gastric pits, which contain the openings of the gastric glands.

GASTRIC CIRCULATION

The stomach is a richly vascular organ, receiving blood through the **right gastric** and **gastroepiploic arteries** from the common hepatic artery, the **left gastric artery** from the coeliac trunk, and the **left gastroepiploic** and **short gastric arteries** from the splenic artery. These vessels form anastomoses at all levels but especially in the submucosa, where a well-developed submucosal plexus is found.

Blood drains from the stomach into the **splenic, superior mesenteric** and **hepatic portal veins** (Figure 15.4).

NERVE SUPPLY OF THE STOMACH

The stomach is innervated by both sympathetic and parasympathetic nerve fibres. The sympathetic supply is derived from the **coeliac ganglia**, while the parasympathetic fibres are carried in the **vagus nerves**. Sympathetic stimulation causes vasoconstriction, reduces peristalsis and brings about contraction of the pyloric sphincter. Parasympathetic stimulation, on the other hand, increases peristalsis and relaxes the pyloric sphincter; it also promotes gastric secretion.

Gastric glands

Gastric glands show some structural, and therefore functional, differences in the various regions of the stomach.

The glands of the **cardiac region** consist almost entirely of mucus-secreting cells. The glands may be simple or branched and are present in relatively small numbers.

The **fundus** and **body** of the stomach contain large numbers of glands with between three and seven openings into each pit. Each gland may be simple or branched and has three different types of cell: mucous neck cells, oxyntic cells and peptic cells (Figure 15.20).

Mucous cells, of the same type as those that line the stomach, are also found in the uppermost region of the gland. Lower down these are replaced by structurally distinguishable **neck mucous cells**; these cells lack the large masses of mucin characteristic of lining cells. Neck mucous cells are also found scattered among the other cell types in deeper regions of the gland. In addition to their secretion of mucus, neck mucous cells also secrete small amounts of pepsinogen.

Oxyntic cells predominate in the middle part of the gland. They secrete hydrochloric acid and intrinsic factor. Oxyntic cells may also be found in small numbers in the basal region. The electron microscope reveals that oxyntic cells have a characteristic deep circular invagination (canaliculus) in their apical cytoplasm; this canaliculus is lined by microvilli.

Enzyme-secreting **peptic** (zymogenic or **chief**) **cells** are found in the basal region of the glands.

The wall of the pyloric region of the stomach is studded with deep

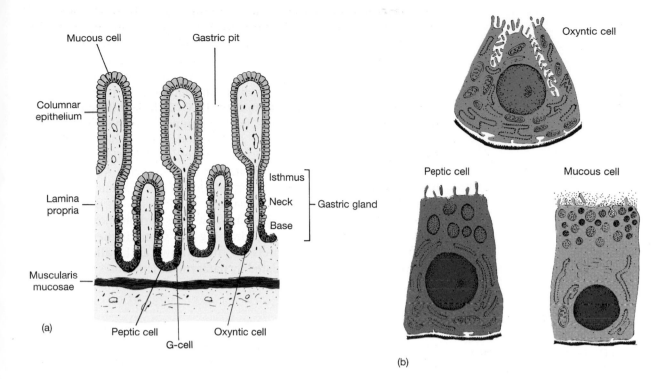

(a)

(b)

Figure 15.20 **(a)** The gastric mucosa, showing the gastric pits, (the gastric pits have been widened for clarity). **(b)** The secretory cells of the gastric glands.

gastric pits containing the openings of glands similar to those of the cardiac region. The cells are predominantly mucus-secreting, although oxyntic cells also occur in small numbers. In addition, the pyloric glands contain **G-cells**, a type of enteroendocrine cell, which secrete the hormone gastrin into the surrounding blood vessels.

Some 15 different types of enteroendocrine cell are found in the epithelial lining of the gastrointestinal tract, some in the intestinal glands, others on the villi.

Gastric juice

Gastric juice contains hydrochloric acid, mucus, a number of pepsins (proteolytic enzymes) and intrinsic factor. The major ions, apart from H^+ and Cl^-, are Na^+, K^+ and HCO_3^-. The total volume of gastric juice secreted each day is of the order of 2–3 L; it is very slightly hypotonic to plasma.

HYDROCHLORIC ACID

The quantity of H^+ secreted by the oxyntic cells is approximately 3 million times that found in plasma, the actual amount being proportional to the rate of secretion. At high rates of secretion, the amount of H^+ in gastric juice is around 150 mmol/L. The presence of such large quantities of acid in gastric juice give it a bactericidal function. In addition, the acid activates pepsins (secreted as inactive pepsinogens by the chief cells) and provides an optimal pH for pepsin activity. Hydrochloric acid also converts ferric iron (Fe^{3+}) to the ferrous (Fe^{2+}) form, which is more soluble in the prevailing (slightly alkaline) pH of the small intestine where it is absorbed.

The precise mechanism of acid secretion is controversial, but it is thought that both H^+ and Cl^- are actively transported into the canaliculi of the oxyntic cells and then pass to the gastric lumen (Figure 15.21).

The H^+ ions are derived from water molecules. The splitting of water molecules also gives rise to OH^- ions, which combine with carbon dioxide (either from plasma or cellular metabolism), with the aid of the enzyme **carbonic anhydrase**, to form HCO_3^-. These diffuse out of the cell in exchange for Cl^-. This Cl^- is then pumped into the canaliculus as the second component of the hydrochloric acid. The presence of hydrochloric acid in the canaliculus creates an osmotic gradient and leads to the withdrawal of water from the cell. A solution of hydrochloric acid is therefore formed inside the canaliculus and is secreted into the lumen of the stomach.

As blood flows through the stomach it loses carbon dioxide and Cl^- and gains HCO_3^-. Venous blood draining the stomach therefore has a higher pH than that which enters, an effect known as the **alkaline tide**.

The oxyntic cells are stimulated by parasympathetic fibres in the vagus nerves, and by the chemical substances gastrin and histamine.

Figure 15.21 Synthesis of hydrochloric acid by an oxyntic cell. H^+ and Cl^- are actively transported into the canaliculus and water follows by osmosis. H^+ is produced by the splitting of H_2O. OH^- also derived from splitting H_2O is resynthesized into H_2O by combining with H^+. H^+ and HCO_3^- are formed from CO_2 and H_2O, which combine under the influence of the enzyme carbonic anhydrase.

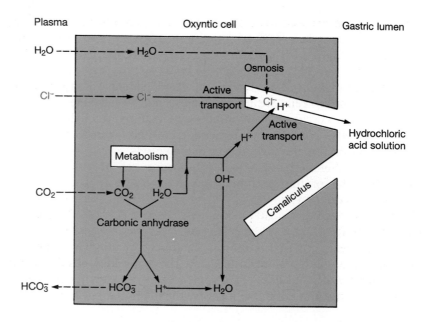

MUCUS

The surface cells of the stomach mucosa secrete an alkaline, viscous mucus which forms a lining layer about 1 mm thick. This affords protection to the mucosal cells from the gastric contents. Mucus is also produced by the neck cells of the gastric glands in the fundus and body, and from most of the cells of the cardiac and pyloric glands. This has a thinner consistency than surface mucus and thus forms a component of gastric juice.

The surface cells have tight cell junctions and a low permeability to H^+. These factors help to protect the underlying tissues from attack by gastric acid and proteolytic enzymes. The cells are replaced every 1–3 days.

Mucous cells are stimulated by parasympathetic fibres in the vagus nerves and directly by mechanical or chemical irritation.

PEPSINS

A number of slightly different pepsins are secreted in inactive form as **pepsinogens** by the peptic cells and, to a much lesser extent, the neck mucous cells. The inactive nature of the enzymes at the time of their secretion prevents the cells from being digested by their own secretory products. Once exposed to the acid in the gastric lumen, the pepsinogen molecules are split and the active pepsins are released.

$$Pepsinogen \xrightarrow{\text{HCl}} pepsin$$

Pepsins act as autocatalysts and are thus able to activate themselves.

$$Pepsinogen \xrightarrow{\text{Pepsin}} pepsin$$

Pepsinogen synthesis occurs continuously, but pepsinogen release only occurs when the cells are stimulated. The pepsinogens are stored within the cells in granules, and are secreted when the cells are stimulated by parasympathetic nerve fibres, histamine or gastrin (weak response).

Pepsins catalyse the hydrolysis of dietary proteins, forming polypeptides and a few free amino acids.

$$Protein \xrightarrow{\text{Pepsin}} polypeptides + amino acids$$

INTRINSIC FACTOR

The oxyntic cells also produce a mucoprotein, intrinsic factor, which is vital for the absorption of vitamin B_{12} from the diet. Vitamin B_{12} is bound to protein in food and is released from it either by cooking or by proteolytic enzymes. Intrinsic factor combines with the free vitamin and protects it from digestion. Absorption of vitamin B_{12} occurs in the ileum, and intrinsic factor is required for the process. Absence of intrinsic factor leads to pernicious anaemia.

> See also **Effects of nutritional deficiencies on erythropoiesis (anaemias)** *(page 336),* in Ch. 11, Blood, Lymphoid Tissue and Immunity.

Control of the secretion of gastric juice

Gastric juice secretion is stimulated by both **intrinsic** and **extrinsic nerve reflexes**, and by the hormone **gastrin**, released from the G-cells of the pyloric glands. A small amount of gastrin is also produced by glands in the duodenum.

Gastrin does not stimulate the production of all of the components of gastric juice equally, exhibiting a much more powerful influence upon acid than upon pepsinogen release.

Parasympathetic stimulation increases the output of acid, mucus, and especially pepsinogen, by the action of acetylcholine upon each of the cell types that produces them.

Histamine stimulates acid secretion, but if histamine H_2 receptors in the stomach are blocked by a drug such as cimetidine, then both parasympathetic stimulation and gastrin fail to stimulate much acid secretion. This supports the suggestion that histamine is involved in the mechanism by which gastrin and acetylcholine stimulate the cells.

Even in a fasting individual, there is a basal rate of gastric secretion, although it consists almost entirely of mucus. Changes in secretion rates are facilitated by a corresponding change in blood flow. In a resting stomach it is about 0.5% of the total cardiac output, whereas in an active stomach it can amount to some 20% of the cardiac output.

Gastric secretion is subdivided into three phases according to where the stimuli originate: the cephalic, gastric and intestinal phases.

CEPHALIC PHASE

The cephalic phase depends upon a range of stimuli that cause secretion of gastric juice before the food arrives in the stomach. It accounts for about 10% of the total secretion associated with a meal. The neural activity that initiates the cephalic phase arises in the brain, in the cerebral cortex, which receives input from taste and smell receptors, or the hypothalamus. Thus, thinking about food or conditioned stimuli such as the clink of cutlery, as well as the taste and smell of food, can bring about the secretion of what is called '**appetite juice**'. There are two mechanisms involved in stimulating secretion: one is neural, the other hormonal. Figure 15.22 shows the neural pathway, which involves the **vagus nerves** from the brain to the gastric glands which, when stimulated, secrete at an increased rate.

Vagal stimulation also extends to the pyloric glands and they respond by releasing **gastrin** into the blood. This effect is mediated via neurones

Figure 15.22 The cephalic phase of gastric secretion.

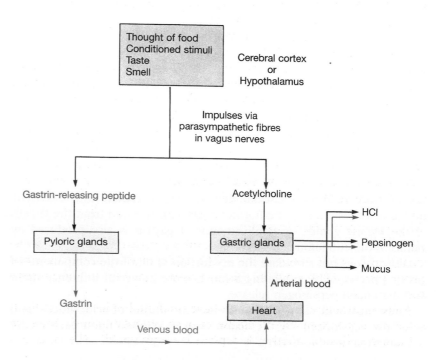

that secrete **gastrin-releasing peptide**. When gastrin returns to the stomach via the circulation it stimulates the gastric glands to release acid and some pepsinogens.

GASTRIC PHASE

The presence of food in the stomach elicits about 80% of the total secretion of gastric juice. The food stretches the stomach wall and this distension stimulates the glands by both **intrinsic** and **extrinsic reflex pathways**. Distension of the pyloric antrum results in the release of gastrin into the blood by an intrinsic reflex. Some substances in the food, known as **secretagogues**, elicit the release of gastrin by an intrinsic reflex. Such substances include alcohol, protein digestion products and caffeine.

INTESTINAL PHASE

As long as food is present in the duodenum it causes the secretion of gastric juice above the basal rate. This effect is hormone-mediated and is at least partly due to the release of gastrin from the duodenal wall.

INHIBITION OF GASTRIC SECRETION

There is a feedback mechanism between acid secretion and gastrin release. If the pH of gastric juice falls, then gastrin release is inhibited. Conversely, if the pH rises then gastrin release is stimulated. A fall in pH is associated with the quantity of food present (the latter tends to neutralize acid) and so a feedback system, reducing further acid secretion, is appropriate and avoids ulcer formation.

The presence of food in the duodenum initiates an **enterogastric reflex**, which is mediated via both intrinsic and extrinsic nerve pathways. The stimuli from the duodenum include distension, protein breakdown products, mechanical irritation and acid.

It is also known that a **hormonal mechanism** is involved in the inhibition of gastric secretion due to the presence of material in the small intestine. Such inhibition may be initiated by a variety of stimuli including acid, fat, protein breakdown products, hypertonic or hypotonic fluids or irritation. The possible hormones involved include secretin, cholecystokinin and gastric inhibitory peptide.

Overall, once food arrives in the duodenum, it reduces both the rate of emptying of the stomach (see *Storage, mixing and emptying functions of the stomach*, below) and the rate of secretion of gastric juice. These mechanisms ensure that food does not enter the small intestine before the gastric digestive processes are complete.

Absorption in the stomach

The amount of food absorbed through the stomach mucosa is inevitably small, partly because most of it is only partially digested at this stage and partly because of the lack of special transport systems in the mucosal cells.

Substances that can be absorbed have small molecules that are lipid-soluble and therefore able to diffuse through cell membranes. One such substance is alcohol, another is **aspirin (salicylic acid)**. The latter is a potential hazard to the stomach wall, because once aspirin leaves the very acid environment in the gastric juice and enters the mucosal cells an increasing number of its molecules dissociate so that it effectively becomes a stronger acid. Since this acid is below the protective layer of mucus it can damage the mucosal cells and lead to bleeding from the lower layers of the stomach wall.

Inflammation and ulceration of the stomach wall

The nature of the stomach's contents render the stomach wall liable to attack by acid and/or proteolytic enzymes. If the balance between the protection offered by the thick mucin lining and the quantity and concentration of gastric juice should alter then the mucosa may be adversely affected, becoming inflamed or ulcerated.

GASTRITIS

Gastritis, or inflammation of the stomach mucosa, may be superficial or severe. Although the cause of gastritis is often not known, both alcohol and aspirin break down the protective barrier of mucus and tight junctions between the mucous cells.

Gastritis may progress to a point where atrophy of the gastric mucosa is complete. In such cases, hydrochloric acid cannot be secreted (**achlorhydria**) and neither can intrinsic factor. A consequence of the lack of hydrochloric acid is that iron is not converted into the ferrous form in which it can be absorbed in the intestine; this leads to the development of **iron-deficiency anaemia**. Lack of intrinsic factor, on the other hand, results in a lack of absorption of vitamin B_{12}, failure of the bone marrow to make sufficient red blood cells and **pernicious anaemia**. This sequence of events also tends to accompany gastrectomy, when part or all of the stomach is surgically removed. Gastritis may, or may not, precede the development of a peptic ulcer.

PEPTIC ULCERS

A peptic ulcer is an area of mucosal breakdown caused by the digestive action of gastric juice. It occurs in the stomach itself (**gastric ulcer**) – in the cardiac region, or in the lesser curvature – or more commonly at the beginning of the duodenum (**duodenal ulcer**). Ulcers occur when there is excessive secretion of gastric juice and/or a reduction in the effectiveness of the mucosal barrier. Smoking, alcohol, coffee, aspirin and stress are all predisposing factors in ulcer formation. A genetic predisposition is also evident. Recent evidence has shown that a cause of ulceration may be the bacterium *Helicobacter pylori*. This organism can not only survive in the very acid conditions found in the stomach but also stimulates a six-fold increase in acid secretion.

Peptic ulcers are characterized by the presence of gnawing pain and in more severe cases, nausea, vomiting and bleeding.

Traditional treatment regimens for ulcers have attempted to both reduce discomfort and effect repair to the damaged area. Antacids reduce the acidity of the stomach, give immediate relief from symptoms, and provide a suitable environment in which it can repair itself. Drugs such as bismuth form a protective coating over the ulcer; the stomach wall is then able to repair itself while being insulated from further damage by acid. The action of bismuth as an antibacterial agent has only recently been appreciated, with the discovery of *Helicobacter*. Antihistamine drugs, such as cimetidine and ranitidine, block H_2 receptors and thereby reduce acid secretion.

The discovery of the link between *Helicobacter* and ulcers has, more recently, led to treatment with antibiotics in combination with bismuth.

Surgical procedures include removal of the damaged part of the stomach and vagotomy. Since vagal stimulation increases gastric secretion, cutting one or both vagus nerves leads to a great reduction in secretion rates and rapid healing of ulcers. Unfortunately, after some months, gastric secretion recommences in the absence of vagal stimulation and another ulcer may develop. A further complication is a loss of gastric motility, which greatly reduces gastric emptying and may lead to varying degrees of pyloric obstruction. Such procedures are becoming less common with the development of more effective drugs.

Storage, mixing and emptying functions of the stomach

The volume of the empty stomach is of the order of 50 mL. As food is swallowed, it passes into the stomach and is laid down in concentric circles in the fundus and body. Filling continues to a maximum volume of about 1 litre and is accompanied by relaxation and stretching of the wall. This ensures that the intragastric pressure does not rise, since this would initiate contractions in the stomach wall that would bring about premature expulsion of the stomach contents into the duodenum.

A patch of longitudinal muscle along the greater curvature, midway between the fundus and the pylorus, generates the basic electrical rhythm, which has a steady frequency of around three bursts per minute. Depolarizations may not reach threshold in an empty stomach, although if they do, feeble contractions in the form of a concentric (peristaltic) wave travelling down in the circular muscle layer towards the pyloric region are initiated every 20 s or so. In hunger, the contractions become more vigorous, since there is a greater number of impulses in each burst of electrical activity and therefore more muscle fibres contract.

When the muscle is stretched by swallowed food, peristaltic contractions are stimulated via both intrinsic and extrinsic pathways to parasympathetic fibres supplying the muscularis externa. About three of these contractions arise every minute at the level of the cardia and travel down towards the pyloric antrum, increasing in force as they go.

The pyloric sphincter is relatively weak and is normally partly open. The peristaltic wave pushes some of the gastric contents through the orifice and into the duodenum. As the wave reaches the orifice it closes and the remainder of the food is forced back into the body of the stomach. By this means the swallowed food is moved around inside the stomach, which breaks it up into smaller pieces and mixes it with gastric juice. As a consequence of these activities, the food develops a pasty consistency and becomes known as **chyme**.

The rate of emptying of the stomach depends on the fluidity of the chyme, the degree of opening of the pyloric orifice, the force of the peristaltic contractions in the wall and inhibitory influences initiated by the arrival of food in the duodenum. All these factors ensure that the stomach empties at a rate that is optimal for the digestion of its contents, both in the stomach and subsequently in the duodenum.

The degree of contraction of the pyloric sphincter is reduced by both parasympathetic activity and gastrin, which increase the aperture of the orifice and allow more chyme to pass through. The force of peristaltic contractions is increased by distension of the stomach wall as well as by gastrin, which can also increase the BER.

A variety of stimuli are initiated by food entering the duodenum and result in reduced peristaltic activity and therefore a reduced rate of gastric emptying. These stimuli include distension of the duodenal wall, acid, digestion products, especially protein breakdown products, and hypo- and hypertonic fluids. Both neural and hormonal components are involved. The neural component is known as the **enterogastric reflex** and involves both intrinsic and extrinsic sympathetic and parasympathetic pathways. The hormone has, in the past, been called enterogastrone, but it is now known that it is actually a group of several duodenal hormones including secretin, cholecystokinin and gastric inhibitory peptide.

Vomiting

The act of vomiting is the forceful expulsion of the contents of the stomach and upper intestine through the mouth. A wide variety of stimuli initiate vomiting, including mechanical irritation of the pharynx, distension of the stomach or duodenum (e.g. by GI tract obstruction) chemical irritation of the GI tract (e.g. due to infection or poisons), morphine, unpleasant sights or odours and motion. Vomiting may also be caused by strong sympathetic stimulation.

The process is regulated by a vomiting centre in the medulla.

Vomiting is usually preceded by symptoms of stress such as an increased heart rate, increased salivation and sweating. Vomiting begins with a sharp intake of breath. This is followed by the opening of the upper oesophageal sphincter, closure of the glottis and the raising of the soft palate. A strong contraction of the diaphragm is accompanied by contraction of the abdominal wall. These contractions squeeze the stomach, thereby raising intragastric pressure. The cardiac sphincter then relaxes and the contents of the stomach are expelled through the mouth.

Strong duodenal contraction can force its contents into the stomach, with the result that bile appears in the vomit.

Prolonged vomiting can result in large losses of water and Na$^+$ and lead to **dehydration**.

Vomiting from the stomach alone will lead to acid depletion and result in **metabolic alkalosis**. On the other hand, vomiting from the intestine may lead to a net loss of alkali and so result in **metabolic acidosis**.

The cardiovascular and renal responses to dehydration are considered in **Control of blood volume** (page 420), in Ch. 12, Circulation of Blood and Lymph, and **Regulation of water balance** (page 501), in Ch. 14, Renal Control of Body Fluid Volume and Composition.

See also **Respiratory and renal regulation of pH in acidosis and alkalosis** (page 511), in Ch. 14, Renal Control of Body Fluid Volume and Composition.

The pancreas

The exocrine part of the pancreas is responsible for the production of several of the major digestive enzymes. About 1200 mL of pancreatic juice is secreted daily.

Structure of the pancreas

The pancreas lies transversely across the abdominal cavity and measures between 12 and 15 cm in length. It has a bulbous 'head' region that fits into the curve of the duodenum, and the main section or 'body' connects with the tapered 'tail', which extends out from the spleen (Figure 15.23). The bulk of the tissue in the organ is composed of pancreatic juice-secreting exocrine cells amongst which are a scattering of hormone-secreting cells, the islets of Langerhans.

> The endocrine aspects of pancreatic function are described in **The islets of Langerhans** (page 632), in Ch. 16, Endocrine Physiology.

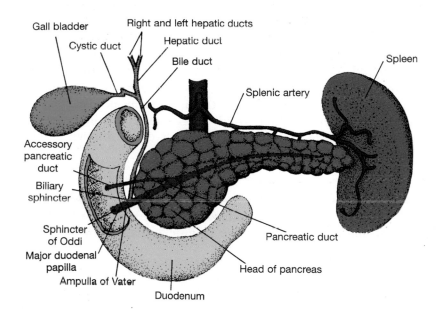

Figure 15.23 The pancreas and neighbouring structures.

The pancreas is covered by a thin connective tissue capsule from which septa arise to penetrate the tissue, dividing it into lobules. Within the lobules, the cells are arranged to form **acini** around a central **intercalated duct** (Figure 15.24). The acinar cells are pyramidal secretory cells, with well-developed endoplasmic reticulum and plentiful zymogen granules. It is these cells that produce the enzyme-rich component of pancreatic juice.

Within the acini the duct cells are cuboidal, but outside they become columnar. The intercalated ducts drain into interlobular ducts and eventually into the centrally located main pancreatic duct, which drains into the duodenum. The other component of pancreatic juice is an alkaline fluid produced by the centroacinar cells and the ductule cells lining the smaller ducts.

The **pancreatic duct** usually fuses with the bile duct just before it

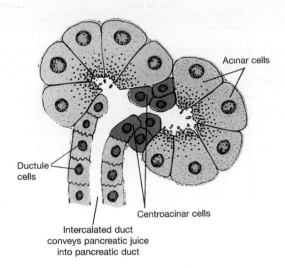

Figure 15.24 A secretory unit of the pancreas, (the lumina are enlarged for clarity). The acinar cell secretes enzymes while the duct cells secrete alkaline fluid.

enters the duodenum, to form a hepatopancreatic ampulla, the **ampulla of Vater**. This opens at the tip of the major duodenal papilla which protrudes into the duodenal lumen (Figure 15.23). The ampulla of Vater and the distal end of the pancreatic duct is surrounded by thickened circular muscle, the **sphincter of Oddi**. In many people there is an **accessory pancreatic duct**, which collects secretions from the lower part of the head of the pancreas. This duct opens through a smaller duodenal papilla.

PANCREATIC CIRCULATION

The blood supply to the pancreas derives primarily from the splenic artery and the **pancreatic-duodenal arteries**. Blood drains from the pancreas into the **hepatic portal**, **splenic** and **superior mesenteric veins**.

NERVE SUPPLY OF THE PANCREAS

The pancreas is innervated by parasympathetic fibres from the **right vagus nerve** and sympathetic fibres from the **coeliac ganglia**. Parasympathetic stimulation increases the secretion of enzyme-rich secretions from the acinar cells.

Pancreatic juice

Pancreatic juice is a watery alkaline fluid, isotonic with plasma and rich in digestive enzymes. Na^+ and K^+ are present in similar concentrations to plasma. The alkalinity of the fluid is due to the presence of a great deal of HCO_3^- which neutralizes the acid chyme passing into the duodenum from the stomach. The total volume of pancreatic juice secreted daily is 1–1.5 L.

HCO_3^- derives from plasma CO_2 which, under the influence of carbonic anhydrase, combines with OH^- from water (Figure 15.25). H^+ is actively transported out into the plasma while HCO_3^- is actively transported out into the duct lumen in exchange for Cl^-. Water passes down

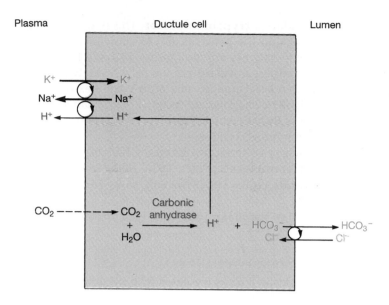

Figure 15.25 Secretion of the ionic component of pancreatic juice. CO_2 diffuses into the secretory cell from the plasma and, under the influence of carbonic anhydrase, combines with H_2O to form H^+ and HCO_3^-. H^+ is expelled from the cell into the plasma and HCO_3^- is passed into the lumen, in exchange for Cl^-. Na^+ is expelled from the cell by the Na^+–K^+ pump, which maintains suitable gradients for the uptake of Na^+ and the removal of H^+ and secretion of HCO_3^-.

an osmotic gradient into the lumen. The active transport of HCO_3^- is actually secondary to the activity of the Na^+–K^+ pump, which creates electrochemical gradients promoting the loss of H^+ and HCO_3^- from the cell.

As the secretion rate of pancreatic juice rises, its HCO_3^- concentration rises and Cl^- concentration falls.

PANCREATIC ENZYMES

The digestive enzymes present in pancreatic juice include ones that break down proteins, carbohydrates and fats.

The **proteolytic enzymes** from the pancreas are secreted in an inactive form. This prevents the enzymes from digesting the cells that produce them. The activation of each proteolytic enzyme is catalysed by a specific enzyme. Thus, trypsinogen is activated to trypsin by enterokinase, which is present on the intestinal villi; trypsin itself then activates chymotrypsinogen, proelastase and procarboxypeptidase. Trypsin can also act as an autocatalyst and bring about the activation of further trypsinogen molecules. These events are summarized in Table 15.4.

In addition to the powerful proteolytic molecules described above, the

Table 15.4 Proteolytic enzymes produced by the pancreas

Inactive form	Activating enzyme	Active form
Trypsinogen	Enterokinase Trypsin	Trypsin
Chymotrypsinogen	Trypsin	Chymotrypsin
Proelastase	Trypsin	Elastase
Procarboxypeptidase	Trypsin	Carboxypeptidase

acinar cells also produce a **trypsin inhibitor**. This is an extra precaution against activation within the pancreas and its subsequent digestion. The actions of proteolytic enzymes are summarized in Table 15.5.

There is also an **alpha-amylase** present which catalyses the hydrolysis of raw starch to release maltose, maltotriose and dextrins.

At least three lipolytic enzymes are secreted by the pancreas. The most important of these is **lipase**, which hydrolyses triglycerides, giving rise to free fatty acids and monoglycerides.

Lastly, the pancreas secretes two enzymes that break down nucleic acids: these are **ribonuclease**, which splits RNA, and **deoxyribonuclease**, which breaks down DNA. In both cases free nucleotides are released.

The actions of all of the major pancreatic enzymes are summarized in Table 15.5.

CONTROL OF SECRETION OF PANCREATIC JUICE

The release of pancreatic juice is regulated by both neural and hormonal mechanisms (Figure 15.26).

Activity in the **parasympathetic fibres** in the vagus nerve to the pancreas increases the production of the enzyme-rich components of the juice. Gastrin has a similar, but much weaker, effect. A small quantity of enzyme-rich fluid is thereby released during the cephalic and gastric phases of gastric secretion.

Once the chyme arrives in the duodenum, it stimulates the release of a much larger volume of pancreatic juice. This is brought about by two hormones, secretin and cholecystokinin.

Secretin is secreted into the blood by enteroendocrine S-cells, located within the epithelial lining of both the duodenum and jejunum, in response to acid. Once secretin reaches the pancreas it stimulates the duct cells to produce copious quantities of the alkaline component of

Table 15.5 Pancreatic enzymes and their actions

Enzyme	Substrates	Products
Trypsin	Proteins and polypeptides	Peptides and amino acids
Chymotrypsin	Proteins and polypeptides	Peptides and amino acids
Elastase	Elastin	Peptides and amino acids
Carboxypeptidase	Polypeptides	Amino acids
α-amylase	Starch	Maltose, maltotriose and dextrins
Lipase	Triglycerides	Fatty acids and monoglycerides
Ribonuclease	RNA	Nucleotides
Deoxyribonuclease	DNA	Nucleotides

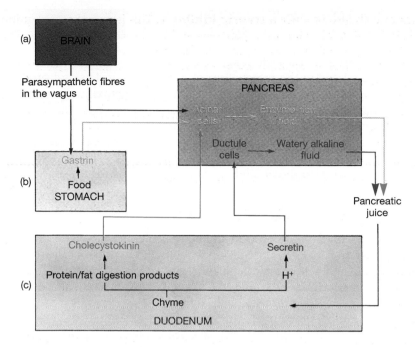

(a) BRAIN

Parasympathetic fibres in the vagus

PANCREAS

Acinar cells → Enzyme-rich fluid

Ductule cells → Watery alkaline fluid

(b) Gastrin ↑ Food STOMACH

Pancreatic juice

(c) Cholecystokinin

Protein/fat digestion products

Secretin

H⁺

Chyme

DUODENUM

Figure 15.26   Control of secretion of pancreatic juice.   **(a)** Cephalic phase.   **(b)** Gastric phase. **(c)** Intestinal phase.

pancreatic juice. This serves to neutralize the acid chyme and provides a suitable pH for the pancreatic enzymes (pH 7.6–9.2).

As soon as fat and protein digestion products appear in the small intestine, they stimulate the release of the hormone **cholecystokinin** from enteroendocrine I-cells in the epithelial lining of the ileum and jejunum. Cholecystokinin reaches the pancreas through the bloodstream and stimulates the acinar cells to release the digestive enzymes. Thus, secretin and cholecystokinin regulate the output of different components of the pancreatic juice. The process of pancreatic secretion continues until the digested chyme has left the small intestine.

Pancreatitis

Pancreatitis, inflammation of the pancreas, is usually due, particularly in its chronic form, either to excess alcohol or to blockage of the ampulla of Vater by a gallstone. In the case of a blockage the accumulation of enzymes within the pancreas becomes so great that trypsin inhibitor fails to prevent the activation of the enzyme. As a result, trypsin is formed, which begins to digest the pancreas itself. It is, therefore, a very painful condition. It is likely that alcohol exerts a toxic influence upon acinar cells, damaging them and causing tissue breakdown .

In either case the pancreas fails to secrete its enzymes into the duodenum. Since the pancreas is the major source of digestive enzymes, lack of them results in severe **nutritional deficiency**, particularly with regard to fats and fat-soluble vitamins and leads to steatorrhoea (see *The malabsorption syndrome*, below). Enzymes may escape into the bloodstream and phospholipases break down pulmonary surfactant and thus contribute to **respiratory distress syndrome**.

The islets of Langerhans may be damaged so that insulin release is reduced or absent. In this case **diabetes mellitus** will develop.

See also **Effects of insulin deficiency (diabetes mellitus)** (page 634), in Ch. 16, Endocrine Physiology.

The liver and gall bladder

The liver carries out a wide range of biochemical activities. It has many functions related to the metabolism of carbohydrates, fats and proteins. It stores iron and several vitamins. It is the site of detoxification of many drugs and poisons and the breakdown of some hormones. The secretion of bile by the liver is important, both for the digestion of fats within the small intestine and for the excretion of bilirubin, a breakdown product of haemoglobin. Bile is stored and concentrated in the gall bladder, which then releases it into the duodenum at a rate optimal for the digestion of fat.

Structure of the liver

The liver is the largest organ in the body, weighing up to 1.8 kg in the adult male and 1.4 kg in the female. It is situated in the upper part of the abdominal cavity beneath the diaphragm and is subdivided into two parts, a **large right** lobe (about five-sixths of the total) and a much smaller **left lobe** (Figure 15.27).

Like the alimentary tract, the liver is almost entirely covered by a layer of peritoneum. Beneath this is a fibrous capsule, which is continuous with areolar connective tissue situated within the substance of the liver. This areolar tissue forms a tree-like structure, which carries branches of the hepatic portal vein, the hepatic artery, bile ducts and lymphatics. These vessels enter and leave the liver through the **porta hepatis**, a short, transverse fissure on the inferior surface of the liver.

LIVER LOBULES

Liver cells are arranged in a large number of minute, polygonal hepatic lobules, approximately 1 mm in diameter. Each lobule consists of a central vein from which radiate sheets of liver cells (**hepatocytes**). At the corners of the lobules are arranged groups of three vessels: a branch of the portal vein, a branch of the hepatic artery and an interlobular bile ductule. These three vessels constitute a **portal triad** (Figure 15.28).

The connective tissue containing these vessels is called a **portal canal** and is separated from the main lobule structure by a single layer of hepatocytes, the **limiting plate**. The portal canal also encloses a variable number of lymph vessels.

Hepatocytes are polygonal cells arranged in sheets (**laminae**) one-cell thick that interconnect with each other. They are rich in glycogen, with a well-developed endoplasmic reticulum and numerous mitochondria. More than one nucleus is often present. The laminae are separated by spaces, or lacunae, which contain **sinusoids** carrying blood from vessels at the periphery of the lobule towards the **central vein**. The sinusoids are composed of fenestrated endothelial cells, which are separated from the hepatocytes by a small space, the **space of Disse** (Figure 15.29). Some of the endothelial cells have relatively large clefts between them, which make the vessel walls highly permeable. Irregular microvilli projecting from the hepatocyte surface occupy this space, and there is little collagen or other supporting material present. Some of the cells

Inferior vena cava

Left lobe

Right lobe

Gall bladder

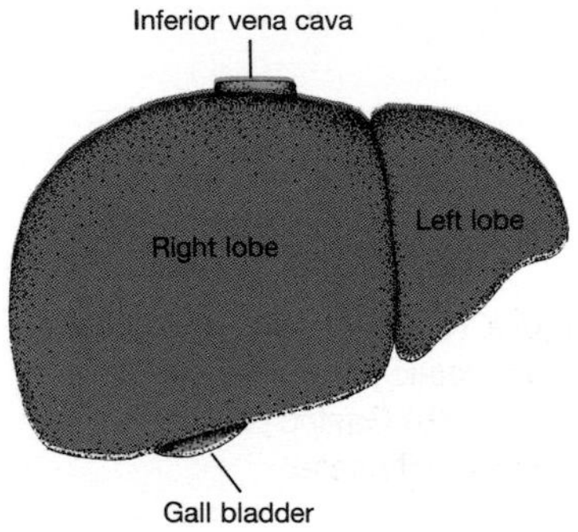

Figure 15.27 Anterior view of the liver.

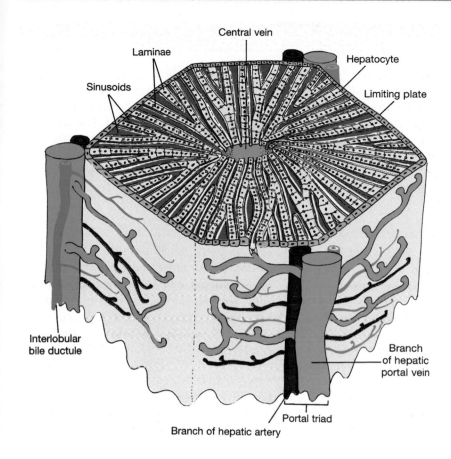

Figure 15.28 A hepatic lobule.

lining the sinusoids are phagocytic, with processes that extend into the sinusoid lumen and between adjacent endothelial cells. These **Kupffer cells** are derived from circulating monocytes and remove damaged erythrocytes and bacteria from the circulation.

Figure 15.29 Hepatocytes and their relationship to sinusoids.

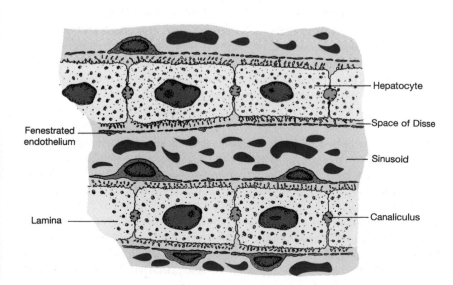

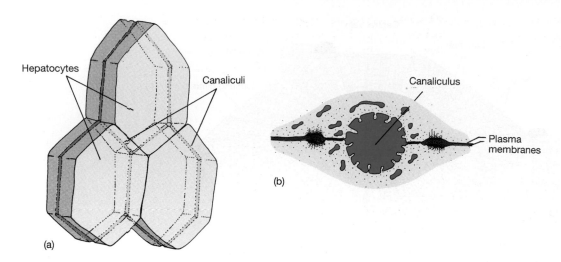

Hepatocytes

Canaliculi

Canaliculus

Plasma membranes

(a)

(b)

Figure 15.30 **(a)** Diagram to show the path of bile canaliculi around and between hepatocytes. **(b)** Ultrastructural appearance of a bile canaliculus in section.

At the abutment of two adjacent hepatocytes, there is a small space, and since spaces between cells are coincidental a system of narrow tubules is formed that is completely enclosed within the hepatocyte sheet (Figure 15.30). These tubules are known as **bile canaliculi** and they carry bile towards the portal triads.

HEPATIC CIRCULATION

About 70% of the blood entering the liver derives from the **hepatic portal vein**, which carries blood from the gut, spleen, pancreas and gall bladder. Within the liver the portal vein branches repeatedly before sending portal venules into the portal triads (Figure 15.28). These venules give rise to branches, the **distributing veins**, which run around the periphery of the lobules. Small **inlet venules** then penetrate the lobule limiting plate and carry blood to the **sinusoids**. The latter drain into the **central vein** of the lobule, which then carries blood down into a larger **sublobular vein**. The sublobular veins gradually converge and fuse to form a variable number of **hepatic veins**, which lead into the inferior vena cava.

The **hepatic artery** carries about 30% of the blood to the liver. Within the liver substance it branches repeatedly, eventually giving rise to distributing branches that carry oxygenated blood around the outside of the lobule. From here arterial blood is passed to the sinusoids, where it mixes with blood from the portal system.

NERVE SUPPLY OF THE LIVER

The liver is supplied with sympathetic and parasympathetic fibres; these also travel in the portal canals. Sympathetic stimulation promotes glycogenolysis and the subsequent release of glucose into the blood. Parasympathetic stimulation increases bile secretion by the hepatocytes.

DRAINAGE OF BILE

At the periphery of the hepatic lobules, the bile canaliculi fuse to form slender intralobular bile ductules which penetrate the limiting plates to enter the interlobular bile ductules of the portal triads (Figure 15.28).

The bile that is carried by the bile ductules leaves the liver in the right or left **hepatic duct**, which shortly fuse to form the **common hepatic duct**. The latter combines with the **cystic duct** from the gall bladder to form the **bile duct**, which drains into the ampulla of Vater and flows into the duodenum when the sphincter of Oddi relaxes (see Figure 15.23).

Secretion of bile by the liver

Bile is a watery fluid containing a variety of substances, but no enzymes. Bile is not, therefore, strictly speaking a digestive juice. It is, however, essential for fat digestion by pancreatic juice because of its ability to prevent fat from forming indigestible globules. Up to 1.5 L of bile is secreted by the liver per day and this is stored in the gall bladder prior to its release into the duodenum.

BILE SALTS

Bile salts are derived from cholesterol and the first stage of their synthesis is the production of two primary bile acids, **chenic acid** and **cholic acid** (Figure 15.31). These acids are conjugated with glycine or taurine in the liver. The four acids thus produced: **glycochenic, taurochenic, glycocholic** and **taurocholic** acids, are secreted in the bile and 75% of them are unchanged as they travel along the small intestine. Nearly all (approximately 95%) of the bile salts are actively reabsorbed in the terminal ileum, where they enter the portal circulation and return to the liver for recycling. This is called the **enterohepatic circulation of bile salts** and means that each bile salt molecule is used over and over again (about 18 times on average).

Two secondary bile acids, **lithocholic acid** and **deoxycholic acid**, are produced in the small intestine by the action of bacteria on the

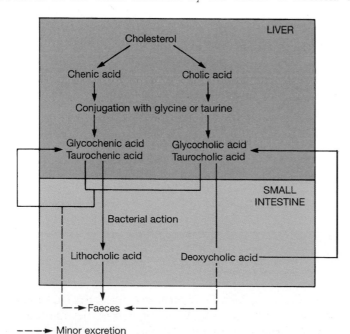

Figure 15.31 Synthesis and fate of bile salts.

conjugated primary bile acids. Deoxycholic acid is mostly absorbed and recycled in the liver, but lithocholic acid is poorly absorbed and is therefore excreted.

Bile salts are the negatively charged dissociation products of the acids. They are effectively hybrid ions with a fatty part derived from cholesterol and a polar end that is hydrophilic. As a result of this structure the ions are able to distribute themselves between fat and water. Thus, the bile salts are able to **emulsify fats**, i.e. they break down the fat droplets entering the small intestine from the stomach into smaller droplets (0.5–1.0 µm in diameter). Other substances aid the emulsification process, including cholesterol, lecithin and the fat digestion products themselves, fatty acids and monoglycerides.

Emulsification is important because it greatly increases the surface area of fat available for digestion by pancreatic lipase. The latter, which is the enzyme responsible for the breakdown of triglycerides, is a water-soluble protein and can therefore only act on the surface of fat droplets.

A second role of bile salts in digestion is that they form **micelles**, minute structures (4–5 nm in diameter) that contain fat digestion products in sufficiently small numbers to be effectively in solution. Micelles are cylindrical structures, the bile salts forming the shell, with their polar ends projecting into the water and the core containing the fat digestion products (free fatty acids and monoglycerides) together with cholesterol, lecithin and fat-soluble vitamins (Figure 15.32).

As bile salts are water-soluble derivatives of cholesterol, they serve to excrete it from the body in this form. A smaller amount of cholesterol is excreted unchanged. Another function of bile salts is that they stimulate bile secretion by the hepatocytes of the liver.

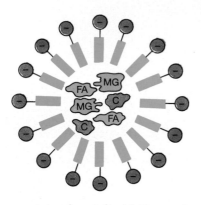

Figure 15.32 A micelle, showing fatty acids (FA), monoglycerides (MG) and cholesterol (C) within a coat of bile salts. Fat-soluble vitamins are also present.

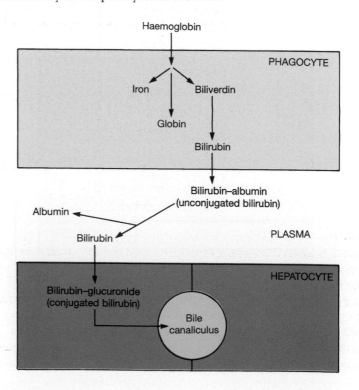

Figure 15.33 Formation of bilirubin and its excretion into bile.

BILIRUBIN

Most of the pigment bilirubin in the bile derives from haemoglobin, although up to 20% comes form other sources such as myoglobin.

Haemoglobin from worn-out red cells is broken down by phagocytic cells, mainly in the spleen. The **bilirubin** released from the phagocytes becomes attached to plasma albumin, in which form (the so-called 'free' form) it is relatively insoluble and cannot cross the glomerular membrane. Bilirubin is split from albumin at the hepatocyte surface and enters the cell (Figure 15.33). Inside the hepatocyte bilirubin is conjugated with glucuronide, which renders it soluble. Most of this **conjugated bilirubin** is actively transported into the bile canaliculi and thence to the bile; some, however, enters the blood via the lymph in the space of Disse.

In the large intestine bacterial action on conjugated bilirubin produces **urobilinogens**, which are colourless. Some of these are absorbed and either returned to the liver or excreted by the kidneys (Figure 15.34). Urobilinogen that remains in the colon becomes converted to stercobilinogen. Following elimination, exposure of urine and faeces to the air oxidizes urobilinogen to urobilin and stercobilinogen to stercobilin, respectively. The colour of stools is due to the presence of conjugated bilirubin that has not been altered by gut bacteria.

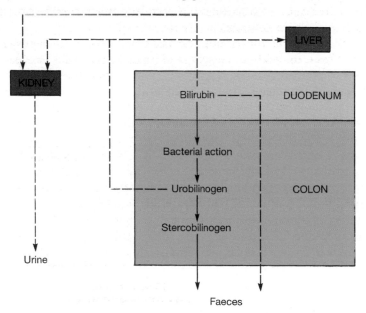

Figure 15.34 Fate of bilirubin. Solid arrows = major route; broken arrows = minor routes.

Jaundice

Jaundice is a condition characterized by a yellow colouration to the skin. It is due to the presence of excess bilirubin in the extracellular fluids, which then accumulates in the skin and deeper tissues.

Jaundice most commonly results either from increased destruction of erythrocytes (**prehepatic or haemolytic jaundice**) or blockage of the bile duct (**posthepatic** or **obstructive jaundice**) (Figure 15.35).

In the first, haemolysis takes place too rapidly for the hepatocytes to excrete all of the bilirubin into the bile. As a result bilirubin accumulates

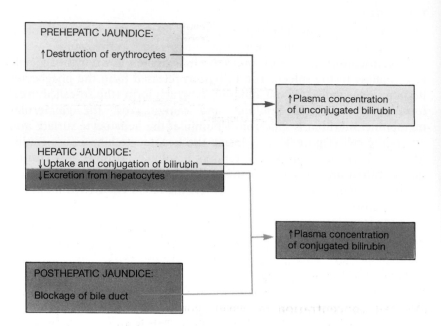

Figure 15.35 The three causes of jaundice and the effects on unconjugated and conjugated bilirubin levels in plasma.

See also **Haemolytic disease of the new-born (erythroblastosis foetalis)** (page 340), in Ch. 11, Blood, Lymphoid Tissue and Immunity.

in the blood. In the second, bilirubin production is normal but it cannot be passed into the intestine so it goes into the blood via the lymphatics.

A third type of jaundice, **hepatic jaundice**, is due to the failure of the liver cells to utilize bilirubin and may be due, for example, to hepatitis or premature birth.

Haemolytic jaundice is characterized by the presence of 'free' (unconjugated) bilirubin in the blood; urine and faeces retain their usual colour. In obstructive jaundice most of the blood's bilirubin is in the conjugated form and, while the urine is dark, the faeces are pale. In hepatic jaundice the liver is unable to take up and conjugate bilirubin so that it is still unconjugated; urine may be dark, but the faeces are pale. If the excretion of conjugated bilirubin from the hepatocytes is impaired then the concentration of conjugated bilirubin in the blood rises.

Jaundice is common in premature babies, since their livers are not yet capable of taking up and conjugating sufficient bilirubin. More serious is the jaundice in erythroblastosis fetalis caused by Rh incompatibility between mother and foetus. In this case, the baby's red cells are broken down by antibodies derived from the mother's blood.

Jaundice itself is not particularly harmful, but it may be a symptom of a more serious condition. For example, gallstones, which block the bile duct and lead to obstructive jaundice, are painful and prevent the passage of bile salts into the duodenum, which significantly reduces fat digestion and absorption.

CONTROL OF BILE SECRETION

Bile acids and other organic constituents are secreted actively by the hepatocytes into the bile canaliculi. To this primary fluid a watery solution containing Na^+ and HCO_3^- is added by the cells lining the bile ducts within the liver.

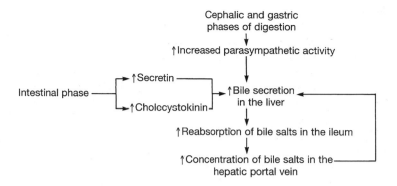

Figure 15.36 Control of bile secretion.

The secretion of bile parallels that of gastric and pancreatic juices, in that **parasympathetic stimulation** increases the bile secretion rate in the cephalic and gastric phases of digestion (Figure 15.36).

After a meal, when bile has been added to the duodenum and subsequently most of the bile salts have been reabsorbed in the ileum, the **bile salt concentration** in hepatic portal venous blood rises. This increase stimulates bile flow from the liver. This is an example of **positive feedback**, i.e. the products of a process promote the release of further product (Figure 15.36).

The **hormones** secretin and cholecystokinin stimulate bile secretion when food enters the duodenum. Secretin promotes a bicarbonate-rich secretion, as it does in the pancreas.

Structure of the gall bladder

The gall bladder is a flask-shaped sac, slate-blue in colour, that lies on the inferior surface of the right lobe of the liver. It is attached to the liver by connective tissue, and its sides are covered by a layer of peritoneum continuous with that covering the liver. The gall bladder measures 7–10 cm long, 3 cm broad and has a capacity of between 30 and 50 mL.

The wall is composed of three layers; the peritoneum, or serous layer, the fibromuscular layer and the mucous layer.

The fibromuscular layer contains fibrous tissue and smooth muscle. The mucous layer is thrown into rugae and is lined by columnar epithelium, which has microvilli. Many capillaries are present beneath this layer. Some of the epithelial cells secrete mucus into the lumen of the gall bladder.

Bile concentration and gall bladder emptying

While bile is stored in the gall bladder, selective reabsorption of some of its constituents occurs. Ions are absorbed, followed by water, but the remaining solutes are not, so that their concentration increases. Overall, the volume of bile may be reduced to as little as one-tenth of its original value. Table 15.6 shows the composition of bile released from the gall bladder into the duodenum.

Bile is delivered to the duodenum by contraction of the gall bladder, which raises the pressure of bile in the bile ducts and causes the sphincter of Oddi to open.

Table 15.6 Composition of bile (as released by the gall bladder) (from Guyton, A. C. and Hall, J. E. (1996) *Textbook of Medical Physiology* W. B. Saunders, Philadelphia)

Substance	Concentration (g/dL)
Water	92.0
Bile salts	6.0
Bilirubin	0.3
Cholesterol	0.3–0.9
Fatty acids	0.3–1.2
Lecithin	0.3
	(meq/L)
Na^+	130
K^+	12
Ca^{2+}	23
Cl^-	25
HCO_3^-	10

The principal stimulus for gall bladder contraction appears to be the hormone **cholecystokinin**. This is released from the duodenum in response to the presence of fat and protein digestion products. As well as causing gall bladder contractions, cholecystokinin causes relaxation of the sphincter of Oddi.

Vagal stimulation increases gall bladder contraction at the same time as promoting secretion of bile from the liver in the cephalic phase, but its physiological role in this connection is probably minor.

Gallstones

Raised levels of cholesterol in the gall bladder caused, for example, by excessive removal of water or bile salts from the bile may lead to the formation of gallstones. Excess cholesterol is often found associated with a diet that is high in fat; individuals with a high fat diet are therefore prone to gallstones. Bacterial infection, too, can lead to the development of gallstones, since inflammation of the gall bladder alters its absorptive characteristics.

Gallstones may exist for several years without any symptoms whatsoever; on the other hand they may enlarge to such an extent that they fill the gall bladder. Smaller stones may block the common bile duct and obstruct the transfer of bile and sometimes pancreatic juice into the duodenum. As a result, fat and possibly carbohydrate digestion are impeded. Impaired fat digestion results in steatorrhoea (see *The malabsorption syndrome*, below).

Gallstones are very painful. They may be removed surgically or destroyed by drugs, ultrasound or lasers.

Metabolic functions of the liver

The hepatic portal vein delivers blood from the gut and other viscera directly to the liver sinusoids. These are in close proximity to the hepatocytes, enabling an easy exchange of substances between the hepatocytes and the blood to occur. The phagocytic Kupffer cells remove bacteria and other debris from the blood draining the gut. The arterial blood supplying the liver mixes with the venous portal blood in the sinusoids.

The hepatocytes extract nutrients and other substances from arterial and portal bloods and carry out a large number of biochemical reactions. Some of the products are used by the hepatocytes themselves but a great number are used elsewhere in the body and are added to the hepatic venous blood draining from the organ.

CARBOHYDRATE METABOLISM

The liver plays a crucial role in maintaining blood glucose levels within narrow limits (normally 4.5–5.0 mmol/L). This is important because all tissues rely on adequate provision of glucose, principally for oxidation, which produces energy. Brain tissue is particularly sensitive to fluctuations in blood glucose level, as glucose is its preferred substrate for energy provision (rather than fat or amino acids).

After a meal, in the absorptive state, there is likely to be a considerable quantity of glucose entering the portal vein from the small intestine. The hepatocytes prevent the blood glucose level from rising too high by absorbing some glucose and converting it to glycogen (**glycogenesis**), a process catalysed by the hormone insulin. The liver also converts glucose to triglycerides (also stimulated by insulin), which can be stored in adipose tissue or oxidized by the liver itself.

In the postabsorptive state, when there is no glucose being absorbed in the gut, the blood sugar level tends to fall. The liver helps to limit this fall by releasing glucose into the blood following the breakdown of glycogen (**glycogenolysis**). This process is catalysed by the hormone adrenaline, as well as by stimulation of the hepatocytes by the sympathetic nervous system.

Glucose is synthesized from amino acids during the postabsorptive state. The production of glucose from non-carbohydrate sources is called **gluconeogenesis** and its effect is to increase the total amount of carbohydrate in the body.

The monosaccharide **galactose**, which is delivered to the liver in the portal vein, is converted into glucose in the hepatocytes. Fructose is largely converted into glucose by the intestinal cells themselves. The term **blood sugar**, therefore, normally means blood glucose, since it accounts for about 95% of all blood sugar (an exception is the hepatic portal vein, where fructose is also present).

> The regulation of blood glucose concentration in the absorptive and postabsorptive states is described in **Regulation of blood glucose concentration** (page 645), in Ch. 16, Endocrine Physiology.

LIPID METABOLISM

Just as hepatocytes take up glucose and fructose from the hepatic portal blood, so also they take up lipids, in the form of **chylomicra**. The triglycerides that are released from the latter are hydrolysed in the liver and the fatty acids produced are either oxidized or used to synthesize other lipids. An excessive amount of fatty acid oxidation in the liver results in an accumulation of breakdown products, **ketoacids** (acetoacetic and beta-hydroxybutyric acids), thereby producing the condition known as **ketoacidosis**. Several types of fat are synthesized in the liver, including cholesterol and its derivatives, phospholipids and lipoproteins. Cholesterol, phospholipids and triglycerides are transported in the blood in the form of lipoproteins (see also *Lipoproteins*, below).

Virtually all the **cholesterol** found in the circulation has been formed in the liver. It is known as endogenous cholesterol, distinguishing it from exogenous cholesterol, which is derived from the diet. A rise in exogenous cholesterol inhibits its formation by the liver, a feedback mechanism that controls plasma cholesterol levels. A diet high in saturated fats does raise plasma cholesterol levels, however, since it is deposited in the liver and stimulates cholesterol formation. Unsaturated fats in the diet reduce cholesterol formation by a mechanism that is not yet understood.

The liver cells also take up lipoprotein and a raised intracellular level of cholesterol inhibits the formation of new cholesterol.

Carbohydrates and amino acids can be converted into lipids in the liver.

PROTEIN METABOLISM

Non-essential amino acids can be synthesized from others in the liver, by the process of transamination (see *Transamination* below).

Many **plasma proteins** are synthesized in the liver, including albumin (about 3 g/d), globulins, complement and clotting factors I, II, V, VII, IX and X.

Amino acids are broken down in the liver, and the reactions include deamination; this is the removal of the amino group (NH_2), which is converted into ammonia (NH_3) and then to urea (NH_2CONH_2) (see *Deamination and Conversion of ammonia to urea*, below). Urea is relatively harmless compared with the toxic ammonia, and the latter's conversion to urea is also employed elsewhere in the body, e.g. to detoxify ammonia produced by gut bacteria in the large intestine.

INACTIVATION OF DRUGS, POISONS AND HORMONES

Hepatocytes are able to inactivate drugs and poisons by rendering them water-soluble for excretion in the bile or urine. Various hormones are inactivated in the liver including the steroids cortisol, aldosterone and the sex hormones, thyroid hormones and antidiuretic hormone.

Storage functions

The liver stores iron and the fat-soluble vitamins A, D, E and K, as well as the water-soluble vitamins B_{12} and folate. It may be noted that vitamin K is not only stored in the hepatocytes, it is also used in the synthesis of clotting factors II, VII, IX and X.

Liver failure

The functions of the blood clotting factors are described on page 328, in Ch. 11, Blood, Lymphoid Tissue and Immunity.

Liver function may be impaired as a result of a number of causes; the physiological consequences are generally predictable in terms of the liver's various functions. The large size of the organ and its large functional reserve means that liver failure only occurs when more than about 80% of its structure has been destroyed.

Acute liver failure results from widespread destruction of hepatic tissue, most often due to viral hepatitis or toxic chemicals or drugs.

A major cause of chronic liver failure is **cirrhosis**. Cirrhosis of the liver is a diffuse disease in which destruction of hepatocytes leads to the development of strands of fibrous tissue and nodules of regenerating cells, which effectively destroy the original structures. Anastomoses develop between the portal and systemic circulations so that substances that are normally metabolized by the hepatocytes enter the systemic circulation. In addition, the pressure exerted by nodules upon branches of the hepatic veins leads to increased portal venous pressure (**portal hypertension**) which is responsible for many of the major manifestations of the disease.

Jaundice accompanies liver failure. If both the uptake and excretion of bilirubin are affected then both unconjugated and conjugated bilirubin levels in the blood rise.

Reduced secretion of bile results in fat malabsorption, with consequent steatorrhoea and fat-soluble vitamin deficiencies.

Blood sugar levels may swing more than usual and diabetes is more common in people with cirrhosis.

Reduced protein synthesis by the hepatocytes leads to a reduction in plasma albumin levels which, in turn, leads to oedema and leakage of fluid into the abdominal cavity (**ascites**). The levels of several other blood proteins, including prothrombin and factors VII, IX and X are also reduced; the ability of the blood to clot is therefore impaired.

The liver is unable to inactivate adrenal oestrogens so that in males testicular atrophy and gynaecomastia (breast enlargement) occurs. Failure of aldosterone metabolism leads to sodium and water accumulation, which contributes to the oedema.

Liver failure is accompanied by a cerebral dysfunction (**hepatic encephalopathy**), which may lead to convulsions, coma and death. It is probably due to the presence in the systemic circulation of nitrogenous substances (possibly ammonia) formed by intestinal bacteria; such substances have passed directly from the portal to the systemic circulations via the anastomoses that have developed within the liver.

Portal hypertension leads to enlargement of the spleen. It may also result in **varicose** veins at other sites, which drain into the portal circulation. Such sites include the lower oesophagus and stomach and the rectum (leading to the development of haemorrhoids). Portal hypertension also contributes to the development of ascites by increasing capillary hydrostatic pressure in the vessels that drain into the hepatic portal vein.

The small intestine

After it leaves the stomach, chyme is mixed with intestinal secretions, bile and pancreatic juice. Digestion is completed and the products are absorbed through the villi of the intestinal wall. Fat is transferred mainly to the lacteals, whereas protein and carbohydrate digestion products are transferred to the blood capillaries in the villi.

The lymphatic system conveys the fat to the venous circulation via the thoracic duct, while the blood draining the small intestine flows first to the liver and then back to the heart in the inferior vena cava.

Waste materials are left in the intestinal lumen and are then passed into the large intestine.

Structure of the small intestine

The small intestine is a muscular tube which, in the living adult, is approximately 5 m long (6–7 m in its relaxed state after death). Length is correlated with height, so that it is generally somewhat longer in men than in women. The small intestine is divided into a number of anatomically recognizable areas: the short, curved **duodenum** (approximately 20 cm long); the **jejunum**, which constitutes about 40% of the total length (2 m); and the **ileum**, which represents the distal 60% (3 m).

The duodenum, which is the widest section of the small intestine, encloses the head of the pancreas and contains the common openings of the bile and pancreatic ducts.

The jejunum has a diameter of about 4 cm and is very vascular, which gives it a reddish appearance.

The ileum has a diameter of about 3.5 cm and a thinner wall than the jejunum.

The jejunum and ileum are connected to the posterior abdominal wall by the mesentery. This is a double layer of peritoneum, between which lie the branches of the blood and lymphatic vessels (lacteals) and nerves which supply the small intestine. Lymph nodes and fat are also present in the mesentery.

Layers of the small intestine wall

A few centimetres from the pylorus, as far as the midpoint of the ileum, the inner surface of the small intestine is thrown into circular folds (**plicae circulares**). These generally extend to between one-half and two-thirds of the circumference of the intestine. They increase the surface area available for absorption, as well as retarding the speed with which chyme passes through the region.

The four layers of the wall of the small intestine differ somewhat from those of the stomach (Figure 15.37).

Figure 15.37 Section through the wall of the duodenum.

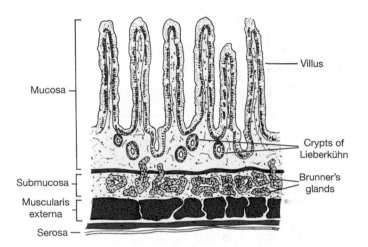

Mucosa

Villus

Crypts of Lieberkühn

Submucosa

Brunner's glands

Muscularis externa

Serosa

The **muscularis externa** contains a thick inner circular layer of smooth muscle, with a much thinner external longitudinal layer. The mucosa is much thicker in the upper than in the lower small intestine and, unlike the stomach, it is studded with minute projections, the villi. These are leaf-like in the upper intestine, becoming finger-like lower down.

VILLI

Villi are 0.5–1.5 mm long and there are between 10 and 40 per square millimetre. Scattered between the villi are small openings of simple tubular intestinal glands, the **crypts of Lieberkühn**.

Each villus consists of a single layer of columnar epithelial cells covering a strip of lamina propria (Figure 15.38). This epithelial covering is constantly renewed by cells arising by cell division in the lower parts of the crypts of Lieberkühn. The new cells migrate slowly over the surface of the villus and are shed from the apex. It has been estimated that as much as 100 g of cells are lost each day from the wall of the alimentary tract and that it takes from 2–4 days to renew the epithelial lining.

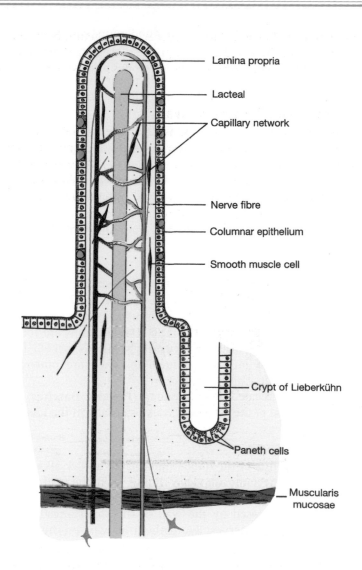

Lamina propria

Lacteal

Capillary network

Nerve fibre

Columnar epithelium

Smooth muscle cell

Crypt of Lieberkühn

Paneth cells

Muscularis mucosae

Figure 15.38 The structure of a villus.

The surface epithelial layer consists mainly of absorptive cells. They are columnar with apical surfaces covered by **microvilli**. The latter are about 1 μm long and there are approximately 600 per cell. Microvilli increase the potential absorptive surface of the small intestine; overall it has a surface area of about 250 m² (the size of a tennis court!). Scattered between the absorptive cells are goblet cells, which are particularly numerous in the epithelium of the ileum.

The lamina propria forms the core of the villus; it contains an extensive capillary network and a central lymph vessel, the **lacteal**. Smooth muscle fibres allow the villus to change its length, and also to move laterally.

BLOOD SUPPLY OF THE SMALL INTESTINE

The **superior mesenteric artery** branches off the abdominal aorta and its branches run between the layers of the mesentery to supply the whole of the small intestine except the duodenum, which receives blood from several different arteries.

The **superior mesenteric vein** drains into the splenic vein, which in turn takes blood to the hepatic portal vein to the liver (see Figure 15.4). The right and left hepatic veins drain into the inferior vena cava.

NERVE SUPPLY OF THE SMALL INTESTINE

The parasympathetic nerve supply to the small intestine is via the **vagus nerves**, whereas the sympathetic fibres travel in the **splanchnic nerves** and synapse in the **coeliac** and **superior mesenteric ganglia**. Both divisions of the ANS connect to the intramural plexus. Parasympathetic stimulation increases intestinal motility and secretion, while sympathetic stimulation brings about vasoconstriction and reduces motility.

Intestinal glands

The **crypts of Lieberkühn** comprise mainly undifferentiated cells, as well as a few Paneth cells of unknown function and enteroendocrine argentaffin cells, like those in the stomach, which secrete hormones.

In the duodenum, the openings of additional glands are found lying between the villi. These are the **Brunner's glands**, which lie in the submucosa below the muscularis mucosae. They are mucous glands which also contain some argentaffin cells.

Solitary and aggregated lymph nodes (**Peyer's patches**) are also found in the mucosa of the intestinal wall, especially in the lower ileum.

Intestinal secretions

The **Brunner's glands** of the duodenum secrete a thick alkaline mucus, which helps to protect the duodenal lining from the acid chyme that passes down from the stomach. These glands are responsive to local factors, to gastrin released by the wall of the small intestine, and are stimulated by the vagus nerves. Sympathetic activity, on the other hand, has an inhibitory effect.

Mucus is also secreted by the goblet cells that are found in large numbers in the mucosal epithelium. These cells are responsive to direct stimulation by the contents of the gut.

The crypts of Lieberkühn secrete an isotonic fluid, at a rate up to about 2 L/d. This juice is essentially extracellular fluid and does not contain enzymes. Digestive enzymes do, however, find their way into the intestinal lumen by an indirect route. The epithelial cells that line the mucosa contain a number of digestive enzymes on their plasma membranes and these cells are constantly sloughed off from the apices of the villi into the lumen of the intestine.

The release of fluid by the crypts of Lieberkühn is primarily under the control of local factors: distension, for example, results in copious secretion by the crypts. Parasympathetic stimulation also increases the rate of secretion, but only two- or three-fold, as will the presence of secretin and cholecystokinin.

The mechanisms involved in the final stages of digestion and the absorption of the products are described in *Digestion and absorption by the small intestinal epithelium*, below. Before this, however, the roles of the pancreas, liver and gall bladder are considered.

Movements of the small intestine

The wall of the small intestine is capable of several different types of movement, the two principal ones being peristalsis and segmentation. Both of these movements are rhythmic and they depend upon the basic electrical rhythm (BER) generated by cells in the longitudinal muscle layer. In the duodenum, BER is around 12 per minute and this reduces to about eight per minute in the terminal ileum.

Both peristalsis and segmentation depend upon the myenteric plexus for their function, although not completely, since pharmacological blocking does not result in total inhibition. The autonomic nervous system serves only to modify these muscular contractions.

The main propulsive movement of the gut is **peristalsis**, which is initiated by distension of the gut wall. The speed of peristalsis is quite slow (0.5–2 cm/s), so that chyme takes between 3 and 5 hours to travel through the small intestine. Intense irritation of the small intestine, for example by pathogens, can cause an unusual form of peristaltic wave (a **peristaltic rush**) which travels more rapidly than usual and for a greater distance, with the result that the contents of the small intestine are rapidly shunted into the colon.

Mixing of the intestinal contents is brought about by **segmentation**. This consists of contractions of short lengths of the circular muscle, about 13 cm long, regularly spaced over a short section of gut, which cause the chyme to be broken up into segments. After a few seconds, the muscle fibres relax and further contraction occurs at points intermediate between the previous ones (Figure 15.39).

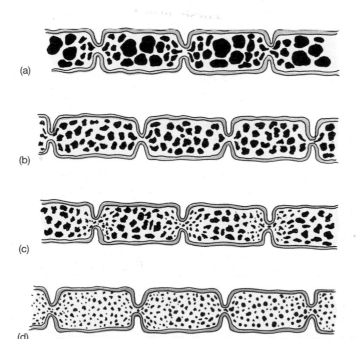

(a)

(b)

(c)

(d)

Figure 15.39 Segmentation contractions in the intestine. **(a)** The intestine is divided into segments by rings of contracting circular muscle. **(b)** The original rings relax and others contract to form new segments. The chyme is mixed with secretions and broken down. **(c)** New contractions at the original points. **(d)** New contractions at the intermediate points.

Thus the segments are alternately split and recombined, which serves to mix the chyme progressively with the various secretions of the small intestine. These contractions travel towards the anus for a short distance and further assist the propulsion of food.

The longitudinal muscle fibres contract over relatively long segments of the gut, causing a reduction in its overall length; 'living' and 'dead' gut lengths are thus very different. Each such contraction, though, is of short duration.

Intestinal motility may be increased by stimulation of the extrinsic parasympathetic fibres, although intrinsic nerve reflexes are generally responsible for most contractile activity. In the **gastroenteric reflex**, for example, distension of the stomach results in increased peristalsis in the small intestine. This is probably mediated by the myenteric plexus, although gastrin may also be involved.

Stimulation of the sympathetic nerve supply inhibits gut motility both directly, by the effect of noradrenaline on the muscle cells, and indirectly, by inhibiting the neurones in the myenteric plexus. The vasoconstriction caused by sympathetic stimulation also tends to reduce activity. Sympathetic fibres are also involved in the **intestino-intestinal reflex**, in which distension of one part of the small intestine results in relaxation of the rest.

The lining of the gut also shows localized activity. The mucosa is thrown into folds by contractions of the muscularis mucosae. These folds serve to increase the surface area of the intestinal lining for the absorption of digested material.

Since the intestinal villi contain smooth muscle fibres they are able to change length and move laterally. These movements are brought about by local reflexes initiated by the presence of chyme. Movements of the villi help to bring fresh material to the mucosal surface and also to promote movements of the lymph within the lacteals and blood within the capillaries.

Gastrointestinal obstruction

Any part of the gut may become obstructed by, for example, a growth, muscular spasm, paralysis, or a variety of other causes. Accumulation of material above the point of obstruction leads to **distension** and subsequent excessive secretion of gastrointestinal fluids. Protein may also be secreted into the gut, leading to a lowering of plasma levels with consequent oedema. Distension results in reflex contraction of the gut wall and may lead to **vomiting**, the precise nature of the vomit being dependent upon the level of the obstruction. This may result in dehydration and electrolyte loss. Accumulation of large amounts of material, particularly in the large intestine, may lead to rupture of the gut wall, with lethal consequences.

Digestion and absorption by the small intestine epithelium

CARBOHYDRATES

The digestion of **starch** begins in the mouth, brought about by the action of **salivary alpha-amylase**, to produce maltose, maltotriose and dextrins. This process continues in the stomach until the salivary amylase is inactivated. It is subsequently continued in the small intestine by the action of pancreatic amylase (Figure 15.40).

Disaccharides in the diet (sucrose, lactose and maltose) are undigested at this stage. These, together with the digestion products of the two alpha-amylases, are finally hydrolysed to monosaccharides by enzymes present on the external surface of the intestinal cell membranes (on the microvilli). Table 15.7 lists these enzymes and their functions.

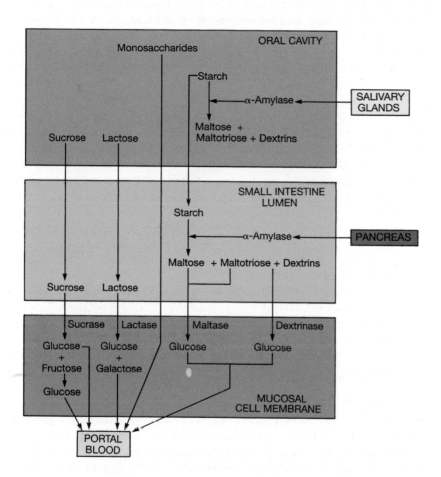

Figure 15.40 Summary of carbohydrate digestion.

Table 15.7 Intestinal epithelial enzymes

Enzyme	Substrate	Product
α-Dextrinase	Dextrins	Glucose
Lactase	Lactose	Glucose and galactose
Maltase	Maltose	Glucose
Sucrase	Sucrose	Glucose and fructose
Peptidases	Polypeptides	Tripeptides and/or dipeptides and/or amino acids

The structures of mono– and disaccharides are described in **Carbohydrates** (page 17), in Ch. 1, Molecules, Ions and Units.

The mechanisms by which substances move across cell membranes is considered in **Movement of substances across the cell membrane** (page 48), in Ch. 2, Cells and the Internal Environment.

Figure 15.41   Absorption of glucose by a surface epithelial cell in the small intestine by secondary active transport. Na^+ is actively extruded from the base and sides of the cell thereby lowering its concentration within the cell. Na^+ diffuses into the cell down its electrochemical gradient, a process facilitated by a carrier protein in the luminal membrane. The carrier also binds glucose and transports it into the cell. Glucose leaves the cell by facilitated diffusion. Fructose is absorbed by facilitated diffusion. Once inside the cell it is converted into glucose.

There are two mechanisms by which **monosaccharides** are absorbed through the wall of the intestine, facilitated diffusion and active transport. Fructose is transported into the intestinal epithelial cells by **facilitated diffusion:** fructose molecules attach to carriers that transport them down a concentration gradient into the cell. Once inside the cell most of the fructose is converted into glucose, and in this form enters the portal blood.

A different carrier from that which carries fructose is used to transport glucose and galactose; it also binds Na^+ (Figure 15.41).

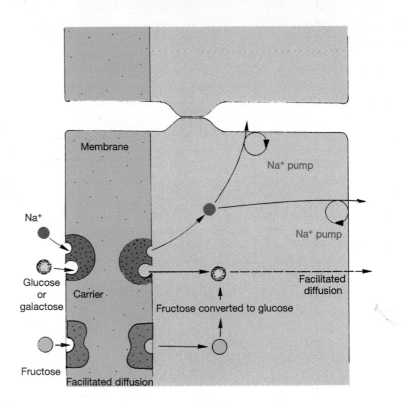

Once they have reached the inner surface of the cell membrane, glucose (or galactose) and Na^+ split off from the carrier. Na^+ is expelled from the cell's lateral surfaces by active transport while glucose (or galactose) passes out by facilitated diffusion. Since the uptake of the sugars is dependent upon the active transport of Na^+, their absorption is said to be by **secondary active transport** and is comparable to the mechanism operating in the proximal convoluted tubule of the kidney.

LIPIDS

Lipid digestion does not begin until the lipid molecules reach the duodenum. Agitation of the lipid in the small intestine, together with the presence of bile salts, serves to bring about the formation of a stable emulsion. The tiny droplets are then digested by **pancreatic lipase** which breaks down triglycerides principally into monoglycerides and free fatty acids (Figure 15.42). Bile salts then contribute to the formation of micelles (see *Bile salts*, below), which contain the digestion products as well as cholesterol, lecithin and fat-soluble vitamins.

The fat digestion products are conveyed to the surface of the intestinal cells as micelles and there the various constituents split up. The monoglycerides and free fatty acids, being highly lipid-soluble, diffuse into the cell, leaving the highly charged bile salts behind. The bile salts are used many times, providing a 'shuttle service' to the absorptive cells before finally being absorbed in the terminal ileum.

Free fatty acids and **monoglycerides** are absorbed mainly in the duodenum and proximal jejunum by **simple diffusion**. Once inside the cells, long-chain fatty acids (more than 10–12 carbon atoms) are reassembled back into triglyceride molecules on the endoplasmic reticulum. They are then packaged by the Golgi apparatus into spherical structures called **chylomicra**, which consist of triglycerides surrounded by a coat of protein, phospholipid, cholesterol and fat-soluble vitamins. These may be as large as 100 nm in diameter. They are released from the

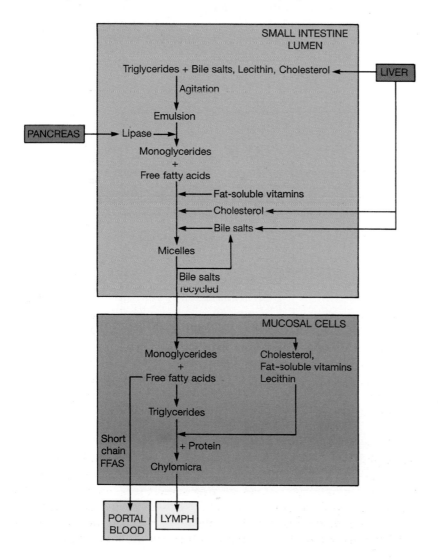

Figure 15.42 Summary of lipid digestion.

base or sides of the intestinal cells by exocytosis and from there they are able to enter the lacteals, rather than the blood capillaries.

Short-chain free fatty acids pass into the portal blood and are not assembled into triglycerides.

PROTEINS

Protein digestion begins in the stomach when **pepsins** in gastric juice catalyse the hydrolysis of protein, liberating polypeptides and a few free amino acids (Figure 15.43). Several **proteolytic enzymes** in pancreatic juice continue this process, leaving a mixture of small peptides and small quantities of free amino acids.

Peptidases are found both on the intestinal cell membranes and within the intestinal cells. Some dipeptides and tripeptides are broken down on the cell surface but most are absorbed intact and broken down within the cell. Virtually all proteins are transported into the blood in the form of amino acids.

Most **peptides** and **amino acids** are absorbed from the intestinal lumen in a manner similar to glucose, i.e. by **secondary active transport**. At least four different carriers are involved. A few molecules are, however, absorbed by facilitated diffusion.

Figure 15.43 Summary of protein digestion.

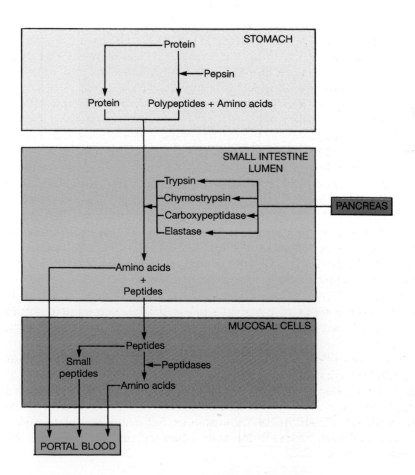

NUCLEIC ACIDS

Nucleic acids are digested in the duodenum by **ribonuclease** and **deoxyribonuclease** in the pancreatic juice. The resulting nucleotides are split at the mucosal surface into phosphoric acid and nucleosides, which are then themselves further split into nitrogenous bases and sugars. The **purines** and **pyrimidines** released at this final stage of digestion are then absorbed by **active transport**.

ABSORPTION OF IONS, WATER AND VITAMINS

Calcium

Ca^{2+} is absorbed by active transport in all parts of the small intestine, especially in the duodenum and jejunum. The process is dependent upon the presence of a Ca^{2+}-binding protein associated with the microvilli, which assists its uptake into the cell, and another to which it binds to traverse the cytoplasm. A Ca^{2+}–ATPase pumps ions out through the basal surface of the cell. The synthesis of the various binding proteins is induced by active vitamin D (1,25-dihydroxycholecalciferol), which in turn requires parathyroid hormone for its activation in the kidney.

Ca^{2+} absorption is aided by the presence of bile acids in the intestinal lumen, but inhibited by fatty acids with which Ca^{2+} forms insoluble soaps.

> See also **Calcium and phosphate absorption by the small intestine** (page 631), in Ch. 16, Endocrine Physiology.

Iron

Most dietary iron is present as ferric ion (Fe^{3+}), in which form it tends to form insoluble complexes with some substances present in the diet, such as tannin and grain fibre, and insoluble salts with anions present in the gut lumen. In the stomach Fe^{3+} is reduced to Fe^{2+} (ferrous iron) in the presence of hydrochloric acid and it is in this form that most of it is absorbed.

Having passed through the stomach, most of the Fe^{2+} is absorbed in the upper part of the small intestine. The mucosal cells of the duodenum and jejunum release a protein, **transferrin**, into the lumen. Two Fe^{2+} ions bind to each transferrin molecule, which then itself binds to a receptor protein on the mucosal cell surface. This complex is then taken up by endocytosis. Once inside the cell, the receptor protein splits off and may be reused, while the Fe^{2+}–transferrin complex travels through the cytoplasm. The Fe^{2+} splits from the transferrin and the latter is secreted back into the gut lumen; Fe^{2+} passes into the blood and binds to plasma transferrin (Figure 15.44).

If excess Fe^{2+} is absorbed it is not passed into the blood in this way, but is instead bound to the protein **apoferritin**, forming **ferritin** within the mucosal cells. Iron stored in this way is lost when the mucosal cells are shed.

Iron passes into the blood stream when plasma levels are low; thus the cellular ferritin is in equilibrium with plasma Fe^{2+}, which is bound to the protein transferrin. The mucosal cells regulate the level of plasma Fe^{2+}, in that when the blood is saturated with Fe^{2+} there is no movement out of the cells. Under these circumstances, Fe^{2+} will accumulate within the cells and then be lost to the body when the cells are shed into the intestinal lumen.

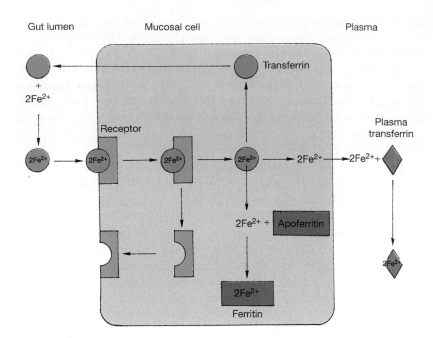

Figure 15.44 The uptake of Fe^{2+} by intestinal mucosal cells. Pairs of Fe^{2+} ions are bound to transferrin in the lumen of the gut. The complex attaches to receptor molecules on the luminal surface of the cell and are taken into the cytoplasm. The transferrin–Fe^{2+} complex then dissociates and the receptor returns to the surface and is reused. Transferrin gives up its Fe^{2+}, which then either passes into the plasma or, if in excess, is stored within the cell as ferritin.

Potassium

K^+ diffuses down an electrochemical gradient out of the intestine and into the blood. The size of this gradient and therefore the rate of K^+ absorption is dependent upon the absorption of water, since the removal of water from the gut increases the K^+ concentration within the gut lumen.

Sodium and chloride

Na^+ is actively transported out of the lumen of the small intestine in association with glucose and amino acids (see above). The quantities involved are very large, some 25–35 g/d, most of which derives from secretions that are added to the alimentary tract. Cl^- diffuses passively along the electrochemical gradient created by Na^+ absorption throughout most of the small intestine, but in the lower ileum and the colon Cl^- is actively absorbed in exchange for HCO_3^-.

Water

Water can diffuse across the wall of the intestine in both directions. It diffuses both into the cells and between them through the tight junctions. The amount of water absorbed depends upon the relative osmolarities of the luminal contents and the blood plasma. Normally, nearly all of the water added to the alimentary tract in secretions (about 7 L) and in the diet (about 2 L) is absorbed.

Vitamins

Most vitamins are absorbed in the upper part of the small intestine; exceptions include vitamins B_{12} and C, both of which are absorbed in the ileum. Many **water-soluble vitamins** are thought to be absorbed in the same way as glucose and most amino acids and small peptides, that is by an active, sodium-linked transport system. Vitamin B_2 appears to be absorbed by facilitated diffusion while B_6 is absorbed by simple diffusion.

Vitamin B_{12} absorption depends upon the presence of intrinsic factor, secreted by the gastric mucosa. Dietary vitamin B_{12} molecules are generally attached to proteins, from which they are split in the stomach. However, they immediately become bound to B_{12}-binding glycoproteins, or **R-proteins**, for which they have a particularly strong affinity. In the duodenum pancreatic proteases cause these complexes to break down and reduces the affinity of the R-proteins for the vitamin so that it is less than that of intrinsic factor. As a result vitamin B_{12} becomes bound to intrinsic factor and it is this form that it is absorbed across the intestinal mucosa. In the absence of intrinsic factor less than 2% of ingested vitamin B_{12} is absorbed.

The absorption of **fat-soluble vitamins** (A, D, E and K) is by simple diffusion.

THE MALABSORPTION SYNDROME

The malabsorption syndrome is caused by a range of conditions that result in the reduced absorption by the intestine of one or more nutrients and therefore lead to symptoms characteristic of deficiency of those nutrients. A major characteristic of malabsorption is **steatorrhoea**, the presence of excess fat in the faeces, which are grey and foul-smelling, and float. The reduced absorption of fat also reduces the absorption of fat-soluble vitamins and so symptoms of their deficiency may occur.

Malabsorption is caused principally by reduced activity of either digestive enzymes, bile salts or intestinal mucosal cells, or lymphatic obstruction.

Reduced activity of digestive enzymes

In pancreatic insufficiency, the enzymes that bring about the hydrolysis of carbohydrates, fats and proteins are reduced so that absorption of all of the major food groups is impaired. However, since salivary amylase and gastric peptidases are still available, between one-half and two-thirds of the products of carbohydrate and protein digestion are still absorbed. Since pancreatic lipase is the sole enzyme able to hydrolyse triglycerides, virtually no fat absorption takes place at all, resulting in steatorrhoea.

Any condition in which the pancreatic ducts are blocked, or pancreatic tissue is destroyed will obviously result in a reduction in the quantity of pancreatic enzymes entering the duodenum. Such conditions include **cystic fibrosis**, in which the ducts are blocked by viscous mucus, and **chronic pancreatitis**, in which pancreatic acini may become atrophied or fibrosed.

Following **gastric resection**, lack of acid and peptidases reduce the efficiency of protein digestion, and the absorption of iron and vitamin B_{12}, leading to anaemia.

Reduced activity of bile salts

Any condition which results in the reduction of bile salts in the small intestine leads to a reduction in fat digestion and absorption by reduced emulsification and micelle formation. **Liver disease** and **biliary tract disease** both reduce micellar solubilization.

Reduced activity of intestinal mucosal cells

Impairment of the intestinal mucosa leads to a reduction in the absorption of foodstuffs. There may be actual destruction of the mucosa as, for example, in **coeliac disease**, when dietary gluten (a protein derived from wheat, oats, barley and rye) causes a severe allergic reaction in the intestinal mucosa of some individuals. There may be loss of the intestinal villi, so that absorption of the breakdown products of digestion is severely restricted, resulting in diarrhoea and malnutrition. Removal of gluten from the diet elicits a rapid recovery in such cases. **Crohn's disease**, which is characterized by inflammation and thickening of segments of the small intestine wall, may also cause mucosal destruction, in addition to intestinal blockage. Temporary impairment of the intestinal mucosa occurs in both **gastrointestinal infections** and **food poisoning**.

Lymphatic obstruction

Blockage of the lymph flow from the gut results in a reduction in the absorption of the products of fat digestion. Lymphatic obstruction can arise within the lymphatic vessels themselves, or by pressure exerted externally by surrounding tissues, e.g. by a tumour.

The large intestine

The large intestine transforms chyme into semi-solid faeces by the absorption of ions and water, and stores them until they are removed by defaecation. It is also able to secrete large quantities of water and electrolytes in response to irritation, e.g. bacterial infection. The colon harbours an extensive population of microorganisms (mainly bacteria) whose presence is necessary for the normal development of lymphoid tissue in the large intestine and thus for resistance to infection. The bacteria synthesize vitamin K, which is necessary for the synthesis of several clotting factors by the liver.

Structure of the large intestine

The large intestine is about 1.5 m long on average (slightly shorter in women than in men) and extends from the end of the ileum to the anus. It may be divided into a number of regions, which are distinguished by both their anatomical structures and positions within the abdominal cavity (Figure 15.45).

The first section is the **caecum**, a blind-ended bulbous sac, approximately 6 cm long and 7.5 cm in diameter, which leads into the ascending colon. The ileum opens into the caecum at right angles, the entrance being guarded by the **ileocaecal valve**, which regulates the passage of digested food material from the small to the large intestine. A short, blind-ended tube, the **vermiform appendix**, protrudes about 9 cm

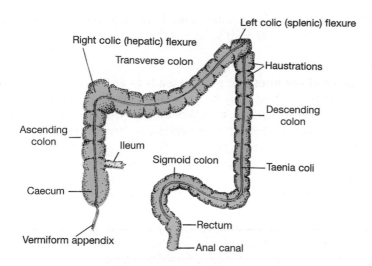

Figure 15.45 The large intestine viewed from the front.

from the outer wall of the caecum; in some herbivores it is considerably larger and is concerned with cellulose digestion, but in humans it is merely vestigial.

The caecum leads directly into the **ascending colon**, which is about 15 cm long and passes up the right side of the abdominal cavity to the lower surface of the liver. Here it bends, at the **right colic (hepatic) flexure**, before passing to the left and forwards for about 50 cm as the **transverse colon**. The latter terminates on the left-hand side of the abdominal cavity, in the vicinity of the spleen, at the **left colic (splenic) flexure**. The **descending colon** passes down for about 25 cm, curving medially and leading into the **sigmoid colon**. This, the last part of the colon, is extremely variable in both length and distribution. The sigmoid colon leads into the **rectum**, which commences near the bottom of the abdominal cavity at the level of the third sacral vertebra. The rectum is about 12 cm long, with a smooth outer wall and an extensively folded mucous membrane (when the cavity is empty). The rectum leads into the narrower **anal canal**, which is usually less than 4 cm long and is characterized by the presence of a mass of muscular sphincters. The **internal anal sphincter** is the thickened upper two-thirds of the circular muscle layer of the anal canal. The **external anal sphincter** is composed of striated muscle and surrounds the whole length of the anal canal. The sphincters seal off the end of the alimentary tract and are therefore normally constricted. Their activity is inhibited during defaecation.

WALL OF THE LARGE INTESTINE

The wall of the large intestine has the same basic structure as that of the small intestine, but there are considerable differences of detail (Figure 15.46).

The outermost layer, the **serosa**, is not present in all parts. Both **muscle layers** are always present, however, and are represented by a thin continuous layer of circular muscle with a longitudinal layer with uneven distribution. In the walls of the caecum and colon, the longitu-

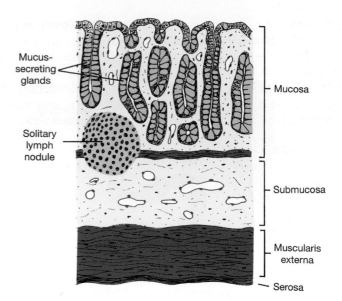

Figure 15.46 Section through the wall of the large intestine.

dinal muscle layer is thickened into three bands (6–12 mm wide), the **taeniae coli**; between these bands the longitudinal layer is much thinner. Towards the lower end of the sigmoid colon the muscle bands coalesce to form a continuous layer, which then extends into the rectum.

The taeniae coli appear to have a shorter length than the rest of the large intestine, so that the wall appears to be puckered, forming a series of pouches or **haustrations**. The circular muscle layer is slightly thickened in the intervals between haustrations.

The submucosa is structurally similar to that of the small intestine, but the mucosa is somewhat different: although it is folded, there are no villi present. The epithelium consists primarily of columnar absorptive cells with scattered goblet cells. There are numerous simple tubular glands that secrete mucus. Solitary lymph nodules are scattered throughout, but are especially numerous in the caecum and vermiform appendix.

BLOOD SUPPLY OF THE LARGE INTESTINE

The blood supply for the bulk of the large intestine is derived from the colic branches of the **superior mesenteric artery**. The left-hand (distal) end of the transverse colon, the descending and sigmoid colons and the rectal area all receive blood from the **inferior mesenteric artery** and the **middle rectal artery**. Blood drains away from the two areas into the corresponding veins, i.e. the **superior** and **inferior mesenteric veins**.

NERVE SUPPLY OF THE LARGE INTESTINE

The large intestine receives its nerve supply from both the sympathetic and parasympathetic systems. The caecum, ascending colon and most of the transverse colon are innervated by sympathetic fibres from the **coeliac** and **superior mesenteric ganglia**, while the parasympathetic supply derives from the vagus nerves.

The left-hand end of the transverse colon and distal parts, as far as the upper half of the anal canal, derive their sympathetic supply from the lumbar region of the spinal cord and from the superior hypogastric plexus. The parasympathetic supply of this part of the gut is derived from the **pelvic splanchnic nerves** (nervi erigentes). Stimulation of these causes peristalsis and defaecation. There are sensory neurones in the nervi erigentes which are stimulated by distension as faeces accumulate.

Secretion in the large intestine

The glands of the large intestine secrete mucus, which protects the intestinal wall and acts as a binding agent for the faeces. Large quantities of water and ions may be produced in response to infection, serving to dilute and flush out the irritants and causing **diarrhoea**.

Mucus secretion is brought about primarily in response to direct tactile stimulation by the intestinal contents, although local reflexes and extrinsic parasympathetic stimulation can also increase mucus production. The latter route is used in **psychogenic diarrhoea**, which may accompany stressful activities.

Absorption in the large intestine

The proximal colon is the main site for the absorption of substances from the chyme, while the distal colon has a storage function.

Na^+ is actively absorbed in the large intestine, a process stimulated by the hormone aldosterone. Na^+ transport in association with glucose or amino acids, as in the small intestine, does not occur.

Cl^- is transported by two methods: one is passive, following Na^+, and the other is active, when Cl^- is exchanged for HCO_3^-.

K^+ absorption may be by active transport. Ca^{2+} ions are absorbed in a similar fashion as in the small intestine, by a vitamin-D-dependent mechanism; Mg^{2+} may be absorbed by the same mechanism.

Water is absorbed up the osmotic gradient created by the absorption of ions and may amount to 500–1000 mL/d.

Urea is metabolized in the colon wall to ammonia, which is subsequently absorbed and then metabolized in the liver. Some of it may be used to synthesize amino acids.

Although the majority of **bile salts** are absorbed in the small intestine, bacteria in the colon deconjugate them, making them more lipid-soluble so that they may be absorbed from this site as well.

Bacterial flora

Although the lumen of the large intestine is sterile at birth, it is quickly invaded by a number of different bacteria; major ones include *Escherichia coli*, *Enterobacter aerogenes* and *Bacteroides fragilis*.

It has been shown that the intestinal lymphoid tissue proliferates as a result of the presence of bacteria in the gut. Immunoglobulins (IgA) are present on the mucosa and help to prevent the passage of harmful organisms into the blood.

The bacteria produce several vitamins, including vitamin K, vitamin B_{12}, thiamine and riboflavin, although only vitamin K is absorbed in sufficient quantities to be physiologically significant.

The bacteria are able to metabolize some cellulose, digestive enzymes and other cellular debris and produce various gases.

Flatus

The main gases of flatus result from bacterial action in the colon. Several of these gases, including carbon dioxide, methane and hydrogen, are odourless. Nitrogen and oxygen, both of which are derived from swallowed air, are also usually present. In addition, small amounts of odoriferous substances are found that impart the characteristic odour; they include ammonia, hydrogen sulphide, indole, skatole and volatile amines.

Some foods form particularly suitable substrates for bacterial action and their presence in the diet therefore results in increased volumes of gas. They include beans, cabbage, cauliflower and onions. Up to 10 L of gas may be present in the large intestine in a day, but only about 600 mL is expelled as flatus, the rest being absorbed by the intestinal wall.

Movements of the large intestine

Chyme enters the caecum through the ileocaecal valve. This valve is normally in a state of tonic contraction, but it opens briefly and a small amount of chyme passes through each time a peristaltic wave arrives.

Various types of movement occur in the colon, including peristalsis, segmentation, haustral shuttling and mass movements. The BER in the colon has a low frequency compared with that in the small intestine and the pacemaker is located half-way along the colon. This may account for the fact that **peristalsis** in the proximal colon moves towards the caecum, rather than the rectum. In the transverse and descending colon, the commonest movements are **segmentation contractions**, which may be stationary or propulsive. **Haustral shuttling** involves apparently random contractions that move the contents backwards and forwards and bring about mixing.

Mass movements occur, usually in the transverse colon, only a few times a day. A length of some 20 cm distal to a distended or irritated site in the colon contracts for about 30 s, so emptying that section of the colon. Mass movements may be brought about reflexly through the myenteric plexus as a result of distension of the stomach or duodenum by ingested food (**gastrocolic** or **duodenocolic reflexes**). This sudden movement of colonic contents can push large amounts of faeces into the rectum and initiate the desire to defaecate.

Movement of chyme through the large intestine is a slow process. Although as much as 75% of the remains of a meal are lost in the faeces within 72 hours, it may take up to a week for the entire meal to pass through the gut.

DEFAECATION

The removal of salts and water from the large intestinal contents renders them increasingly solid, so that by the time they have reached the rectum they are in a semi-solid state and have formed the faeces.

The **faeces** consist of the indigestible remains of food, such as cellulose and other dietary fibre, and other substances associated with them:

fat; ions and water; digestive enzymes; mucus; cells from the lining of the alimentary tract; and bile pigments, which give colour to the faeces.

The presence of faeces in the rectum initiates the **defaecation reflex**, as well as a desire to defaecate. The reflex involves the stimulation of sensory neurones, which travel from the rectum to the sacral segments of the spinal cord, and the parasympathetic fibres in the nervi erigentes, which stimulate peristalsis in the descending and sigmoid colon, the rectum and anal canal (Figure 15.47). This contraction may be sufficiently powerful to empty the colon from the splenic flexure onwards with one peristaltic wave. There is also a weaker intrinsic reflex, mediated by the myenteric plexus.

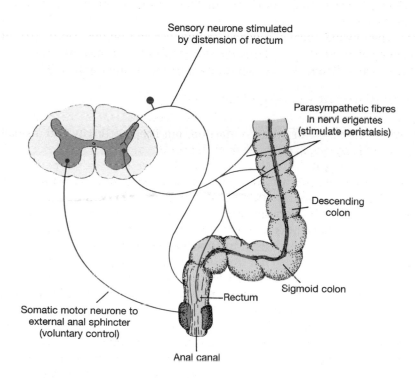

Sensory neurone stimulated by distension of rectum

Parasympathetic fibres in nervi erigentes (stimulate peristalsis)

Descending colon

Sigmoid colon

Rectum

Somatic motor neurone to external anal sphincter (voluntary control)

Anal canal

Figure 15.47 Pathways of the defaecation reflex.

When the peristaltic wave reaches the internal anal sphincter, it relaxes. However, defaecation also depends upon the state of contraction of the external anal sphincter. Voluntary relaxation of this sphincter enables the faeces to be voided. The afferent signals transmitted via the spinal cord to the cerebral cortex also usually result in voluntary contraction of the abdominal muscles and deep inspiration to lower the diaphragm and raise the intra-abdominal pressure and assist evacuation.

Constipation and diarrhoea

Constipation is the infrequent elimination of hard, relatively dry faeces. It is most often due to voluntary inhibition of the defaecation reflex. If this behaviour is continued over a long period of time the reflex weakens, exacerbating the problem. The presence of hard faeces in the rectum causes discomfort and may, when voided, cause damage to the anal canal.

Constipation in an individual with normally regular bowel habits may be a symptom of an intestinal disease – cancer of the colon, for example.

Diarrhoea is due to the rapid movement of faeces through the large intestine and results in the production of liquid faeces. A common cause is infection by bacteria or virus. The organisms irritate the wall of the distal ileum and the large intestine, which respond by increasing secretion rates; motility also increases. As a result, large quantities of fluid are propelled through the gut and expelled as liquid faeces. It may also occur in inflammatory conditions such as Crohn's disease and colitis (especially ulcerative colitis), which stimulate increased intestinal movement.

Anxiety states may give rise to psychogenic diarrhoea, when stimulation of the distal colon by the parasympathetic system increases secretion rates and intestinal motility.

Diarrhoea can be life-threatening, since it can bring about severe loss of water and electrolytes (particularly Na^+ and HCO_3^-) from the body. In severe cases, therefore, water and electrolyte replacement form an important part of treatment.

Metabolic fate of absorbed food

The products of carbohydrate, lipid and protein digestion enter the circulation (via the lymph in the case of lipids) and pass to the cells where they are utilized in a variety of ways.

Overall, metabolism can be subdivided into **anabolism** (synthesis) and **catabolism** (breakdown). In anabolic reactions, large molecules are assembled from smaller ones; they include the synthesis of proteins from amino acids, glycogen from glucose and triglycerides from fatty acids and glycerol. Catabolic reactions are the reverse, breaking down large molecules into smaller ones. In cells, the principal catabolic reaction is oxidation.

> Oxidation and other types of chemical reactions are described in **Chemical reactions** (page 27), in Ch. 1, Molecules, Ions and Units.

Carbohydrate metabolism

GLUCOSE UPTAKE AND GLYCOGEN SYNTHESIS IN THE LIVER

Glucose molecules diffuse into hepatocytes and are then converted into glucose-6-phosphate by the enzyme glucokinase. In this form glucose cannot escape back into the blood. Glucose-6-phosphate is then converted into glycogen, the form in which carbohydrate is stored, by the process of **glycogenesis**. Glycogen can also be formed from non-carbohydrate sources such as lactate, pyruvate, glycerol and some amino acids; this process is termed **gluconeogenesis**. Glucose uptake and glycogen formation are both regulated by insulin.

GLUCOSE RELEASE FROM THE LIVER

Glycogen breakdown in the liver (**glycogenolysis**) is stimulated by the hormones adrenaline and glucagon and results in the production of glucose-6-phosphate. Free glucose is split from glucose-6-phosphate by enzymes (**phosphatases**) in the liver cells and it is then able to pass out into the blood and thus be taken up by other tissues.

GLUCOSE UPTAKE BY THE TISSUES

Glucose is taken up by the extrahepatic tissues and also combines with phosphate to form glucose-6-phosphate. This reaction (**phosphorylation**) is catalysed in one direction only by the enzyme **hexokinase**. As a result, glucose is effectively 'trapped' within the cells. In muscle, glucose can be converted to glycogen. Glucose is taken into most cells by facilitated diffusion, a process that is stimulated by the hormone insulin. Glucose can also be taken up by the cells of adipose tissue, in which case it may be stored as triglyceride; conversion of glucose to fatty acids can also take place in the liver. The fatty acids then circulate and can be stored in adipose tissue.

GLUCOSE OXIDATION

Each molecule of glucose is broken down in three stages, although each stage is itself subdivided into a number of smaller steps. Initially, glucose is split into two molecules of pyruvate by the process of **glycolysis**; pyruvate is then broken down to release carbon dioxide and several other metabolites in the **citric acid cycle**; **oxidative phosphorylation** completes the process, giving rise to water and adenosine triphosphate (ATP), the cell's chemical energy store.

Glycolysis

The first stage of glucose catabolism is glycolysis, which, since it occurs in the absence of oxygen, is described as **anaerobic**, and which takes place within the cytosol of the cell (Figure 15.48).

Anaerobic glycolysis involves the splitting of a molecule of glucose (a six-carbon molecule) through a series of enzyme-driven reactions to give rise to two molecules of **pyruvate** (a three-carbon molecule). These reactions liberate energy, some of which is stored in two molecules of ATP. Four hydrogen atoms are also liberated; two of them are used to reduce the oxidized form of the electron acceptor **nicotinamide adenine dinucleotide** (NAD^+) to NADH and the other two become H^+.

In the continuing absence of oxygen, or if the build up of pyruvate inside the cell is too rapid, pyruvate is converted to **lactate**. This occurs in active skeletal muscle cells during exercise.

> ATP, NAD and FAD are covered in **Nucleotides** (page 26), in Ch. 1, Molecules, Ions and Units.

The citric acid cycle

The next stage in the oxidation of **pyruvate** to **carbon dioxide** and **water** involves the conversion of pyruvate to **acetyl coenzyme A** (acetyl-CoA), which then enters a cycle of chemical reactions called the citric acid, or Krebs, cycle, named after Hans Kreb (1900–1981) (Figure 15.48). These reactions take place inside the mitochondria of the cell. For each molecule of glucose, two molecules of acetyl-CoA enter the citric acid cycle. When each molecule of pyruvate is converted to acetyl-CoA, one carbon atom is removed and forms a molecule of CO_2. Within the citric acid cycle, acetyl-CoA (a two-carbon compound) combines with oxaloacetate (a four carbon compound) to form citrate (a six-carbon compound), which is then converted back to oxaloacetate through a number of intermediate steps; the two carbon atoms lost in this process are oxidized to CO_2 (Figure 15.49).

Figure 15.48 Oxidation of glucose. **Anaerobic glycolysis:** Glucose is broken down in the cytosol to form two molecules of pyruvate; two molecules of ATP are synthesized. **Citric acid cycle:** Pyruvate enters a mitochondrion and is converted into acetyl-CoA, with the production of two CO_2 molecules. The two molecules of acetyl-CoA enter the citric acid cycle and, with the addition of six water molecules, are broken down in a series of steps with the production of two molecules of ATP, four CO_2 molecules, six H^+ ions and the reduced electron acceptors NADH and $FADH_2$. **Oxidative phosphorylation:** Electrons from these compounds are then passed along the electron transport chain to O_2, which then combines with H^+ to form 12 water molecules. Concurrently, 34 molecules of ATP are generated by the phosphorylation of ADP.

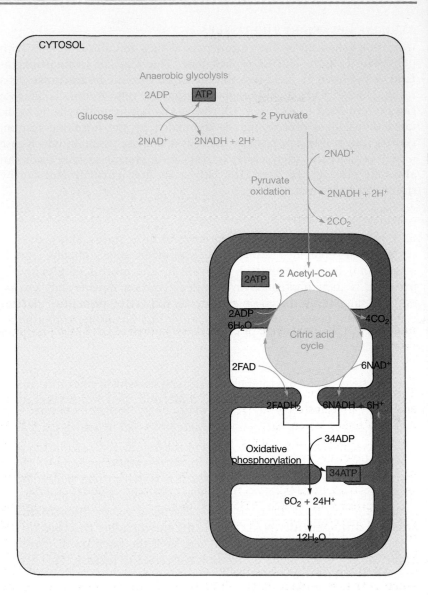

Acetyl-CoA molecules are thus effectively used up. Electrons that are also released during the cycle combine with the electron acceptors **NAD⁺** and **flavin adenine dinucleotide (FAD)**, reducing them to NADH and $FADH_2$. The breakdown of the two pyruvate molecules liberates six NADH and two $FADH_2$ molecules. In addition, six hydrogen atoms are released and two molecules of ATP are produced directly by the combination of ADP and phosphate. A total of six water molecules is also used up in the citric acid cycle.

Ignoring the fact that most H^+ and electrons (e^-) are temporarily incorporated into acceptors, the first part of the process of glucose catabolism can be summarized thus:

$$C_6H_{12}O_6 + 6H_2O \longrightarrow 6CO_2 + 24H^+ + 24e^-.$$

The energy stored in the electron acceptors is used to form more ATP

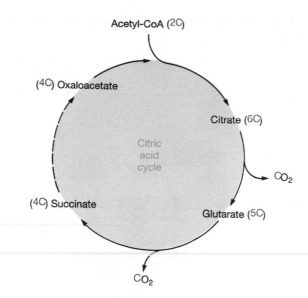

Figure 15.49 The breakdown of acetyl-CoA in the citric acid cycle. The two-carbon acetyl-CoA enters the cycle and combines with four-carbon oxaloacetate to form six-carbon citrate. This then loses two of its carbon atoms as CO_2 molecules and is converted, through a number of intermediate steps (indicated by a broken line), back to oxaloacetate.

molecules in the next stage of the process, known as oxidative phosphorylation.

Oxidative phosphorylation

The electrons taken up by NADH and $FADH_2$ in glycolysis and the citric acid cycle are transferred to oxygen, their energy being incorporated into ATP molecules when ADP and phosphate are combined. Each NADH molecule provides the energy to form three ATP molecules and each $FADH_2$ molecule gives rise to two. This process is carried out by a series of molecular complexes, known as the **electron transport chain**, which form an integral part of the inner membrane of mitochondria.

The process by which ATP is synthesized is dependent upon the passage of electrons down the electron transport chain and the pumping of H^+ out of the mitochondrial matrix into the intermembrane space between the inner and outer membranes. H^+ is liberated during anaerobic glycolysis and the conversion of pyruvate to acetyl-CoA and also when NADH is broken down, since when H atoms are split from the NADH molecule they dissociate into H^+ (a proton) and an electron.

Electrons are passed from molecule to molecule along the electron transport chain (Figure 15.50). As each molecule receives an electron it is reduced and when it passes it on to the next molecule in the chain it is oxidized. Each molecule of the chain has a lower energy level than the preceding one and is anchored in a particular position in the membrane; as the electrons are passed down the chain energy is released at each step. The final electron acceptor is oxygen, and this combines with H^+ to form water. In all, 12 water molecules are formed, but since six were used in the citric acid cycle, the complete breakdown of one glucose molecule yields only six overall.

The second part of the process of glucose catabolism can be summarized:

$$6O_2 + 24H^+ + 24e^- \longrightarrow 12H_2O.$$

Figure 15.50 The electron transport chain. Electrons, from hydrogen atoms, are passed from molecule to molecule, losing a small amount of energy at each step. Some of the energy is used to synthesize ATP (see Figure 15.51); the remainder is lost as heat.

Figure 15.51 The formation of ATP by oxidative phosphorylation. Electrons (e⁻) are pumped out of the mitochondrial matrix by the protein complexes of the electron transport chain. The energy released is used to pump H⁺ into the intermembrane space. The H⁺ gradient so developed enables the ions to diffuse back through ATP synthetase channels, their energy enabling the conversion of ADP to ATP.

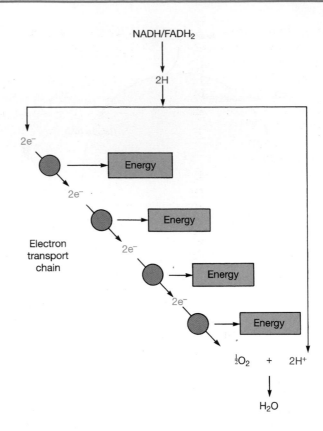

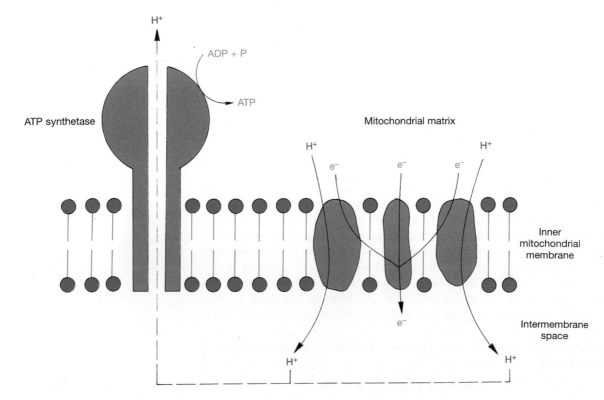

This energy derived from the electrons is used to pump H^+ out of the matrix and thereby create an electrochemical gradient across the inner mitochondrial membrane (Figure 15.51).

The H^+ gradient represents a store of potential energy, which is exploited when the H^+ ions diffuse back into the matrix. As H^+ diffuses down its gradient its energy is used to convert ADP to ATP. The mechanism by which this is brought about probably involves a conformational change in one or more of the enzymes (known as synthetases or synthases) which form part of the inner membrane. The transport of electrons is therefore coupled to the movement of H^+ and the synthesis of ATP.

Summary of ATP synthesis in glucose oxidation

For each glucose molecule metabolized by the cell, 34 molecules of ATP are liberated during oxidative phosphorylation, two are liberated during anaerobic glycolysis and two come from the citric acid cycle. A total of 38 ATP molecules therefore represents the maximum energy yield from a single molecule of glucose.

Not all the energy released during glucose breakdown is stored as ATP: about one-third is lost from the body as heat. The overall equation for glucose breakdown in the presence of oxygen is therefore:

$$C_6H_{12}O_6 + 6O_2 \longrightarrow 6CO_2 + 6H_2O + 38\,ATP + HEAT.$$

Lipid metabolism

During digestion, triglyceride molecules from the diet are hydrolysed principally to monoglycerides and free fatty acids. Once inside the intestinal epithelial cells, these digestion products combine to resynthesize triglycerides. Short-chain fatty acids are delivered directly to the portal blood.

CHYLOMICRA

Triglyceride molecules combine with phospholipid, cholesterol and protein inside the cells of the intestinal mucosa to form small spherical particles called **chylomicra**; these are then passed into the lacteals and delivered to the general circulation via the thoracic duct. Chylomicra cause the plasma to appear cloudy for an hour or two after eating.

Most of the fat is removed from the blood in adipose tissue and in the liver. **Lipoprotein lipase** in the capillary endothelial cells in adipose tissue and liver breaks down the triglycerides of chylomicra, which adhere to the endothelial surface. The fatty acids that are released pass into cells at these sites and reform triglycerides with intracellular glycerol. The chylomicron remnants remain in the blood and interact with high-density lipoprotein particles, which increases their cholesterol content. They are then taken up by the liver and broken down to release free fatty acids and glycerol, free cholesterol and amino acids.

LIPOGENESIS

Fatty acids are synthesized by the condensation of two-carbon units in a reversal of the oxidation pathway. The process takes place in the cytosol with the growing fatty acid molecule being transformed into an acyl-carrier protein. The reactions are enzyme-catalysed and occur in a number of steps, beginning with acetyl-CoA, which has been transported out of the mitochondria, and usually lead to the formation of palmitic acid (16 carbons). The latter can then be converted into stearic and oleic acids (both of which have 18 carbons) by enzymes in the smooth endoplasmic reticulum. Fatty acids are subsequently combined with glycerol, either within mitochondria or on the endoplasmic reticulum, forming triglycerides.

LIPOLYSIS

Fat stored within adipose cells is broken down (lipolysis), in a reaction which is catalysed by **lipases**, to fatty acids which pass into the blood where they combine with albumin. These are referred to as **'free' fatty acids**, distinguishing them from those which are combined with other substances such as glycerol and cholesterol.

LIPOPROTEINS

Lipid is mainly transported as lipoprotein, most of which is formed in the liver. Several classes of lipoprotein have been identified: they are very-low-density lipoprotein (**VLDL**), intermediate-density lipoprotein (**IDL**), low-density lipoprotein (**LDL**) and high-density lipoprotein (**HDL**). Lipoprotein density increases with increase in the cholesterol and phospholipid content and decrease in the triglyceride content. Thus, VLDLs contain relatively large amounts (about 60%) of triglycerides and 40% cholesterol and phospholipid, while HDLs contain very little triglyceride (5%) and about 50% cholesterol and phospholipid. The largest amount of cholesterol is found in LDLs (Table 15.8).

VLDLs are the major source of plasma triglycerides in the post-absorptive state. They enter the circulation from the liver and interact with HDLs before being digested at endothelial surfaces to release triglyceride, which is taken up by the cells. The triglyceride content of the VLDLs is thus reduced and their cholesterol content increased so that they become IDLs. Approximately half of these are taken up by the liver and the other

Table 15.8 Lipid content of lipoproteins (modified from Berne, R. and Levy, M. (1993) *Physiology*, 3rd edn, C. V. Mosby, St Louis) VLDL = very low density lipoproteins; IDL = intermediate density lipoproteins; LDL = low density lipoproteins; HDL = high density lipoproteins

Name	Triglyceride (%)	Cholesterol (%)	Phospholipid (%)
VLDL	60	6	8
IDL	30	30	22
LDL	7	50	20
HDL	5	19	30

half become LDLs, although the mechanism by which this occurs is not understood. LDLs are the major source of circulating cholesterol and virtually all cells have **LDL receptors**. Attachment of an LDL complex to a cell surface precedes its uptake, subsequent digestion and release of cholesterol and phospholipids. Therefore cholesterol uptake varies according to the rate of production of LDL receptors.

High levels of cholesterol in the circulation may lead to the formation of atheromatous plaques in the walls of blood vessels. HDLs appear to be able to help prevent the deposition of cholesterol. It is suggested that they may absorb cholesterol and transfer it to IDLs and LDLs prior to transport back to the liver. Whatever the mechanism, it is well established that a high HDL:LDL ratio results in a reduced risk of cardiovascular disease.

The primary role of HDL seems to be to act as a facilitator in the movement of plasma lipids. It contains apoprotein-C, an activator for lipoprotein lipase, which is required for the removal of fatty acids from both VLDLs and chylomicra.

> Atheromatous plaques are described in **Ischaemic heart disease** (page 390), in Ch. 12, Circulation of Blood and Lymph.

FATTY ACID OXIDATION

Within the tissues, fatty acids are broken down and release energy. Fatty acids in the cytosol are attached to CoA, forming **acyl-CoA** (Figure 15.52). The acyl group is then separated off and transported into a mitochondrion where, on the matrix side of the inner membrane, it combines with another CoA molecule, reforming acyl-CoA. Each molecule of acyl-CoA is then oxidized to form one molecule of **acetyl-CoA** and one of acyl-CoA, which is shorter by two carbon atoms than the original. This is accompanied by the reduction of **NAD⁺** and **FAD** to NADH and FADH₂ and the production of H⁺. This process is repeated until the fatty acid molecule has been broken down completely. The acetyl-CoA molecules formed by this sequence of events enter the **citric acid cycle** and **electron transport chain** and are broken down in exactly the same way as those formed during glucose metabolism; **ATP** is again liberated primarily during oxidative phosphorylation.

Repeated removal of carbon atoms thus leads to the formation of several acetyl-CoA molecules from each fatty acid molecule. A six-carbon fatty acid gives rise to three acetyl-CoA molecules, each of which generates 17 ATP molecules in the citric acid cycles and electron transport chain, a total of 51 ATP molecules. One ATP molecule is broken down during the formation of each acyl-CoA molecule, so that a net gain of 48 ATP molecules occurs when a six-carbon fatty acid is completely oxidized. It may be recalled that complete oxidation of glucose liberates 38 ATP molecules. Obviously, the actual amount of energy liberated during the breakdown of a fatty acid depends upon its size and the numbers of acetyl-CoA molecules that it can form; one molecule of stearic acid ($CH_3(CH_2)_{16}COOH$), for example, can yield 146 molecules of ATP.

Additional energy release occurs due to the oxidation of glycerol in the tissues. On separation from fatty acids, glycerol is converted to phosphoglyceraldehyde, which is an intermediate compound in anaerobic glycolysis.

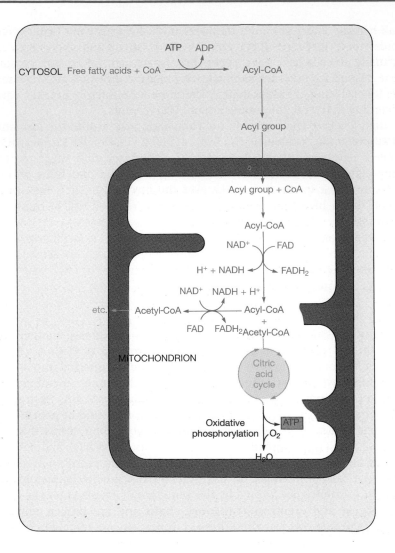

Figure 15.52 Oxidation of a fatty acid. The molecule combines with CoA to form acyl-CoA in the cytosol. The acyl group is then split off and enters the mitochondrion, combining with another CoA and reforming acyl-CoA The latter is split into a further acyl-CoA molecule, which is two C atoms shorter, and acetyl CoA, which enters the citric acid cycle. NAD$^+$ and FAD are both reduced during this process. Acyl-CoA continues to lose C atoms until the whole molecule has been broken down.

KETOACIDOSIS

The products of fat oxidation may appear in the urine in certain conditions, such as low-carbohydrate and/or high-fat diets; diabetes mellitus, when carbohydrate metabolism is impaired; and in starvation. These substances include **acetoacetic acid**, **beta-hydroxybutyric** (β-**hydroxybutyric**) acid and **acetone** and are collectively known as **ketone bodies**. They are formed in the liver when triglycerides are being catabolized and result from an accumulation of **acetyl-CoA** that is not oxidized in the citric acid cycle. Two molecules of acetyl-CoA combine to form a single molecule of acetoacetic acid and most of this is converted into beta-hydroxybutyric acid and a very small amount into acetone. Under normal circumstances these molecules are rapidly conveyed to the tissues and metabolized. However, in the absence of carbohydrate metabolism, oxaloacetate, one of its products to which acetyl-CoA must bind in order to enter the citric acid cycle, is absent. The resultant accumulation of ketone bodies, which may be 30 times normal, produces ketoacidosis and leads to metabolic acidosis.

The immediate consequence of ketoacidosis is that the blood buffers the excess H^+ and, if its limit is exceeded, the blood becomes more acid and the pH is lowered. As a result of this, more H^+ is excreted into the urine. The raised acidity also stimulates ventilation, and acetone, which smells of pear drops or hay, can be smelt on the breath. Ketones have a deleterious effect on the brain and can lead to coma.

CONVERSION OF CARBOHYDRATES AND AMINO ACIDS INTO FATTY ACIDS

Fatty acids can be formed from both carbohydrates and some amino acids, particularly when either are present in excess. A small amount of carbohydrate conversion occurs in adipose tissue, but most is in the liver, as is all amino acid conversion. In both cases acetyl-CoA is formed which is then converted into fatty acids.

Protein metabolism

Amino acids are absorbed from the gut into the blood and pass to the tissues. The blood's amino acid concentration is maintained within narrow limits and a fall in the level results in the rapid breakdown of cellular protein and the release of amino acids into the circulation. These functions are regulated by the hormone cortisol.

PROTEIN SYNTHESIS

Within the cells, some amino acids are synthesized into structural proteins, while others are oxidized with the release of energy. Growth hormone, insulin and testosterone all promote the uptake of amino acids from the blood into cells.

Having entered a cell, the amino acids are used to synthesize proteins under the direction of nuclear DNA and messenger RNA. This protein may form a permanent structure or may simply represent a store of amino acids that can be liberated when required. Amino acids are not stored as discrete units.

> The mechanism of protein synthesis is described in detail on page 61, in Ch. 2, Cells and the Internal Environment.

AMINO ACID CATABOLISM

Deamination

Amino acids that have not been taken up by cells and synthesized into proteins or other nitrogen-containing compounds are broken down, mainly in the liver, to keto acids and ammonia, by the process of deamination (Figure 15.53). This involves the removal of the amino group ($-NH_2$) from the amino acid molecule to form a keto ($-CO$) acid and ammonia (NH_3).

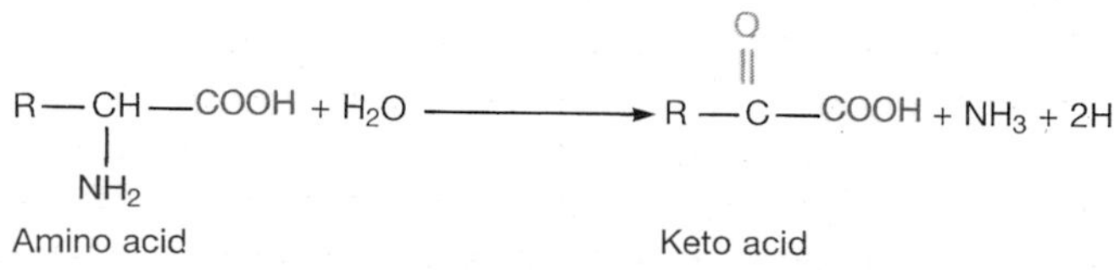

$$R-\underset{\underset{\text{Amino acid}}{NH_2}}{CH}-COOH + H_2O \longrightarrow R-\overset{\overset{O}{\|}}{\underset{\text{Keto acid}}{C}}-COOH + NH_3 + 2H$$

Figure 15.53 Deamination of amino acids. The amino group ($-NH_2$) from the amino acid is replaced by a keto group ($-CO$), and the amino group is converted into ammonia (NH_3), with the addition of hydrogen from water.

Conversion of ammonia to urea

Ammonia is converted into the less toxic urea in a series of steps known as the **ornithine cycle** (Figure 15.54). Using the energy from the breakdown of ATP, ammonia is incorporated into carbamoyl phosphate, which enters the ornithine cycle. Further nitrogen is obtained from aspartic acid. The two nitrogen-containing groups are then combined with a molecule of carbon dioxide (derived from HCO_3^-), to form urea ($CO(NH_2)_2$), which diffuses out of the liver cells and is eventually excreted in urine.

Figure 15.54 Ammonia (NH_3) from an amino acid is incorporated into a carbamoyl phosphate molecule and taken into the ornithine cycle. It is combined with $-NH_2$ from aspartic acid to form urea, which is then excreted in the urine.

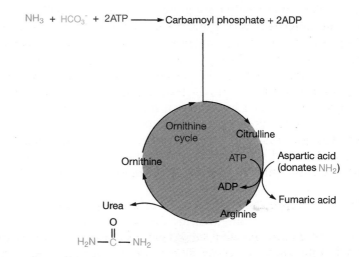

Keto acid oxidation

The keto acids produced by deamination in the liver can be oxidized by most body tissues, after they have been converted into a substance that is able to enter the citric acid cycle. The precise compounds formed depends upon the particular keto acids; they include pyruvic acid, acetyl-CoA and the ketone body acetoacetate. Once these compounds have entered the citric acid cycle, they are oxidized to carbon dioxide and water. Overall, the quantity of ATP molecules formed by the oxidation of 1 g of protein is less than the equivalent number produced in glucose oxidation.

TRANSAMINATION

Non-essential amino acids can be formed by the process known as transamination. Amino groups are transferred to alpha-keto acids, thereby forming new amino acids. Pyruvic acid, formed in carbohydrate oxidation, is converted into alanine by this method (Figure 15.55). Glutamine, which is present in large quantities in the tissues, is a major source of amino groups.

Respiratory quotient and respiratory exchange ratio

A measure of food utilization is '**respiratory quotient**', or **RQ**. This is the ratio of the volume of carbon dioxide produced to the volume of

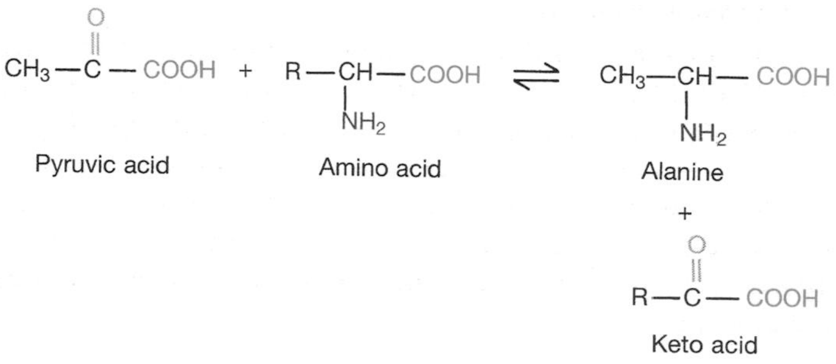

Figure 15.55 Transamination of amino acids. The amino group and a hydrogen atom from one amino acid are exchanged with the oxygen from a keto acid (pyruvic acid), which therefore becomes an amino acid (alanine).

oxygen consumed within a given period of time. The average RQ of carbohydrate is 1.0, while that of fat is 0.7. Protein has an average RQ of 0.8. The reason for these discrepancies is that fat and protein metabolism gives rise to large numbers of hydrogen atoms which combine with oxygen to form water; as a result, less carbon dioxide is formed. Thus, for example:

Glucose $\quad C_6H_{12}O_6 + 6O_2 \longrightarrow 6CO_2 + 6H_2O \qquad\qquad RQ = 6/6 = 1.0$

Palmitic $\quad C_{15}H_{31}COOH + 23O_2 \longrightarrow 16CO_2 + 16H_2O \qquad RQ = 16/23 = 0.7$
acid

Alanine $\quad 2C_3H_7O_2N + 6O_2 \longrightarrow (NH_2)_2CO + 5CO_2 + 5H_2O \quad RQ = 5/6 = 0.83.$

RQ is a measure of the metabolism of foods by the tissues. The '**respiratory exchange ratio**' (R) is the ratio of carbon dioxide output by the lungs to the amount of oxygen taken in and used up. It therefore measures the overall metabolic activity of the whole body. An R value of 0.9, for example, would indicate that rather more carbohydrate than fat was being metabolized. As R falls towards 0.7, more fat is being utilized by the tissues.

METABOLIC RATE

The metabolic rate is the total amount of energy consumed by an individual per hour. In a laboratory, food samples can be burned and all their energy is liberated as heat. Within the body, food is catabolized and some energy is liberated as heat, some is used as work and some is stored as ATP. Eventually, all the energy released in the body is converted to heat. Measuring the rate of heat production by the body therefore provides a direct measurement of metabolic rate. It can be measured more easily indirectly, however, by measuring oxygen consumption and assuming that each litre of oxygen metabolized with a mixed diet liberates 20.1 kJ of heat.

Metabolic rate depends upon both the total amount and the type of food that is consumed. If carbohydrates, lipids and proteins are burned completely they yield 17.22, 39.06 and 22.18 kJ/g respectively.

In the body, similar values are found for carbohydrate and fat, but protein oxidation is incomplete, since it leads to the formation not only of carbon dioxide and water but also of urea and other nitrogenous compounds. The energy actually released by protein is thus 17.16 kJ/g.

Joules are explained in **Energy** (page 29), in Ch. 1, Molecules, Ions and Units.

Basal metabolic rate

Since metabolic rate changes with diet, with time and also with activity, the most useful comparative measurement is obtained when the body is at rest. It is therefore measured when the individual has been resting at a comfortable temperature for 12–14 hours after a meal. This is 'basal metabolic rate' (BMR). BMR is related to size and sex and an 'average' young man has one of about 250 kJ/h, a young woman 220 kJ/h. BMR is very high in children and falls rapidly until the age of 20 or so; after that it falls more slowly. Apart from the age-related fall, an individual's BMR remains constant over long periods of time and 85% of subjects studied have been shown to have BMRs that are less than 10% above or below the mean for their age, sex and weight.

Metabolic rate and activity

Although BMR remains constant, actual energy expenditure (MR) varies greatly with differing levels of activity so that, for example, a 55 kg women may use only 3.77 kJ of energy every minute while lying in bed, but up to 25.0 kJ/min while participating in strenuous sport (Table 15.9).

Table 15.9 Average energy expenditure at different levels of exertion (kJ/min) (Reproduced with permission from Lentner, C. (ed.) (1981) *Geigy Scientific Tables*, Vol. 1 Ciba-Geigy

Activity	65 kg man	55 kg woman
Bed-rest	4.52	3.77
Sitting	5.82	4.82
Standing	7.32	5.73
Walking (4.9 km/h)	15.5	12.6
Walking (4.9 km/h with a 10 kg load)	16.7	14.2
Office work (sedentary)	7.5	6.7
Domestic work (cooking/light cleaning/window cleaning)	8.8–18.0	7.1–14.6
Light industry (printing/tailoring/ electrical/chemical industries)	9.6–17.2	7.9–13.4
Building industry	13.4–25.1	
Light sports (golf/sailing/bowls/billiards)	10.5–21.0	8.3–16.7
Moderate sports (dancing/horse-riding/swimming/tennis)	21.0–31.5	16.7–25.1
Strenuous sports (athletics/rowing/ soccer)	≥31.5	≥25.0

Endocrine physiology

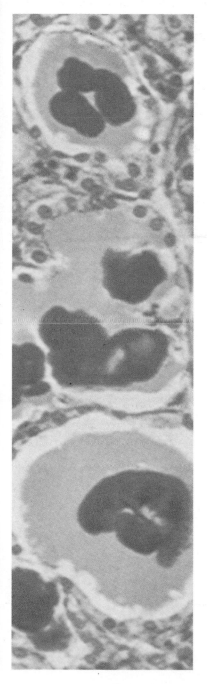

16

The body's activities are regulated by two types of mechanisms: neural and hormonal. Generally, hormonally-induced responses are slower than those initiated by neurones so that there may be a long delay between the application of a stimulus to an endocrine gland and the final manifestation of hormone action; the duration of the hormone action itself may also be very long. Neural responses are generally very rapid and of short duration.

General features of hormones and endocrine glands

Characteristics of hormones

The general structures of glands are described in **Glands** (page 77), in Ch. 3, Tissues.

Hormones are chemical messengers most of which are secreted directly into the blood by endocrine glands (Figure 16.1). Table 16.1 lists the hormones secreted by endocrine glands. In addition, there are a number that are produced by other structures, including gut hormones and erythropoietin, which is produced in the kidney. Hormones regulate

Figure 16.1 Locations of the major endocrine glands.

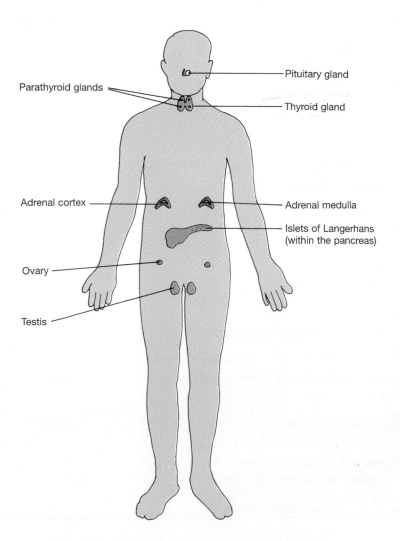

Parathyroid glands

Pituitary gland

Thyroid gland

Adrenal cortex

Adrenal medulla

Islets of Langerhans (within the pancreas)

Ovary

Testis

Table 16.1 Hormones secreted by endocrine glands

Name (Alternative name)		Site of release	Chemical nature
Adrenocorticotrophic hormone (ACTH) (Corticotrophin)	Trophic hormones	Anterior pituitary gland (adenohypophsis)	Polypeptide (39 aa)
Thyroid stimulating hormone (TSH) (Thyrotrophin)			Glycoprotein
Follicle stimulating hormone (FSH)			Glycoprotein
Luteinizing hormone (LH)			Glycoprotein
Prolactin (PRL)			Polypeptide (198 aa)
Growth hormone (GH) (Somatotrophin)			Polypeptide (191 aa)
Antidiuretic hormone (ADH (Arginine vasopressin) (AVP)		Posterior pituitary (neurohypophysis)	Peptide (9 aa)
Oxytocin			Peptide (9 aa)
Thyroxine (T_4)		Thyroid gland	Iodinated tyrosine derivative
Tri-iodothyronine (T_3)			Iodinated tyrosine derivative
Calcitonin (Thyrocalcitonin)			Polypeptide (32 aa)
Parathyroid hormone (PTH) (Parathormone)		Parathyroid gland	Polypeptide (84 aa)
Insulin		Islets of Langerhans	Protein (51 aa)
Glucagon			Polypeptide (29 aa)
Adrenaline (Epinephrine)		Adrenal medullae	Catecholamine
Noradrenaline (Norepinephrine)			Catecholamine
Aldosterone	Mineralocorticoids	Adrenal cortices	Steroid
Deoxycorticosterone			Steroid
Cortisol (Hydrocortisone)	Glucocorticoids		Steroid
Corticosterone			Steroid
Dehydroepiandrosterone (DHEA)	Androgen		Steroid
Oestrogens – principally oestradiol		Ovaries	Steroid
Progestogens – principally progesterone			Steroid
Inhibin			Protein
Andrgens – principally testosterone		Testes	Steroid
Inhibin			Protein
Human chorionic gonadotrophin (HCG)		Placenta	Glycoprotein
Human chorionic somatomammotrophin (HCS) (Human placental lactogen) (HPL)			Protein (191 aa)
Oestrogens – principally oestriol			Steroid
Progesterone			Steroid

The functions of gastrin are described in **Control of the secretion of gastric juice** (page 553), and the functions of secretin and CCK in **Control of secretion of pancreatic juice** (page 562) and **Bile concentration and gall bladder emptying** (page 571), in Ch. 15, Digestion and Absorption of Food.

See also **Neurotransmitters in the autonomic nervous system** (page 277), in Ch. 9, Autonomic and Somatic Motor Activity, and **Neurotransmitters in the brain** (page 178), in Ch. 5, The Brain.

See **Biological molecules** (page 16), in Ch. 1, Molecules, Ions and Units.

See **Protein synthesis** (page 61), in Ch. 2, Cells and the Internal Environment.

many of the biochemical reactions taking place within cells and consequently exert influences upon a range of cellular processes, including metabolic rate, growth and the uptake, synthesis and secretion of materials. They do not initiate new reactions but modify the rates of those already taking place.

Hormones may be classified as either 'general' or 'local'. General hormones are secreted into the bloodstream and usually exert an influence some distance from their origin: adrenaline, oestrogen and growth hormone, for example. Local hormones include those which act on tissues which are close to their point of origin. The hormones produced by the wall of the gut fall into this category and include gastrin, secretin and CCK.

Some hormones affect all, or most, tissues in the body, e.g. thyroxine and growth hormone, while others have specific 'target' cells. Adrenocorticotrophic hormone, for example, only acts on specific cells in the adrenal cortex.

There is some overlap between hormones and neurotransmitters. Noradrenaline is a neurotransmitter of the sympathetic nervous system and is also widely distributed in the brain stem, particularly in the medulla oblongata, and at other sites within the central nervous system; it is also released into the circulation by the cells of the adrenal medullae.

Some nerve endings release hormones rather than neurotransmitters: for example, ADH is released by nerve endings in the posterior pituitary into the blood stream. The secretion of hormones from nerve endings into the blood is termed **neurocrine release**.

The term **paracrine release** is used to describe the secretion of hormones into the interstitial fluid that surrounds them, and their diffusion to cells that lie close by. Somatostatin, which is produced by cells in the islets of Langerhans in the pancreas, inhibits the release of both insulin and glucagon from nearby cells in this way.

Hormones fall into three broad chemical groups (Table 16.1):
- **amines**, which derive from the amino acid tyrosine, e.g. hormones produced by the thyroid gland and adrenal medullae;
- **proteins, glycoproteins and peptides**, e.g. hormones produced by the pituitary gland;
- **steroids**, which derive from cholesterol, e.g. hormones produced by the adrenal cortices, the ovaries and testes.

Synthesis, storage and secretion of hormones

Proteins and peptides are synthesized on the endoplasmic reticulum under the direction of mRNA. Initially, large molecules (**preprohormones**) are formed, which are passed to the Golgi apparatus of the cell; during this process the preprohormone is firstly shortened to a **prohormone** and then to the **hormone** itself, which is then stored in secretory vesicles or granules.

Since the assembly of protein hormones from amino acids is regulated by mRNA, which is transcribed from part of a DNA molecule, it has been possible to transfer human hormone-directing genes into bacteria, which then become capable of synthesizing human hormones. In this way the large-scale manufacture of human insulin and growth hormone has become possible.

The use of hormones extracted from human tissues in replacement therapy has been linked with the spread of infectious disease, e.g. **Creutzfeldt–Jakob disease** (**CJD**) the human equivalent of 'mad cow disease') has been contracted by patients receiving human pituitary gland extracts.

Steroid hormones are synthesized from the precursor cholesterol, which is present in large quantities within the cell. Steroid hormones are not stored, but instead are both synthesized and released when the gland is stimulated.

Amines are synthesized from tyrosine via a number of enzyme-catalysed steps. Catecholamines are stored in granules, whereas thyroid hormones are stored as part of much larger protein molecules in large follicles within the gland.

Since the synthesis of both amines and steroids is dependent upon a large number of enzyme-driven steps and each enzyme is itself synthesized under the direction of a different gene, there is a great potential for genetic error; many congenital hormone deficiencies have been identified.

Proteins and catecholamines are released by the exocytosis of the granules that contain them; this process is accompanied by the uptake of Ca^{2+}. Steroid and thyroid hormones leave the cytoplasm through the plasma membrane.

Hormones do not become fully functional until after they have been released from the cells that synthesize them. Thus, in the ovaries, testosterone produced by theca cells is taken up by granulosa cells and converted to oestrogen.

> Ovarian structure is described in **Ovaries** (page 649), in Ch. 17, Sex and Reproduction.

Alternatively, precursor molecules may be converted to those with a higher activity in another tissue. In this way, 7-dehydrocholesterol, which is converted in the skin to vitamin D_3 by the action of sunlight, is then activated in the liver and kidneys to 1,25-dihydroxycholecalciferol, which functions as a hormone. Activation can also take place in the blood. Angiotensinogen, which is released by the kidneys, is converted to angiotensin I and then angiotensin II, the active form, by enzymes from the kidneys and the lungs.

Regulation of hormone secretion

Most hormones are secreted continuously by exocytosis, but at variable rates, depending upon the factors which stimulate or inhibit them.

> See **Endocytosis and exocytosis** (page 51), in Ch. 2, Cells and the Internal Environment.

Most hormone release is regulated via **negative feedback** mechanisms (Figure 16.2). A stimulus promotes the release of hormone by an endocrine gland. The hormone then brings about a physiological response, which tends to reverse the stimulus, which leads to a reduction in hormone output. That is, the response has a negative feedback effect on the rate of secretion of the hormone. In this way, hormone levels in the blood remain relatively low.

In a small number of cases **positive feedback** mechanisms operate in the control of hormone secretion. For example, the preovulatory surge of oestrogen (from the ovaries) leads to rises in LH and FSH (from the

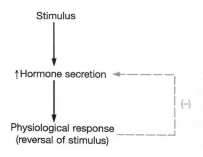

Stimulus

↑Hormone secretion

Physiological response
(reversal of stimulus)

(−)

Figure 16.2 The negative feedback control mechanism for the regulation of hormone output.

adenohypophysis), which stimulate a further increase in oestrogen. This type of regulation occurs over a narrow response range.

Some hormone release is stimulated by **neural activity**. The release of oxytocin from the posterior pituitary is in response to suckling the nipple and relies upon the passage of nerve impulses between the breast and the hypothalamus (see Figure 17.20). Many hormones show a pattern of changes in blood concentration which is repeated daily (circadian rhythm) or over longer periods. Circadian rhythms depend upon rhythm generators in the brain and continue in the absence of normal dark–light cycles, though often with a modified time base (see Figure 16.20).

The time taken between the receipt of a stimulus by an endocrine gland and the final manifestation of hormone action differs between hormones. In the case of thyroxine, for example, there is a delay of 2–3 days following its introduction into the circulation before a rise in metabolic rate is observed. This delay is termed the **latent period** of hormone action. It then takes another 8 or so days before it exerts its maximum effect. Other hormones act almost instantaneously and exert influences that are comparatively short-lived. Adrenal medullary hormones are released within the first second following sympathetic stimulation. They are also absorbed and/or destroyed very quickly so that the duration of their effects last for a maximum of only 3 minutes.

The sensitivity of a particular tissue to a hormone depends upon the presence of **receptors** to which hormone molecules can attach. Such receptors render a tissue a 'target' for hormone action. Most hormone receptors are on the surface membranes, although some are within the target cells. There may be up to 100 000 receptors per cell, each with a molecular weight of up to 200 000 and they are highly specific. The numbers of receptors on the surface or within particular cells are variable and their formation is dependent upon the presence of hormone. Generally, hormone binding results in a reduction in the number of receptors present (**down-regulation**). Repeated exposure of tissues to hormones therefore results in fewer receptors and a diminished response. Conversely, some hormones increase the number of receptors present (**up-regulation**), which increases the sensitivity of the target cells. The positions of receptors are determined by the permeability characteristics of cell membranes. Membranes are very permeable to steroid and thyroid hormone molecules but relatively impermeable to peptides, proteins and catecholamines. As a consequence, the receptors for proteins/peptides and catecholamines are found on the surfaces of target cells while those for steroids and thyroid hormones are located within the nuclei.

Cellular mechanisms of hormone action

Hormones combine with target cell receptors using a 'lock and key' mechanism (Figure 16.3). They may either (1) combine with membrane receptors and activate changes within the cytoplasm or (2) enter the cell and combine with receptors primarily within the nucleus, to form complexes that react with DNA.

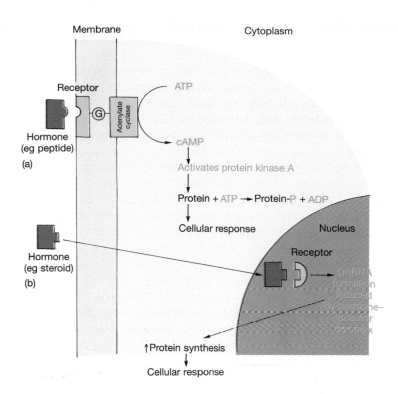

Figure 16.3 Cellular actions of hormones. **(a)** Some hormones react with receptors on the cell surface and activate a second messenger (cAMP). **(b)** Other hormones enter the cytoplasm and then (usually) the nucleus before combining with a receptor protein. This complex then increases mRNA synthesis.

COMBINATION WITH MEMBRANE RECEPTORS

Protein or peptide hormones and the catecholamines combine with surface receptors, which are linked through the membrane to intracellular enzyme systems by G-proteins (Figure 16.3). In the most common of these, the enzyme **adenylate cyclase** is activated within the cell, which leads to the formation of the nucleotide **cyclic AMP** (cAMP) from ATP.

cAMP is known as a **second messenger** or **intracellular hormone mediator**, since it transfers the influence of the hormone into the cell. It brings about the activation of **protein kinase A**, which phosphorylates specific proteins in the cell. In this way a few molecules of cAMP can initiate the formation of a large number of enzymes in a metabolic pathway. The specific actions depend upon the particular enzymes present in a cell, so that the same messenger (cAMP) is able to initiate different responses in different cells. The effects of cAMP include enzyme activation, increasing membrane permeability, initiation of muscle contraction or relaxation, promotion of protein synthesis and causing the secretion of cellular products. cAMP is rapidly hydrolysed within cells by the enzyme **cyclic nucleotide diesterase**, which converts it to the inactive form 5'-AMP, preventing a build-up of the active molecule.

Some hormones, such as insulin and catecholamines, inhibit adenylate cyclase so that levels of intracellular cAMP fall and protein phosphorylation reduces.

Another, less common, intracellular hormone mediator is **cyclic guanosine monophosphate** (cGMP), which is formed from guanosine

See **Nucleotides** (page 26), in Ch. 1, Molecules, Ions and Units.

triphosphate by the action of guanylyl cyclase. cGMP acts as a second messenger for atrial natriuretic peptide, released by the cells of the atrium when they are stretched.

Ca^{2+} is also able to act as a second messenger. Combination of a hormone with its receptor activates a G protein, which opens Ca^{2+} channels and allows the entry of ions. Inside the cell, Ca^{2+} combines with the protein **calmodulin** and activates it. The Ca^{2+}–calmodulin complex increases or decreases the activity of a specific enzyme pathway within target cells; it also activates myosin kinase, which causes the contraction of smooth muscle, a response brought about by a number of hormones.

Some hormones combine with membrane receptors leading to the activation of **phospholipase C**. This initiates the breakdown of phospholipid (phosphatidyl inositol biphosphate) in the membrane into diglyceride and inositol triphosphate which exerts second messenger effects.

COMBINATION WITH RECEPTORS IN THE NUCLEUS

Steroid hormones enter the cytoplasm and most pass into the nucleus before combining with protein receptors to form complexes. These complexes then combine with DNA, initiating the transcription of specific genes, thereby producing mRNA and leading to the synthesis of the corresponding proteins (usually one or more enzyme molecules). Thyroid hormones also enter the nucleus before combining with receptors.

Transport of hormones by the blood

Of those hormones that are carried in the blood, catecholamines and proteins/peptides circulate as free hormones, but steroids and thyroid hormones are attached to specific plasma globulins; there is an equilibrium between the free and the bound molecules.

Free hormone + Plasma protein $\rightleftharpoons$ Hormone–protein complex
('bound' hormone)

Although the total hormone concentration in plasma comprises the free hormone plus the bound hormone, only the free hormone is physiologically active because it can bind to receptors on or within its target cells. As the free hormone is used up by the target cells, it is replaced in the blood by dissociation of the bound form, The latter therefore provides a circulating store of hormone. The equilibrium reaction is pH-sensitive so, should the pH of plasma change, the reaction can be 'pushed' in one direction or the other, changing the concentration of free hormone.

The length of time that hormones remain in the blood is closely correlated with their binding characteristics. Thyroxine, which is 99.95% bound to plasma proteins, has a **half-life** of 6 days (i.e. after 6 days its concentration is half what it was on the first day); that of aldosterone, only 15% of which is bound, is 25 minutes; insulin, which is not bound at all, has a half life of between 8 and 9 minutes. Protein binding therefore produces a circulating store of hormones and retains them in the circulation for long periods of time.

Inactivation of hormones

Just as hormones are continuously secreted, so they are continuously removed from the circulation. Some hormones taken up by target cells are metabolized, while thyroid and steroid hormones are broken down in the liver and the products excreted in the bile or urine. Liver insufficiency can therefore result in the accumulation of any of these hormones, with accompanying symptoms of hormone excess. Less than 1% of hormone molecules are excreted in urine and faeces.

Endocrine glands

The endocrine glands lack common embryological origins, but nevertheless share certain characteristics. All contain at least one type of secretory cell and all are highly vascular. Since, with the exception of the hypophysis and the adrenal medullae, they are stimulated to action by blood-borne chemicals, they can be transplanted from their original position within the body and, provided they are reconnected to the circulation, still function effectively. Removal or hypofunction of the gland results in a deficiency state, but this can be reversed by administration of glandular extracts. Hyperfunction of a gland reveals the actions of hormones in an exaggerated form.

The pituitary gland (hypophysis)

The pituitary gland is about 1 cm long, 1–1.5 cm wide and 0.5 cm deep, weighs about 500 mg and lies at the base of the brain in a small depression in the sphenoid bone. The gland consists of two functionally independent parts. The anterior portion (**adenohypophysis**) is derived from the roof of the embryonic mouth cavity and is composed of epithelial tissue. It is divided into three regions, the **pars distalis, pars intermedia** and **pars tuberalis**. The posterior pituitary (**neurohypophysis**) is a downgrowth from the floor of the hypothalamus and consists, therefore, of neural tissue. It is divided into two regions, the **pars nervosa** and the **infundibulum**, or stalk (Figure 16.4).

The pituitary receives blood through the **superior** and **inferior hypophysial arteries**. The superior vessels give rise to a number of **capillary plexuses**, which drain into several long and short veins that run over the surface of the pituitary stalk; these constitute a **portal system**, which supplies the **sinusoids** of the pars distalis. The inferior vessels primarily supply the neurohypophysis.

Adenohypophysis

The bulk of the adenohypophysis is formed from the pars distalis. It contains clumps and cords of cells separated by blood-filled sinusoids. Two types of cell are found: **chromophils**, which take up stain, and **chromophobes**, which do not. The former can be divided into at least five different types of cell, on the basis of their specific staining reactions, which correlate with the production of particular hormones. Up to 40% of the cells are classified as **somatotrophs**, which secrete growth

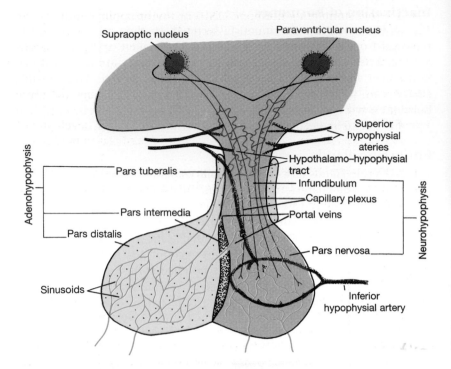

Figure 16.4 The pituitary gland and its blood supply.

hormone, and about 20% as **corticotrophs**, which secrete ACTH; the other types (**thyrotrophs, gonadotrophs and mammotrophs**) each constitute less than 5% of the total number of cells present.

The adenohypophysis secretes two groups of hormones:

- those that regulate other endocrine tissues, the so-called trophic hormones;
- those that regulate non-endocrine tissues. These include growth hormone and prolactin.

Growth hormone (GH) or somatotrophin, as well as promoting growth in children, also controls a number of metabolic pathways in both adults and children. **Prolactin** (PRL) promotes the production of milk by the mammary glands of lactating women.

In addition, the adenohypophysis synthesizes a prohormone, **pro-opiomelanocortin** (**POMC**). This molecule is cleaved into several active fragments, including the trophic hormone ACTH, and the opiate beta-endorphin (β-endorphin). In the pars intermedia POMC is broken down in a different way, giving rise to **melanocyte stimulating hormone** (**MSH**). MSH causes skin darkening in amphibians and reptiles, but only does so in humans when present in excessively high concentrations.

See **Prolactin** (page 675), in Ch. 17, Sex and Reproduction.

TROPHIC HORMONES

The four trophic hormones are responsible for the growth and development of a number of endocrine glands, as well as their maintenance in adulthood. They also directly regulate hormone output from the target glands.

- Thyroid stimulating hormone (TSH) or thyrotrophin stimulates the thyroid to release thyroxine (T₄) and tri-iodothyronine (T₃).
- Adrenocorticotrophic hormone (ACTH) or corticotrophin stimulates the adrenal cortices to release glucocorticoids.

Two hormones influence the reproductive organs and are therefore called gonadotrophic hormones or **gonadotrophins:**
- **Follicle stimulating hormone** (**FSH**) promotes the development of ovarian follicles and oestrogens in females and sperm production in males.
- **Luteinizing hormone** (**LH**) promotes the development of the corpus luteum and oestrogens and progesterone in females, and testosterone production in males.

Further details of the actions of trophic hormones are covered with their target glands.

Effects of deficiency of adenohypophysial hormones (panhypopituitarism)

In adults panhypopituitarism is usually due to destruction of the adeno-hypophysis by a tumour and results in atrophy of the target endocrine glands, with resulting hypothyroidism, reduction in adrenal glucocorticoid release and loss of sexual function. In children, one of the principal manifestations is dwarfism, which is accompanied by failure of the gonads to mature. Ischaemic necrosis of the gland (Sheehan's syndrome), usually caused by postpartum haemorrhage, was once a relatively common cause of hypopituitarism, but with better obstetric care it is now much less common.

Hypothalamic regulation of adenohypophysial hormone secretion

The release of hormones by the pars distalis is regulated directly by the hypothalamus. A number of hypothalamic neurones have axons that terminate near a capillary plexus at the top of the pituitary stalk. These axon terminals store hypothalamic releasing and inhibiting hormones. When the neurones are stimulated the hormones are released into the portal blood vessels on the surface of the pituitary stalk and are transported to the pars distalis, where they stimulate the release of adenohypophysial hormones. Discrete groups of hypothalamic neurones produce specific **releasing** (or **inhibiting**) **hormones** that, in turn, promote the release (or inhibition) of specific anterior pituitary hormones. Table 16.2 lists the hypothalamic regulatory hormones and Figure 16.5 shows the relationships between the hypothalamus, adenohypophysis and target endocrine glands. The hormones released by the target glands generally exert negative feedback on either or both the adenohypophysis and the hypothalamus and reduce the output of both hypothalamic regulatory hormones and the corresponding adenohypophysial hormones.

GROWTH HORMONE

Growth hormone (GH), or somatotrophin, is a large polypeptide consisting of 191 amino acids. It is structurally similar to, and shares certain lactogenic properties with, prolactin. GH is required for growth and development in children and its absence leads to dwarfism.

Table 16.2 Hypothalamic regulatory hormones

Name	Adenohypophysial hormone
Thyrotrophin releasing hormone (TRH)	Thyrotrophin
Corticotrophin releasing hormone (CRH)	Corticotrophin
Gonadotrophin releasing hormone (GnRH)	{ Follicle stimulating hormone { Luteinizing hormone
Growth hormone releasing hormone (GHRH) Growth hormone inhibiting hormone (somatostatin) (GHIH) }	Growth hormone
Prolactin releasing hormone (PRH) Prolactin inhibiting hormone (PIH) }	Prolactin

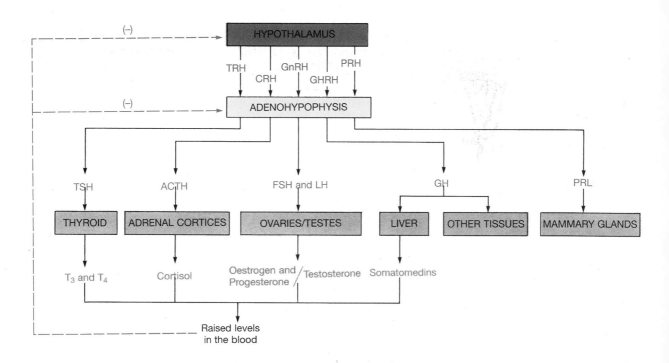

Figure 16.5 Relationships between the hypothalamus, adenohypophysis and target organs.

Growth-promoting actions of growth hormone

The growth of infants and children is largely under the control of GH. Although plasma levels rise and fall throughout the day, in children the basal level is about 6 ng/mL, while in adults it is less than 3 ng/mL. Levels continue to fall throughout life, so that in the very old there is about a quarter as much GH present as in the very young.

GH causes growth in most tissues. It promotes mitosis, thereby increasing cell numbers (**hyperplasia**) and an increase in cell size (**hypertrophy**). It also causes differentiation of cells in, for example, bone and muscle.

The growth-promoting actions of GH on bone and cartilage are not due to the action of the hormone itself, but to the presence of a number of small proteins, **somatomedins**, many of which are formed in the liver under the direction of the hormone. There is a latent period of about 12 hours following GH release before growth commences, during which molecules of somatomedin begin to be synthesized. They are transported in the blood attached to plasma proteins which gives them a relatively long half-life of about 20 hours; the half-life of GH is only 20 min. Generally, plasma levels of somatomedin are much more stable than levels of GH, which can rise and fall rapidly.

Osteoblasts also synthesize somatomedins and it is highly probable that these are more important than circulating somatomedins in promoting bone growth.

Metabolic actions of growth hormone

In addition to its growth-promoting effects, the hormone exerts a number of metabolic actions (Figure 16.6).

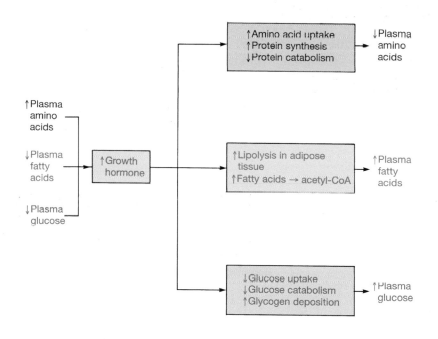

Figure 16.6 The metabolic effects of growth hormone.

• **Increased uptake of amino acids from the blood by most cells**. Within the cells it promotes the transcription of DNA to form mRNA molecules and increases the rate of mRNA translation, thereby increasing the rate of protein synthesis. It also reduces the rates of catabolism of proteins and amino acids within cells. Overall, GH brings about a reduction in the concentration of amino acids in the plasma. Its actions are described as 'protein-sparing'.

• **Increased rate of lipolysis in adipose tissues and the release of fatty acids into the blood**. In all tissues it promotes the breakdown of fatty acids to acetyl-CoA with the release of energy. Under the influence of GH, therefore, fat is used as a source of energy, rather than carbohydrate or protein.

- **Reduced uptake of glucose by cells and decreased rate of utilization as a source of energy**. In the liver particularly, the reduced ability of the cells to utilize glucose leads to an excess, which is deposited as glycogen.

Regulation of growth hormone secretion

Over and above the decrease in basal levels of GH with increasing age, the amounts rise and fall on an hourly basis and are influenced by feeding, stress and physical exercise. In an adult the basal level may be as low as 1.5 ng/mL and may rise as high as 50 ng/mL in starvation conditions. A decrease in plasma glucose is a particularly potent stimulus for the release of GH; a fall in plasma fatty acids and a rise in amino acid levels, especially arginine, produces a similar, though less powerful response.

Hypoglycaemia stimulates the hunger centre within the hypothalamus, resulting in feelings of hunger and the desire to eat. Cells in this region secrete **growth hormone releasing hormone** (**GHRH**); this passes into the portal blood vessels, which transport it down to the adenohypophysis, and stimulates the release of GH into the circulation (Figure 16.7). A second hypothalamic hormone, **growth hormone inhibiting hormone** (**GHIH**), also called somatostatin, is inhibited at the same time.

Other stimuli that promote the release of GH include stressors such as cold, fright and muscular exercise. In response to these stimuli, GH shifts the balance towards fat rather than carbohydrate breakdown. Cortisol,

Figure 16.7 The regulation of growth hormone secretion. A number of stimuli promote the release of GHRH and suppress that of GHIH by the hypothalamus, which results in an increase in the release of GH by the adenohypophysis. GH causes the liver to release somatomedins into the circulation, which then stimulate the growth of cartilage and bone. At the same time they, and GH, suppress GHRH and promote GHIH production by the hypothalamus, which leads to a reduction in GH output. GH probably acts directly on tissues other than cartilage and bone.

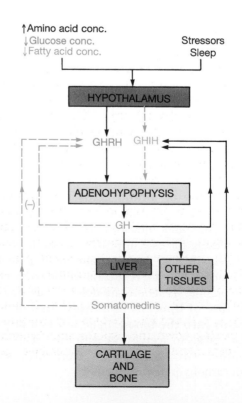

another hormone released during stress, has a similar action. GH release also occurs at the beginning of periods of deep sleep and is inhibited during REM sleep.

A rise in plasma GH and the presence of somatomedins in the circulation suppresses further GH release. This is probably mediated by a reduction in GHRH and an increase in GHIH.

Effects of growth hormone deficiency (pituitary dwarfism)

Lack of GH most often occurs in conjunction with lack of the other adenohypophysial hormones as panhypopituitarism. In about a third of cases in children, dwarfism is due to lack of GH alone so that, although growth is inhibited, there is normal puberty. This type of dwarfism can be cured completely by the administration of GH. Hyposecretion of GH in adults does not result in a specific deficiency state.

Effects of growth hormone excess (gigantism and acromegaly)

Excessive amounts of GH in children stimulate growth of the epiphyses of the long bones, leading to a final height of up to 9 feet (**gigantism**). Hyperglycaemia may cause destruction of the insulin-secreting cells of the pancreas and lead to diabetes. GH-producing cell tumours may grow to such a size that they cause the rest of the gland to be destroyed, leading to panhypopituitarism.

In adults, since the epiphyses of the long bones are already fused, bone growth is largely confined to the hands, feet and face and leads to a characteristic elongated, pronounced jaw and forehead in the condition known as **acromegaly** ('enlarged extremities'). The internal organs also enlarge and there may be increased convex curvature of the vertebral column.

Neurohypophysis

The pars nervosa, which forms the bulk of the neurohypophysis, contains a rich network of unmyelinated nerve fibres. Their cell bodies lie in the hypothalamus, in the supraoptic and paraventricular nuclei, and the fibres themselves pass to the pituitary via the infundibulum in the **hypothalamo-hypophysial tract**. Within the pars nervosa the nerve endings lie close to a network of vascular sinusoids. Lying between and surrounding the neural elements are numerous **pituicytes**, stellate cells with branching processes that provide support.

Antidiuretic hormone (**ADH**), which is also known as arginine vasopressin, and oxytocin are both stored in and released by the neurohypophysis. The hormones are synthesized by nerve cell bodies in the hypothalamus, the supraoptic nucleus producing ADH and the paraventricular nucleus oxytocin. Both hormones migrate slowly down the insides of their axons to the nerve endings in the pars nervosa, where they are stored. Both hormones are transported in association with protein molecules (**neurophysins**) which form part of the hormone precursor molecules. Transit time is approximately 10 hours.

The hormones are released into the blood by exocytosis as a result of nerve impulses passing down the hypothalamo-hypophysial tract; the process is Ca^{2+}-dependent and closely resembles neurotransmitter release.

See **Oxytocin** (page 676), in Ch. 17, Sex and Reproduction.

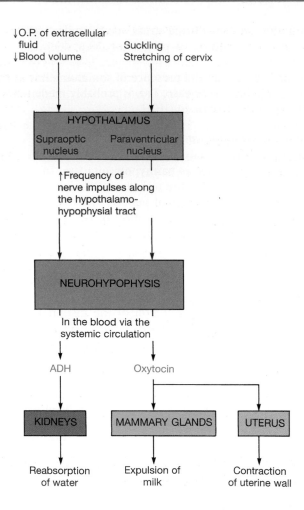

Figure 16.8 Relationships between the hypothalamus, neurohypophysis and target organs.

Synthesis and release of the hormones are, therefore, separate processes that occur in different places; synthesis takes place in the hypothalamus, secretion in the neurohypophysis. Figure 16.8 summarizes the relationships between the hypothalamus, the neurohypophysis and the target organs.

Both hormones circulate in the blood unattached to carrier proteins and are rapidly removed from the circulation, mainly by the kidneys. Approximately half the hormone molecules disappear from the blood in less than 1 minute, but the remainder takes up to 3 further minutes to be removed.

ANTIDIURETIC HORMONE (ADH)

ADH is a small peptide containing nine amino acids. Its primary effect is the production of a small quantity of urine (antidiuresis). ADH molecules bind to receptors on the luminal surfaces of cells in the collecting ducts of the kidneys. This induces adenyl cyclase activity and the formation of cAMP which, in turn, leads to the phosphorylation of a membrane protein and an increase in the permeability of the cells to water and urea. An increased quantity of water is therefore reabsorbed

The role of ADH in the regulation of water reabsorption by the kidney tubules is described in **Regulation of water balance** (page 501), in Ch. 14, Renal Control of Body Fluid Volume and Composition, and the rise in blood pressure caused by ADH in **Control of blood volume** (page 420), in Ch. 12, Circulation of Blood and Lymph.

from the tubules back into the blood, thereby raising the osmotic pressure of the urine and reducing its output (see Figure 14.17).

ADH also exerts a stimulatory influence upon smooth muscle and, through its action on the walls of arterioles, raises arterial blood pressure. It is this influence that gives rise to the alternative name, arginine vasopressin. The hormone does not usually bring about a marked rise in pressure, however, because baroreceptor reflexes reduce both cardiac output and peripheral resistance.

ADH increases the release of ACTH in response to CRH-RH and thereby assists ACTH in its response to stress.

Effects of ADH deficiency (diabetes insipidus)

Lack of ADH results in a reduction in the volume of water reabsorbed by the kidneys and renders them unable to produce concentrated urine. This condition is known as diabetes insipidus and is characterized by the production up to 15 L of dilute urine per day and excessive thirst.

Effects of ADH excess (inappropriate secretion of ADH)

Excess ADH release leads to excessive reabsorption of water with the production of a reduced volume of highly concentrated urine, accompanied by a reduction in plasma Na^+ (hyponatraemia). The latter is thought to be due to high levels of atrial natriuretic peptide secreted in response to the expanded plasma volume.

It is this hyponatraemia that produces the symptoms of headache, drowsiness, nausea, altered mental state and coma.

See also **Atrial natriuretic peptide and the regulation of sodium and potassium balance** (page 507), in Ch. 14, Renal Control of Body Fluid Volume and Composition.

The thyroid gland

The thyroid gland lies just below the larynx and consists of two lateral lobes, each measuring about 5 cm by 3 cm and 2 cm deep, connected by an isthmus which is approximately 1.25 cm across; in adults it weighs less than 30 g (Figure 16.9).

The gland is covered by a connective tissue capsule from which project septae or trabeculae that divide it into lobules. Each lobule is subdivided into 20–40 roughly spherical follicles, separated by a connective tissue stroma containing a rich network of capillaries, lymphatics and nerves.

Each follicle consists of a single layer of epithelial cells resting on a basal lamina, enclosing a central cavity containing a variable amount of viscous colloid. The colloid consists of a protein, **thyroglobulin**, and contains the principal thyroid hormone, **thyroxine** (T_4) and smaller amounts of **tri-iodothyronine** (T_3). The follicular cells vary in height, being columnar when active and flattened when inactive.

Scattered between the follicular epithelial cells, lying on the basement membrane, are a number of parafollicular, or **C-cells**, which secrete **calcitonin** (thyrocalcitonin).

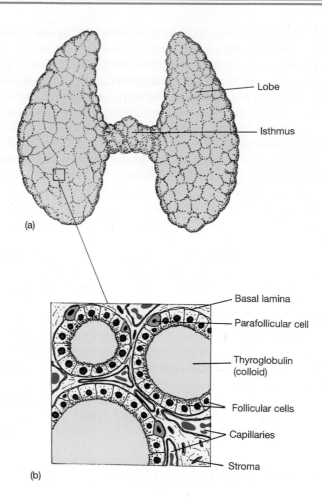

Figure 16.9 The thyroid gland.
(a) External appearance.
(b) A small section of thyroid tissue showing the follicles.

TRI-IODOTHYRONINE (T_3) AND THYROXINE (T_4)

Both T_3 and T_4 are synthesized in the thyroid gland by the iodination of the amino acid **tyrosine**. The follicular cells actively take up iodide (I^-) from the blood; the thyroid contains the highest concentration of I^- in the body.

Each tyrosine molecule has either one I^- ion added to it, forming **monoiodotyrosine**, or two, forming **di-iodotyrosine**. One monoiodotyrosine and one di-iodotyrosine molecule are then linked, forming a molecule of T_3, or two di-iodotyrosines are joined, forming T_4. T_3 and T_4 are conjugated with a large glycoprotein, also synthesized by the follicular cells, forming **thyroglobulin** (mol. wt 660 000). Only three or four T_4 molecules are formed within each thyroglobulin and overall only about one-tenth as much T_3. The iodination of tyrosine, hormone synthesis and the conjugation of hormones forming thyroglobulin all take place within the follicular cells (Figure 16.10).

The follicular cells take up small amounts of colloid by pinocytosis. Membrane-bound colloid vesicles then fuse with lysosomes and hydrolysis of thyroglobulin releases free hormones. These then diffuse into the blood. Monoiodotyrosine and di-iodotyrosine released at the same time are metabolized within the cell and the I^- is reused.

T_3 and T_4 are carried largely bound to plasma proteins, principally thyroid hormone binding globulin; only about 0.3% of T_3 and 0.03% of T_4 is transported free. T_4 is bound more tightly than T_3 and its plasma half-life is about 6 days, whereas that of T_3 is only 1 day. In the tissues most T_4 is converted to T_3, which is the physiologically active hormone.

Metabolic actions of T_3 and T_4

The primary physiological effect of the thyroid hormones is to increase basal metabolic rate in most tissues. Hormone molecules enter target cells and combine with protein receptors within the cells' nuclei, which have a much greater affinity (up to six times) for T_3 than for T_4. The combination of hormone and receptor initiates mRNA synthesis and leads to the formation of Na^+-K^+-ATPase, which increases oxidation.

Following the introduction of a single large dose of T_4 there may be a time lag of 2–3 days before a rise in metabolic rate is observed. After this latent period there is a steady rise in BMR, which peaks at 10–12 days and then drops so slowly that an appreciably raised BMR may still be observed after 60 days.

The thyroid hormones appear to be necessary for protein synthesis and therefore growth but, when present in excess, protein breakdown predominates and growth is retarded. They are also required for the development and growth of the skeleton in infancy and in childhood.

In the presence of low levels of T_3 and T_4 there is an increase in insulin-promoted glycogen synthesis in muscle; in excess the hormones stimulate glycogenolysis. The hormones also stimulate the absorption of glucose from the gut lumen and enhance its uptake by adipose tissue and muscle.

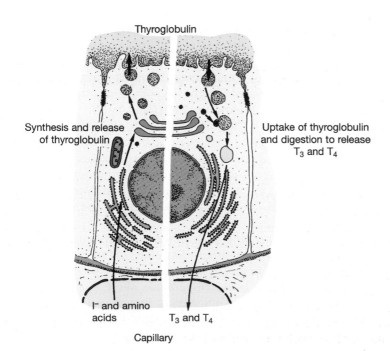

Thyroglobulin

Synthesis and release of thyroglobulin

Uptake of thyroglobulin and digestion to release T_3 and T_4

I⁻ and amino acids

T_3 and T_4

Capillary

Figure 16.10 Thyroid cell function. **Left-hand side:** I⁻ and amino acids are removed from the blood by follicular cells and used to synthesize thyroglobulin, which is stored within the colloid in the centre of the follicles. **Right-hand side:** thyroglobulin is removed from the follicles and digested, releasing T_3 and T_4, which diffuse into the blood.

The hormones promote lipolysis in adipose tissue, increased oxidation of free fatty acids and a reduction in plasma cholesterol by increasing its uptake by the adrenal cortices, gonads and liver.

Other actions of T_3 and T_4

T_3 and T_4 exert a number of physiological influences upon the body as a whole; they include:

- increasing the number of adrenergic receptors in the walls of blood vessels and therefore enhancing the effects of catecholamines;
- development and maintenance of the nervous system, and when present in high concentrations increasing the rate of neural functions;
- increasing the excitability of heart muscle, which leads to an increased heart rate and raised cardiac output; the hormones also enhance the effect of adrenaline on the heart; small increases in thyroid hormone concentration may increase the strength of each beat, but high concentrations reduce it, due to increased protein breakdown;
- increasing gastrointestinal motility and the rate of secretion of digestive juices – high concentrations therefore often result in diarrhoea;
- maintenance of sexual function: in men their absence leads to loss of sex drive (**libido**); in women, lack of hormone leads to either excessive menstrual bleeding or irregular periods – the mechanisms underlying these conflicting observations have yet to be clarified;
- maintenance of water content and secretions in the skin.

Regulation of T_3 and T_4 synthesis and secretion

The release of T_3 and T_4 is regulated by thyroid stimulating hormone (TSH), which is synthesized by the adenohypophysis. TSH promotes the uptake of I^- by the thyroid follicular cells, iodination of tyrosine and the formation of T_3 and T_4, and the storage and breakdown of thyroglobulin. Under the influence of TSH, follicular cells take up droplets of thyroglobulin from the colloid, digest it and release T_3 and T_4 into the circulation.

TSH secretion is regulated by the hypothalamic trophic hormone **thyrotrophin releasing hormone** (**TRH**) and by the plasma levels of the two thyroid hormones. TRH, a tripeptide, is released in small pulses by cells in the hypothalamus, passes through the portal vessels of the pituitary stalk to the adenohypophysis and stimulates the release of stored TSH. This then passes to the thyroid and brings about the release of T_3 and T_4. In addition to exerting their metabolic influences, these two hormones suppress TSH (and possibly TRH) output and thereby reduce their own (Figure 16.11).

Somatostatin and dopamine both inhibit TSH, as do glucocorticoids when present in high concentrations. Extreme cold increases T_3 production but not, apparently, that of T_4. Late in gestation, the foetus develops the ability to maintain its body temperature; there is a sudden rise in foetal TSH output with an accompanying increase in T_4. These levels remain elevated for some weeks or even months before returning to those observed in adults.

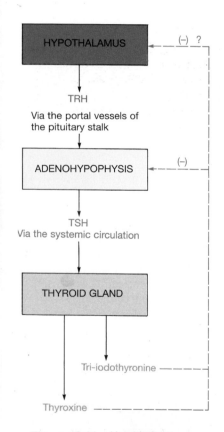

Figure 16.11 Hypothalamo-hypophysial regulation of thyroid hormone secretion. The hormones inhibit the adenohypophysis and possibly the hypothalamus.

I⁻ availability also regulates hormone production. When I⁻ is only present in small amounts, hormone production is proportional to the amount of available ion. When present in excessive amounts, however, I⁻ inhibits the production of thyroid hormones.

Effects of T_3 and T_4 deficiency (cretinism and myxoedema)

Lack of dietary iodine, once a relatively common occurrence in some areas (e.g. Derbyshire), results in an inability of the thyroid to form hormones; as a result, thyroidal suppression of TSH is removed. TSH stimulates the thyroid, which enlarges but is unable to produce sufficient hormones. The end result is an enlarged thyroid gland, which is evident as a greatly swollen neck, or **goitre**.

Hypothyroidism is characterized by a reduction in the basal metabolic rate with a slowing of mental and physical functions, low heart rate and increased weight, although suppression of appetite prevents gross obesity. There is usually cold intolerance and an increase in plasma cholesterol concentration. Coarse dry skin, brittle nails and loss of head and eyebrow hair are also observed. There is a reduction in gastrointestinal motility, resulting in constipation. In long-standing conditions there may be deposition of proteoglycans in the interstitial spaces, producing swelling (**myxo-edema**). This is manifested as a swollen larynx, resulting in a hoarse voice, a thickened tongue, increase in heart size and non-pitting subcutaneous oedema.

> Proteoglycons are described in **Areolar (loose) connective tissue** (page 80), in Ch. 3, Tissues.

In young children hypothyroidism, termed **cretinism**, leads to dwarfism and mental retardation.

Effects of T_3 and T_4 excess (Graves disease)

A goitre may also be present in hyperthyroidism, but in this case the gland is secreting hormones. Graves disease is an autoimmune disease caused by antibodies, which are formed against TSH receptors in the gland, called **long-acting thyroid stimulator** (**LATS**). These antibodies mimic the effects of TSH and promote oversecretion of the hormones. TSH levels are usually reduced due to the negative feedback effects of the large amounts of T_3 and T_4 in the blood.

The increased levels of T_3 and T_4 raise the basal metabolic rate, which results in weight loss, even in the presence of normal dietary intake, nervousness and emotional instability, fatigue, heat intolerance, sweating, increased heart rate, and increased bowel movements (though not necessarily diarrhoea). A characteristic staring appearance (**exophthalmos**) is due to the infiltration of the orbital soft tissues with extracellular fluids and mucopolysaccharides. Exophthalmos , however, is not caused by excess T_3 and T_4, but by the presence of autoantibodies.

CALCITONIN

Calcitonin is a 32-amino acid peptide synthesized and released by the parafollicular or C-cells of the thyroid follicular epithelium (Figure 16.9). It is a regulator of blood Ca^{2+} and a rise in the latter promotes calcitonin release. Calcitonin reduces osteoclast activity and therefore bone resorption, which lowers blood Ca^{2+}. It also decreases the formation of osteoclasts. In the kidneys, the hormone promotes a minor increase in Ca^{2+}

and PO_4^{3-} excretion. Calcitonin has a half-life in the circulation of about 5 minutes.

In adults the physiological effects of calcitonin are minor because osteoclast activity is small, so that its reduction has little overall effect on Ca^{2+} metabolism. Calcitonin deficiency or excess, therefore, does not have much influence upon Ca^{2+} and PO_4^{3-} metabolism.

The parathyroid glands

There are usually four small glands, each weighing less than 50 mg, which are usually located beneath the capsule of the thyroid, on its rear surface (Figure 16.12). Each gland is enclosed by a fibrous capsule and contains two types of cell: chief cells, which secrete parathyroid hormone, and oxyphil cells, which are thought to be immature chief cells.

Figure 16.12 **(a)** Location of the parathyroid glands. **(b)** Chief cells secrete parathyroid hormone; oxyphil cells are probably immature chief cells.

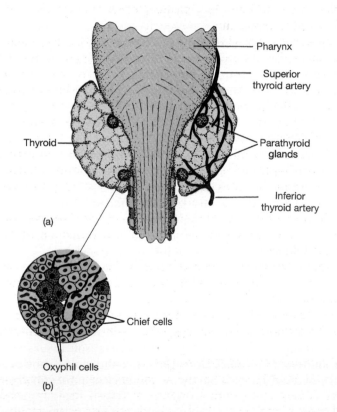

PARATHYROID HORMONE (PTH)

Parathyroid hormone (PTH), or parathormone, is a polypeptide consisting of 84 amino acids and is the primary regulator of blood Ca^{2+} and PO_4^{3-} levels (Figure 16.13).

A reduction in blood Ca^{2+} stimulates the chief cells, in the presence of Mg^{2+}, to both synthesize and secrete PTH; a rise in blood Ca^{2+} suppresses

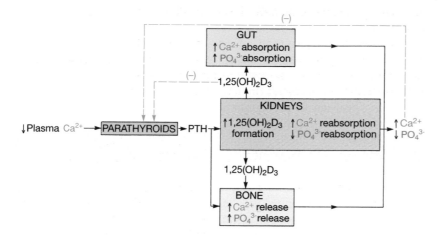

Figure 16.13 Regulation of blood Ca^{2+} and PO_4^{3-} concentrations by PTH and $1,25(OH)_2D_3$. Note that the release of PO_4^{3-} from bone and its absorption from the gut tends to raise plasma levels but, because the kidneys increase its excretion, the net effect is to lower plasma PO_4^{3-}.

PTH release. The glands also contain receptors for active vitamin D, 1,25-dihydroxycholecalciferol ($1,25(OH)_2D_3$) which, when present in large quantities, also suppresses PTH release. Once in the circulation PTH has a half-life of only a few minutes.

PTH appears to raise blood Ca^{2+} in two stages. The first, rapid, stage is brought about by the action of lacunar osteocytes in the haversian systems of compact bone. These cells cause the removal of Ca^{2+} from their immediate fluid environment which, in turn, allows exchangeable Ca^{2+} (from $CaHPO_4$) to dissolve out of the bone matrix, a process that also requires the presence of $1,25(OH)_2D_3$. This is followed by a slower phase in which osteoclasts, formed from precursor cells under the influence of PTH, actively resorb Ca^{2+} and PO_4^{3-} from the non-exchangeable fraction (hydroxyapatite – $Ca_{10}(PO_4)6OH_2$). Osteoclast activity enables bone to be remodelled, repairing fractures and changing its shape under mechanical stress.

PTH decreases the reabsorption of PO_4^{3-} in the proximal convoluted tubules of the kidneys and increases Ca^{2+} reabsorption in the distal convoluted tubules.

This action, therefore, promotes a rise in blood Ca^{2+} concentration and a fall in PO_4^{3-} concentration. PTH also stimulates the conversion of 2,5-hydroxycholecalciferol to $1,25(OH)_2D_3$ in the kidneys. The latter promotes the absorption of Ca^{2+} in the gut. In the proximal tubules PTH reduces the reabsorption of Na^+ and HCO_3^- which promotes diuresis.

See **Bone** (page 89), in Ch. 3, Tissues.

See **Renal regulation of calcium and phosphate balance** (page 508), in Ch. 14, Renal Control of Body Fluid Volume and Composition.

Effects of PTH deficiency (hypoparathyroidism)

A reduction in PTH leads to the condition known as **hypoparathyroidism**. It may result from a number of causes, including inadvertent surgical removal of the parathyroid glands during thyroidectomy. Lack of PTH reduces the Ca^{2+}-releasing effects of osteocytes and osteoclasts so that blood Ca^{2+} levels fall (hypocalcaemia). This results in increased nerve and muscle excitability and tetany. The laryngeal muscles are often affected and should their contraction cause blockage of the respiratory tract, then death may ensue. Sensory neurones are also affected and pricking sensations may be felt in the lips, fingers and toes.

Effects of PTH excess (hyperparathyroidism)

Excessive amounts of PTH are most often due to the presence of a benign tumour and results in raised Ca^{2+} (hypercalcaemia) and lowered PO_4^{3-} (hypophosphataemia). Since the Ca^{2+} has been obtained from bone, then bone weakness (**osteitis fibrosa cystica**) may ensue; this is characterized by fractures of the long bones and compression fractures of the spine. Localized brown tumours, or bone cysts, are formed by the PTH-regulated activities of groups of osteoclasts.

Raised blood Ca^{2+} exerts a number of influences on the CNS and leads to depression, mental aberration, fatigue, constipation and anorexia.

In the kidneys, the raised Ca^{2+} reduces the distal nephrons' ability to form concentrated urine so that polyuria and dehydration ensue. High levels of Ca^{2+} in the kidneys may lead to the formation of kidney stones comprising calcium oxalate or calcium phosphate.

Raised levels of Ca^{2+} are associated with excessive secretion of gastrin and HCl in the stomach, which gives a predisposition to peptic ulcers.

Regulation of blood calcium and phosphate concentrations

The maintenance of a stable blood Ca^{2+} concentration is essential for the effective operation of a wide range of activities. Ca^{2+} is required in: the process of neurotransmitter release from the endings of neurones; muscle contraction; modulation of cell metabolism in connection with hormone action; secretion by a variety of glands, including salivary, pancreatic and gastric; blood clotting; imparting hardness to bone; and as a stabilizer of nerve and muscle cell membranes.

The adult body contains approximately 1 kg of calcium, most of it in the bone matrix, in the form of hydroxyapatite. In extracellular fluid it exists in three main forms, as free Ca^{2+} (50%), bound to proteins (40%) and as calcium salts such as citrate and lactate (10%). Only the free Ca^{2+} is able to pass between compartments in the body and it is this fraction whose concentration is regulated. The relative proportions of bound and free Ca^{2+} are pH-dependent: if blood pH rises then some of the free Ca^{2+} becomes bound, so that its effective concentration is lowered. This can arise following hyperventilation and may result in tetany.

About 1000 mg of dietary calcium is taken into the body each day of which about 350 mg is absorbed from the gut. A total of 190 mg is secreted back into the gut lumen and may be lost in the faeces, so that the net amount absorbed is only 160 mg. This amount is excreted by the kidneys, keeping the total amount within the body constant.

Extracellular Ca^{2+} levels are maintained within narrow limits (around 2.5 mmol/L) by regulating the balance of its absorption in the intestine, its removal from (resorption) and deposition in (accretion) bone, and its excretion through the kidneys. Short term regulation of plasma Ca^{2+} is achieved mainly by the actions of PTH on bone and kidneys. Long-term regulation is due primarily to the effect of PTH upon the synthesis of

1,25-dihydroxycholecalciferol (1,25(OH)$_2$D$_3$) and the latter's influence upon the intestinal absorption of Ca^{2+} (Figure 16.13).

While PTH and 1,25(OH)$_2$D$_3$ increase the entry of Ca$_3$(PO$_4$)$_2$ from both bone and the intestine into the blood, the kidneys promote Ca^{2+} reabsorption and PO$_4^{3-}$ excretion so that overall, while Ca^{2+} level rises, that of PO$_4^{3-}$ falls.

The physiological importance of PO$_4^{3-}$ is primarily as part of the phosphate buffer system that operates within cells and in the blood, as well as in the lumen of the nephrons of the kidneys. In the body fluids, PO$_4^{3-}$ combines with H$^+$, forming HPO$_4^{2-}$ and H$_2$PO$_4^-$.

PTH is the primary regulator of plasma PO$_4^{3-}$ concentration.

See **Buffers** (page 15), in Ch. 1, Molecules, Ions and Units.

Calcium and phosphate absorption by the small intestine

Dietary calciferol (vitamin D$_2$) and cholecalciferol (vitamin D$_3$), which is formed in the skin by the action of sunlight, are converted to 25-hydroxycholecalciferol in the liver (Figure 16.14).

This is then activated in the kidneys by PTH to 1,25(OH)$_2$D$_3$ which promotes the absorption of Ca^{2+} by the intestinal epithelium. Activation of vitamin D by PTH is influenced by the body's requirement for Ca^{2+} so that a fall in plasma Ca^{2+} results in increased activation of the vitamin and, over a number of days, an increase in Ca^{2+} and PO$_4^{3-}$ absorption from the gut. Both Ca^{2+} and PO$_4^{3-}$ are absorbed by active transport in the duodenum and jejunum and by facilitated diffusion in the ileum; due to its longer length, the latter is quantitatively more important.

Bone calcium and phosphate

Most of the calcium in bone is in the form of hydroxyapatite (Ca$_{10}$(PO$_4$)6OH$_2$); about 1% is in the form of CaHPO$_4$ which can be exchanged with extracellular fluid relatively easily. Each day approximately 550 mg of Ca^{2+} is exchanged between bone and extracellular fluid.

PTH and 1,25(OH)$_2$D$_3$ stimulate the removal of Ca^{2+} from bone, in response to a fall in plasma Ca^{2+}, by promoting the resorption of exchangeable bone and the transport of Ca^{2+}, along with PO$_4^{3-}$, into the plasma (see *Parathyroid hormone*, above). Osteoclasts, formed under the influence of PTH, bring about a longer-term (hours to days) response in which there is breakdown of hydroxyapatite, which releases more Ca^{2+} and PO$_4^{3-}$. Bone reabsorption and accretion are normally balanced so that there is no overall change in bone mass. However, an extreme systemic lack of Ca^{2+} may lead to the release of ions from bones through this mechanism.

Calcitonin has been shown to reduce osteoclast activity and therefore reduce Ca^{2+} removal from bone in children. In adults, however, the actions of calcitonin are minor.

Role of the kidneys

The kidneys promote Ca^{2+} reabsorption and PO$_4^{3-}$ excretion so that while Ca^{2+} levels rise, PO$_4^{3-}$ falls.

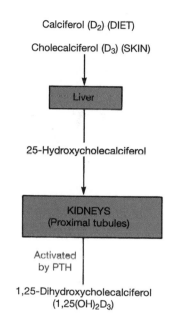

Calciferol (D$_2$) (DIET)

Cholecalciferol (D$_3$) (SKIN)

Liver

25-Hydroxycholecalciferol

KIDNEYS
(Proximal tubules)

Activated by PTH

1,25-Dihydroxycholecalciferol
(1,25(OH)$_2$D$_3$)

Figure 16.14 Activation of vitamin D$_2$ in the diet and D$_3$ formed in the skin to 1,25-dihydroxycholecalciferol. The liver, kidneys and parathyroid hormone (PTH) are all required for this process.

See **Renal regulation of calcium and phosphate balance** (page 508), in Ch. 14, Renal Control of Body Fluid Volume and Composition.

The islets of Langerhans

The hormone-secreting islets of Langerhans are located within the pancreas, which is located behind and below the stomach and is enclosed partially by the curve of the duodenum. The bulk of the pancreas is composed of exocrine cells that secrete pancreatic juice, among which are scattered approximately 1 million islets of Langerhans.

They are particularly numerous in the tail region. Each islet is composed of 2000–3000 cells, but even so the total mass of tissue only represents less than 2% of the whole pancreas (Figure 16.15).

The exocrine structure of the pancreas is described in **Structure of the pancreas** (page 559), in Ch. 15, Digestion and Absorption of Food.

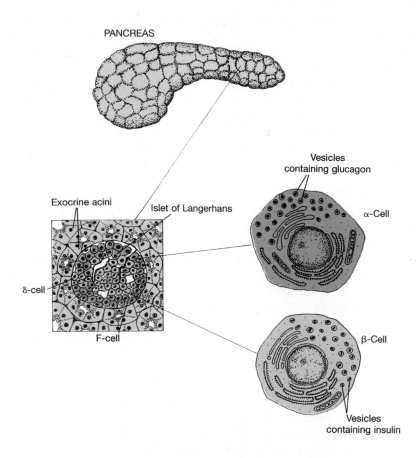

Figure 16.15 The pancreas, illustrating the appearance of a single islet of Langerhans, with details of alpha- and beta-cells.

Each islet is a compact mass of epithelial cells with an extensive network of capillaries. Four different cell types have been identified:

- Most numerous are the **beta-** or **B-cells**, which secrete insulin; they represent up to 70% of the cells present in the islets.
- Glucagon-secreting **alpha-** or **A-cells** make up 20–30%.
- **Delta-** or **D-cells**, which secrete somatostatin, make up the bulk of the rest.
- In addition, small numbers of **F-** or **PP-cells** secrete pancreatic polypeptide.

INSULIN

Insulin is a small protein consisting of an alpha chain of 21 amino acids, linked to a beta chain of 30 amino acids by two disulphide bridges. It is derived from a much larger precursor, **preproinsulin**, which is synthesized on the endoplasmic reticulum of the beta-cells. Preproinsulin passes into the cytosol, losing part of its length to form **proinsulin**, a single chain of 73 amino acids. During the process of packaging the hormone into secretory granules, the chain becomes folded, the connecting piece linking the alpha and beta chains is lost and the insulin molecule is formed.

Regulation of insulin secretion

A variety of stimuli promote the release of insulin into the blood, most important of these being a rise in glucose concentration in the blood. Raised amino acid (especially arginine) levels also stimulate insulin secretion, and raised fatty acid levels have a weaker action. The gastrointestinal hormones gastrin, secretin, cholecystokinin and gastric inhibitory peptide all promote insulin release, as do the hormones glucagon, growth hormone and cortisol; oestrogen and progesterone have a much smaller stimulatory influence. Vagal (parasympathetic) stimulation of the pancreas increases insulin release, whereas sympathetic action reduces it.

Metabolic actions of insulin

Insulin is released into the blood by a process of exocytosis. It is carried by the blood to the tissues, where it binds to specific insulin receptors on the surfaces of the cells of virtually all tissues except liver and brain. Glucose binding activates membrane receptors, leading to the formation of protein kinase, which in turn promotes the movement of protein carriers from the cytosol to the plasma membrane. Glucose is then taken into the target cell by a process of facilitated diffusion.

Within the cell, glucose is rapidly phosphorylated and enters a variety of metabolic pathways. In muscles it may be converted into glycogen or

See **Active transport and facilitated diffusion** (page 50), in Ch. 2, Cells and the Internal Environment.

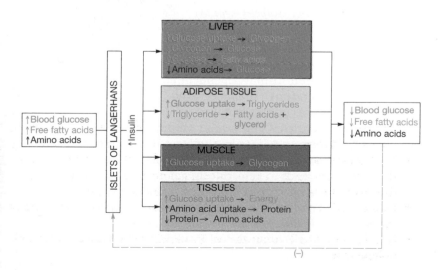

Figure 16.16 Regulation of the secretion and metabolic actions of insulin.

is broken down to liberate energy; in adipose tissue it is converted into fatty acids (Figure 16.16).

Insulin does not directly promote glucose uptake by the liver in the same way as in other tissues. It increases glucokinase activity in hepatocytes, which speeds up the phosphorylation of glucose, effectively trapping it within the cells and creating a steep glucose gradient, which favours its uptake by diffusion. At the same time it promotes glycogen synthesis. Insulin also inhibits phosphorylase, an enzyme that brings about glycogenolysis, so that release of glucose from the liver is reduced.

The overall action of insulin on carbohydrate metabolism is to increase glycogen deposition within the liver while lowering blood glucose levels.

Since the utilization of glucose is increased, that of fat decreases. Insulin is therefore said to promote fat 'sparing'. In the liver, insulin promotes the synthesis of fatty acids; these are then transported to adipose tissue, where they are stored. In the cells of adipose tissue insulin inhibits the action of hormone-sensitive lipase, which normally causes the hydrolysis of stored triglycerides (lipolysis) and thereby lowers free fatty acid concentration in the blood. Insulin also promotes glucose uptake and the formation of alpha-glycerophosphate (α-glycerophosphate) which is then converted to glycerol and to triglycerides in adipose tissue.

Insulin promotes the uptake of amino acids from the blood in many tissues. It increases mRNA translation and therefore promotes protein synthesis. Catabolism of protein is inhibited. In the liver, gluconeogenesis is depressed which further prevents protein breakdown and promotes protein formation. Blood amino acid concentration therefore falls.

Overall, insulin enables glucose to be used as a substrate for the production of energy. It promotes the uptake of glucose by many tissues and allows its subsequent breakdown to release energy. It swings the body's metabolic processes away from protein and fat as energy sources and towards glucose.

Effects of insulin deficiency (diabetes mellitus)

Diabetes mellitus is the most common of all endocrine diseases. It exists in two principal forms: type I, or insulin-dependent diabetes, which represents approximately one-quarter of all cases, and the more common type II, or non-insulin-dependent form.

In **insulin-dependent diabetes**, the pancreatic beta-cells are perceived as 'non-self' by the immune system. As a consequence they are attacked and destroyed and insulin production falls. Lack of insulin leads to a rise in glucose release by the liver and its underutilization by non-hepatic tissues with resulting hyperglycaemia. Ketone body production by hepatic cells leads to ketoacidosis, a potentially fatal condition.

In **non-insulin-dependent diabetes**, insulin deficiency is due to defective insulin receptors. It is a condition often precipitated by obesity and pregnancy. Both glucagon and insulin are present, but the activity of glucagon is much higher than that of insulin. Hyperglycaemia develops, but not ketoacidosis.

The **manifestations of diabetes** are many and can be understood in terms of a reduction in the effects of insulin on carbohydrate, fat and protein metabolism. There is reduced uptake of glucose by the cells of many tissues. Glycogenolysis and gluconeogenesis in the cells of the liver increase. Glucose accumulates in the blood, causing hyperglycaemia which results in glucose in the urine (glucosuria) and causes excessive fluid loss by the kidneys (polyuria) by the process of osmotic diuresis. Without treatment, the resultant dehydration can reduce blood volume, leading to circulatory failure, reduced cerebral blood flow, coma and death. The reduced blood pressure to the kidneys reduces or may even stop urine production, so that waste products such as urea accumulate in the blood (uraemia) and exacerbate coma.

See **Osmotic diuresis** (page 507), in Ch. 14, Renal Control of Body Fluid Volume and Composition.

In severe type I diabetes, in the absence of insulin, lipolysis is stimulated, leading to the release of free fatty acids. These are oxidized in the liver to acetyl-CoA which, in the absence of insulin, is unable to enter the Krebs cycle. Instead it is converted to acetoacetic, beta-hydroxybutyric acids and acetone, the so-called ketone bodies. The accumulation of these strong keto acids in the plasma causes metabolic acidosis. Some acetone is given off by the lungs and has a characteristic 'pear drops' or 'new-mown hay' odour. Keto acids appear in the urine (ketonuria). Some H^+ replaces K^+ in the cells and excessive amounts of K^+ may be lost in the urine. Lowering of the pH of the blood stimulates the respiratory centres, causing rapid, deep breathing (Kussmaul respiration) which results in excessive loss of CO_2. Failure of energy production and acidosis further contributes to the development of coma.

See **Ketoacidosis** (page 602), in Ch. 15, Digestion and Absorption of Food, and **Increased arterial H$^+$ concentration** (page 460), in Ch. 13, Respiration.

Protein breakdown occurs, leading to muscle wasting, and reduced protein synthesis impairs wound healing.

Diabetics usually have increased susceptibility to infection, probably due to the hyperglycaemia encouraging the proliferation of microorganisms.

Overall, therefore, nutrient levels in the blood rise, but the cells are unable to make use of them. There is, therefore, 'starvation in a sea of plenty'.

Effects of insulin excess

Excess insulin may result from the presence of an islet cell adenoma or, more commonly, to an insulin overdose; it leads to hypoglycaemia. The symptoms are primarily behavioural and may resemble drunkenness or mental aberration. The low level of blood glucose stimulates increased sympathetic activity with increase in heart rate, sweating and vasoconstriction in the skin. If blood glucose levels remain low the cells of the brain are not able to take in sufficient for their needs and hypoglycaemic coma may ensue.

GLUCAGON

Glucagon is a short polypeptide, consisting of a single chain of 29 amino acids, released by the alpha-cells of the islets of Langerhans. It is released primarily in response to a fall in blood sugar, but also a rise in amino-acid level (Figure 16.17), sympathetic stimulation and rises in the levels of gastrointestinal hormones (except secretin, which exerts an inhibitory

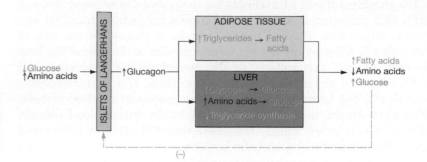

Figure 16.17 Regulation of the secretion and metabolic actions of glucagon.

influence). Glucagon secretion is inhibited by raised blood glucose and insulin.

Glucagon activates adenyl cyclase in the membranes of hepatocytes, leading to the formation of cyclic AMP. This, in turn, leads to an increase in the rate of conversion of glycogen to glucose (glycogenolysis) and a rise in blood glucose concentration. Glycogen synthesis is inhibited.

In the presence of increased levels of amino acids in the blood, glucagon promotes gluconeogenesis, in which amino acids are converted to glucose and blood amino acid levels fall.

Glucagon activates adipose cell lipase which increases lipolysis and, therefore, blood fatty acid concentration; it also inhibits triglyceride synthesis (lipogenesis) in the liver.

Effects of glucagon excess

Glucacon-secreting tumours are found occasionally, mostly in post-menopausal women. The effects of excess glucagon result in increased glycogenolysis and gluconeogenesis, leading to mild diabetes but without ketoacidosis. High levels of glucagon may contribute to the hyperglycaemia that is observed in uncontrolled diabetes.

SOMATOSTATIN

Somatostatin is a short peptide (14 amino acids) produced by the delta-cells of the islets of Langerhans. It has a very short half-life, only remaining in the blood for 3 minutes. Stimuli for its release include raised blood glucose, amino acid or fatty acid levels and increased amounts of gastrointestinal hormones.

Somatostatin depresses release of both insulin and glucagon by the pancreas. It reduces gut motility and also the secretion of digestive juices and the absorption of digestion products. Its action may extend the time period in which food, especially fat, is digested and assimilated.

PANCREATIC POLYPEPTIDE

Pancreatic polypeptide is a relatively small molecule consisting of 36 amino acids. Its release is stimulated by hypoglycaemia but it is also secreted in response to the ingestion of food, gastrointestinal secreta-gogues and cholinergic stimulation. It also inhibits exocrine secretion by the pancreas.

The adrenal glands

The two adrenal glands are located one on top of each kidney. Each gland is a flattened pyramid with a base measuring about 5 cm across, is about 1 cm thick and weighs approximately 10 g.

Each gland (Figure 16.18) is bounded by a capsule and contains two easily distinguishable areas, the outer cortex and the inner medulla. The cortices and medullae of the adrenal glands have different embryological origins and are functionally separate glands.

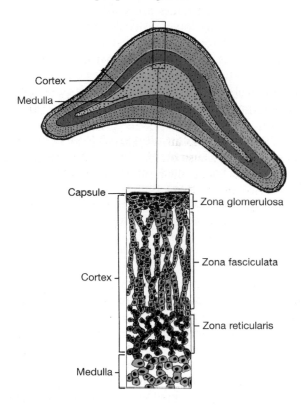

Figure 16.18 Section through an adrenal gland. (**Inset**) Histological appearance of adrenal tissue.

The adrenal cortices

The cortex constitutes approximatcly 80–90% of each gland (by volume). It contains three layers, or zones: the zona glomerulosa, the zona fasciculata and the zona reticularis.

The outermost layer, the **zona glomerulosa**, consists of columnar epithelial cells containing small numbers of lipid droplets. Cells are arranged in clusters separated by thin connective tissue septae that extend inwards from the capsule. This layer produces aldosterone and a small amount of deoxycorticosterone. These hormones are described as **mineralocorticoids** because they regulate the minerals Na^+ and K^+.

The middle layer, the **zona fasciculata**, comprises 80% of the cortex. It consists of long columns of pale, polyhedral cells one or two cells thick, separated by capillaries. The cells contain large numbers of large lipid droplets containing cholesterol esters, precursors of the hormones cortisol and corticosterone. These are termed **glucocorticoids** because of their actions on carbohydrate metabolism, although they also exert a number of other effects.

The innermost layer of the cortex, the **zona reticularis**, has an irregular boundary with the medulla. It consists of anastomosing networks of small cells, which contain fewer lipid droplets than those of the middle layer. This layer synthesizes small quantities of sex hormones, principally the male hormone (androgen) **dehydroepiandrosterone** (DHEA).

Synthesis of adrenocortical hormones (corticosteroids)

All of the adrenocortical hormones are synthesized from cholesterol, a major component of plasma low-density lipoprotein which is taken up by the adrenal cells by receptor-mediated endocytosis. Cholesterol is stored within the cells as cholesterol esters within lipid droplets. When the cell is stimulated, the enzyme cholesterol esterase causes the liberation of free cholesterol from storage; cholesterol is then converted enzymatically into the appropriate hormone, which is then released into the blood.

Since the cortical hormones are all derived from cholesterol they are structurally similar and because of this they exert overlapping functions. Cortisol, for example, has a mild mineralocorticoid action, which is about 500 times less potent than that of aldosterone. However, since cortisol is usually present in much higher concentrations than aldosterone, its mineralocorticoid activity is of some importance.

ALDOSTERONE AND DEOXYCORTICOSTERONE (MINERALOCORTICOIDS)

Both mineralocorticoids are present in the plasma in approximately the same concentrations (0.05–0.2 ng/mL), but aldosterone exerts an influence approximately 15 times that of deoxycorticosterone.

The release of aldosterone from the cells of the zona glomerulosa is mediated primarily by the action of the renin–angiotensin system and also in response to a rise in plasma K^+ and, to a much lesser extent, a fall in Na^+ (see Figure 14.18). ACTH induces only a transient increase in aldosterone output by a direct stimulatory mechanism. It does, however, maintain the adrenal cortex as a whole, and in its absence the zona glomerulosa regresses so that other stimuli do not function as effectively. Most aldosterone circulates unbound to protein and is metabolized in the liver.

Aldosterone promotes Na^+ reabsorption, K^+ secretion and some water reabsorption in the kidneys, salivary glands and sweat glands.

Effects of aldosterone deficiency (Addison's disease)

Lack of aldosterone secretion decreases Na^+ and water retention, leading to a reduced blood volume and dehydration. Since Na^+ is not reabsorbed by the kidneys, K^+ and H^+ are not secreted in exchange, so that hyperkalaemia and metabolic acidosis occur.

Effects of aldosterone excess

Benign aldosterone-secreting tumours of the adrenals (**Conn's**

Low density lipoproteins are described in **Lipid metabolism** (page 599), in Ch. 15, Digestion and Absorption of Food.

See also **Role of aldosterone in the regulation of sodium and potassium balance and blood volume (**page 505), in Ch. 14, Renal Control of Body Fluid Volume and Composition. The actions of aldosterone salivary glands are described in **Salivation** (page 544), in Ch. 15, Digestion and Absorption of Food, and the actions of aldosterone on sweat glands in **Acclimatization of sweating** (page 319), in Ch. 10, The Skin and the Regulation of Body Temperature.

syndrome) occur rarely and cause excessive loss of K⁺, with a consequent reduction in plasma levels (hypokalaemia) and Na⁺ and water retention, leading to hypertension.

More commonly, excessive aldosterone release is caused by high levels of renin released in response to conditions such as renal ischaemia or reduced effective plasma volume as in cardiac failure (**secondary hyperaldosteronism**).

CORTISOL AND CORTICOSTERONE (GLUCOCORTICOIDS)

The plasma concentration of cortisol is up to 30 times that of corticosterone (i.e. 180 ng/mL compared to 6 ng/mL). Cortisol is responsible for about 95% of glucocorticoid activity.

Cortisol (hydrocortisone) is released in response to ACTH from the adenohypophysis (Figure 16.19), a rise in plasma ACTH being followed 15–30 minutes later by a rise in cortisol.

ACTH activates adenyl cyclase in the cells of the zona fasciculata of the adrenal cortex which leads to the formation of cyclic AMP, with the consequent synthesis of cortisol from cholesterol. Rising plasma cortisol levels exert a negative feedback effect on the hypothalamus and adenohypophysis. Plasma cortisol levels are, however, far from constant, rising and falling between seven and 15 times each day, being generally low during sleep and rising to a particularly high level about 1 hour after waking (Figure 16.20).

Against this background of episodic release of cortisol, physical and mental stressors both act as potent stimuli for its rapid release (see *Cortisol and stress*, below).

A total of 75–80% of all cortisol molecules circulate bound to an alpha-globulin, transcortin; about 15–20% are bound to albumin and only 5% circulate unbound. It has a half-life of 70–90 minutes in the circulation and is metabolized mostly in the liver.

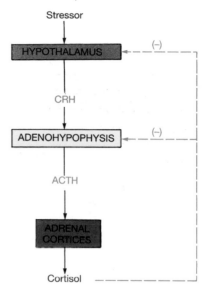

Figure 16.19 Relationships between the hypothalamus, adenohypophysis and adrenal cortices.

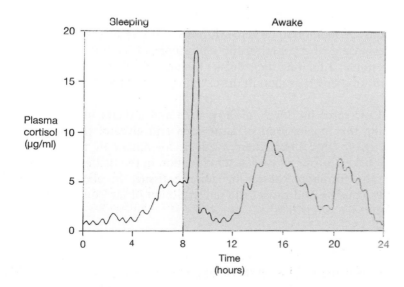

Figure 16.20 24-hour cycle of cortisol release.

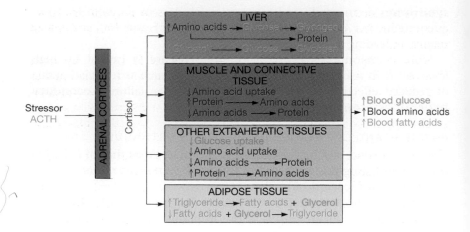

Figure 16.21 Role of cortisol in the regulation of glucose, amino acid and fatty acid metabolism.

Metabolic actions of cortisol

Cortisol raises blood sugar levels through a number of mechanisms (Figure 16.21).

- It facilitates the degradation of protein in muscles and connective tissue into amino acids and its subsequent conversion into glucose and glycogen in the liver. This process (gluconeogenesis) is of particular importance when fasting for long periods, since blood glucose and glycogen stored in the liver are used up within about the first 24 hours.
- Cortisol inhibits the uptake of glucose by cells by antagonizing insulin-stimulated glucose uptake and therefore decreases the utilization of exogenous glucose.
- Cortisol enhances glucagon release by the islets of Langerhans, which then promotes glycogenolysis in the liver.

Cortisol causes the amino acid concentration of plasma to rise. It achieves this by:

- reducing the conversion of amino acids into protein in all tissues, except the liver, where they are taken up and used for gluconeogenesis, in addition to protein synthesis;
- decreasing the extrahepatic utilization of amino acids by, for example, inhibiting their uptake by muscle cells;
- breaking down protein in the extrahepatic tissues.

Cortisol increases the levels of fatty acids and glycerol in the blood by increasing the mobilization of fatty acids and glycerol (lipolysis) from adipose tissue; this makes them available for uptake by the liver to be used to make glucose, as well as for oxidation in the tissues. Cortisol also retards the formation of fat by adipose tissue. In addition, cortisol increases appetite and causes the redistribution of fat from the extremities to the face and trunk.

Other actions of cortisol

Cortisol is also required for the maintenance of cardiovascular function and responsiveness. In its absence, excessive vasodilation can occur and there is a reduction in blood pressure. It also improves myocardial function and is thought to increase the number of beta-adrenoceptors in cardiac muscle.

Although its mineralocorticoid potential is about 500 times less than that of aldosterone, plasma concentrations are so much higher (up to 180 ng/mL compared to 0.2 ng/mL) that cortisol's effects are quantitatively of some importance. However, cortisol is not released in response to changes in body fluid volume or composition, since the cells of the zona fasciculata are not sensitive to angiotensin II.

When present in high concentrations, cortisol inhibits the body's immune responses, through a number of mechanisms. Cortisol:

- stabilizes lysosomal membranes, which prevents the release of the proteolytic enzymes whose actions lead to cellular destruction;
- decreases capillary permeability so that fewer leucocytes are able to gain access to inflamed areas;
- depresses the phagocytic activities of neutrophils;
- suppresses T lymphocyte activity, including formation of some of the proteins that support the inflammatory process, e.g. interleukin-1;
- stimulates the synthesis of anti-inflammatory proteins;
- inhibits the synthesis of proinflammatory substances;
- reduces the numbers of eosinophils and lymphocytes in the blood;
- slows down wound repair.

Cortisol influences the activities of the central nervous system. It modulates perception and emotions, although such influences are generally only recognizable in clinically altered states. Thus, for example, a sudden rise in cortisol induces a temporary euphoria followed by depression.

Effects of cortisol deficiency (Addison's disease and ACTH deficiency)

Two types of insufficiency are found; both are rare. Primary insufficiency (**Addison's disease**) is, in most cases, thought to be due to autoimmune destruction of cortical tissues and includes symptoms of aldosterone, as well as cortisol deficiency. Secondary insufficiency, due to lack of ACTH, only involves cortisol deficiency since aldosterone secretion is not directly regulated by ACTH.

Reduced levels of cortisol reduce the amount of glucose in the circulation and depress protein and fat breakdown. General weakness and dizzy spells commonly occur and there is an inability to withstand any sort of stress. Lack of cortisol in the blood removes inhibition of the hypothalamus, with the result that large quantities of ACTH are released into the blood. ACTH exhibits some MSH-like properties and, when present in large quantities, tends to increase skin pigmentation.

Effects of cortisol excess (Cushing's syndrome)

Excessive secretion of cortisol can be due either to the presence of a tumour in the adrenal cortex, or increased release of ACTH from the adenohypophysis.

Excess cortisol promotes a rise in blood sugar by reducing its uptake by the tissues, leading to 'adrenal diabetes'. Cortisol also encourages the removal of amino acids from the tissues and their deposition in the liver. As a result, there is muscle wasting, particularly in the limbs, and a breakdown of collagen, especially in the skin, which may tear subcutaneously, giving rise to purplish striae. Loss of protein from bones renders them fragile.

Cortisol causes the mobilization of fat from adipose tissue and its deposition in the face ('moon face'), abdominal wall and upper back ('buffalo hump').

Since cortisol is present in such large quantities, its mineralocorticoid properties become quantitatively even more important, causing Na⁺ and water retention, which leads to hypertension, and K⁺ loss, which promotes muscle weakness.

Excessive amounts of cortisol also suppress immune responses and their manifestations and render individuals particularly susceptible to infection.

Cortisol and stress

Stress can be defined as a psychophysiological state caused by a **stressor**. Precise identification of a stressor is, however, difficult. Physiological stressors are essentially 'strong' stimuli such as hypoglycaemia, hypotension, intense heat or cold. Psychological stressors include bereavement, anxiety, fear and restraint against one's will.

The nature of the stressor affects the type of response, so that physical trauma may elicit an inflammatory response where fear does not.

Hans Selye distinguished between local adaptive responses specific to a stressor, e.g. inflammation, and those due to any stressor, which he called '**the general adaptation syndrome**' (**GAS**).

GAS is divided into three phases: the alarm reaction, the stage of resistance and the stage of exhaustion (Figure 16.22).

In **the alarm reaction**, the body's resistance to stress initially falls and then rises above normal. It is accompanied by a sharp rise and then a fall in plasma cortisol concentration.

The stage of resistance reflects a period during which physiological responses are combating the stressor and plasma cortisol levels, though raised, are not particularly high.

The exhaustion stage is reached if the stressor persists after the

Figure 16.22 Selye's general adaptation syndrome. AR = alarm reaction; SR = stage of resistance; SE = stage of exhaustion.

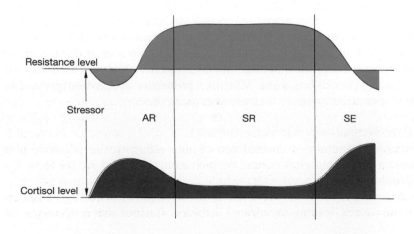

resistance stage. In this stage the body's resistance falls again and cortisol levels rise.

Cortisol is essential for life and its absence produces susceptibility to stress. Exactly how cortisol offers resistance to stressors is far from clear, but at least some of its actions can be seen in this context. The metabolic shift away from carbohydrate towards the oxidation of fat spares the body's limited stores of carbohydrate and draws upon the much larger stores of fat in adipose tissue. This is particularly appropriate in situations where a person may not feel like eating or is unable to move and gain access to food. Cortisol contributes to the maintenance of arterial blood pressure and thereby the avoidance of vascular shock.

ANDROGENS

The zona reticularis secretes small quantities of the androgen dehydroepiandrosterone (DHEA). DHEA is converted into **testosterone**, the primary male sex hormone, in the extra-adrenal tissues. Adrenal androgens are secreted in larger amounts during foetal development, as well as in early puberty, which suggests a growth-promoting role during this period. In men it has little effect, since much larger amounts are produced by the testes. In women, however, it thought to stimulate the growth of axillary and pubic hair. The sex drive in women has been attributed to the adrenal androgens.

The adrenal medullae

The medullae contain large epithelial cells arranged in rounded clusters or short cords around venules or capillaries. The medullary cells have a special affinity for stains containing chromium salts and are identified as chromaffin cells; they are, as a consequence, easily distinguishable from those of the cortex. The chromaffin cells synthesize the catecholamines adrenaline and noradrenaline; hormones which have a sympathomimetic effect.

ADRENALINE AND NORADRENALINE (CATECHOLAMINES)

The adrenal medullae are effectively modified sympathetic ganglia. Preganglionic sympathetic fibres innervate medullary cells and stimulate them to release their hormones directly into the blood. The two hormones synthesized and released by the adrenal medullae, adrenaline (known in the US as epinephrine) and noradrenaline (norepinephrine) are both catecholamines and are derived from tyrosine. Noradrenaline also functions as a postganglionic neurotransmitter in the sympathetic nervous system.

Preganglionic sympathetic fibres release acetylcholine, which depolarizes the membranes of the medullary cells and increases their permeability to Ca^{2+}. This causes exocytosis of stored granules of catecholamines into the blood. About 80% of the hormone liberated is adrenaline and 20% noradrenaline. Since each preganglionic fibre is in contact with several cells then relatively large quantities are released.

Many tissues contain alpha- and beta-adrenoceptors, which are varyingly sensitive to catecholamines. The precise consequence of the release of adrenomedullary hormones therefore depends upon the type of

See **Vascular shock** (page 421), in Ch. 12, Circulation of Blood and Lymph; see also **The autonomic nervous system and stress** (page 284), in Ch. 9, Autonomic and Somatic Motor Activity.

See **Sympathomimetic actions of adrenaline and noradrenaline** (page 281), in Ch. 9, Autonomic and Somatic Motor Activity.

See also **Adrenergic receptors** (page 281), in Ch. 9, Autonomic and Somatic Motor Activity.

receptors present in particular tissues. Adrenaline combines strongly with beta-adrenoceptors and less strongly with alpha-receptors, while noradrenaline combines strongly with alpha-adrenoceptors but only weakly with beta-adrenoceptors.

The physiological activities of the medullary hormones mirror those of the sympathetic nervous system and structurally the medullae are considered to be an extensions of that system.

In summary, adrenaline and noradrenaline prepare the body for the performance of physical activity, the so-called 'fright, fight or flight' response.

Noradrenaline brings about vasoconstriction in the skin, gut, kidneys, genitalia and mucous membranes, causing a rise in systolic and diastolic blood pressures. In skeletal muscle it also promotes constriction, but adrenaline exerts a more powerful vasodilating influence which lowers total peripheral resistance and diastolic blood pressure. Adrenaline causes an increase in the rate and strength of the heart beat, whereas noradrenaline exerts a less powerful influence on the force of contraction. Noradrenaline alone brings about slowing of the heart as a result of reflex action resulting from the rise in systemic blood pressure.

In the respiratory tract both hormones bring about bronchodilation, with adrenaline exerting the stronger influence.

Both hormones promote relaxation of the smooth muscle of the gut wall and of the urinary tract, with adrenaline exerting a stronger influence. Noradrenaline, in particular, causes contraction of both gastrointestinal and urinary sphincters.

In addition, both hormones bring about pupillary dilation by stimulating contraction of the radial muscles of the iris.

The metabolic actions of adrenaline are much more powerful than those of noradrenaline. The amounts of glucose and free fatty acids in the blood are increased, thereby providing a ready source of energy to perform physical activity. Adrenaline promotes gluconeogenesis and glycogenolysis in the liver, thereby increasing the amount of available glucose. It also induces glycogenolysis in skeletal muscle but, since muscle cells lack the enzyme glucose-6-phosphatase, glucose is not released into the blood. Adrenaline also increases the catabolism of glucose and can increase metabolic rate by up to 15%.

Adrenaline has several effects on the CNS, which noradrenaline does not show to any strong extent. These include the feelings of fear and anxiety, tremor and increased ventilation.

Effects of catecholamine excess (phaeochromocytoma)

Tumours of the adrenal medullae are relatively rare. They result in persistent secretion of catecholamines leading to the development of hypertension, due to increased peripheral vasoconstriction and increased cardiac output. Palpitations and tachycardia are also observed, as well as feelings of anxiety. Sweating is a common symptom.

Hypertension may be continuous, but often its occurrence is episodic as hormones are added to the circulation in sudden spurts due, for example, to pressure being exerted on the adrenals as a result of postural changes.

Regulation of blood glucose concentration

Glucose is only one of a number of possible sources of energy in most tissues, but it is the only source in nervous tissue, the retina and the germinal epithelium of the ovaries and testes. Failure to maintain glucose homoeostasis may have serious consequences and can, particularly because of its requirement by the brain, lead to coma and in extreme cases to death.

Should glucose levels become very high, then its high osmotic pressure in extracellular fluid may cause cellular dehydration. Its presence in high concentrations in plasma results in its loss in the urine which, in addition to representing loss of energy from the body, results in osmotic diuresis with loss of water and ions (see *Effects of insulin deficiency (diabetes mellitus)*, above).

The maintenance of a stable blood sugar concentration is brought about by the actions of a number of hormones that are detailed individually in other sections of this chapter.

Blood glucose rises after a meal, in the **absorptive state**, but then falls during the period between meals, the **postabsorptive state**.

Absorptive state

After a meal, when the products of digestion are being absorbed, glucose is added to the blood and its concentration rises to as high as 7 mmol/L. This absorptive state may last for up to 4 hours and is a period of relative carbohydrate excess. During this period a number of physiological mechanisms act to reduce the levels of glucose in the blood.

The rise in blood glucose directly stimulates the release of **insulin** from the islets of Langerhans of the pancreas. Insulin promotes the uptake of glucose by most tissues and its deposition as glycogen in the cells of the liver. The latter is particularly important as about two-thirds of the absorbed glucose is deposited as glycogen. Insulin also inhibits the release of glucose from the liver. At the same time, insulin inhibits triglyceride breakdown, thereby reducing the supply of fat to the tissues. By these means blood glucose concentration is prevented from rising excessively during the absorptive state.

Postabsorptive state

After the absorption of food has taken place, there is a relative lack of glucose and its concentration in the blood falls to 3–5 mmol/L. A fall in blood glucose stimulates the islets of Langerhans to release glucagon. **Glucagon** promotes glycogenolysis in the liver and the release of glucose into the blood. Glucagon also promotes gluconeogenesis in the liver, converting amino acids, lactate and glycerol to glucose. It also promotes the mobilization of fat (lipolysis) from adipose tissue.

Hypoglycaemia stimulates the hypothalamus which, in turn, causes sympathetic stimulation of the adrenal medullae and the release of catecholamines. **Adrenaline**, like glucagon, stimulates glycogenolysis and gluconeogenesis in the liver and promotes lipolysis.

A rapid fall in blood glucose or prolonged fasting stimulates receptors in the hypothalamus, which causes the release of GHRH, with the subsequent release of growth hormone by the adenohypophysis. **Growth hormone** depresses glucose utilization by the tissues and promotes the deposition of glycogen. It therefore reduces the removal of glucose from the blood stream and helps to maintain a stable level. The hormone also transfers the balance of energy production within the tissues from glucose towards fatty acids, by increasing triglyceride breakdown in adipose tissue.

Long term fasting stimulates the hypothalamus to release CRH which leads to the release of corticotrophin by the adenohypophysis. As a result cortisol output from the adrenal cortex increases. **Cortisol** promotes the formation of glucose from amino acids within the liver and decreases its usage by the tissues.

17

Sex and reproduction

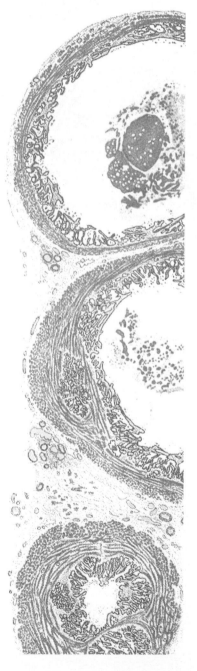

Female sex organs (genitalia)

The organs specific to the female sex (**primary sexual characteristics**) comprise two ovaries, two fallopian tubes, the uterus, the vagina and the external genitalia (Figures 17.1, 17.2). The breasts (mammae) containing rudimentary mammary glands are present in both sexes, but only in women do they develop and become functional, during lactation.

Figure 17.1 The internal female organs viewed from the front.

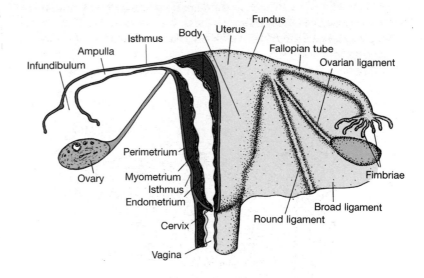

Figure 17.2 External female genitalia. The positions of the underlying greater vestibular glands and bulbs of the vestibule are also shown.

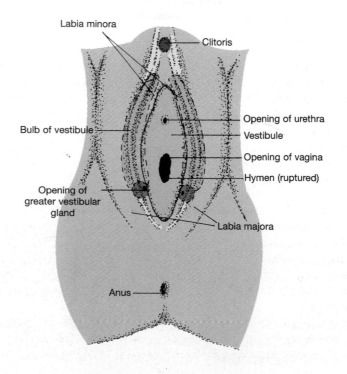

Ovaries

The ovaries have two principal functions: the production of eggs (ova) and the synthesis and secretion of sex hormones (oestrogens and progesterone).

Each ovary is a grey-pink ovoid body about 3 cm long, with a scarred and wrinkled appearance as a consequence of ovulation. The ovaries are held in place by the **ovarian** and **broad ligaments** on the rear wall of the abdominal cavity, although their precise position is variable, particularly after pregnancy, which displaces them.

The surface of each ovary is covered with a single layer of cuboidal epithelium (germinal epithelium), beneath which lies a cortex containing numerous **ovarian follicles**, each of which contains an immature egg (**oocyte**) (Figure 17.3). In the centre of the organ is a medulla of fibrous tissue containing blood vessels and nerve fibres.

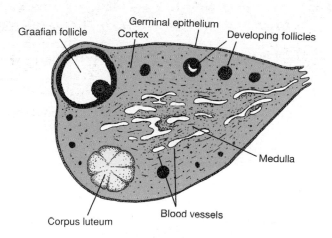

Figure 17.3 Section through an ovary.

At birth the ovaries contain about 2 million oocytes. Thereafter the number reduces through life: at puberty there are about 300 000 and by the end of the reproductive period (menopause) there are few, if any, oocytes still left. Usually, one oocyte matures approximately every 28 days. If ovulation occurs 13 times per year and proceeds uninterrupted by pregnancy for the entire reproductive period (say 35 years), then only about 455 oocytes will mature and be released at ovulation; the rest gradually degenerate.

OOGENESIS

The lengthy process of ova production (**oogenesis**) begins in the foetus with the development of primary oocytes from primitive germ cells (**oogonia**). Thereafter, development is suspended until puberty. Secondary oocytes are produced just before ovulation, but it is only if such an oocyte is fertilized that the final stage of development to the ovum occurs.

Early in foetal life, the oogonia divide repeatedly by mitosis (Figure 17.4). However, by the third month, proliferation of the germ cells ceases. The oogonia develop into **primary oocytes** which become

See **Mitosis** (page 55), in Ch. 2, Cells and the Internal Environment.

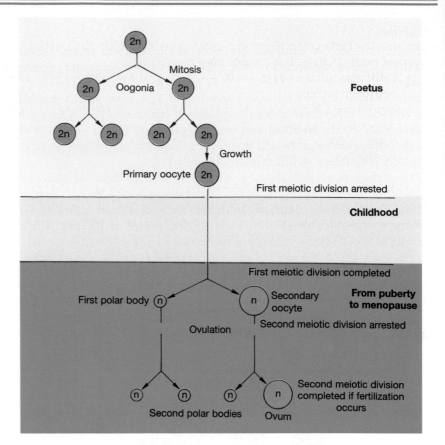

Figure 17.4 Summary of oogenesis. Oogonia divide early in fetal life and develop into primary oocytes. The cells are the usual diploid (2n). The first meiotic division is halted until just before ovulation (after puberty) when haploid (n) cells are produced containing two chromatids per chromosome: the secondary oocyte and the first polar body. After fertilization, the second meiotic division is completed producing an ovum and the second polar body (haploid cells with single chromosomes).

See **Meiosis** (page 57), in Ch. 2, Cells and the Internal Environment.

surrounded by a layer of flattened cells, forming a primordial follicle. The primary oocytes begin to divide by meiosis, the mechanism by which their chromosome number is halved. Division is halted, however, late in prophase I and the cells remain in this form until puberty.

The cells have 46 chromosomes, each with two chromatids.

During the follicular phase of the ovarian cycle, several of the primordial follicles mature. Just before ovulation of one of them, the first meiotic division (started at the very least some 10–14 years earlier) is completed, resulting in two daughter cells, containing 23 chromosomes, each with two chromatids. One daughter cell (**secondary oocyte**) receives nearly all the nutritious cytoplasm, the other (smaller) daughter cell is called the **first polar body**. The secondary oocyte starts the second meiotic division but is arrested in metaphase II.

If fertilization occurs, the second meiotic division is completed, producing daughter cells with 23 chromosomes with a single chromatid. In the same way as in the first meiotic division, the cytoplasm is unevenly divided so that the **second polar body** is small and the sister cell, the **ovum**, is much larger. The first polar body divides at the same time, producing two second polar bodies. All the polar bodies eventually disintegrate. From each fertilized primary oocyte, therefore, only one ovum is produced. This contrasts with the equivalent process in men (spermatogenesis) in which each primary spermatocyte produces four spermatozoa.

OVARIAN CYCLE

The ovarian cycle comprises the events occurring within the ovaries on average every 28 days. It is divided into three phases:

- **follicular phase** (days 1–10) – a period of follicular growth and oestrogen secretion;
- **ovulatory phase** (days 11–14) – terminates in the release of an oocyte from one ovary;
- **luteal phase** (days 14–28) – during which the corpus luteum synthesizes progesterone and oestrogens.

The duration of the luteal phase is remarkably constant (14 days), whereas the length of the whole ovarian cycle can vary from 21–40 days. These events are under hormonal control (see *Hormonal regulation of the ovarian and menstrual cycles*, below).

Each oocyte is surrounded by a single layer of flattened cells, the whole constituting a **primordial follicle**. Under the influence of follicle stimulating hormone (FSH), 10–25 primordial follicles begin to develop each month. The flattened cells become cuboidal and divide forming the **stratum granulosum** and the oocyte enlarges becoming surrounded by a thick membrane (**zona pellucida**) (Figure 17.5).

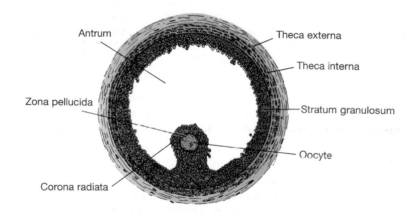

Figure 17.5 Mature (graafian) follicle from an ovary.

The connective tissue stroma surrounding the follicle differentiates into two layers: the **theca interna** and **theca externa**. Under the influence of luteinizing hormone (LH), the theca interna synthesizes male hormones (androgens), which are then converted into oestrogens by the granulosa cells. The granulosa and theca cells secrete very small amounts of progesterone. Inhibin, a protein hormone, is also secreted by the granulosa cells.

A fluid-filled cavity (**antrum**) appears within the stratum granulosum and the follicle enlarges further, largely by expansion of the antrum. The mature (**graafian**) follicle measures 1–1.5 cm in diameter and forms a bulge on the surface of the ovary. At **ovulation**, the follicle ruptures, releasing the oocyte and its surrounding sphere of granulosa cells (**corona radiata**) into the abdominal cavity.

Of the several follicles which begin to develop, usually all but one degenerate after about 7 days, becoming **atretic follicles**. Occasionally two oocytes are released, leading to the possibility of two fertilizations resulting in non-identical (**fraternal**) twins.

Following ovulation, the follicular cells enlarge forming a yellow body (**corpus luteum**), which synthesizes progesterone as well as oestrogens and inhibin.

If fertilization does not occur, the corpus luteum degenerates after about 12 days and becomes a white body (**corpus albicans**).

Fallopian (uterine) tubes

The fallopian tubes, whose openings lie close to the ovaries, transport the ovulated oocyte from the vicinity of the ovary to the uterus; fertilization can occur during this process.

The distal end of each tube is dilated into the **ampulla**, the principal site of fertilization, and terminates in the funnel-shaped **infundibulum**, fringed with ciliated, finger-like processes (**fimbriae**) (Figure 17.1). Around the period of ovulation, the fimbriae move over the surface of the ovary, the cilia create currents in the peritoneal fluid; these actions draw the oocyte from the peritoneal cavity into the fallopian tube.

The fallopian tubes, whose inner surfaces are thrown into folds, are some 10 cm in length and are lined with columnar secretory and ciliated cells. The secretory cells produce a fluid that moistens and nourishes the oocyte (and sperm, should they be present). The cilia beat towards the uterus, thereby aiding transport of the oocyte. A much more powerful propulsive action, however, is peristalsis by smooth muscle in the wall of the tube.

See **Peristalsis** (page 535), in Ch. 15, Digestion and Absorption of Food.

The proximal end of each tube, at the entrance to the uterus, is a constricted region called the **isthmus**. The fallopian tubes are held in position by part of the broad ligament and, unlike the ovaries, are covered by visceral peritoneum.

Uterus

The uterus lies in front of the rectum and above and slightly behind the bladder in the pelvis (Figure 17.6).

Figure 17.6 Midline section of the female pelvis.

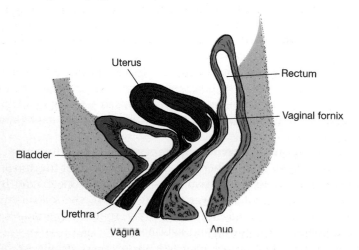

It is a muscular, thick-walled hollow organ which, in women who have not been pregnant, resembles an inverted pear, being 7–8 cm long and about 5 cm wide. It is usually larger after pregnancy.

The regions of the uterus are: 1) the **fundus**, which lies above the junction with the fallopian tubes; 2) the **body**, the main section; 3) the **isthmus**, a narrower section above 4) the **cervix** or neck, which projects into the vagina (Figure 17.1).

The uterine wall (Figure 17.1) comprises an outer layer of visceral peritoneum (**perimetrium**); a thick middle layer of smooth muscle (**myometrium**) and an inner mucous membrane (**endometrium**) comprising a layer of simple columnar epithelium with a connective tissue lamina propria beneath.

The endometrium is further subdivided into a superficial layer (**stratum functionalis**) and a **stratum basalis**. The stratum functionalis undergoes structural changes during the menstrual cycle and is shed during menstruation. Tubular **uterine glands** composed of columnar epithelium traverse the endometrium and open on to its surface. The mucosa of the upper two-thirds of the cervix contains glands that secrete alkaline mucus.

The uterus is supported inferiorly by the pelvic floor muscles and is held in position by various ligaments including the **round ligament**, which attaches it to the anterior abdominal wall.

UTERINE BLOOD SUPPLY

The **uterine arteries** arise from the internal iliac arteries in the pelvis and branch into several **arcuate arteries** in the myometrium. **Radial arteries** connect the arcuate arteries with **straight** and **coiled arteries** in the endometrium (Figure 17.7). The coiled arteries supply the stratum functionalis, whereas the straight arteries supply the stratum basalis. There is an extensive network of veins, some of which are enlarged into **sinuses**, in the endometrium.

MENSTRUAL CYCLE

The endometrial lining of the uterus undergoes cyclical changes each month which, like the events of the ovarian cycle, are regulated by hormones (see *Hormonal regulation of the ovarian and menstrual cycles*, below).

During the **menstrual phase** (days 1–5) the stratum functionalis is detached from the stratum basalis and, together with blood (50–150 ml in total) , constitutes the menstrual flow (**menses)** through the vagina.

The **proliferative phase** (days 6–14) is a period of regeneration of the stratum functionalis, stimulated by oestrogens.

The **secretory phase** (days 15–28) corresponds to the luteal phase of the ovarian cycle in which progesterone is secreted. The spiral arteries develop, the tubular glands become coiled and secrete glycogen into the uterine cavity. The endometrium becomes prepared for implantation by a fertilized ovum. If this does not occur, the corpus luteum degenerates and the subsequent fall in progesterone causes the spiral arteries to kink and constrict strongly. The resultant ischaemia causes the stratum functionalis to degenerate. At around day 28, the spiral arteries relax, blood

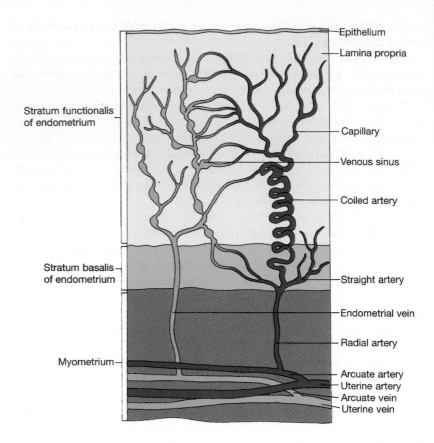

Epithelium
Lamina propria

Stratum functionalis
of endometrium

Capillary

Venous sinus

Coiled artery

Stratum basalis
of endometrium

Straight artery

Endometrial vein

Radial artery

Myometrium

Arcuate artery
Uterine artery
Arcuate vein
Uterine vein

Figure 17.7 Blood vessels of the uterine wall.

rushes into them and detaches the stratum functionalis, initiating the menstrual phase.

Dysmenorrhoea

The mechanism by which the spiral arteries constrict prior to menstruation involves prostaglandins. Women who have painful periods (cramps) usually produce increased amounts of prostaglandins, which cause uterine contractions and vasoconstriction elsewhere, which can cause headache, nausea and vomiting.

Endometriosis

Endometriosis is a condition in which endometrial tissue escapes from the uterine lining into the peritoneal cavity via the fallopian tube(s). The tissue most commonly lodges on the ovaries or linings of the fallopian tubes (causing sterility), but may also lodge in the wall of the colon. The tissue initiates inflammation and fibrosis and is subject to the monthly structural changes which are under hormonal control. Symptoms include pelvic pain, dysmenorrhoea and uterine or rectal bleeding.

Vagina

The vagina is a thin-walled tube, about 9 cm long, which runs from the cervix to the exterior of the body and which lies between the bladder and the rectum (Figure 17.6). It is penetrated by the penis during copulation, delivers the menstrual flow to the outside and acts as a birth canal during delivery of a baby.

The vaginal wall comprises an outer layer of connective tissue (**adventitia**), a middle layer of **smooth muscle** and an inner **mucosa**, lined by non-keratinized stratified squamous epithelium.

The epithelial cells contain stored glycogen, which is oxidized anaerobically by glycolysis to lactic acid; the resultant acid pH (3.5–4.0) offers resistance to invading microorganisms and sperm.

The mucosa does not contain glands, so that vaginal lubrication is dependent on mucus secreted by cervical glands or the external vestibular glands. The anterior and posterior walls of the vagina are normally in contact with each other.

The top of the vagina surrounds the cervix as a fold (**vaginal fornix**; Figure 17.6). The hymen is an incomplete partition across the vagina at its external opening (Figure 17.2). This vascular extension of the mucosa can be ruptured and bleed during the first sexual intercourse or during sporting activities or the insertion of a tampon or speculum.

> Glycolysis (page 595), in Ch. 15, Digestion and Absorption of Food; see also **Innate (non-specific immunity)** (page 355), in Ch. 11, Blood, Lymphoid Tissue and Immunity.

External genitalia (vulva)

The external genitalia comprise the mons pubis, the labia, the vestibule and the clitoris (Figure 17.2).

The **mons pubis** is the rounded, fat-containing area overlying the junction of the two pubic bones (pubic symphysis). After puberty, the mons pubis is covered with pubic hair.

The **labia majora** (Latin, 'larger lips') are two folds of skin containing fat, which run from the mons pubis and protect and enclose the thinner, more delicate, hair-free **labia minora** ('smaller lips'), which produce sebum that lubricates the vagina.

The **vestibule** is the area lying within the labia minora, which contains the external opening of the vagina lying posterior to the urethral orifice. One pea-sized **greater vestibular (Bartholin's) gland** lies either side of the vaginal opening and secretes mucus into the vestibule (Figure 17.2). These glands are the female counterpoint of the male bulbourethral glands.

The **bulbs of the vestibule** lie on either side of the vaginal orifice (Figure 17.2). Each bulb has a posterior, dilated end lying next to the greater vestibular gland, and a tapered anterior end next to the clitoris. The bulbs are the homologue of the male corpus spongiosum and become engorged with blood during sexual excitement.

The junction of the labia minora forms a hood (**prepuce**) over the **clitoris**, which lies immediately anterior to the vestibule. The clitoris is richly supplied with mechanoreceptors sensitive to touch and contains erectile tissue homologous to the corpora cavernosa in the male penis.

Breasts (mammae)

The two rounded breasts lie are attached to the thoracic pectoral muscles. Each breast is surmounted by a pigmented **nipple**, which lies slightly below the centre of each breast and is surrounded by a ring of pigmented skin (**areola**). The areola becomes larger and darker during pregnancy and the colour remains dark thereafter.

Erection of the nipples is caused by contraction of smooth muscle fibres within it, stimulated by cold, touch or sexual excitement.

Internally, each breast is subdivided into 15–20 lobes arranged radially from the nipple. The lobes are separated by interlobar connective tissue, which forms suspensory ligaments that support the breasts and attach them to the overlying skin and underlying muscle fascia. Adipose tissue, which in non-lactating women forms the bulk of the tissue, surrounds the lobes (Figure 17.8).

Figure 17.8 A breast with lactating mammary glands.

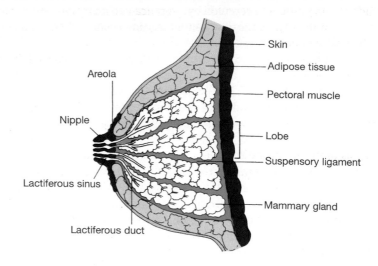

MAMMARY GLANDS

The mammary glands are modified sweat glands, compound alveolar in type, which lie within the lobes of the breasts.

The **secretory cells** vary in height from cuboidal to columnar depending on their secretory activity. They are surrounded by **myoepithelial cells** (basket cells), stellate, contractile cells that lie between the secretory cells and the basement membrane.

In non-pregnant women (and in men) the mammary glands are relatively underdeveloped. It is only during late pregnancy and during lactation that the glands develop fully and produce firstly colostrum and later milk (see *Lactation*, below).

Each lobe contains a **lactiferous duct** which drains the milk from the mammary glands and conveys it to the nipple, in response to suckling by the infant. Just below the areola, each duct has a dilated region (**lactiferous sinus**) where milk accumulates.

Glandular structures are described on page 77 in Ch. 3, Tissues.

Ovarian hormones

Ovarian hormones include two classes of steroids: oestrogens and progestogens, and a protein, inhibin.

See also **Cellular mechanisms of hormone action** (page 612), in Ch. 16, Endocrine Physiology.

Oestrogens

The ovaries produce two oestrogens, principally **oestradiol** and also **oestrone**. A much weaker hormone, **oestriol**, is synthesized from the other two in the liver and therefore also appears in the circulation. Oestrogens are secreted by the developing follicles and after ovulation by the corpus luteum.

Once released into the circulation, most oestrogen molecules become bound to albumin and oestrogen-binding globulin.

Oestrogens are essential for the development and maintenance of female organs and the secondary sexual characteristics (see *Puberty*, below). The hormones have some specific anabolic actions: promoting the growth of bones and closure of the epiphysial discs; growth of the epithelial linings of the fallopian tubes, uterus and vagina. They increase metabolic rate slightly.

Oestrogens increase the ciliary activity and contractility of the fallopian tubes and the excitability of uterine muscle. They stimulate the secretion of thin cervical mucus, which is less of a barrier to sperm than the thicker mucus that otherwise prevails. Oestrogens induce the synthesis of progesterone receptors in endometrial cells.

The hormones increase the vascularity and thickness of the skin and they promote salt and water retention by the kidneys, bone deposition by osteoblasts and lower blood cholesterol.

The liver inactivates oestradiol and oestrone by converting them to oestriol, as well as conjugating them with glucuronides and sulphates. About 20% of these salts are excreted in the bile, 80% in the urine.

> See also **Ossification and growth of long bones** (page 93), in Ch. 3, Tissues.

Progestogens

The major progestogen, **progesterone**, is secreted in very small amounts by both the granulosa and thecal cells of developing follicles and in much higher quantities by the corpus luteum. A second progestogen, **17-alpha-hydroxyprogesterone**, is also produced, albeit in extremely small quantities, and has the same actions as progesterone.

Progesterone circulates in the blood bound to albumin and progesterone-binding globulin, is rapidly converted into **pregnanediol** in the liver and has a half life of only about 5 minutes in the circulation.

Glandular secretion by the oestrogen-primed endometrium is stimulated by progesterone; it decreases myometrial and fallopian tube contractility and renders cervical mucus thick and sticky. All these actions are suitable preparation and support for early pregnancy, should it occur.

Progesterone has a thermogenic effect and causes a rise in body temperature of about 0.5°C after ovulation.

Inhibin

Inhibin is secreted throughout the ovarian cycle: by the granulosa cells during the follicular phase and by the corpus luteum in the luteal phase. Its name refers to its inhibitory action on the release of FSH by the adenohypophysis.

Figure 17.9 Changes in the plasma hormone levels during the ovarian and menstrual cycles.

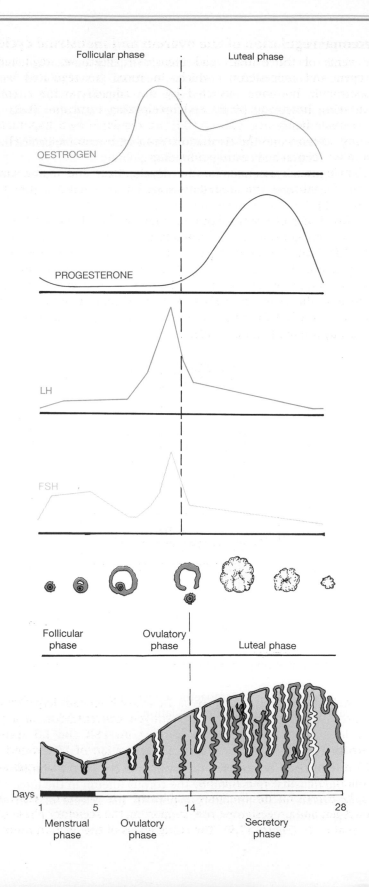

Hormonal regulation of the ovarian and menstrual cycles

The events of the ovarian and menstrual cycles are regulated by oestrogen and progesterone which, in turn, are regulated by the gonadotrophic hormones secreted by the adenohypophysis: **follicle stimulating hormone (FSH)** and **luteinizing hormone (LH)**. Like other trophic hormones, FSH and LH are regulated by a hypothalamic releasing hormone, **gonadotrophin releasing hormone (GnRH)**, and by negative feedback by ovarian hormones.

See also **Hypothalamic regulation of adenohypophysial hormone secretion** (page 617), in Ch. 16, Endocrine Physiology.

Following the degeneration of the corpus luteum, the plasma concentrations of oestrogens and progesterone are low and menstruation occurs (Figure 17.9).

The low levels of ovarian hormones means that their negative feedback effect on gonadotrophic hormone secretion is also low, and the levels of FSH and LH therefore rise. These hormones stimulate follicular development and oestrogen secretion which, in turn, stimulates growth of the endometrium. During this period oestrogen exerts an inhibitory influence on the secretion of LH and FSH: LH concentration stays fairly constant, whereas FSH concentration falls because its secretion is also inhibited by inhibin (Figure 17.10).

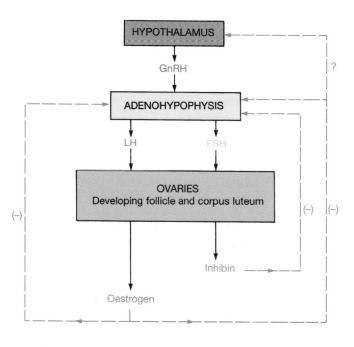

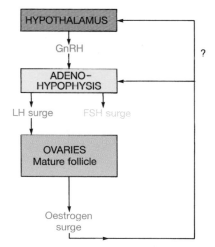

Figure 17.10 Negative feedback regulation of FSH and LH secretion via the adenohypophysis, and possibly the hypothalamus as well.

As one follicle reaches maturity in the ovary it releases large amounts of oestrogen which raises plasma oestrogen concentration to a point where it effects a positive feedback effect on FSH and LH secretion (Figure 17.11). The surge in plasma concentration of LH around days 12–13 is the trigger for ovulation to occur and for the transformation of the follicle into the corpus luteum.

As the corpus luteum becomes established, the plasma concentrations of oestrogen and progesterone rise, supporting the secretory phase of the menstrual cycle (Figure 17.9). The rising levels of the ovarian hormones

Figure 17.11 Positive feedback regulation of FSH and LH secretion initiated by the high plasma concentration of oestrogen produced by a mature ovarian follicle via the adenohypophysis, and possibly the hypothalamus as well. The LH surge then stimulates ovulation and the formation of the corpus luteum.

exert a negative feedback effect on gonadotrophin release, and inhibin further suppresses FSH secretion. In the absence of fertilization, the corpus luteum degenerates (possibly by producing a prostaglandin which destroys it); the plasma concentrations of oestrogen and progesterone consequently fall and the cycle repeats itself.

CONTRACEPTIVE PILLS AND IMPLANTS

'**The pill**' is an oral contraceptive that contains synthetic oestrogens and progestogens. The pill is taken daily for 21 days, during which the high doses of hormones suppress the levels of FSH and LH by negative feed-back so that ovulation does not occur. Withdrawal of the pill for 5 or 7 days results in an endometrial bleed stimulated by a fall in progestogen levels.

The '**mini-pill**' contains progestogen only, which changes the consistency of the cervical mucus and prevents sperm from entering the uterus.

An **implant** is available that consists of several tubes filled with crystals of progestogen. The tubes are placed surgically under the skin in the forearm, where they release the hormone at a constant low level for 5 years.

The 'morning-after pill' contains a high dose of a synthetic oestrogen which prevents implantation and is used as a postcoital contraceptive.

Female puberty

In young girls, the levels of both the ovarian hormones and the trophic hormones that regulate their output are very low. Research has shown that the hypothalamus is capable of releasing gonadotrophin releasing hormone, but that for some unknown reason it does not do so. Around the age of 8 years, however, GnRH secretion begins to rise and so the hypothalamus secretes increasing amounts of the trophic hormones LH and FSH. These then stimulate the ovaries to secrete greater quantities of oestrogens and the hormone-dependent changes of puberty begin.

There is an increase in height due to increased osteoblast activity in bones, the internal and external female sex organs enlarge and the **secondary sexual characteristics** develop. These include: development of the ductile system of the breasts; fat deposition, particularly in the breasts, buttocks and thighs; growth of pubic and axillary hair (although this is caused by adrenal androgens). The whole process of puberty normally takes several years before the first menstrual period (**menarche**) occurs, after which women enter the (potential) reproductive or child-bearing period.

Menopause

Menopause, popularly called the 'change of life', is the term applied to the period of time during which ovarian function reduces to a low level of activity and ovulation ceases. It may last from a few months to a few years and usually occurs between 45 and 55 years of age.

The small number of follicles remaining in the ovaries at the menopause have become relatively unresponsive to gonadotrophins. This results in very low levels of ovarian sex hormones and high levels of

FSH and LH which are no longer suppressed by negative feedback.

The combined effect of low steroids and high gonadotrophins can induce a number of physical and mental changes over several years. These include mood changes, fatigue, dyspnoea and 'hot flushes' (intense vasodilation, particularly of the face) and night sweating. The menstrual periods and ovulation both eventually cease.

Following the menopause, the ovaries reduce in size and few if any primary oocytes remain. Oestrogen output virtually ceases. The effects of oestrogen deficiency include: a reduction in the total amount of adipose tissue and its more even distribution; a reduction in size of the uterus, vagina and breasts; a thinning and drying of the epithelial linings of the fallopian tubes, uterus and vagina; thinning of the skin; and increased incidence of osteoporosis and arteriosclerosis.

Hormone replacement therapy (**HRT**), which uses low doses of oestrogen, reduces the menopausal symptoms and subsequent changes resulting from oestrogen deficiency. The rate of bone loss is reduced, thereby reducing osteoporosis, and cholesterol levels fall, thereby reducing the incidence of arteriosclerosis. There is possibly an increased risk of breast cancer.

As the female libido is thought to be caused by adrenal androgens, the menopause does not affect it.

See also **Lack of bone salt (osteoporosis and osteomalacia** (page 95), in Ch. 3, Tissues; arteriosclerosis is explained in **Ischaemic heart disease** (page 390), in Ch. 12, Circulation of Blood and Lymph.

Hypogonadism from birth (female eunuchism)

Hypogonadism due to surgical removal of the ovaries in an adult woman results in the same changes as the menopause. If ovaries are absent or underfunction from birth, however, then the female organs remain infantile and the secondary sexual characteristics do not develop. In addition, the action of oestrogen in closing the epiphysial discs is reduced, so that such young women become as tall as or taller than men.

Female hypergonadism

Tumours of the granulosa or thecal cells secrete oestrogens and cause irregular endometrial bleeding as well as development of the secondary sexual characteristics.

An **ovarian teratoma** is a cyst comprising fibrous tissue surrounding atrophied ovarian tissue. The cyst wall may contain a variety of tissues and organs including nervous tissue, muscle, skin, bone, teeth, intestine, lung and thyroid. Active thyroid tissue can produce symptoms of hyperthyroidism.

Female sexual responses

Sexual sensations can be initiated by tactile stimulation of a variety of 'erogenous zones', particularly the clitoris and vagina, from where sensory signals pass into the sacral segments of the spinal cord through the pudendal nerve, and thence to spinal reflex arcs and to the sensory cortex.

Sexual sensations are conveyed via the anterolateral system (page 218), in Ch. 7, Sensory Processing.

The bulbs of the vestibule and the clitoris are innervated by parasympathetic neurones in the nervi erigentes from the sacral region of the spinal cord. Stimulation of these neurones causes vasodilation and erection of the tissues. Parasympathetic neurones also stimulate the greater vestibular glands which respond by increasing mucus secretion into the vestibule.

The vaginal mucosa and breasts also become engorged with blood and the nipples become erect by smooth muscle contraction.

During the female **orgasm** or climax, the uterus and vagina undergo rhythmic contraction and the heart rate and blood pressure increase. These events are stimulated by increased sympathetic activity.

There is widespread tonic contraction of skeletal muscles. The muscles in the vestibular and anal area contract rhythmically.

These intensely pleasurable experiences are followed by a period of calm relaxation (**resolution**). Unlike the male orgasm, the female orgasm does not have a refractory period, so that more than one orgasm can follow in rapid succession. Female orgasm is not necessary for conception to occur, although some of the actions might facilitate the transport of sperm through the uterus into the fallopian tubes.

Male sex organs (genitalia)

The organs specific to the male sex (**primary sexual characteristics**) comprise two testes, the penis, a system of ducts that transport spermatozoa in testicular fluid from the testes to the penis and a number of accessory glands that secrete fluids into the ducts (Figure 17.12). The mixture of fluids ejaculated from the penis is known as **semen**.

Testes

The testes are contained within the **scrotum**, which lies outside the abdomen, suspended at the root of the penis. As a result, the testes are maintained at a temperature around 34°C rather than at the core body temperature of 37°C, which would kill the sperm. The scrotum is a loose sac of heavily pigmented skin and fascia, overlying a layer of smooth muscle (**dartos muscle**), which contracts in response to cold or sexual excitement, wrinkling and reducing the surface area of the scrotum. The **cremaster muscle**, skeletal muscle that connects the testis to the abdominal wall, also contracts in the cold, raising the testes nearer to the abdomen.

In the foetus, the testes begin to develop within the abdominal cavity near the kidneys. The descent of the testes usually starts about 2 months before birth and is complete by about 1 month after birth. **Undescended testes** (**cryptorchidism**) cannot produce viable sperm and have an increased risk of testicular cancer. The condition can be corrected by the administration of testosterone or by surgical intervention.

Each testis is ovoid and measures approximately 2.5 cm by 4.5 cm. It has a connective tissue capsule connected to intratesticular septa that

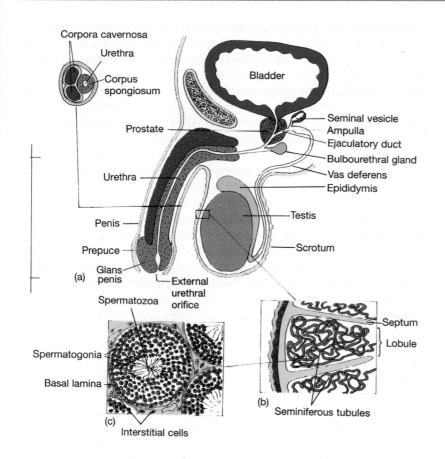

Figure 17.12 **(a)** Midline section of the male pelvis showing the location of the male organs. (**Inset**) A cross-section through the penis showing the relationships between the corpora cavernosa, the corpus spongiosum and the urethra. **(b)** An enlarged section of the testis showing a lobule containing seminiferous tubule(s). **(c)** An enlarged cross-section of a seminiferous tubule containing developing spermatozoa.

incompletely divide it into 200–300 wedge-shaped lobules. Each lobule contains one or more highly convoluted **seminiferous tubules**, lined by cells that produce spermatozoa (Figure 17.12). Between the seminiferous tubules, the **interstitial cells** (**Leydig cells**) produce male hormones (androgens) and inhibin, a hormone also synthesized by the ovaries.

The seminiferous tubules contain tall cells (**sustentacular** or **Sertoli cells**), which extend from the basal lamina to the lumen. These cells nurture the developing spermatozoa, secrete testicular fluid in which the spermatozoa leave the testes and remove cellular debris produced during spermiogenesis.

Another important role played by the sustentacular cells is that they form the **blood–testis barrier**. The barrier comprises tight junctions between the cells, which prevent any antigenic membrane proteins from the developing sperm gaining access to blood vessels surrounding the seminiferous tubules. This prevents an autoimmune reaction being mounted against the sperm.

SPERMATOGENESIS

The process by which primordial male germ cells (**spermatogonia**) produce mature germ cells (**spermatozoa**) is called **spermatogenesis**. It is the equivalent of oogenesis in females.

Spermatogenesis begins at puberty in the seminiferous tubules and continues throughout life. The process takes about 74 days. Estimates vary, but the two testes probably produce over 100 million sperm per day.

The primordial spermatogonia, which lie in the outermost few layers of the seminiferous tubules, divide by mitosis, producing a clone. Some of these cells differentiate into **primary spermatocytes**; others remain as primordial spermatogonia, providing a source of future spermatozoa (Figure 17.13).

As development proceeds, successive generations of cells are pushed towards the centre of the seminiferous tubules.

The primary spermatocyte enlarges and undergoes the first meiotic division, forming two **secondary spermatocytes** (23 chromosomes, each with two chromatids), which undergo the second meiotic division producing **spermatids** (23 chromosomes, each with one chromatid). Spermatids then differentiate into spermatozoa (**spermiogenesis**), during which process they lose cytoplasm and develop a tail. All the descendants of the same spermatogonium remain attached to each other by cytoplasmic bridges until the final stage, when spermatozoa are formed. This reduces the possibility of immature antigenic sperm passing through the blood–testis barrier.

See **Mitosis** (page 55), in Ch. 2, Cells and the Internal Environment.

See **Meiosis** (page 57), in Ch. 2, Cells and the Internal Environment.

Figure 17.13 Summary of spermatogenesis. Spermatogonia divide after puberty and develop into primary spermatocytes (diploid cells, 2n). The primary spermatocytes undergo the first meiotic division which produces secondary spermatocytes which are haploid (n) and each chromosome contains two chromatids. The second meiotic division produces spermatids (haploid cells with single chromosomes), which then mature into spermatozoa by the process called spermiogenesis.

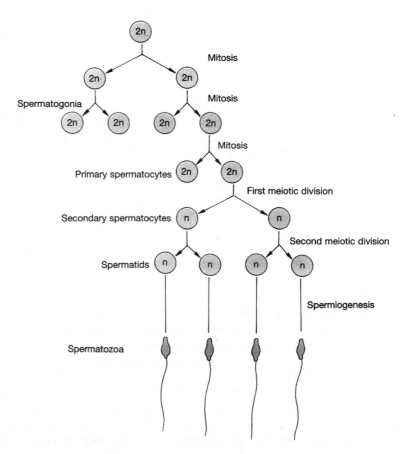

A spermatozoon comprises a head, midpiece and tail (flagellum) (Figure 17.14).

The **head** comprises a nucleus containing DNA with an enzyme-filled vesicle (**acrosome**) at the tip. The acrosome enables the sperm to penetrate the ovum (see *Fertilization*, below).

The **midpiece** contains mitochondria which produce energy, principally for movement.

The **flagellum** contains contractile filaments capable of producing a whip-like movement, propelling sperm at a velocity of 1–4 mm/min.

After ejaculation sperm are viable for only 1–2 days at body temperature. Once inside the female genital tract they are activated by a process called **capacitation** (takes 1–10 h), which is essential if fertilization is to occur. The sperm head membrane becomes weaker and also more permeable to Ca^{2+}, which therefore enters the cell and causes the activity of the flagellum to change from a weak, undulating motion to a more forceful whip-like action. The Ca^{2+} also facilitates enzyme release from the acrosome.

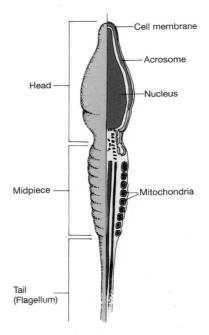

Figure 17.14 A mature spermatozoon (sperm).

Epididymis, vas deferens and urethra

The spermatozoa are conveyed from each testis to the exterior by a series of ducts: the epididymis, vas deferens and urethra.

The spermatozoa produced in the testis are conveyed from the efferent ductules, lined by ciliated columnar epithelium, into the duct of the **epididymis**, a coiled tube some 6 m long. The epididymis, which has a head, body and tail region, lies next to the testis, posterolaterally. The duct is lined with pseudostratified epithelium. Some of the cells secrete glycoproteins into the lumen, which is then adsorbed on to the surface of the spermatozoa. During their passage through the duct of the epididymis (about 20 days) the spermatozoa mature and become mobile. During ejaculation, the smooth muscle in the wall of the duct of the epididymis contracts from the tail upwards, pushing the spermatozoa into the vas deferens.

The **vas deferens** (ductus deferens) is approximately 45 cm long and conveys testicular fluid containing spermatozoa from the epididymis into the ejaculatory duct in the pelvic cavity. This fluid makes up about 10% of the total volume of semen. The vas is lined by columnar, non-ciliated epithelium. It has a dilated end (**ampulla**) which joins with the duct of the seminal vesicle, forming a common duct, the **ejaculatory duct**, which, in turn, joins the urethra in the prostate gland (Figure 17.12). During ejaculation, the smooth muscle in the wall of the vas undergoes peristalsis, thereby transporting sperm into the urethra.

The **urethra** is about 20 cm long, originates at the base of the bladder and conveys semen and urine to the exterior.

See also **Urethra** (page 477), in Ch. 14, Renal Control of Body Fluid Volume and Composition.

Accessory glands

The two seminal vesicles, two bulbourethral glands and the prostate gland (Figure 17.12) collectively secrete fluid, which constitutes 90% of semen.

Each **seminal vesicle** lies between the posterior surface of the bladder and the rectum and is about 5 cm long. The vesicles are single tubes lined with secretory cells, which produce about 60% of the volume of semen. The viscous, pale yellow fluid contains fructose and other nutrients, fibrinogen and prostaglandins. The prostaglandins cause the cervical mucus to become more receptive to the spermatozoa and possibly cause peristaltic contractions in the uterus and fallopian tubes, propelling the sperm towards the fallopian tubes.

The **prostate gland** encircles the top of the urethra, beneath the bladder. It is about 4 cm across, 3 cm high and 2 cm deep. The secretory tissue is contained in follicles within the gland that connect with 12–20 excretory ducts. The smooth muscle in the capsule of the prostate contracts during ejaculation. The thin, white fluid secreted by the prostate gland (about 30% of the total volume of semen) is alkaline and therefore reduces the acidity of fluid from the vas and also counteracts the acidity of the vagina. Sperm are optimally motile at pH 6–6.5. The fluid also contains a clotting enzyme, which, when mixed with fibrinogen in the fluid from the seminal vesicles, produces fibrin. This causes the semen to coagulate which gives it greater adherent properties. Profibrinolysin in prostatic fluid becomes fibrinolysin (plasmin), which breaks down fibrin in the semen in 15–20 min. The motility of the spermatozoa after this is much greater.

The prostate gland often hypertrophies after the age of 45–50, occluding the urethra and causing difficulty with micturition and an increased incidence of bladder infection.

The yellow, spherical **bulbourethral glands** lie on either side of the membranous urethra and measure about 1 cm in diameter. They secrete mucus into the semen before ejaculation.

> Fibrinolysis is described on page 331 in Ch. 11, Blood, Lymphoid Tissue and Immunity.

Penis

The penis, like the testes, lies externally, beneath the abdomen. The tip of the penis is enlarged, forming the **glans penis**, which is covered by the **foreskin** (**prepuce**), unless this has been surgically removed (**circumcision**). The penis contains three longitudinal columns of erectile tissue: the **corpus spongiosum**, which surrounds the urethra and is continuous with the glans penis; and the two **corpora cavernosa**, which lie side by side in front of the corpus spongiosum (Figure 17.12). The erectile tissue consists of a sponge-like network of trabeculae, containing connective tissue and smooth muscle fibres, which enclose vascular spaces connected to blood vessels. During erection the vascular spaces become engorged with blood and the penis becomes hard rather than flaccid and therefore adapted for penetration.

Testicular hormones

The male sex hormones (androgens) produced by the interstitial cells of Leydig, in the testes, comprise the steroids **testosterone, dihydrotestosterone** and **androstenedione**.

Testosterone is converted within most target cells to the more potent hormone dihydrotestosterone.

> See also **Cellular mechanisms of hormone action** (page 612), in Ch. 16, Endocrine Physiology.

The major androgen, testosterone, is mostly carried in the blood bound to albumin or gonadal steroid-binding globulin, where it remains for 30–60 min.

Androgens are essential for the development and maintenance of male organs and the secondary sexual characteristics (see *Male puberty*, below). They are anabolic steroids whose principal actions are caused by an increase in protein synthesis. They also raise basal metabolic rate by up to 15% and are responsible for the sex drive (libido). In men who have inherited a baldness trait, testosterone causes hair loss from the top of the head.

The inactivation of testosterone is similar to that of oestrogens. The liver converts testosterone to androsterone and dehydroepiandrosterone and conjugates them with glucuronide or sulphate. These salts are then excreted in the bile or the urine.

The interstitial cells also secrete the protein inhibin, which, like its counterpart in women, inhibits the secretion of FSH from the adenohypophysis.

Hormonal regulation of testosterone secretion

The adenohypophysial hormones **FSH** and **LH** regulate the activities of both male and female gonads. The names, however, relate to female follicles and the corpus luteum rather than to male structures, although LH is also known as **interstitial cell stimulating hormone (ICSH)** in men.

LH stimulates the interstitial cells in the testes to secrete testosterone, which in turn exerts a strong negative feedback effect on the hypothalamus and a weaker action on the adenohypophysis (Figure 17.15).

Spermatogenesis is initially stimulated by both FSH and testosterone, and probably maintained by testosterone alone. FSH output is inhibited by inhibin, not by testosterone.

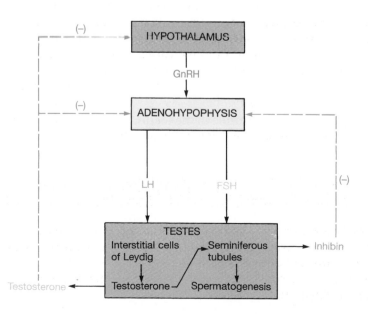

Figure 17.15 The relationships between the hypothalamus, the adenohypophysis and the testes.

Male puberty

The development of the male organs during foetal development is caused by testosterone secreted in response to placental HCG (see *Placenta*, below).

A few weeks after birth, the interstitial cells reduce in number and the hormone levels fall correspondingly until the onset of puberty. During childhood, the plasma levels of the gonadotrophic hormones are also very low, for unknown reasons. It is likely that a contributory factor is that the hypothalamus is highly sensitive to the negative feedback action of testosterone. Towards puberty, which generally occurs later in boys than in girls, the sensitivity of the hypothalamus reduces, so that the secretion of GnRH increases, causing an increase in gonadotrophin secretion, which in turn increases the concentration of circulating testosterone.

The raised plasma testosterone levels at the onset of puberty stimulate the growth of the penis, testes and scrotum, as well as the accessory organs. The hormone has a strong anabolic effect and also promotes physical growth and development of organs other than sex organs. This gives rise to male **secondary sexual characteristics**: growth and increased strength of bone and muscle; enlargement of the larynx, with an accompanying deepening of the voice; growth of facial, pubic and axillary hair and body hair in general. Testosterone stimulates sebaceous gland secretion, which can cause acne.

The pelvis narrows and lengthens. Growth of the long bones ceases after closure of the epiphyses, an event which is generally later in boys than girls. Testosterone also has a mild salt and water retaining action on the kidneys.

Sebaceous glands are described on page 313 in Ch. 10, The Skin and the Regulation of Body Temperature.

Male hypergonadism

Excessive amounts of testosterone are produced rarely by testicular tumours. If the interstitial cells are involved then precocious puberty is induced in young boys, with early closure of the epiphyses and consequent small stature. Tumours of the seminiferous tubules can contain tissues such as hair, teeth, skin, bone, nerve, muscle or even placental tissue. The production of placental oestrogens can cause breast development (**gynaecomastia**).

Male hypogonadism

In the absence of testosterone in the foetus, female organs develop.

Testosterone deficiency prior to puberty results in male **eunuchism**, in which the primary sexual characteristics remain infantile and the secondary sexual characteristics do not develop. The bones and muscles are relatively weak and closure of the epiphyses is delayed, so that the overall height can increase. Facial and body hair does not develop and balding does not occur. The larynx remains small, so that the voice is high-pitched.

Male **castration** after puberty results in some diminution of sexual characteristics, but they remain more developed than they were before puberty.

Male sexual responses

Sexual arousal can be stimulated by a multitude of cerebral stimuli (e.g. auditory, visual, olfactory, emotion and erotic thoughts) as well as by mechanical stimulation, particularly of the glans penis. The sensory fibres relay in the sacral region of the spinal cord. Parasympathetic stimulation via the nervi erigentes of the small arteries, which supply the vascular spaces in the penis, is increased; sympathetic tone is simultaneously reduced. Engorgement of the vascular spaces results in erection of the penis, a process aided by compression of the venous drainage.

Parasympathetic stimulation of the bulbourethral and urethral glands increases the secretion of lubricating mucus, which flows out along the urethra during sexual intercourse (coitus).

When sexual stimulation becomes very intense, the balance of autonomic activity changes, so that sympathetic activity becomes dominant. Fibres from the upper lumbar segments of the spinal cord innervate the genital organs involved, as well as the internal sphincter of the bladder.

Prior to the expulsion of semen to the exterior (**ejaculation**), the various fluids that constitute semen are collected together in the urethra, a process called **emission**. Emission and ejaculation constitute the male **orgasm**. Firstly the vas deferens contracts, propelling the sperm in testicular fluid into the urethra. Secondly the coat of the prostate gland contracts, and lastly the seminal vesicles contract so that the fluids mix together with the mucus secreted by the bulbourethral glands. The internal sphincter of the bladder contracts, preventing urine leaving or semen entering.

The distended urethra stimulates mechanoreceptors, which convey sensory impulses along the pudendal nerves. This conveys a sensation of fullness and also stimulates rhythmic contractions both of the internal genital ducts and of skeletal muscles that compress the erectile tissue at the base of the penis. These muscle contractions are supported by thrusting movements of the pelvic and trunk muscles, all of which cause ejaculation of the semen out of the penis and (if heterosexual intercourse is taking place) deep into the vagina or cervix.

There are some similarities between the male and female orgasm: local rhythmical contractions and generalized muscular contraction; a rise in heart rate and blood pressure; and feelings of intense pleasure followed by a period of relaxation. A major difference, however, is that there is a latent period in men during which a second erection is not possible. The length of this period is extremely variable, from a few minutes to several hours.

Pregnancy

Pregnancy covers the period from conception (fertilization of the oocyte) until the baby is born. The developing baby (conceptus) starts life as a **pre-embryo** (weeks 1–2), becomes an **embryo** (weeks 3–8) and later a

foetus (week 9 onwards). The period of intrauterine development (**gestation**) is measured from the first day of the last menstrual period, i.e. 2 weeks before ovulation. Gestation is usually 40±2 weeks.

Fertilization

The secondary oocyte together with the corona radiata is released into the peritoneal cavity at ovulation (see *Ovarian cycle*, above). The small cell mass enters the fallopian tubes and is moved along it, principally by peristalsis at first, later by the much weaker ciliary action alone (see *Fallopian (uterine) tubes*, above). The oocyte is viable 12–24 hours after ovulation. It remains within the fallopian tube for up to 4 days.

Semen, containing as many as 250 million spermatozoa, is deposited in the upper vagina during sexual intercourse (copulation or coitus). Spermatozoa have been detected in the distal fallopian tube only 5 minutes after ejaculation. It is unlikely, however, that such progress is due to their swimming action alone, rather that they 'surf' over the mild myometrial contractions that occur about 80% of the time. Their frequency is about three contractions per minute, travelling towards the fallopian tubes. One possible cause of infertility is the reduction or absence of these myometrial contractions. Of the 250 million sperm in the ejaculate, however, as few as 50 may reach the oocyte.

Only one spermatozoon actually fertilizes the oocyte. The sperm head binds to receptors on the outer surface of the zona pellucida that surrounds the cell. The acrosomal enzymes in the sperm head (Figure 17.4) then digest a hole through the zona pellucida and the sperm enters the space immediately surrounding the egg. Several sperm bind to the zona pellucida, but the first one to penetrate it fuses with the egg. Contractile elements in the egg draw the sperm head into the cytoplasm. The fertilized egg (**zygote**) immediately secretes substances that prevent other sperms entering and trigger the second meiotic division (see *Oogenesis*, above). Within 24 hours the male and female chromosomes have become surrounded by a membrane, forming pronuclei that move to the centre of the cell, and the chromosomes replicate. The cell divides by mitosis, but without growth, several times, forming a cluster of 16 or 32 cells, called a **morula**.

Should the daughter cells separate during these early cell divisions, then development to term would produce identical siblings, most often twins, but occasionally triplets or quadruplets.

Implantation and early development

The morula enters the uterus where it floats freely for about 3 days, during which time its cells continue to divide. During the next few days the **blastocyst** develops; a hollow sphere of cells with an inner cell mass which will give rise to the foetus and an outer **trophoblast**, which forms the placenta (Figure 17.16).

Around 7 days after ovulation, the blastocyst begins to implant into the endometrium, assisted by proteolytic enzymes secreted by the trophoblast. By about 11 days after ovulation, implantation is complete.

Rarely, implantation takes place in sites other than the uterus: the fallopian tube or even the abdominal cavity. Such **ectopic pregnancy**

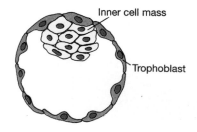

Figure 17.16 A blastocyst. The inner cell mass develops into the fetus; the trophoblast becomes the placenta.

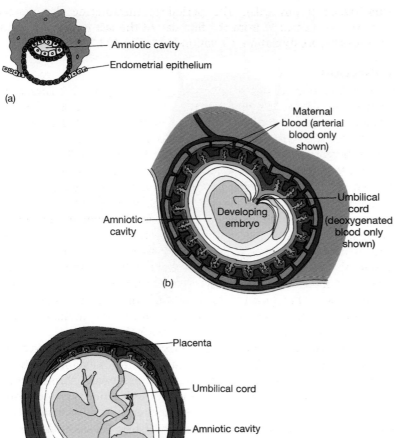

(a)

Amniotic cavity

Endometrial epithelium

Maternal blood (arterial blood only shown)

Amniotic cavity

Developing embryo

Umbilical cord (deoxygenated blood only shown)

(b)

Placenta

Umbilical cord

Amniotic cavity

Developing foetus

Uterus

(c)

Figure 17.17 Various stages of development of the conceptus. **(a)** Early implanted blastocyst. **(b)** 1-month embryo. **(c)** 3-month foetus.

cannot be sustained and is either followed by spontaneous abortion or surgical removal.

The **amniotic cavity**, containing **amniotic fluid**, develops within the inner cell mass (Figure 17.17).

The embryo and then the foetus float in amniotic fluid, attached by the umbilical cord to the placenta.

The corpus luteum remains the main source of progesterone during the first 6–8 weeks. Under the influence of progesterone the cells of the endometrium store large quantities of glycogen, fats and minerals and maintain the embryo until the placenta has developed, after about 5 weeks.

Placenta

Cords of tissue grow out of the outermost layer of the trophoblast

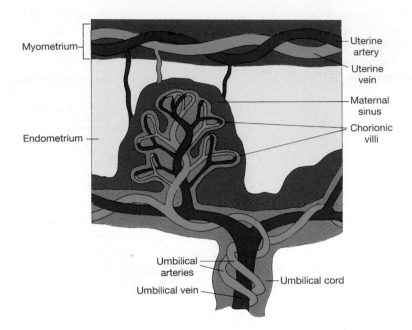

Figure 17.18 The placenta. Fetal blood in the chorionic villi is surrounded by sinuses containing maternal blood.

For Po$_2$ values in the lungs see Table 13.5 and Figure 13.11, in Ch. 13, Respiration.

(**chorion**) into the endometrium, digesting cells and using their contents as nutrient sources. Capillaries grow out from the developing embryo and, by the 16th day after fertilization, blood is flowing through them. At the same time sinuses containing the mother's blood develop around the cords. Thus foetal blood is contained in chorionic villi surrounded by sinuses containing maternal blood (Figure 17.18). The maternal sinuses are supplied by the uterine artery and drained by uterine veins.

The developing embryo is linked to the developing placenta by an **umbilical cord**, which contains two coiled **umbilical arteries**, carrying deoxygenated blood from the embryo to the placenta, and a single vein carrying oxygenated blood back. The placenta is fully grown by the end of the third month of gestation.

Initially the surface area of the interface between the mother's and the embryo's circulations is minute and even at the end of pregnancy it is still only a few square metres. The minimum thickness of the membranes separating the bloods is about 3.5 μm; it is, however, thin enough to enable two-way diffusion of molecules, but (usually) thick enough to prevent cells leaking across in either direction.

Transfer of oxygen from the maternal sinuses (Po$_2$ around 6.7 kPa) to the foetal circulation results in a mean Po$_2$ of 4.0 kPa in oxygenated foetal blood towards the end of pregnancy. This is a much lower value than that found in postnatal oxygenated blood.

Foetal haemoglobin concentration, however, is 50% greater than that of maternal blood and has a 20–30% higher capacity for oxygen.

The Po$_2$ of foetal blood is up to 0.4 kPa higher than that of maternal blood and its extreme solubility in the placental membrane allows rapid gas transfer. The CO_2 transferred into the mother's blood stimulates her respiratory centre and promotes rapid ventilation, which leads to its removal.

The transfer of carbon dioxide from the foetus's to the mother's blood renders the former alkaline, which favours the uptake of oxygen by foetal blood; this is the converse of the Bohr effect.

The cells lining the chorionic villi take up glucose from the mother's circulation by facilitated diffusion. The foetus uses glucose preferentially as an energy source. Amino acids, Ca^{2+}, PO_4^{3-} and vitamin C are all absorbed actively, whereas fatty acids, ketones, K^+, Na^+ and Cl^- all transfer by diffusion.

The waste products urea, uric acid and creatinine all diffuse from the foetal into the maternal blood.

> The Bohr effect is explained in **Oxyhaemoglobin dissociation curve** (page 452), in Ch. 13, Respiration.

Foetal monitoring

There are three principal methods by which the wellbeing of the foetus is investigated: ultrasound, amniocentesis and chorionic villus sampling.

Ultrasound is a technique in which sound waves in the high-frequency range (20 000–80 000 Hz) are transmitted into the uterus. Since sound travels at different speeds in different tissues, a moving picture is generated on a television screen from the reflected sound waves.

Amniocentesis is a process by which amniotic fluid is withdrawn by syringe, usually after the 14th week of pregnancy to reduce the risk of damaging the foetus. Both the fluid itself and any foetal cells floating in it can be used for the diagnosis of genetic diseases.

The removal of a small amount of tissue from a **chorionic villus** is another way of obtaining foetal cells. In this case, a small tube is inserted into the mother's vagina through the cervical canal to the placenta. The risk to the foetus is therefore less than amniocentesis, and so this technique is usually carried out earlier, between 8 and 10 weeks of pregnancy.

Hormonal regulation of pregnancy

Once the embryo has embedded in the uterine wall, the trophoblast releases **chorionic gonadotrophin** (**HCG**), a glycoprotein similar in structure to LH, into the mother's bloodstream. HCG acts like LH and maintains the integrity of the corpus luteum, which therefore continues to secrete **progesterone** and **oestrogen**. These two hormones maintain the endometrium and provide a suitable environment for the further development of the embryo.

HCG appears in the maternal circulation around the third week of gestation (one week after fertilization). The detection of this hormone is used in **pregnancy tests**. HCG peaks around 10 weeks of gestation and then falls to a low level by about 16 weeks, which is maintained until the end of pregnancy. Even in the early stages of its growth the placenta secretes small quantities of oestrogen (principally oestriol) and progesterone and by the time that the HCG level falls there is sufficient placental oestrogen and progesterone in the mother's circulation to maintain pregnancy. The levels of circulating oestrogen and progesterone then continue to rise until parturition (Figure 17.19). The foetal adrenal cortices produce androgens, which are converted into oestriol by the placenta.

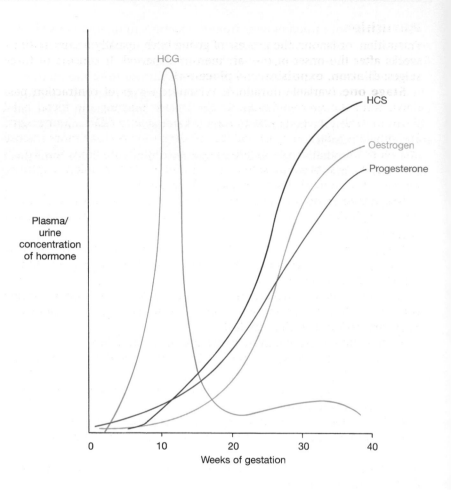

Figure 17.19 Plasma levels of oestrogen, progesterone, human chorionic somatomammotrophin and human chorionic gonadotrophin (HCG) during pregnancy.

The placenta secretes **human chorionic somatomammotrophin (HCS)**, also known as human placental lactogen (HPL), which appears in the maternal circulation about six weeks after fertilization. Levels rise steadily throughout pregnancy and flatten towards parturition. HCS has weak growth-promoting activity but since it is present in high concentrations it may make a contribution to maternal (but probably not foetal) development. HCS promotes the production of somatomedins by the placenta and these may contribute to foetal growth. HCS also has lactogenic activity, but the influence of prolactin is much stronger.

There is a two- to three-fold increase in the size of the mother's pituitary gland, largely due to hypertrophy of mammotrophs; somatotrophs decrease in numbers leading to a decrease in GH production. FSH and LH secretion is also low, while TSH is generally unchanged from non-pregnant levels. ACTH may be suppressed by the high levels of oestrogen and progesterone, but aldosterone output rises as pregnancy proceeds.

The effectiveness of insulin is reduced during pregnancy, possibly as a result of the actions of HCS and GH, with the result that maternal plasma glucose concentration rises. This increases the availability of glucose for the foetus. At full term the foetus is using 5 mg/kg/min of glucose, which is about twice that used by the mother.

Parturition

Parturition, or labour, the process of giving birth, usually occurs at 40 ± 2 weeks after the onset of the last menstrual period. It consists of three stages: **dilation**, **expulsion** and **placental**.

Stage one (variable duration): Peristaltic waves of contraction pass down from the uterine fundus to the cervix, pushing the foetal head down towards the cervix and causing the opening to dilate. Contractions are initially 15–30 min apart and last 10–30 s; they become more intense and more frequent as labour progresses. During the previous few weeks the cervix has become softer and thinner. The amnion ruptures, releasing the amniotic fluid ('breaking the water').

Stage two (1 hour or less): The foetus passes through the cervix and out through the vagina. The contractions last for about 1 minute, occurring every 2–3 min.

Stage three (10 minutes): Uterine contractions 1) cause the placenta to separate from the endometrium and be ejected and 2) seal off the raw surface and limit bleeding.

Oxytocin and prostaglandins are both known to stimulate uterine contraction, but the sequence of events that initiates labour is not clear. There are various contributory factors:

- stretching of uterine muscle increases its contractility;
- the foetus releases various chemicals including cortisol and oxytocin;
- the ratio of progesterone to oestrogen falls, which increases uterine muscle contractility;
- the number of oxytocin receptors in the uterus increases;
- prostaglandins are secreted by the uterus, stimulated by oxytocin.

From about 30 weeks onwards, irregular uterine contractions (**Braxton Hicks contractions**) occur.

Lactation

During pregnancy the milk-secreting tissues and the duct systems in the breasts develop and additional fat is deposited. Oestrogen, progesterone, glucocorticoids, GH, insulin, prolactin and HCS are all thought to play a part.

For the first 2–3 days after birth, a clear fluid, **colostrum**, is produced, which has a similar composition to milk without the fat and which contains IgG antibodies.

Milk secretion follows and is maintained by the hormone prolactin. Milk expulsion or 'let-down' is regulated by the hormone oxytocin. The release of both of these hormones is stimulated by suckling.

See also **Antibodies** (page 362), in Ch. 11, Blood, Lymphoid Tissue and Immunity.

PROLACTIN

Prolactin (PRL) is a polypeptide comprising 198 amino acids, synthesized by the adenohypophysis. It promotes milk secretion during lactation. The basal level of PRL in the plasma is about 10 ng/ml with a half-life of 20 min. During pregnancy the levels rise from about the fifth week until birth when they may be 10 times the basal level. Even though levels are so high, milk is not produced, because of the inhibitory influences of oestrogen and progesterone. The removal of these influences at birth enables PRL to promote copious secretion of milk.

After birth, the basal plasma PRL falls over a few weeks to non-pregnant levels, but suckling by the infant causes a rapid surge, lasting about 1 hour, of up to 20 times the basal level.

Unusually, prolactin output is regulated largely by a hypothalamic inhibiting hormone (PIH or dopamine). The hypothalamic stimulating hormone, prolactin releasing hormone (PRH), exerts a lesser influence.

PIH is released from the hypothalamus into the portal vessels and is carried to the adenohypophysis where it suppresses the release of PRL

Figure 17.20 Suckling-induced reflex release of prolactin. Prolactin exerts a negative feedback effect on the fall in the release of prolactin inhibiting hormone (PIH) by the hypothalamus.

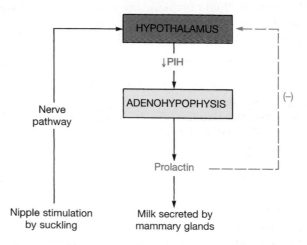

(Figure 17.20).

Suckling initiates a neurocrine reflex which inhibits PIH release, leading to a rise in the rate of secretion of PRL into the blood. Prolactin itself stimulates the release of PIH, so reducing further secretion of PRL ('short loop' inhibition).

Lack of PRL leads to an inability to lactate.

PRL exerts an inhibitory influence on the production of GnRH, so that in excess it can cause a cessation of menstrual cycles (amenorrhoea) and infertility in women and a reduction in testosterone output and sperm production in men.

OXYTOCIN

See also **Neurohyophysis** (page 621), in Ch. 16, Endocrine Physiology.

Oxytocin, like ADH, is a peptide consisting of nine amino acids which is synthesized in the hypothalamus and secreted from the neurohypophysis.

Oxytocin has two principal physiological effects: milk ejection from the breasts of lactating mothers, and uterine contraction during parturition.

Suckling of the nipple by the infant stimulates a neurocrine reflex, in which sensory impulses are propagated up to the brain and motor impulses stimulate the release of stored oxytocin from the neurohypophysis (Figure 17.21).

Oxytocin is carried in the blood to the breasts, where it induces contraction of the myoepithelial cells, which lie outside the milk-

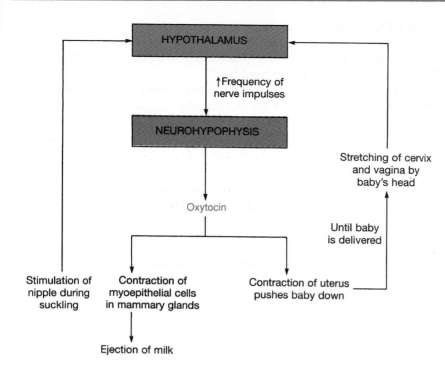

Figure 17.21 Reflex release of oxytocin during suckling and parturition.

secreting alveoli. Milk is thereby expelled.

Stretching of the cervix during parturition induces reflex release of oxytocin which stimulates uterine contraction. A positive feedback cycle is initiated whereby cervical stretching initiates oxytocin release, which in turn enhances uterine contraction, which pushes the baby further down and increases cervical stretching. Once the baby is delivered, the cycle is broken.

Recommended further reading

General books on physiology and related sciences

Alberts, B., Bray, D., Lewis, J. et al. (1989) *Molecular Biology of the Cell*, 2nd edition, Garland, New York.

Berne, R. M. and Levy, M. N. (1992) *Physiology*, 3rd edn, C. V. Mosby, St Louis, MO.

Brown, A. M. and Stubbs, D. W. (eds) (1988) *Medical Physiology*, Churchill Livingstone, Edinburgh.

Brown, T. A. (1992) *Genetics: A Molecular Approach*, 2nd edn, Chapman & Hall, London.

Burkitt, H. G. et al. (1993) *Wheater's Functional Histology*, 3rd edn, Churchill Livingstone, Edinburgh.

Chandrasoma, P. and Taylor, C. (1991) *Concise Pathology*, Appleton Lange, Norwalk, CT.

Darnell, J., Lodish, H. and Baltimore, D. (1990) *Molecular Cell Biology*, 2nd edn, Scientific American Books, New York

Devlin, T. M. (1992) *Textbook of Biochemistry with Clinical Corrections*, 3rd edn, Wiley-Liss, New York.

Elseth, G. D. and Baumgardner, K. D. (1994) *Principles of Modern Genetics*, West, New York.

Fawcett, D. W. (1994) *Bloom and Fawcett: A Textbook of Histology*, 12th edn, Chapman & Hall, London.

Ganong, W. F. (1995) *Review of Medical Physiology*, 17th edn, Appleton and Lange, Norwalk, CT.

Gelehrter, T. D. and Collins, F. S. (1990) *Principles of Medical Genetics*, Williams & Wilkins, Baltimore, MD.

Guyton, A. C. and Hall, J. E. (1996) *Textbook of Medical Physiology*, 9th edn, W. B. Saunders, Philadelphia, PA.

Hinwood, B. (1993) *A Textbook of Science for the Health Professions*, 2nd edn, Chapman & Hall, London.

Netter, F. (1964–91) *The CIBA Collection of Medical Illustrations*, CIBA-Geigy, Basle.

Passmore, R. and Robson, J. S. (eds) (1985) *A Companion to Medical Studies*, Blackwell, Oxford.

Rang, H. P., Dale, N. M. and Ritter, J. M. (1995) *Pharmacology*, 3rd edn, Churchill Livingstone, Edinburgh.

Williams, P. L., Warwick, R., Dyson, M. and Bannister, L. H. (1995) *Gray's Anatomy*, 38th edn, Churchill Livingstone, Edinburgh.

Journals

Annual Review of Physiology
British Medical Bulletin
News in Physiological Science
Physiological Reviews
Recent Advances in Physiology
Scientific American

Circulation

Berne, R. M. and Levy, M. N. (1992) *Cardiovascular Physiology*, 6th edn, C. V. Mosby, St Louis, MO.

Smith, J. J. and Kampine, J. P. (1990) *Circulatory Physiology — The Essentials*, Williams and Wilkins, Baltimore, MD.

Endocrine and reproductive physiology

Asterita, M. E. (1985) *The Physiology of Stress*, Plenum Publishing Co., London.

Greenspan, F. S. (1991) *Basic and Clinical Endocrinology*, 3rd edn, Appleton Lange, Norwalk, CT.

Griffin, E. G. and Ojeda, S. R. (1992) *Textbook of Endocrine Physiology*, 2nd edn, Oxford University Press, Oxford.

Selye, H. (1978) *The Stress of Life*, 2nd edn, McGraw-Hill, New York.

White, D. A. and Baxter, M. (eds) (1994) *Hormones and Metabolic Control*, 2nd edn, Edward Arnold, Sevenoaks.

Yen, S. S. C. and Jaffee, R. B. (1991) *Reproductive Endocrinology*, 3rd edn, W. B. Saunders, Philadelphia, PA.

Exercise physiology

Åstrand, P.-O. and Rodahl, K. (1986) *Textbook of Work Physiology*, 3rd edn, McGraw-Hill, New York.

Brooks, G. A. and Fahey, T. D. (1987) *Fundamentals of Human Performance*, Macmillan, Basingstoke.

Jones, D. A. and Round, J. M. (1990) *Skeletal Muscle in Health and Disease: A Textbook of Muscle Physiology*, Manchester University Press, Manchester.

McArdle, W. D., Katch, F. I. and Katch, V. L. (1986) *Exercise Physiology: Energy Nutrition and Human Performance*, 2nd edn, Lea & Febiger, Philadelphia, PA.

Newsholme, E. A., Leech, A. R. and Duester, G. (1994) *Keep On Running: The Science of Training and Performance*, John Wiley & Sons, New York.

Rosenbaum, D. A. (1991) *Human Motor Control*, Academic Press, New York.

Rothwell, J. C. (1994) *Control of Human Voluntary Movement*, 2nd edn, Chapman & Hall, London.

Immunity

Benjamini, E. and Leskowitz, S. (1991) *Immunology: A Short Course*, Wiley-Liss, New York.

Brostoff, J., Scadding, G. K., Male, D. and Roitt, I. M. (1991) *Clinical Immunology*, Gower, Aldershot.

Kirkwood, E. M. and Lewis, C. J. (1989) *Understanding Medical Immunology*, 2nd edn, John Wiley & Sons, Chichester.

Stites, D. P. and Terr, A. I. (1991) *Basic and Clinical Immunology*, 7th edn, Appleton and Lange, Norwalk, CT.

Neurophysiology and related anatomy

Borden, G. J., Harris, K. S. and Raphael, L. J. (1994) *Speech Science Primer: Physiology, Acoustics, and Perception of Speech*, 3rd edn, Williams & Wilkins, Baltimore, MD.

Brodal, P. (1992) *The Central Nervous System: Structure and Function*, Oxford University Press, Oxford.

Carpenter, M. B. (1991) *Core Text of Neuroanatomy*, 4th edn, Williams & Wilkins, Baltimore, MD.

Fitzgerald, M. J. T. (1992) *Neuroanatomy, Basic and Clinical*, 2nd edn, Baillière Tindall, London.

Holmes, O. (1993) *Human Neurophysiology: A Student Text*, 2nd edn, Chapman & Hall, London.

Kruk, Z. L. and Pycock, C. J. (1991) *Neurotransmitters and Drugs*, Chapman & Hall, London.

Martinez, J. L. Jr and Kesner, R P. (1991) *Learning and Memory: A Biological View*, 2nd edn, Academic Press, New York.

Wall, P. D. and Melzack, R. (eds) (1989) *Textbook of Pain*, 2nd edn, Churchill Livingstone, Edinburgh.

Nutrition, digestion and metabolism

Bender, D. A. (1993) *Introduction to Nutrition and Metabolism*, UCL Press, London.

Davenport, H. W. (1982) *Physiology of the Digestive Tract*, 5th edn, Year Book Medical Publishers, Chicago, IL.

Sanford, P. A (1982) *Digestive System Physiology*, Edward Arnold, Sevenoaks.

Walker, A. F. (1992) *Human Nutrition*, Cambridge University Press, Cambridge.

Renal physiology

Lote, C. J. (1994) *Principles of Renal Physiology*, 3rd edn, Chapman & Hall, London.

Selden, D. W. and Giebisch, G. H. (eds) (1992) *The Kidney, Physiology and Pathophysiology*, 2nd edn, Raven Press, New York.

Vander, A. J. (1991) *Renal Physiology*, 4th edn, McGraw-Hill, New York.

Respiration

Levitsky, M. G. (1991) *Pulmonary Physiology*, 3rd edn, McGraw-Hill, New York.

Mines, A. H. (1992) *Respiratory Physiology*, 3rd edn, Raven Press, New York.

Nunn, J. F. (1987) *Applied Respiratory Physiology*, Butterworths, Oxford.

Royal College of Physicians (1971) *Smoking and Health Now*, Pitman Medical and Scientific, London.

Widdicombe, J. and Davies, A. (1983) *Respiratory Physiology*, Edward Arnold, London.

Index

Page numbers appearing in *italic* refer to tables, page numbers appearing in **bold** refer to figures.